D1209039

Biomarkers in
Cancer Screening
and Early
Detection

TRANSLATIONAL ONCOLOGY

SERIES EDITORS

ROBERT C. BAST, MD

Vice President for Translational Research
The University of Texas MD Anderson Cancer Center
Houston, TX, USA

MAURIE MARKMAN, MD

Senior Vice President for Clinical Affairs
Cancer Treatment Centers of America

Clinical Professor of Medicine
Drexel University College of Medicine
Philadelphia, PA, USA

ERNEST HAWK, MD, MPH

Vice President, Division of OVP, Cancer Prevention and Population Sciences
The University of Texas MD Anderson Cancer Center
Houston, TX, USA

Biomarkers in Cancer Screening and Early Detection

EDITED BY

Sudhir Srivastava, Ph.D, MPH

WILEY Blackwell

This edition first published 2017 © 2017 by John Wiley & Sons, Inc.

Registered office: John Wiley & Sons, Ltd, The Atrium, Southern Gate, Chichester, West Sussex, PO19 8SQ, UK

Editorial offices: 9600 Garsington Road, Oxford, OX4 2DQ, UK
The Atrium, Southern Gate, Chichester, West Sussex, PO19 8SQ, UK
111 River Street, Hoboken, NJ 07030-5774, USA

For details of our global editorial offices, for customer services and for information about how to apply for permission to reuse the copyright material in this book please see our website at www.wiley.com/wiley-blackwell.

The right of the author to be identified as the author of this work has been asserted in accordance with the UK Copyright, Designs and Patents Act 1988.

All rights reserved. No part of this publication may be reproduced, stored in a retrieval system, or transmitted, in any form or by any means, electronic, mechanical, photocopying, recording or otherwise, except as permitted by the UK Copyright, Designs and Patents Act 1988, without the prior permission of the publisher.

Designations used by companies to distinguish their products are often claimed as trademarks. All brand names and product names used in this book are trade names, service marks, trademarks or registered trademarks of their respective owners. The publisher is not associated with any product or vendor mentioned in this book.

Limit of Liability/Disclaimer of Warranty: While the publisher and author(s) have used their best efforts in preparing this book, they make no representations or warranties with respect to the accuracy or completeness of the contents of this book and specifically disclaim any implied warranties of merchantability or fitness for a particular purpose. It is sold on the understanding that the publisher is not engaged in rendering professional services and neither the publisher nor the author shall be liable for damages arising herefrom. If professional advice or other expert assistance is required, the services of a competent professional should be sought.

Library of Congress Cataloging-in-Publication Data

Names: Srivastava, Sudhir, 1954– editor.
Title: Biomarkers in cancer screening and early detection / edited by Sudhir Srivastava.
Description: Chichester, West Sussex ; Hoboken, NJ : John Wiley & Sons, Ltd, 2017. |
 Series: Translational oncology | Includes bibliographical references and index. |
Identifiers: LCCN 2017022050 (print) | LCCN 2017022586 (ebook) | ISBN 9781118468838 (pdf) |
 ISBN 9781118468821 (epub) | ISBN 9781118468807 (cloth)
Subjects: | MESH: Biomarkers, Tumor | Early Detection of Cancer
Classification: LCC RC270 (ebook) | LCC RC270 (print) | NLM QZ 241 | DDC 616.99/4075–dc23
LC record available at https://lccn.loc.gov/2017022050

A catalogue record for this book is available from the British Library.

Wiley also publishes its books in a variety of electronic formats. Some content that appears in print may not be available in electronic books.

Cover image: (Left) © Alexander Raths/Shutterstock; (Top Right) © WLADIMIR BULGAR/Gettyimages; (Bottom Right) © LAGUNA DESIGN/Gettyimages

Cover design by Wiley

Set in 9.5/12pt MinionPro by Aptara Inc., New Delhi, India
Printed and bound in Malaysia by Vivar Printing Sdn Bhd

10 9 8 7 6 5 4 3 2 1

This book is dedicated to my mother, the late Kamla Srivastava, and to my mother-in-law, the late Madhuri Gopal, who raised, nurtured and disciplined me with love and respect.

Contents

List of Contributors

Lokesh Agrawal
Cancer Diagnosis Program, Division of Cancer Treatment and Diagnosis, Bethesda, MD, USA

Jaffer A Ajani
Professor, Department of GI Medical Oncology, The University of Texas MD Anderson Cancer Centre, Houston, TX, USA

Melinda C Aldrich
Department of Thoracic Surgery and Division of Epidemiology, Vanderbilt University Medical Centre, Nashville, TN, USA

Peter J Allen
Department of Surgery, Memorial Sloan-Kettering Cancer Center, New York, NY, USA

Karen S Anderson
Center for Personalized Diagnostics, Biodesign Institute, Arizona State University, Tempe, AZ, USA

Robert C Bast, Jr.
Department of Experimental Therapeutics, University of Texas MD Anderson Cancer Center, Houston, TX, USA

Pamela L Beatty
Department of Immunology, University of Pittsburgh School of Medicine, PA, USA

Harry B Burke
Biomedical Informatics and Medicine Departments, F. Edward Herbert School of Medicine, Uniformed Services University of the Health Sciences, Bethesda, MD, USA

Sandra Cascio
Department of Immunology, University of Pittsburgh School of Medicine, PA, USA

Fondazione RiMED, Palermo, Italy

Amitabh Chak
Gastroenterology Division, Case Western Reserve University, University Hospitals of Cleveland, Cleveland, OH, USA

Daniel W Chan
Department of Pathology, John Hopkins University School of Medicine, Baltimore, MD, USA

Center for Biomarker Discovery and Translation, John Hopkins Medical Institutions, Baltimore, MD, USA

Qiongrong Chen
Postdoctoral fellow, Department of GI Medical Oncology, The University of Texas MD Anderson Cancer Centre, Houston, TX, USA

Barbara A Conley
Cancer Diagnosis Program, Division of Cancer Treatment and Diagnosis, Bethesda, MD, USA

Stephen A Deppen
Department of Thoracic Surgery, Vanderbilt University Medical Centre, Nashville, TN, USA

Albert Dobi
Center for Prostate Disease Research, Department of Surgery, Uniformed Services University of the Health Sciences, Rockville, MD, USA

Barbara K Dunn
National Cancer Institute, Division of Cancer Prevention, Chemoprevention Agent Development Research Group, Bethesda, MD, USA

Elena Elimova
Postdoctoral fellow, Department of GI Medical Oncology, The University of Texas MD Anderson Cancer Center, Houston, TX, USA

Olivera J Finn
Department of Immunology, University of Pittsburgh School of Medicine, PA, USA

Anna K Füzéry
Department of Laboratory Medicine and Pathology, University of Albert, Edmonton, AB, Canada

Alberta Health Services, Edmonton, AB, Canada

Aniruddha Ganguly
Cancer Diagnosis Program, Division of Cancer Treatment and Diagnosis, Bethesda, MD, USA

Sharmistha Ghosh
Cancer Biomarkers Research Group, Division of Cancer
Prevention, National Cancer Institute, Rockville, MD, USA

William M Grady
Clinical Research Division, Fred Hutchinson Cancer
Research Center, Seattle, WA, USA

Department of Medicine, University of Washington School
of Medicine, Seattle, WA, USA

William E Grizzle
Department of Pathology, University of Alabama at
Birmingham, Birmingham, AL, USA

Eric L Grogan
Veterans Affairs, Tennessee Valley Healthcare System,
Nashville Campus, Department of Thoracic Surgery
Medical Centre, Nashville, TN, USA

Kishore Guda
General Medical Sciences-Oncology, Case Western Reserve
University, University Hospitals of Cleveland, Cleveland,
OH, USA

Mohamed Hassanein
Division of Allergy, Pulmonary and Critical Care Medicine,
Vanderbilt-Ingram Cancer Centre, TN, USA

Jennifer Inra
Division of Population Sciences, Dana-Farber Cancer
Institute, Boston, MA, USA

Division of Gastroenterology, Brigham and Women's
Hospital and Harvard Medical School, Boston, MA, USA

J Milburn Jessup
Cancer Diagnosis Program, Division of Cancer Treatment
and Diagnosis, Bethesda, MD, USA

Jacob Kagan
Division of Cancer Prevention, National Cancer Institute,
Bethesda, MD, USA

Benjamin A Katchman
Center for Personalized Diagnostics, Biodesign Institute,
Arizona State University, Tempe, AZ, USA

Andrew M Kaz
Clinical Research Division, Fred Hutchinson Cancer
Research Center, Seattle, WA, USA

Research and Development Service, VA Puget Sound Health
Care System, Seattle, WA, USA

Department of Medicine, University of Washington School
of Medicine, Seattle, WA, USA

Kelly Y Kim
Cancer Diagnosis Program, Division of Cancer Treatment
and Diagnosis, Bethesda, MD, USA

Barnett S Kramer
National Cancer Institute, Division of Cancer Prevention,
Bethesda, MD, USA

Karl E Krueger
Division of Cancer Prevention, National Cancer Institute,
National Institutes of Health, Rockville, MD, USA

Jocelyn Lee
Cancer Biomarkers Research Group, Division of Cancer
Prevention, National Cancer Institute, Rockville, MD, USA

Tracy Lively
Cancer Diagnosis Program, Division of Cancer Treatment
and Diagnosis, Bethesda, MD, USA

Karen H Lu
Department of Gynecologic Oncology, University of Texas
MD Anderson Cancer Center, Houston, TX, USA

Yanxin Luo
Department of Colorectal Surgery, The Sixth Affiliated
Hospital, Sun Yat-Sen University, Guangzhou, P.R. China

Clinical Research Division, Fred Hutchinson Cancer
Research Center, Seattle, WA, USA

Upender Manne
Department of Pathology and Comprehensive Cancer
Center, University of Alabama Birmingham, AL, USA

Sanford D Markowitz
Oncology Division, Case Western Reserve University,
University Hospitals of Cleveland, Cleveland, OH, USA

Pierre P Massion
Division of Allergy, Pulmonary and Critical Care Medicine,
Vanderbilt-Ingram Cancer Centre, Veterans Affairs,
Tennessee Valley Healthcare System, Nashville Campus,
TN, USA

Tawnya C McKee
Cancer Diagnosis Program, Division of Cancer Treatment
and Diagnosis, Bethesda, MD, USA

Sarfraz Memon
Cancer Diagnosis Program, Division of Cancer Treatment
and Diagnosis, Bethesda, MD, USA

Suresh Mohla
Tumour Biology and Metastasis Branch, Division of Cancer
Biology, National Cancer Institute, National Institutes of
Health, Bethesda, MD, USA

Nathan Nobis
Morehouse School of Medicine and Morehouse College, Atlanta, GA, USA

Christos Patriotis
Cancer Biomarkers Research Group, Division of Cancer Prevention, National Cancer Institute, National Institutes of Health, Bethesda, MD, USA

Molly Perencevich
Division of Population Sciences, Dana-Farber Cancer Institute, Boston, MA, USA

Division of Gastroenterology, Brigham and Women's Hospital and Harvard Medical School, Boston, MA, USA

Balananda-Dhurjati Kumar Putcha
Department of Pathology, University of Alabama, Birmingham, AL, USA

David F Ransohoff
Department of Medicine, Lineberger Comprehensive Cancer Centre, University of North Carolina at Chapel Hill, Chapel Hill, NC, USA

Temesgen Samuel
Centre for Cancer Research and Department of Pathobiology, Tuskegee University, Tuskegee, AL, USA

Shashwat Sharad
Center for Prostate Disease Research, Department of Surgery, Uniformed Services University of the Health Sciences, Rockville, MD, USA

Yu Shyr
Professor, Department of Biostatistics, Vanderbilt University School of Medicine, Nashville, TN, USA

Archana Simmons
Department of Experimental Therapeutics, University of Texas MD Anderson Cancer Center, Houston, TX, USA

Steven J Skates
Massachusetts General Hospital and Harvard Medical School, Boston, MA, USA

Heath D Skinner
Assistant Professor, Department of Radiation Oncology, The University of Texas MD Anderson Cancer Centre, Houston, TX, USA

Stephen Sodeke
Tuskegee University National Centre for Bioethics in Research and Health Care, Tuskegee, AL, USA

Shumei Song
Assistant Professor, Department of GI Medical Oncology, The University of Texas MD Anderson Cancer Center, Houston, TX, USA

Brian S Sorg
Cancer Diagnosis Program, Division of Cancer Treatment and Diagnosis, Bethesda, MD, USA

Taduru Sreenath
Centre for Prostate Disease Research, Department of Surgery, Uniformed Services University of the Health Sciences, Rockville, MD, USA

Sudhir Srivastava
Cancer Biomarkers Research Group, Division of Cancer Prevention, National Cancer Institute, National Institutes of Health, Bethesda, MD, USA

Shiv Srivastava
Centre for Prostate Disease Research, Department of Surgery, Uniformed Services University of the Health Sciences, Rockville, MD, USA

Sapna Syngal
Division of Population Sciences, Dana-Farber Cancer Institute, Boston, MA, USA

Division of Gastroenterology, Brigham and Women's Hospital and Harvard Medical School, Boston, MA, USA

Eva Szabo
Lung and Upper Aerodigestive Cancer Research Group, Division of Cancer Prevention, National Cancer Institute, National Institutes of Health, Bethesda, MD, USA

Ian M Thompson
CHRISTUS Santa Rosa Medical Center, San Antonio, TX, USA

Magdalena Thurin
Cancer Diagnosis Program, Division of Cancer Treatment and Diagnosis, Bethesda, MD, USA

James Tricoli
Cancer Diagnosis Program, Division of Cancer Treatment and Diagnosis, Bethesda, MD, USA

Roopma Wadhwa
Postdoctoral fellow, Department of GI Medical Oncology, The University of Texas MD Anderson Cancer Centre, Houston, TX, USA

Paul D Wagner
Cancer Biomarkers Research Group, Division of Cancer Prevention, National Cancer Institute, National Institutes of Health, Rockville, MD, USA

Sam C Wang
Department of Surgery, Memorial Sloan-Kettering Cancer Center, New York, NY, USA

Wendy Wang
Cancer Biomarkers Research Group, Division of Cancer Prevention, National Cancer Institute, National Institutes of Health, Rockville, MD, USA

Malgorzata Wojtowicz
Lung and Upper Aerodigestive Cancer Research Group, Division of Cancer Prevention, National Cancer Institute, National Institutes of Health, Bethesda, MD, USA

Elisa C Woodhouse
Tumour Biology and Metastasis Branch, Division of Cancer Biology, National Cancer Institute, National Institutes of Health, Bethesda, MD, USA

Fei Ye
Associate Professor, Department of Biostatistics, Vanderbilt University School of Medicine, Nashville, TN, USA

Matthew R Young
Cancer Biomarkers Research Group, Division of Cancer Prevention, National Cancer Institute, National Institutes of Health, Rockville, MD, USA

Preface

Despite the recent decline in cancer incidence rates, long-term mortality rates remain unchanged. One of the most important factors for increased survival of cancer is detection at an early stage. Clinical assays that detect the early events of cancer through the use of molecular signatures or biomarkers offer an opportunity to intervene and prevent cancer progression. Molecular signatures of the phenotype of a cell that aids in early cancer detection and risk assessment will likely play an important role in screening and early detection. Although new information and technologies are clearly the driving force in biomarker discovery, translating new findings into clinical application remains a major challenge.

Tumor development is a complex process requiring coordinated interactions between numerous proteins, signaling pathways and cell types. As a result of extensive studies on the molecular pathogenesis of cancer, several novel regulatory pathways and networks have been identified. The steps in these pathways have delineated a number of unique events in cells, marked by morphological and histological changes and altered expression of genes and proteins. During the transformation of a normal cell into a cancer cell, the cell signature changes, and these changes become unique signals of their presence and inherent features. By reading these signals accurately, we can improve the early detection and diagnosis of individual cancers. After decades of using basic research in an attempt to unravel the underlying cellular and molecular mechanisms of cancer, the scientific community has uncovered novel candidate targets for the early detection of cancer. By the time a tumor is detected, several molecular changes have already occurred. Diagnostic assays to detect these changes using BIOMARKERS have considerable potential for early detection.

Discovering cancer biomarkers is a relatively easy process based on the number of papers published every year on this subject. However, translating these discoveries into useful clinical assays will be very difficult. To date, fewer than 25 cancer biomarkers have been approved by the US Food and Drug Administration (FDA) and most of these are for monitoring the response to therapy. In the field of biomarkers, much of the biomarker research remains "stuck" at the discovery phase. A number of explanations have been given for the lack of cancer biomarkers being moved into clinical use. These include the high performance standards needed to make a biomarker clinically useful, the complex biology of tumors, a flawed discovery process, lack of validation or a validation process that is cumbersome and expensive, regulatory requirements, and an academic system that does not reward translational research.

Biomarker research requires a knowledge-driven environment in which investigators generate, contribute, manage and analyze data available from a variety of sources and technological platforms. The goal is a continuous feedback loop to accelerate the translation of data into knowledge. Collaboration, data sharing, data integration and standards are integral to achieving this goal. Only by seamlessly structuring and integrating data sources will the complex and underlying causes and outcomes of cancers be revealed, and effective prevention, early detection and personalized treatments, be realized. There is a general consensus that if markers from the early stages of the tumor may be identified, then treatment is likely to be more successful.

Screening tools are needed that exhibit the combined requirements of high SENSITIVITY and high SPECIFICITY for early-stage cancers which are widely accepted, affordable and safe. Significant improvement in our basic understanding of the biology of cancer initiation and progression has shown that oncogenes and tumor suppressor gene mutations can be identified in bodily fluids that drain from an organ affected by the tumor. In this book, a number of chapters discuss the various aspects of biomarkers, from discovery to development to validation to clinical utility and clinical use. Clinical utility refers to the ability to make clinical decisions and improve outcomes.

The chapters in the book are organized into three sections: Section I lays the foundation for biomarker discovery, development and validation. Section II discusses organ-specific topics relevant to the clinical needs in early detection, the natural history of the disease and associated evidence in support of biomarker research, an overview of the current state-of-the art in biomarker research, current progress toward bringing these biomarkers into clinical use and the future of biomarker-based screening and early detection for the respective organ types. Section III addresses the current screening strategies for select organ types, and dis-

cusses deficiencies with the present practice and identifies clinical needs that may benefit from biomarker-based approaches.

It is hoped that readers will appreciate the complexities of biomarker research, especially for detection and screening and be inspired or inspire others to take the challenging tasks of biomarker discovery, development and validation. In the era of precision medicine, biomarkers have an important role to play by only not identifying disease-specific molecular changes, but also in identifying targets for precision treatments. Early detection and precision medicine are inseparable approaches and will jointly inform the future course of actions in the clinical management of diseases. The use of biomarkers (for instance in triaging patients who are likely to benefit and who will not benefit from subsequent diagnostic work-ups) will not only benefit clinical management, but will also be an important part of health economics in which the cost to the society and medical care will be optimized, reduced and improved.

PART I
Foundations of Biomarker Research

CHAPTER 1

Nuts and Bolts of Biomarker Research

Sharmistha Ghosh[1] and Sudhir Srivastava[2]

[1]Cancer Biomarkers Research Group, Division of Cancer Prevention, National Cancer Institute, Rockville, MD, USA

[2]Cancer Biomarkers Research Group, Division of Cancer Prevention, National Cancer Institute, National Institutes of Health, Bethesda, MD, USA

What is a biomarker?

A biomarker is a particular characteristic, or a molecular fingerprint, which indicates manifestation of a physiological state, and which can be objectively quantified to distinguish a normal state from a pathological condition (e.g., cancer) or a response to a therapeutic intervention. The National Cancer Institute (NCI) of the National Institutes of Health (NIH) defines biomarker as: "A biological molecule found in blood, other body fluids, or tissues that is a sign of a normal or abnormal process, or of a condition or disease. A biomarker may be used to see how well the body responds to a treatment for a disease or condition. Biomarkers are also called molecular markers and signature molecules." [1]

As a normal cell undergoes a complex process of transformation into a cancerous state, it is hoped that measurable characteristics can be analyzed to derive a meaningful clinical decision – either directly, from the early-stage tumor before it is palpable or detectable by sensitive screening technologies available at this time, or as a result of an immunological response to the tumor. The characteristics include a broad range of biochemical entities such as nucleic acids (e.g., DNA, mRNA, long and small [short] non-coding RNA), proteins, post-translationally modified proteins (e.g., phosphoproteins, glycoproteins, methylated proteins, glycolipids), sugars, lipids and small metabolites, as well as whole circulating cells or biophysical characteristics of tissues.

Failure to detect an identifiable molecular marker may not be a negative predictor of malignancy, and a positive test for a molecular marker may not always be a positive predictor of malignancy. However, an ideal biomarker should indicate a reliable positive or negative correlation with the presence of the disease, which means that the clinical test for the biomarker should have high sensitivity (true positive rate – that is, the ability to correctly identify individuals with the disease) and specificity (true negative rate – that is, the ability to correctly identify individuals without the disease). The clinical value of a biomarker test is based on its positive predictive value (PPV), or how likely it is for test-positive individuals to actually have the disease, and its negative predictive value (NPV), or how likely it is for test-negative individuals to not have the disease. These again depend on the prevalence of the disease in the population of interest. Biomarkers also need to be easily accessible (e.g., by non-invasive methods for screening purposes), quantifiable, analyzable, and interpretable.

Biomarkers in Cancer Screening and Early Detection, First Edition. Edited by Sudhir Srivastava.
© 2017 John Wiley & Sons, Inc. Published 2017 by John Wiley & Sons, Inc.

Why biomarker research is imperative

The development of cancer is preceded by numerous germline and somatic mutations, structural changes in chromosomes, and other genetic and epigenetic changes, which transform normal cells into benign tumors and, progressively, into malignant and metastatic forms. Cancer is a heterogeneous, multigenic group of diseases; the heterogeneity lies not only at the biochemical level (genes, proteins, metabolites), but also at the tissue and population level (e.g., [2–10]). The enormous complexity makes cancer detection, diagnosis, and treatment quite challenging. Although cancers diagnosed at earlier stages have a much better prognosis compared with cancers diagnosed at later stages, it is noteworthy that many cancer patients are diagnosed at a stage at which the cancer is too far advanced to be cured.

Currently, recommendations for early detection of cancer in average-risk individuals are available for colorectal, cervical, breast, endometrial (in menopausal women) and prostate cancers, and in high-risk individuals in the case of lung cancer. There has been a substantial increase in "cancer" incidence as a result of screening, but without a proportional decrease in mortality despite treatment. This implies that screening identifies a large reservoir of indolent cancers (overdiagnosis) [11], which would have never become symptomatic without screening, and did not require any treatment. However, because it is not known at this time which lesions are indolent, many individuals are put through intensive treatments unnecessarily, which often causes anxiety as well as substantial physical and financial harm. An extensive discussion on existing screening modalities, recommendations, and the consequences and complexities involved is beyond the scope of this chapter. A shared decision-making discussion between the patients and their physicians, based on existing data, and also taking into consideration an individual patient's values and philosophies on healthcare, is important [12].

The ability to identify tumors that are destined to progress, and which are associated with morbidity and mortality at an early stage, will allow effective treatment interventions and reduce deaths. Identification of tumor-specific molecular signatures is imperative for a new approach to early detection, diagnosis, prognosis, disease classification and risk prediction. It will also help to implement appropriate treatment decisions and therapeutic interventions, to monitor treatment response and efficacy (i.e., a measurable effect on a clinical end point), and to overcome drug resistance in a precise, patient-specific approach. Such practice of tailored "personalized medicine", based on the molecular portraits of tumor cells, allows physicians to inform individual patients of the expected outcomes – for example, whether treatments or surveillance approaches will be beneficial, and when to stop treatment based on response to drug(s). An illustration of several windows of clinical relevance in the management of cancer during its course of development is shown where different biomarker profiles can be applied to each of these windows for optimal management of cancer (Figure 1.1).

A few biomarkers discussed in this section underscore their utilization as clinical tools for facilitating diagnosis and treatment of tumors. Germline mutations in the high-penetrance genes breast cancer 1 (*BRCA1*) and breast cancer 2 (*BRCA2*), which are associated with hereditary susceptibility to breast and ovarian cancers, somatic mutations in phosphatidylinositol-4,5-bisphosphate 3-kinase catalytic subunit alpha (*PIK3CA*) gene in colorectal tumors which can act as predictive biomarker for adjuvant aspirin therapy, and metastatic melanoma patients who harbor v-raf murine sarcoma viral oncogene homolog B $(BRAF)^{V600E}$ mutations in tumors and are treated with the BRAF inhibitor vemurafenib are some well-known examples [14–16]. Another example is a translocation occurring between the breakpoint cluster region (*BCR*) gene on chromosome 22 and the Abelson (*ABL*) tyrosine kinase gene on chromosome 9 in chronic myelogenous leukemia (CML), where the fusion product BCR-ABL is implicated in disease pathogenesis. Imatinib, a drug that effectively treats CML, was developed against the BCR-ABL fusion product.

Protein-based biomarkers, such as overexpression of human epidermal growth factor receptor 2 (HER2; also known as ERBB2) in breast tumors, serve as a marker for prognosis of breast cancer, as well as an effective target for treatment with

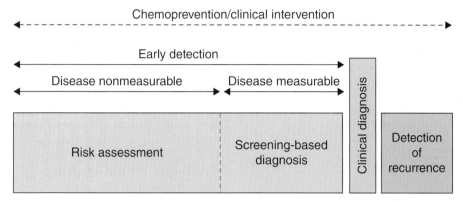

Figure 1.1 Biomarker application in the clinic. A long window of opportunity for chemoprevention or any clinical intervention is divided into sub-windows, based on whether a risk assessment is made when the disease is non-measureable, or an early diagnosis is made based on screening for measurable characteristics of the tumor, or a clinical diagnosis is made when the disease is symptomatic or has recurred. Adapted from [13]. For a color version of this figure please see color plate section.

trastuzumab, a HER2-specific monoclonal antibody [17, 19]. Levels of cancer antigen 25 (CA 125) in serum can be indicative of disease progression and treatment response in ovarian cancer, but this is not definitive because of high false-positive rate [20, 21]. A recently discovered biomarker, fibulin-3, in plasma and effusions of mesothelioma patients, may be promising for early detection, diagnosis and prognosis of pleural mesothelioma, if validated in well-designed prospective studies [22]. The prostate-specific antigen (PSA) is widely used as a prostate cancer screening marker, although its reliability as a screening tool is controversial. After reviewing all evidence, the US Preventive Services Task Force recommends against PSA testing for screening purposes (Grade D Recommendation since 2011), because the estimated harms outweigh benefits [23, 24]. However, PSA remains a good biomarker for the monitoring and management of patients with advanced prostate cancer.

Biomarker discovery can also start in the clinic, following a reverse course to the bench. Recently, the genome sequencing of bladder tumor of an exceptional responder to everolimus treatment showed that a loss-of-function mutation in tuberous sclerosis complex 1 (*TSC1*) had high correlation with everolimus sensitivity [25]. This demonstrates that unconventional individual patient information can be extracted to discover biomarkers of drug sensitivity, which will help the identification of specific subsets of patients

who would respond to particular treatments, or provide a novel insight into the molecular mechanisms. Therefore, molecular characterization of tumors is the key to early detection, diagnosis, prognosis and development of effective treatments.

Existing screening techniques are incapable of distinguishing benign and indolent cancers from aggressive ones, and even the histopathological criteria are insufficient for this. Biomarkers, in conjunction with existing screening and imaging techniques, can also become very important diagnostic tools. Despite the widely available colonoscopy, a diagnostic screening method that can detect precancerous polyps and early-stage colon cancer, only about 40% of newly diagnosed colon cancers are localized. This is primarily because of noncompliance to colonoscopy, and missed cancers due to technical or other reasons. Among asymptomatic patients, the rate of missed cancers in the hands of experienced operators range from 2–6%; the highest being on the right side of the colon [26, 27].

Non-invasive biomarker tests may have a higher probability of population-wide compliance, and can help reduce cancer burden and improve clinical outcomes by identifying individuals at moderate or high risk who must have colonoscopy. Recently, a multi-target stool DNA testing with significantly higher sensitivity (detects more cancers in average-risk, asymptomatic individuals), but lower specificity (namely, more false positive results) compared with the well-known fecal immunochemical test, has been reported. However, whether this new test has a role in colorectal cancer screening is beyond the scope of this study [28].

This chapter aims to provide a comprehensive outline of a systematic approach to biomarker development designed to cope effectively with the US regulatory system, under which the products are brought to the market, and also to provide an insight into the various available tools that support the discovery and development of biomarkers. Subsequent chapters of this book will focus on biomarkers for early detection, diagnosis, prognosis and risk assessment (excluding genome-wide association studies) of cancer.

A systematic approach to developing clinically useful biomarkers: important tools and infrastructure to address the challenges

Successful translation of promising biomarkers from the bench to the clinic has been relatively rare [29]. Although a few molecular biomarkers have been approved by the US Food and Drug Administration (FDA) for various clinical purposes [30], none is suitable for population screening. Most biomarkers do not progress beyond the discovery stage, and it is important to understand "why" there is this disappointingly slow pace before one can think of developing effective strategies for biomarker development.

Historically, biomarker discovery efforts have been piecemeal, silo-oriented, unorganized, and lacking a systematic approach. Biomarker discovery and validation are also attributed to a host of technological and methodological problems. To name a few, there has been a lack of adequate numbers of trained personnel to collect and process biospecimens, a lack of well-annotated samples, a lack of standardized protocols or quality control, a lack of blinding of researchers and randomization of animals or patient samples, and a lack of supporting tools. All these problems are further compounded by technological limitations of detecting low-abundance signals in limited amounts of biospecimens. This has produced a patchwork of standards, a lack of reproducible data and, often, conflicts and confusion. Numerous publications,

albeit published in reputable journals with rigorous peer review standards, exemplify how problems with study design, statistical deficiencies (such as overfitting of data), and lack of validation (analytic validity or clinical validity of a biomarker test) can lead to misinterpretation of the data and wrongful conclusions [31]. These are all significant impediments in the development of clinically useful biomarkers.

NCI's Early Detection Research Network and the five-phase schema

Given the challenges and costs involved in developing and validating biomarkers, it is difficult, or even impossible, for a single institution or agency to undertake the work single-handedly. Validated biomarkers, however, may prove useful to many stakeholders. Therefore, for a concerted effort to accelerate the development of systematic, evidence-based discovery of cancer biomarkers, which is a highly complex process in itself, it is beneficial to recognize the power of large, well-planned organizational structures (consortia), where technological and intellectual resources are shared and integrated towards a common goal. By leveraging the strengths of multidisciplinary, multisite partners, and by sharing costs, consortia are more likely to take on challenges that individual stakeholders cannot meet [32–36]. The team environment of consortia also has the benefits of better quality control, effective validation of results, effective utilization of scientific and financial resources, ans can develop the best standardized practices, help with troubleshooting problems, and draw inspiration from team members.

The Early Detection Research Network (EDRN) of the NCI (http://edrn.nci.gov/), launched in 2000, is the first comprehensive network created to scrupulously discover and validate biomarkers for early detection of cancer. Since its inception, the EDRN has made significant progress in developing a dynamic organized infrastructure for identifying candidate biomarkers, accommodating rapidly evolving technologies, and conducting multicenter validation studies and building resources, while also fostering public-private partnerships (PPPs) with industries, and developing collaborations with other government agencies and designated cancer centers.

Table 1.1 FDA approved diagnostic tests.

Biomarker	Clinical utility	Year of approval	EDRN principal investigator/ industrial partner
%[-2]proPSA	Reduce the number of unnecessary initial biopsies during prostate cancer screening. Also, appears to be highly associated with increased risk of aggressive disease.	2012	D. Chan/Beckman Coulter
PCA3 (in urine)	Biopsy or re-biopsy decisions in patients at risk for prostate cancer.	2012	J. Wei/Gen-Probe
OVA1™ (5 analytes in blood: CA 125, prealbumin, apolipoprotein A-1, beta2 microglobulin, and transferrin)	Prediction of ovarian cancer risk in women with pelvic mass.	2010	D. Chan/ Vermillion
Risk of ovarian malignancy (ROMA) (algorithm with CA125 and HE4 blood tests for pelvic mass malignancies)	Prediction of ovarian cancer risk in women with pelvic mass.	2011	S. Skates/Fujirebio Diagnostics
Combined panel of blood DCP (approved by FDA in 2007) and AFP-L3 (approved by FDA in 2005)	Risk assessment for development of hepatocellular carcinoma.	2011	J. Marrero/Wako Diagnostics

The valuable resources developed by EDRN that are worth mentioning include development of common data elements (CDEs), standard operating procedures (SOPs), diagnostic assays that are in use in the community, ten standard biospecimen reference sets, and a strong bioinformatics base, in collaboration with the Jet Propulsion Laboratory (JPL) of the National Aeronautics and Space Administration (NASA). The infrastructure gives researchers with promising biomarkers a platform to assess them accurately for translating discovery into clinical use. A total of five EDRN-developed or -supported biomarker-based diagnostic tests have been approved by the FDA (Table 1.1), and many diagnostic tests are currently in use in (CLIA) laboratories (Table 1.2). The EDRN Biomarker Database (BMDB) tracks all of EDRN's research progress, as well as related entities such as protocols and publications. Relevant information is available from the National Cancer Institute at http://edrn.nci.nih.gov/.

All studies follow the recommended five-phase schema [37] and the Prospective Sample Collection Retrospective Evaluation (PRoBE) guidelines [38], which address the methodological and biostatistical challenges that were not considered in the past,

and evaluate the step-by-step evidence necessary to allow a thorough assessment of promising new biomarkers for diagnostic, screening, and prognostic purposes, and validate their applications in clinical settings before proclaiming use as clinical tools. The phases of biomarker development, which are analogous to the drug development process, are as follows (Table 1.3):

Phase 1: Preclinical Exploratory. The first step in biomarker development often begins with exploratory preclinical studies, which aim to identify unique characteristics or molecular signatures of tumor tissues, compared with normal tissues to develop biomarkers, with great discriminatory ability (i.e., correctly distinguish cancer from non-cancer).

Phase 2: Clinical Assay Development and Validation. Because tissues should not be procured using invasive mechanisms for screening purposes, the idea is to conduct biomarker assays using non-invasively obtained samples, such as blood, urine, saliva and so on. Clinical assays that can distinguish subjects with cancer from those without cancer are developed, optimized and validated in this phase, using non-invasively obtained biosamples. However, it is

Table 1.2 CLIA certified diagnostic tests.

Biomarker assay	Clinical utility	EDRN principal investigator/CLIA laboratory
MiPS (Mi prostate score urine test), Multiplex analysis of T2-ERG gene fusion, PCA3 and serum PSA	Detection of prostate cancer	A. Chinnaiyan/Gen-Probe
IHC and FISH for T2-ERG fusion	Detection of prostate cancer	A. Chinnaiyan/Roche
GSTP1 methylation	Repeat biopsies in prostate cancer	D. Sidransky/ OncoMethylome
Mitochondrial deletion	Detection of prostate cancer	National Institute of Standards and Technology (NIST)/Mitomics
Proteomic panel	Detection of lung cancer	W. Rom/Celera
Aptamer-based markers	Detection of lung cancer	W. Rom/Somalogic
80-gene panel	Detection of lung cancer	A. Spira/Allegro
Vimentin methylation in stool	Detection of colon cancer	S. Markowitz/Labcorp
Galectin-3 ligand	Detection of advanced adenomas and colon cancer	R. Bresalier/BG Medicine
GP73	Risk of hepatocellular carcinoma	T. Block/Beckman Coulter
8-gene panel for Barrett's esophagus	Progression prediction	Stephen Meltzer/ Diagnovus

not known at this stage whether the biomarker can be used for early detection. EDRN's standard biospecimen reference sets, which use common sets of biospecimens from well-characterized and matched cases and controls, have been carefully developed and annotated to overcome many of the logistic and design-related issues in preliminary and advanced biomarker validation.

Phase 3: Retrospective Longitudinal Repository Studies. In this phase, the ability of the biomarker to detect preclinical disease and its promise as a screening tool for early detection (how long before a patient's clinical diagnosis the biomarker could be detected in the biospecimen)

are evaluated by analyzing samples from case patients before their clinical diagnosis.

Phase 4: Prospective Screening Studies. If a biomarker shows promise as a screening tool in Phase 3, a prospective screening study is conducted, where the screen is applied to a relevant population to determine the operating characteristics of the screening test. Screen-positive individuals go through diagnostic procedures to determine the stage or nature of the cancer. A small-scale assessment of costs and survival benefits associated with screening is also done.

Phase 5: Cancer Control Studies. This phase evaluates whether screening reduces the burden of

Table 1.3 The five phases of biomarker development.

Phase	Purpose
Phase 1: Preclinical exploratory	Promising directions identified. It is established that the biomarker is able to distinguish between cancer cases and control subjects.
Phase 2: Clinical assay and validation	Clinical assay detects established disease.
Phase 3: Retrospective longitudinal	Biomarker detects disease early before it becomes clinical and a "screen positive" rule is defined.
Phase 4: Prospective screening	Extent and characteristics of disease detected by the test and the false referral rate are identified.
Phase 5: Cancer control	Impact of screening on reducing the burden of disease on the population is quantified.

Adapted from [37].

cancer on the population, and if there is a net benefit. Even if the biomarker detects disease early, it may not have an overall benefit for the screened population because of:

a ineffective treatments;

b poor compliance or difficulties with implementing the screening program in community practice;

c economic or morbidity-associated costs of screening itself and of the diagnostic work-up of false-positive individuals; and/or

d overdiagnosis of cancers, which would not have been detected without screening and may have caused no harm or death.

The four key components of the PRoBE study design relate to clinical context and outcomes, criteria for measuring biomarker performance, the biomarker test itself, and the study size (Pepe et al. 2008).The design also has greater implications (e.g., use in biomarker discovery, creating valuable biorepositories), as indicated by the authors.

The biospecimen-based assessment modality pathway

Based on the evidentiary framework proposed in the two seminal studies mentioned earlier [37, 38] and a systematic approach of the translational biomarker research taken by EDRN, the Translational Research Working Group (TRWG) of the NCI drafted a biospecimen-based assessment modality pathway (BM Pathway) [39], which sketches out the necessary elements in biomarker development, and also provides a framework for understanding key scientific and regulatory challenges, and guidance on how to meet the challenges and facilitate biomarker development with a programmatic and operational perspective. Such a tool is geared towards maximum effectiveness and efficiency of translational research activity. The five main phases of the BM pathway (Figure 1.2), which also overlaps significantly with phases 2 through 4 of the schema described earlier [37], are as follows:

1 *Credentialing:* The exploratory data need to be scrutinized and prioritized, to evaluate how well the key questions on clinical validity, clinical need, practicality of assay development, and so on, are addressed.

2 *Supporting tools:* Reproducible assays, standard reagents, biorepositories are some important tools. The biospecimens used for biomarker research need to be properly preserved, well annotated and clinically relevant.

3 *Creation of modality:* An assay conducted on a limited number of biospecimens to define the patient subset needs to be further validated, and correlation with clinical outcomes needs to be established using a large number of retrospectively collected specimens.

4 *Preclinical development:* The development of tests underscores the importance of systematically cataloged information on a wide range of biomarkers, even the ones that individually do not show a robust association with clinical phenomena. Clinically important tests often include a group of genes instead of individual biomarkers (e.g., Oncotype DX Breast Cancer Assay that helps treatment decisions). A prospective study will determine the performance characteristics of the test, and establish a statistically significant correlation with predetermined endpoint(s).

5 *Clinical trials:* It is important to conduct randomized controlled clinical trials before implementation of the biomarker test in clinical settings.

In addition, interactions between the BM pathway and developmental pathway for new targeted therapeutic agents where a diagnostic target can also be a therapeutic target need to be considered [39]. Although this is, theoretically, a cost-effective process, it involves logistical complications and coordination challenges, because these are often developed by different research entities with different organizational structures and business policies, such as academia and industry. However, a merger of the two pathways seems inevitable, with the advent of high-throughput 'omics' technologies, such as genomics, proteomics and metabolomics, where the generated "big data", coupled with sophisticated computational and bioinformatics methods, provides an insight into the underlying biological functions and processes [40–43]. Currently, the trend is shifting from a single biomarker to a more systematic pathway, and network-based panel of biomarkers for both diagnostic and therapeutic use.

The Cancer Genome Atlas (TCGA) (https://cancergenome.nih.gov/abouttcga), launched in 2005, uses the latest sequencing and analysis methods to characterize mutational landscapes

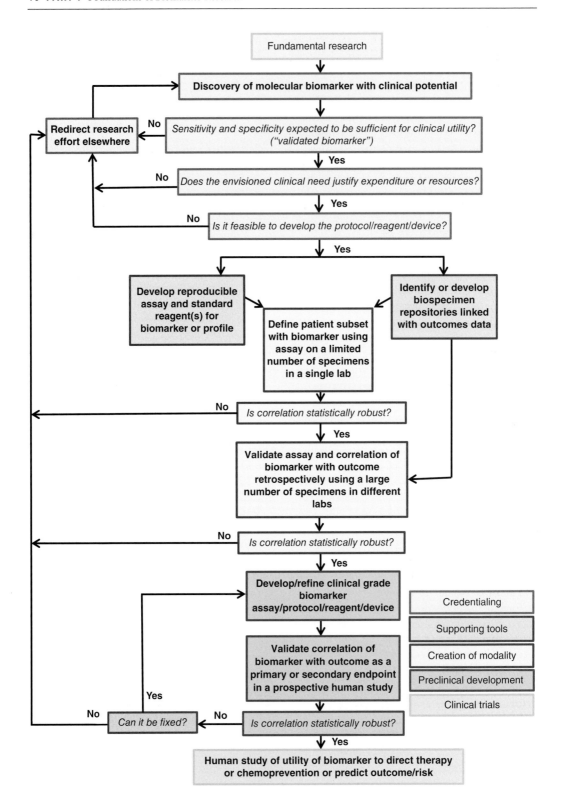

in various tumor types, and to identify molecular abnormalities that influence pathophysiology, affect outcome and constitute therapeutic targets. In a recently published article by the TCGA Pan-Cancer Group, the authors write that "Given the rate at which TCGA and International Cancer Genome Consortium projects are generating genomic data, there are reasonable chances of identifying the 'core' cancer genes and pathways and tumor-type-specific genes and pathways in the near term." [44]

Regulatory systems in the United States

To bring any diagnostic product to the market, the biomarker discovery and development process must meet the requirements set by the regulatory agencies in the United States. The Centers for Disease Control and Prevention, in partnership with the Centers for Medicare and Medicaid Services (CMS), support the Clinical Laboratory Improvement Amendments of 1988 (CLIA) to ensure that Federal standards are applied to all US clinical laboratories that test human specimens for health assessment, or to diagnose, prevent, or treat disease. The FDA regulates all medical devices, including *in vitro* diagnostic products. All procedures in nonclinical studies used to support a product that is submitted to the FDA for approval must follow Good Laboratory Practices (US FDA Bioresearch Monitoring Good Laboratory Practice: http://www.fda.gov/ICECI/EnforcementActions/Bioresearch Monitoring/ucm133789.htm).

The regulations are subject to modification and evolution in the light of new trends in medical research. With the growing popularity of omics-based tests, which are highly complex in themselves, and considering some recent publicized cases of unreliable or falsified tests that may have caused harm to patients [45, 46], Federal regulators have focused on implementing rigorous standards for such tests, in order to prevent premature omics assays from entering the market and guide treatment decisions. In a recent article [47], the NCI, in collaboration with investigators representing areas of expertise relevant to omics-based test development, has defined an omics-based test as "an assay composed of or derived from multiple molecular measurements and interpreted by a fully specified computational model to produce a clinically actionable result." The FDA needs a more dynamic process for updating the regulatory policies, to keep pace with the newly developed clinical tests based on rapidly evolving modern technologies.

The changing landscape of biomarker research

Biomarker research requires continued investment in quality control, in strong technological, statistical and bioinformatics infrastructure, and in developing biospecimen repositories for generating high-quality data that meet US regulatory requirements.

The increasing use of systems biology and bioinformatics as pivotal tools for analysis and interpretation of biological functions has become increasingly popular. Systems approaches encompassing large sets of components have unraveled a range of cellular functions and networks [48–52], so it is

Figure 1.2 Biospecimen-Based Assessment Modality (BM) Pathway. The BM pathway is depicted as a flowchart, a schematic process representation widely used in engineering. The origin of the process is at the top. Fonts in bold indicate activity steps. Fonts in italics indicate conditional tests or decision steps. Unidirectional arrows represent the direction of the activity sequence and the direction of transfer of supporting tools from their parallel development paths to the main path of modality development. For each activity or decision point, it is understood that there are many more variations that can occur, and that not all steps may occur in each instance. The pathway does not address the ways in which insights gained from late-stage clinical trials can influence the development process. Biospecimen-based assessment devices can be used for screening, early detection, diagnosis, prediction, prognosis, or response assessment. The pathways are conceived, not as comprehensive descriptions of the corresponding real-world processes, but as tools designed to serve specific purposes, including research program and project management, coordination of research efforts, and professional and lay education and communication [39]. For a color version of this figure please see color plate section.

conceivable that the availability of fully sequenced genomes and omics-based "big data" has brought mathematical and computational tool-based resolutions to cancer pathogenesis within reach. It certainly has the potential to comprehend extremely complex, nonlinear biological networks, and to provide a cogent and coherent understanding of the cellular functionalities. The Systems Biology Workbench (SWB; http://sbw.sourceforge.net/) is a useful collection of tools for simulation, analysis, and visualization of biochemical networks.

Although it may be game-changing to harness and use big data in the clinic, the existing electronic health record data systems [42] are not equipped to handle large volume of data, such as whole genome sequencing of patients, where each patient sequencing generates between 5–10 gigabytes of data. Therefore, ancillary systems supporting the use of omics-based research in the clinic need to be developed in parallel. Because of the gaining momentum of such information fusion in the field of biology, it will be also useful to bridge the gap between biologists and computer scientists, and to invest in training more young investigators to handle mathematical and computational tools.

Furthermore, there are economic considerations in the implementation and utilization of a new biomarker-based healthcare approach. Unraveling the pathogenic processes of cancer and tumor development using modern technological tools to meet the demands of "personalized medicine" results in increased complexities and, often, may result in more laboratory tests. So, what does this mean for the already escalating healthcare costs in the United States? In a microeconomic analysis of personalized medicine [53], the authors analyzed the cost-effectiveness of different types of tests from a payer perspective, and showed that, depending on the test, it may be cost-saving or cost-creating, or may even be cost-neutral per patient. Although the cost estimates are based on treatment costs in the United States, the results could be widely applicable. Also, guidelines need to be established and post-market surveillance strategies need to be enforced before such tests are implemented in the clinic in order to ensure that preferential use of "personalized" tests is not driven by any financial interests.

Last, but not least, a paradigm shift in funding and administrative approaches in academia

nationwide is warranted, to show support for collaboration-driven research. Although the concept of team science is not new, and substantial investments have been made in this direction, it is still not a widely acceptable practice in biomedical research. Investigators often believe that working independently results in increased productivity and drives competitive research; however, their resistance to collaborations often also stems from the fact that building a large collaborative network requires major investment of time, could be difficult to organize, may involve geographical barriers, and may require additional finances.

In addition, collaborative efforts are likely deterred by the fact that the current system rewards individual accomplishments over collaborative efforts, in the form of awarded grants or tenure in academia. If collaborative efforts are rewarded by recognizing multi-author publications in grant applications, alongside individual work of the investigators, inculcating the significance of collaborations in young minds at the graduate level (e.g., encourage multi-advisor thesis), and revising promotion and tenure policies in support of team-based interdisciplinary research, it may encourage the investigators to invest their time and efforts in forming strong collaborative networks. It is worth mentioning that the NIH, and several institutions, have been taking strides in this direction by emphasizing the value of team science. However, significant progress remains to be achieved.

References

1. Biomarkers Definitions Working Group (2001). Biomarkers and surrogate endpoints: preferred definitions and conceptual framework. *Clinical Pharmacology & Therapeutics* **69**, 89–95.
2. Anderson K, Lutz C, van Delft F W, Bateman C M, Guo Y, Colman S M, Kempski H, Moorman A V, Titley I, Swansbury J, Kearney L, Enver T, Greaves M (2011). Genetic variegation of clonal architecture and propagating cells in leukaemia. *Nature* **469**, 356–61.
3. Chapman P B, Hauschild A, Robert C, Haanen J B, Ascierto P, Larkin J, Dummer R, Garbe C, Testori A, Maio M, Hogg D, Lorigan P, Lebbe C, Jouary T, Schadendorf D, Ribas A, O'Day S J, Sosman J A, Kirkwood J M, Eggermont A M, Dreno B, Nolop K, Li J, Nelson B, Hou J, Lee R J, Flaherty K T, McArthur G A, B-S Group (2011).

Improved survival with vemurafenib in melanoma with BRAF V600E mutation. *New England Journal of Medicine* **364**, 2507–16.

4. Gerlinger M, Rowan A J, Horswell S, Larkin J, Endesfelder D, Gronroos E, Martinez P, Matthews N, Stewart A, Tarpey P, Varela I, Phillimore B, Begum S, McDonald N Q, Butler A, Jones D, Raine K, Latimer C, Santos C R, Nohadani M, Eklund A C, Spencer-Dene B, Clark G, Pickering L, Stamp G, Gore M, Szallasi Z, Downward J, Futreal P A, Swanton C (2012). Intratumor heterogeneity and branched evolution revealed by multiregion sequencing. *New England Journal of Medicine* **366**, 883–92.

5. Ljungman M, Lane D P (2004). Transcription – guarding the genome by sensing DNA damage. *Nature Reviews Cancer* **4**, 727–37.

6. Navin N, Kendall J, Troge J, Andrews P, Rodgers L, McIndoo J, Cook K, Stepansky A, Levy D, Esposito D, Muthuswamy L, Krasnitz A, McCombie W R, Hicks J, Wigler M (2011). Tumour evolution inferred by single-cell sequencing. *Nature* **472**, 90–4.

7. Shah S P, Morin R D, Khattra J, Prentice L, Pugh T, Burleigh A, Delaney A, Gelmon K, Guliany R, Senz J, Steidl C, Holt R A, Jones S, Sun M, Leung G, Moore R, Severson T, Taylor G A, Teschendorff A E, Tse K, Turashvili G, Varhol R, Warren R L, Watson P, Zhao Y, Caldas C, Huntsman D, Hirst M, Marra M A, Aparicio S (2009). Mutational evolution in a lobular breast tumour profiled at single nucleotide resolution. *Nature* **461**, 809–13.

8. Shibata D, Schaeffer J, Li Z H, Capella G, Perucho M (1993). Genetic heterogeneity of the c-K-ras locus in colorectal adenomas but not in adenocarcinomas. *Journal of the National Cancer Institute* **85**, 1058–63.

9. Sottoriva A, Spiteri I, Shibata D, Curtis C, Tavare S (2013). Single-molecule genomic data delineate patient-specific tumor profiles and cancer stem cell organization. *Cancer Research* **73**, 41–9.

10. Xu X, Hou Y, Yin X, Bao L, Tang A, Song L, Li F, Tsang S, Wu K, Wu H, He W, Zeng L, Xing M, Wu R, Jiang H, Liu X, Cao D, Guo G, Hu X, Gui Y, Li Z, Xie W, Sun X, Shi M, Cai Z, Wang B, Zhong M, Li J, Lu Z, Gu N, Zhang X, Goodman L, Bolund L, Wang J, Yang H, Kristiansen K, Dean M, Li Y, Wang J (2012). Single-cell exome sequencing reveals single-nucleotide mutation characteristics of a kidney tumor. *Cell* **148**, 886–95.

11. Esserman L J, Thompson I M Jr, Reid B (2013). Overdiagnosis and overtreatment in cancer: an opportunity for improvement. *JAMA* **310**, 797–8.

12. Elmore J G, Kramer B S (2014). Breast cancer screening: toward informed decisions. *JAMA* **311**, 1298–9.

13. Hassanein M, Rahman J S, Chaurand P, Massion P P (2011). Advances in proteomic strategies toward the early detection of lung cancer. *Proceedings of the American Thoracic Society* **8**, 183–8.

14. Davies H, Bignell G R, Cox C, Stephens P, Edkins S, Clegg S, Teague J, Woffendin H, Garnett M J, Bottomley W, Davis N, Dicks E, Ewing R, Floyd Y, Gray K, Hall S, Hawes R, Hughes J, Kosmidou V, Menzies A, Mould C, Parker A, Stevens C, Watt S, Hooper S, Wilson R, Jayatilake H, Gusterson B A, Cooper C, Shipley J, Hargrave D, Pritchard-Jones K, Maitland N, Chenevix-Trench G, Riggins G J, Bigner D D, Palmieri G, Cossu A, Flanagan A, Nicholson A, Ho J W, Leung S Y, Yuen S T, Weber B L, Seigler H F, Darrow, T L, Paterson H, Marais R, Marshall C J, Wooster R, Stratton M R, Futreal P A (2002). Mutations of the BRAF gene in human cancer. *Nature* **417**, 949–54.

15. Flaherty K T, Puzanov I, Kim K B, Ribas A, McArthur G A, Sosman J A, O'Dwyer P J, Lee R J, Grippo J F, Nolop K, Chapman P B (2010). Inhibition of mutated, activated BRAF in metastatic melanoma. *New England Journal of Medicine* **363**, 809–19.

16. Nazarian R, Shi H, Wang Q, Kong X, Koya R C, Lee H, Chen Z, Lee M K, Attar N, Sazegar H, Chodon T, Nelson S F, McArthur G, Sosman J A, Ribas A, Lo R S (2010). Melanomas acquire resistance to B-RAF(V600E) inhibition by RTK or N-RAS upregulation. *Nature* **468**, 973–7.

17. Baselga J (2006). Targeting tyrosine kinases in cancer: the second wave. *Science* **312**, 1175–8.

18. Druker B J (2004). Imatinib as a paradigm of targeted therapies. *Advances in Cancer Research* **91**, 1–30.

19. Yeon C H, Pegram M D (2005). Anti-erbB-2 antibody trastuzumab in the treatment of HER2-amplified breast cancer. *Investigational New Drugs* **23**, 391–409.

20. Kabawat S E, Bast R C Jr, Bhan A K, Welch W R, Knapp R C, Colvin R B (1983). Tissue distribution of a coelomic-epithelium-related antigen recognized by the monoclonal antibody OC125. *International Journal of Gynecologic Pathology* **2**, 275–85.

21. Spitzer M, Kaushal N, Benjamin F (1998). Maternal CA-125 levels in pregnancy and the puerperium. *Journal of Reproductive Medicine* **43**, 387–92.

22. Pass H I, Levin S M, Harbut M R, Melamed J, Chiriboga L, Donington J, Huflejt M, Carbone M, Chia D, Goodglick L, Goodman G E, Thornquist M D, Liu G, de Perrot M, Tsao M S, Goparaju C (2012). Fibulin-3 as a blood and effusion biomarker for pleural mesothelioma. *New England Journal of Medicine* **367**, 1417–27.

23. Marcus P M, Kramer B S (2012). Screening for Prostate Cancer with Prostate-Specific Antigen: What's the Evidence? *American Society of Clinical Oncology Educational Book* **32**, 96–100.

24. McNaughton-Collins M F, Barry M J (2011). One man at a time – resolving the PSA controversy. *New England Journal of Medicine* **365**, 1951–3.

25. Iyer G, Hanrahan A J, Milowsky M I, Al-Ahmadie H, Scott S N, Janakiraman M, Pirun M, Sander C, Socci N D, Ostrovnaya I, Viale A, Heguy A, Peng L, Chan T A, Bochner B, Bajorin D F, Berger M F, Taylor B S, Solit D B (2012). Genome sequencing identifies a basis for everolimus sensitivity. *Science* **338**, 221.

26. Bressler B, Paszat L F, Chen Z, Rothwell D M, Vinden C, Rabeneck L (2007). Rates of new or missed colorectal cancers after colonoscopy and their risk factors: a population-based analysis. *Gastroenterology* **132**, 96–102.

27. Rex D K, Rahmani E Y, Haseman J H, Lemmel G T, Kaster S, Buckley J S (1997). Relative sensitivity of colonoscopy and barium enema for detection of colorectal cancer in clinical practice. *Gastroenterology* **112**, 17–23.

28. Imperiale TF, Ransohoff DF, Itzkowitz SH, Levin TR, Lavin P, Lidgard GP, Ahlquist DA, Berger BM (2014). Multitarget Stool DNA Testing for Colorectal-Cancer Screening. *New England Journal of Medicine* **370**, 1287–97.

29. Nass S J, Moses H L (eds, 2007). *Cancer Biomarkers: The Promises and Challenges of Improving Detection and Treatment.* National Academies Press, Washington, DC.

30. Dunn B K, Wagner P D, Anderson D, Greenwald P (2010). Molecular markers for early detection. *Seminars in Oncology* **37**, 224–42.

31. Diamandis E P (2010). Cancer biomarkers: can we turn recent failures into success? *Journal of the National Cancer Institute* **102**, 1462–7.

32. Chin-Dusting J, Mizrahi J, Jennings G, Fitzgerald D (2005). Outlook: finding improved medicines: the role of academic-industrial collaboration. *Nature Reviews Drug Discovery* **4**, 891–7.

33. Croft SL (2005). Public-private partnership: from there to here. *Transactions of the Royal Society of Tropical Medicine and Hygiene* **99** Suppl 1, S9–14.

34. Kettler H, White K, Jordan S (2003). *Valuing Industry Contributions to Public-Private Partnerships for Health Product Development.* The Initiative on Public-Private Partnerships for Health, Global Forum for Health Research, Geneva, Switzerland.

35. Nishtar S (2004). Public-private 'partnerships' in health – a global call to action. *Health Research Policy and Systems* **2**, 5.

36. Schwartz K, Vilquin J T (2003). Building the translational highway: toward new partnerships between academia and the private sector. *Nature Medicine* **9**, 493–5.

37. Pepe M S, Etzioni R, Feng Z, Potter J D, Thompson M L, Thornquist M, Winget M, Yasui Y (2001). Phases of biomarker development for early detection of cancer. *Journal of the National Cancer Institute* **93**, 1054–61.

38. Pepe M S, Feng Z, Janes H, Bossuyt P M, Potter J D (2008). Pivotal evaluation of the accuracy of a biomarker used for classification or prediction: standards for study design. *Journal of the National Cancer Institute* **100**, 1432–8.

39. Srivastava S, Gray J W, Reid B J, Grad O, Greenwood A, Hawk E T, Translational Research Working Group (2008). Translational Research Working Group developmental pathway for biospecimen-based assessment modalities. *Clinical Cancer Research* **14**, 5672–7.

40. Hanash S (2004). Integrated global profiling of cancer. *Nature Reviews Cancer* **4**, 638–44.

41. Souchelnytskyi S (2005). Proteomics of TGF-beta signaling and its impact on breast cancer. *Expert Review of Proteomics* **2**, 925–35.

42. Sreekumar A, Poisson L M, Rajendiran T M, Khan A P, Cao Q, Yu J, Laxman B, Mehra R, Lonigro R J, Li Y, Nyati M K, Ahsan A, Kalyana-Sundaram S, Han B, Cao X, Byun J, Omenn G S, Ghosh D, Pennathur S, Alexander D C, Berger A, Shuster J R, Wei J T, Varambally S, Beecher C, Chinnaiyan A M (2009). Metabolomic profiles delineate potential role for sarcosine in prostate cancer progression. *Nature* **457**, 910–4.

43. Tainsky M A (2009). Genomic and proteomic biomarkers for cancer: A multitude of opportunities. *Biochimica Et Biophysica Acta – Reviews on Cancer* **1796**, 176–193.

44. Kandoth C, McLellan M D, Vandin F, Ye K, Niu B, Lu C, Xie M, Zhang Q, McMichael J F, Wyczalkowski M A, Leiserson M D, Miller C A, Welch J S, Walter M J, Wendl M C, Ley TJ, Wilson R K, Raphael B J, Ding L (2013). Mutational landscape and significance across 12 major cancer types. *Nature* **502**, 333–9.

45. Buchen L (2011). Cancer: Missing the mark. *Nature* **471**, 428–32.

46. Samuel Reich E (2011). Cancer trial errors revealed. *Nature* **469**, 139–40.

47. McShane L M, Cavenagh M M, Lively T G, Eberhard D A, Bigbee W L, Williams P M, Mesirov J P, Polley M Y, Kim K Y, Tricoli J V, Taylor J M, Shuman D J, Simon R M, Doroshow J H, Conley B A (2013). Criteria for the use of omics-based predictors in clinical trials. *Nature* **502**, 317–20.

48. Chen KC, Calzone L, Csikasz-Nagy A, Cross FR, Novak B, Tyson JJ (2004). Integrative analysis of cell cycle control in budding yeast. *Molecular Biology of the Cell* **15**, 3841–62.

49. Duarte N C, Herrgard M J, Palsson B O (2004). Reconstruction and validation of Saccharomyces cerevisiae iND750, a fully compartmentalized genome-scale metabolic model. *Genome Research* **14**, 1298–309.

50. Feist A M, Henry C S, Reed J L, Krummenacker M, Joyce A R, Karp P D, Broadbelt L J, Hatzimanikatis V, Palsson B O (2007). A genome-scale metabolic reconstruction for Escherichia coli K-12 MG1655 that accounts for 1260 ORFs and thermodynamic information. *Molecular Systems Biology* **3**, 121.

51. Klipp E, B Nordlander, R Kruger, P Gennemark, S Hohmann (2005). Integrative model of the response of yeast to osmotic shock. *Nat Biotechnol* **23**, 975–82.

52. Tyson J J, Chen K, Novak B (2001). Network dynamics and cell physiology. *Nature Reviews Molecular Cell Biology* **2**, 908–16.

53. Davis J C, Furstenthal L, Desai A A, Norris T, Sutaria S, Fleming E, Ma P (2009). The microeconomics of personalized medicine: today's challenge and tomorrow's promise. *Nature Reviews Drug Discovery* **8**, 279–86.

CHAPTER 2

Cancer Genome Methylation: Biology, Biomarker and Therapeutic Opportunities

Shashwat Sharad, Taduru Sreenath, Shiv Srivastava, and Albert Dobi

Center for Prostate Disease Research, Department of Surgery, Uniformed Services University of the Health Sciences, Rockville, MD, USA

Introduction

Epigenetic alterations, such as DNA methylation and histone modifications, are among the most common known molecular alterations in human neoplasia [1–3]. The term "epigenetics" was coined by Conrad Waddington (1905–1975) in the 1940s. Epigenetic modifications control gene expression through covalent modifications (methylation, acetylation) of DNA or chromatin without altering the genomic sequences. Global alterations in the whole genome, through epigenetic machinery including DNA methylation, histone modifications, nucleosome positioning and higher order of chromatin architecture, are the hallmarks of the cancer epigenome [4].

Over 70% of the CpG nucleotides present in the human genome are methylated. These DNA sequences are found in small 500–2000 bp stretches, termed CpG islands [5, 6], and these areas are frequently located in and around the transcription-start sites in most human genes. X-chromosome inactivation, genomic imprinting, inactivation of transposable elements are examples of robust DNA methylation controlled gene regulation. Defects in imprinted epigenetic marks are key factors causing dysfunction of various cellular signaling pathways [7]. Thus, epigenetic alterations, along with genomic DNA sequence alterations, play critical roles in tumor development and progression [8–10].

Alterations in the epigenome may lead to genetic mutations and likewise, genetic mutations in epigenetic regulators may also lead to an altered epigenome [4, 7]. Indeed, epigenetic alterations play crucial roles in tumorigenesis [4,9,10]. Abnormalities in epigenetic patterns are much more widespread than individual gene alterations in cancer cells [11]. Within the cancer genome, there are several hot spots for aberrant epigenetic modulations leading to gene silencing or activation, chromatin deregulation, and activation of aberrant cell renewal mechanisms [12]. Analysis of cancer genomes from cancer patients facilitate better understanding of epigenetic aberrations, which has great potential in the detection and treatment in all types of cancers. In this chapter, we discuss features of DNA methylation in the cancer genome, and its utility as biomarker or therapy target.

Biomarkers in Cancer Screening and Early Detection, First Edition. Edited by Sudhir Srivastava.
© 2017 John Wiley & Sons, Inc. Published 2017 by John Wiley & Sons, Inc.

DNA methylation mechanisms

DNA methylation is one the most characterized modifications within the genome, and is catalyzed by DNA methyltransferases (DNMTs). Gene or promoter sequences are modified by the addition of a methyl group to the carbon-5' position of cytosine residue within the context of CpG nucleotides by DNA methyltransferases. Although promoters of tissue-specific genes are enriched in CpG sequences (CpG islands), these sequences are largely unmethylated under normal conditions. Promoters lacking CpG islands are less prone to methylation-specific inhibition of gene expression. In addition to promoters and intergenic regions, methylation of CpG sequences is also found within transcribed regions of the mammalian genome [12]. Disruptions of global methylation patterns in all of these regions is frequently observed in cancer cells (Figure 2.1).

Focal methylation alterations in an imprinted locus can cause developmental anomalies and demethylation of classical satellite DNA can cause chromosome instability and fatal defects in cellular immunity [13]. However, more needs to be learned about the factors and conditions that trigger *de novo* methylation. Most of the experimental data on biological functions related to genomic methylation patterns of higher vertebrates came from phenotypic assessment of mammals that resulted from the mutational studies of DNMT genes.

In mammals, there are three families of DNMTs; DNMT1, DNMT2 and DNMT3 (Figure 2.2). Only DNMT1 and DNMT3s have direct DNA methyltransferase activity. The DNMT3 family consists of three members; DNMT3A, DNMT3B and DNMT3L. The normal function of DNMT1 is mainly in the maintenance of DNA methylation, whereas DNMT3A and DNMT3B are shown to regulate DNA methylation in response to developmental signals [14]. Elevated levels of DNMT1 and DNMT3 mRNAs have been detected in human tumors [15, 16]. DNMT3A and DNMT3B catalyze DNA methylation in a *de novo* fashion, while DNMT1 maintain existing DNA methylation patterns [4, 17, 18].

DNA methylation and cancer

The genomic methylation patterns of cancer tissues are distinct from corresponding normal tissues, and the specific differences are under evaluation for diagnostic or prognostic purposes. In cancer cells, abnormal methylation of promoter regions deregulates gene expression mainly through transcriptional silencing while, in the gene body, this happens by transcriptional activation or altered

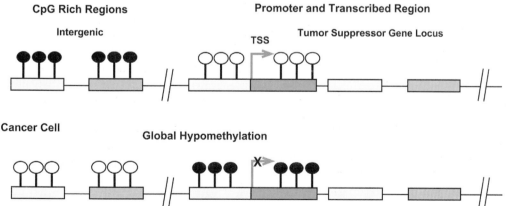

Figure 2.1 Global hypomethylation: The diagram represents the hypo- and hyper-methylation of tumorsuppressor gene loci and intergenic regions, respectively, within the genome. In cancer cells, hypomethylation of intergenic CpG sequences and aberrant hypermethylation of tumor suppressor gene loci are hallmarks of the cancer epigenome. For a color version of this figure please see color plate section.

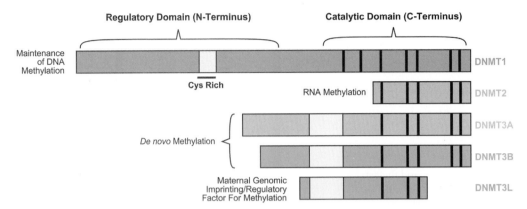

Figure 2.2 DNA Methyltransferases. Schematic diagram of the three main DNA methyltransferase families mammalian; DNMT1; DNMT2 and DNMT3. The DNMT1 is the largest enzyme (≈ 200 kDa), composed of a C-terminal catalytic domain and a large N-terminal regulatory domain with several functions. The DNMT2 (391 aa) lacks the N-terminal domain. The DNMT3 family belongs to three enzymes, DNMT3A (912 aa), DNMT3B (865 aa) and DNMT3L (387 aa). The N-terminus of DNMT3A and 3B are divergent, as opposed to the C-terminus, which is highly similar. The DNMT3L is closely related to C-terminus of DNMT3A and 3B, but lacks the DNA cytocine-methyltransferase motifs (modified figure from [16]). For a color version of this figure please see color plate section.

splicing (Figure 2.3) [19]. During cancer initiation and progression, significant alterations in the DNA-methylation landscape are apparent, such as global DNA hypomethylation to activate oncogenes, hypermethylation of tumor suppressor genes to silence gene expression [20]. Transcriptional regulation of genes by DNA methylation occurs either through direct interference with, or enhanced recruitment of, transcription factor binding to promoter sequences, or through indirect mechanisms affecting the recruitment of chromatin remodeling enzyme complexes [21].

Several genes involved in pathways, such as cell-cycle control and apoptosis, DNA repair,

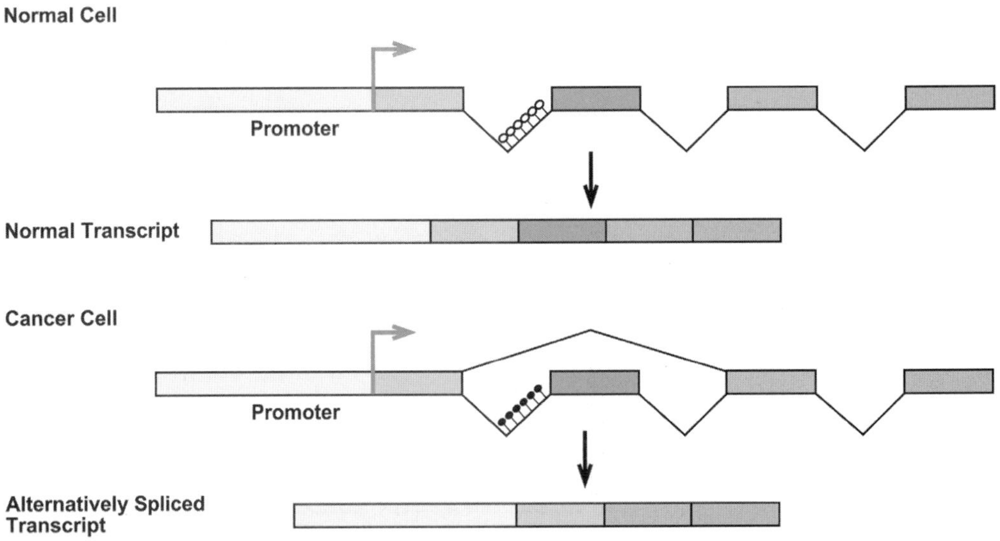

Figure 2.3 Alternatively spliced transcript. The schematic diagram represents the intronic hypo- and hyper-methylation in normal or cancer cells by creating alternatively spliced transcripts. Alternatively, alterations of methylation patterns may also result in gene silencing and altered chromatin structure. For a color version of this figure please see color plate section.

adhesion and metastasis, transformation and signal transduction, have been identified as targets for methylation. Global loss of methylcytosine throughout the genome is associated with cancer progression and metastasis in various tumor types, including prostate, bladder, colorectal, cervical, hepatocellular, and brain tumors [20]. Silencing of specific tumor suppressor genes, or activation of oncogenes through altered methylation, is commonly associated with the cancer initiation, progression, invasion, and metastasis [22].

Remarkably, genes are differentially methylated in cancer in a stage-dependent manner: in bladder and prostate cancer, Glutathione S-transferase P (*GSTP1*), Retinoic acid receptor beta (*RARβ*), Tazarotene-induced gene-1 (*TIG1*) and Adenomatous polyposis coli (*APC*); in lung cancer, RAS association domain family 1 isoform A (*RASSF1A*), *p16*, Fragile histidine triad protein (*FHIT*), and H-Cadherin(heart) (*CDH13*); in colorectal cancer, Vimentin (VIM), GATA binding protein 4 (*GATA4*), NDRG family member 4 (*NDRG4*); and in kidney cancer, von Hippel-Lindau tumor suppressor, E3 ubiquitin protein ligase (*VHL*), *p16*, *p14*, *APC*, *RASSF1A* and tissue inhibitor of metalloproteinase-3 (*TIMP3*) genes have been widely studied as targets for hypermethylation [reviewed in ref. 23].

Methylation silencing of DNA repair genes is a potential causal link between epigenetic silencing and mutation in cancer [24]. Loss of function mutations of the DNA mismatch repair genes *hMLH1* or *hMLH2* (human mutS homolog 1 and 2) are known to be associated with early development of endometrial and colon cancers [24]. DNA hypermethylation silences a DNA repair gene, O6-methylguanine-DNA methyltransferase (*MGMT*), contributing to genomic instability through mutations in tumor protein p53 (*TP53*) and Kirsten rat sarcoma viral oncogene homolog (*K-RAS*) [25].

Silencing of genes involved in cell cycle control, such as cyclin-dependent kinase inhibitor 2A (*CDKN2A (p14^{ARF} and p16^{INK4a})*, *CDKN1A* (*p21*), may also directly contribute to tumorigenesis [26]. Furthermore, methylation silencing of genes regulating cell adherence and migration may also contribute to oncogenesis. Among

these genes, *CHD1*, *TIMP3*, *RASSF1A* and members of the secreted frizzled-related protein family (*SFRP1*, *SFRP2*, *SFRP4*, and *SFRP5*), controlling the Wnt pathway, are frequently silenced by epigenetic mechanisms without inactivating genomic rearrangements or mutations [27].

In hormonally driven cancers, epigenetic silencing of genes involved in the negative control of hormone receptor levels may lead to gain of function. For example, the androgen inducible prostate transmembrane protein androgen induced 1 (*PMEPA1*) gene is predominantly expressed in normal prostate epithelial cells. PMEPA1, as an androgen-induced protein, maintains the androgen receptor protein levels in prostate epithelium by recruiting androgen receptor to the NEDD4-1 E3 ubiquitin ligase, and facilitating the proteasomal-mediated degradation of PMEPA1 through a tight negative feedback mechanism. However, in two-thirds of prostate cancers, the expression of *PMEPA1* is either decreased or lost due to DNA methylation. Thus, loss of *PMEPA1* results in enhanced androgen signaling and increased tumor growth (Figure 2.4) [28–30].

Recently recognized hypermethylation of regulatory sequences of microRNAs (MIR) can significantly contribute to tumorigenesis [31–34] through downregulation of protective miRNAs, which results in the overexpression of DNMTs, further facilitating promoter DNA hypermethylation in cancer [35, 36]. In addition to specific gene promoter regions and enhancers, DNA methylation can also affect various microRNA loci, leading to downstream activation of oncogenes [36,37]. Whole-genome evaluation of cancer-associated epigenetic alterations recently revealed direct activation of oncogenic microRNAs (oncomirs) by DNA hypomethylation [38]. Oncomir activation has been reported in lung adenocarcinoma, in chronic lymphocytic leukemia, pancreatic cancer and hepatocellular carcinoma, and is expected to be found in other cancers. Genome-scale evaluation of global DNA methylation patterns in lethal metastatic prostate cancers revealed intriguing stability of hyper- and hypo-methylated patterns, within metastatic sites of an individual, suggesting such genomic modifications as drivers events in cancer progression [39, 40].

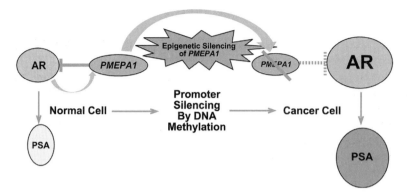

Figure 2.4 Silencing of the PMEPA1 gene disrupts a negative control over AR, leading to enhanced AR activity and resulting in elevated levels of PSA. Silencing of the PMEPA1 gene leads to enhanced AR activity in prostate cancer, by eliminating a negative regulatory control of AR protein levels. PMEPA1 facilitates AR protein degradation, which can be monitored by the detection of PSA, a tightly AR-regulated gene. For a color version of this figure please see color plate section.

Overall, the identification of cancer-specific global, as well as gene-specific hypo- or hypermethylation patterns, has a promise as biomarkers for susceptibility, early detection, prognosing progression, or monitoring treatment response.

DNA methylation as cancer biomarker

The biomarker utility of altered DNA methylation suggested by gene-specific and genome-wide approaches has been recognized as promising tool, not only for assessing cancer risk, but also in early diagnosis, molecular staging of tumors, and monitoring drug response [41]. Several epigenetically altered genes in various cancers have been identified through global assessment of the cancer epigenome by The Cancer Genome Atlas (TCGA, http://cancergenome.nih.gov), The Encyclopedia of DNA Elements (ENCODE, http://www.genome.gov/encode) and the MethylCancer initiatives (http://methycancer.psych.ac.cn).

However, a potential DNA methylation-based cancer biomarker should over-perform or complement existing cancer biomarkers [42]. Successfully developed DNA methylation-based cancer biomarkers have to meet rigorous validation criteria, including specificity, sensitivity, reproducibility, minimally invasive sample access, clinical performance and cost effectiveness [43, 44]. Recognizing that none of the single cancer biomarkers show perfect performance, monitoring a panel

of DNA methylation biomarkers appears to be the feasible approach.

Along these lines, gene methylation panels, alone or combined with other biomarkers, have advanced to clinical application stages for detection of colorectal cancer (*NDRG4*, *BMP3* and *VIM*) [45–47], predicting bladder cancer recurrence (*SOX1*, *IRAK3*, and *L1-MET*) [48], detection of prostate cancer (*GSTP1*, *APC* and *RASSF1*) with a sensitivity of 68% and specificity of 64% [49], and staging of cervical cancer (*p16*, *RARB*, *DAPK BRCA1* and *HIC1*) [50], highlighting just a few examples among emerging DNA methylation-based cancer biomarkers. Epigenetic marks of *p16*, *CDH13*, *RASSF1A* and *APC* genes have been evaluated in sequential blood samples of patients with non-small cell lung carcinoma for assessing progression-free survival [51]. As a consequence of aberrant epigenetic marks, the concept of "epigenetic therapy" has emerged for cancer treatment to reverse the epigenetic silencing of protective genes by using DNA demethylating agents.

DNA hypermethylation of CpG islands is being considered for complementing current risk assessment and diagnostic tools [52]. One of the most widely studied methylation marker for diagnostic application is the *GSTP1*, with 92% sensitivity and 85% specificity in the context of prostate cancer. Similarly, detection of the *p16*, *MGMT*, *DAPK* and *RASSF1A* panel of hypermethylated genes in sputum may reveal subjects with high risk for lung cancer [53]. Furthermore, studies have revealed that methylation marks of *TFPI2 or GATA4* in stool DNA can be used for early detection of colorectal cancer [54].

As a marker for prognostic stratification, *RASSF1A* inactivation by promoter methylation has been shown to indicate poor prognosis in patients with different types of cancers [55, 56]. Similarly, *P16* and *CDH13* methylation in patients with non-small cell lung cancer are associated with early recurrence [51]. Towards developing prognostic cancer biomarkers, DNA hypermethylation of gene panels has been shown to predict overall survival in patients diagnosed with acute myeloid leukemia [57]. Similarly, hypomethylation of histone H3lysine4 (H3K4me2) and acetylated histone H3lysine18 can predict clinical recurrence in prostate, lung, kidney, breast and pancreatic cancer patients [58–61].

Several studies have shown strong associations of DNA methylation marks with diagnosis, clinical outcome or chemosensitivity, suggesting that cancer patients may indeed benefit from the clinical application of DNA methylation biomarkers (Tables 2.1 and 2.2).

Recently, Food and Drug Administration USA approved *NDRG4* and *BMP3* methylation [45] as a new test Cologuard that screens for colorectal cancer with more than 90% specificity and sensitivity. The Epi proColon (Septin9) has become a CLIA-level blood test for colorectal cancer screening,

Table 2.1 Diagnostic and prognostic methylation biomarkers in cancer.

Cancer type	Methylation biomarker marker
Colon/colorectal cancer	SEPT9*, P16 ink4a, MGMT, MLH1, VIM^
Prostate cancer	GSTP1^, RASSF1^, APC^
Bladder	SOP, VIM
Lung cancer	P16 ink4a
Breast cancer	GSTP1, BRCA1, SEPT9
Large B Cell lymphoma brain	GSTP1
Endometrial cancer	MLH1
Ovarian cancer	MLH1, BRCA1
Head and neck cancer	SEPT9
Brain tumor	MGMT

Actively investigated epigenetic biomarker (*FDA approved and ^CLIA level).

Table 2.2 Clinically approved epigenetic test for cancer.

Cancer type	Test	Epigenetic marker
Colon/colorectal cancer	Cologuard*	Detection of NDRG4 and BMP3 methylation
Colon/colorectal cancer	Epi proColon^	Detection of methylated Septin9
Colon/colorectal cancer and precancerous adenomas	ColoSure^	Detection of methylated vimentin
Prostate, lung and colon	MDxHealth^	Epigenetic assay

*FDA approved; ^CLIA level.

with 68% sensitivity and 80% clinical specificity. Colorectal cancer is curable in more than 90% of cases if diagnosed at early localized stages. The Septin9 assay is based on detecting aberrantly methylated DNA in blood plasma. This tumor-associated methylation pattern is now being used to detect specifically cell-free DNA shed into the blood stream by tumor cells [62].

Although the methylated vimentin- based assay Colosure has not obtained FDA clearance or approval, it is currently a CLIA-level non-invasive test that detects colorectal cancer and precancerous adenomas [63]. MDxHealth developed and commercialized advanced epigenetic tests (sensitivity of 74% and specificity of 63%) through its US-based CLIA-accredited, CAP-certified laboratory facility. These DNA-based technologies utilize the Methylation-Specific-PCR platform to improve cancer diagnosis and treatment. Methylation-specific PCR can directly measure the methylation status, and can help in minimizing false positive results by distinguishing methylated from unmethylated DNA. These epigenetic tests assist clinicians in repeat biopsy and potential treatment decisions.

Epigenetic therapeutics in cancer

DNA methylation and histone modifications have been investigated in epigenetic therapeutics and cancer management. Although targeted reversal of epigenetic alterations is challenging, selective reversal of epigentically silenced genes may be reasonably achievable by compounds modulating genes

Table 2.3 Therapeutic drugs targeting cancer epigenome in various cancers.

Cancer type	Methylation inhibitors
Prostate cancer	Azacytidine, flavonoids
Acute myeloid leukemia	Azacytidine, decitabine,* zebularine
Breast cancer	Decitabine, procaine
Head and neck cancer	Decitabine
Lung cancer	Decitabine
Urinary bladder cancer	Decitabine
Solid tumors	Decitabine, hydralazine
Cervical cancer	Hydralazine
Myelodysplastic syndromes	Azacytidine, decitabine, zebularine

Actively Investigated DNA Methyl transferace inhibitor as treatment response (*FDA approved and rest at CLIA level).

that control DNA methylation, histone acetylation, and histone methylation [20]. Some of these are already being used clinically, with encouraging results highlighting the potential of epigenetic therapy and facilitating the development of novel drugs targeting the altered epigenetic program in cancer (Table 2.3).

Methylation of a mismatch repair gene, hMLH1, in ovarian and colon cancer cells can contribute to chemoresistance to chemotherapeutic agents. Early studies have indicated that treatment with a DNA demethylating agents, such as 5-aza-2′-deoxycytidine, can lower the threshold of chemoresistance by reactivating hMLH1 expression [64, 65]. Similar pioneering studies have indicated chemosensitization by DNA demethylating agents in leukemia cells resistant to cytochrome c-dependent apoptosis mediated by apoptotic peptidase activating factor 1 (APAF-1) [66, 67]. These findings have provided strong rationale for the potential clinical utility of DNA demethylating agents.

Over the last decade, two promising compounds, azacitidine and decitabine, have been developed as DNA demethylating agents, and have been approved by the Food and Drug Administration (FDA) clinical for their efficacy in hematological malignancies, especially in the pre-leukemic disorder and myelodysplastic syndrome [68–72]. Also, histone deacetylase (HDAC) inhibitors, another epigenetic-modifying group, are being used in clinical practice. HDAC enzymes may reverse abnormal gene silencing in cancer through DNMTs. HDAC inhibitors, such as vorinostat (also known as, suberoylanilide hydroxamic acid – SAHA) and romidepsin (also known as depsipeptide or FK228) are potent anti-tumor agents, and have been approved by the FDA for treating cutaneous T-cell lymphoma [73, 74]. Moreover, HDAC inhibitors may be synergistic with current anti-cancer treatments in lowering drug resistance [75], suggesting that HDAC inhibitors may, indeed, be useful in overcoming resistance to chemotherapy, providing new opportunities in addressing drug resistance as a major concern in cancer treatment. In summary, azacitidine and decitabine can modify multiple cellular pathways through gene reactivation, and can sensitize cancer cells, complementing current chemotherapeutic treatment approaches [20].

Recently, novel compounds have been developed (e.g. the DOT1L inhibitor EPZ004777) which inhibit H3K79 methylation and prevent transcription of genes facilitating the apoptosis of mixed lineage leukemia (MLL) translocation harboring cancer cells. DOT1L inhibitors selectively eliminate cells harboring the MLL gene translocation, and interfere with the expression of MLL-associated genes by inhibiting H3K79 methylation [76].

Another recently developed epigenetic drug is the bromodomain inhibitor JQ1 (GSK525762) [77,78], which inhibits the transcriptional activator function of C-MYC oncogene that is overexpressed in a majority of cancers [79]. These compounds target epigenetic components with improved therapeutic efficacy, compensating for specific genetic defects. The presence of multiple genetic and epigenetic abnormalities present within the cancer genome suggests that future approaches may indeed need to be developed that combine epigenetic with non-epigenetic anti-cancer strategies [80].

Conclusion and perspectives

The role of altered epigenetic landscape has been well recognized in tumorigenesis. Most studied, and perhaps most understood, among epigenetic alterations is the methylation of CpG sequences. Endeavors addressing cancer epigenomes will

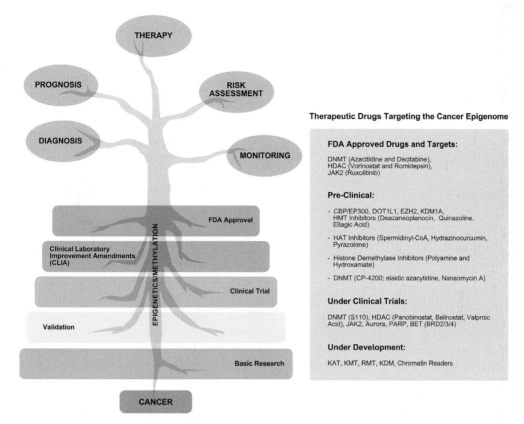

Figure 2.5 Cancer epigenome: biomarkers and therapeutic targets. The model represents the process of developing epigenetic biomarkers for diagnosis, prognosis, risk assessment, treatment response monitoring and therapeutic targets in cancer. FDA approved, pre-clinical and currently evaluated therapeutic drugs and targets are shown in the right panel. For a color version of this figure please see color plate section.

provide in-depth information on common patterns, as well as tumor type-associated epigenetic signatures of malignancies. Further insights into the epigenetics of intratumoral heterogeneity and tumor-tumor microenvironment interactions will lead to refined therapeutic strategies. We have increasing understanding of the relation of epigenetic alterations to causal changes during tumor initiation and progression. This advancement is significant, as it reveals epigenetic hallmarks of cancer consistent with the currently understood global hallmarks of cancer [8]. As a result of better understanding of cancer-associated epigenetic alterations, translational research efforts have resulted in the development of clinically useful biomarker panels for cancer risk assessment, diagnosis, prognosis, and tools for monitoring treatment response. Recognizing that there has been significant progress broader than what we can capture in this chapter, we have highlighted here advancements in the fields of leukemia, colorectal, lung, breast and prostate cancer research and clinical applications (Figure 2.5).

The rapidly emerging area of clinical applications includes targeting the cancer epigenome to decrease chemoresistance or compensating for oncogenic activations in the context of enhancing standard cancer therapy regiments. Major challenges in therapeutic application of epigenetic drugs are posed by tumor heterogeneity, adaptation of tumor cells to genetic and epigenetic selection pressure and moderate selectivity to causal pathways of cancer cells, resulting in treatment side effects. Thus, the most promising direction is to synergize epigenetic therapy with current and emerging therapeutic strategies.

In conclusion, remarkable progress in understanding the role of epigenetic alterations in cancer has resulted in measurable progress in developing epigenetic biomarkers of cancer risk assessment, diagnosis, prognosis, tools for monitoring treatment response and drugs targeting the cancer epigenome, in combination with standard cancer therapies. Epigenetic biomarkers of cancer and therapeutic approaches will increasingly contribute to the clinical practice of cancer care.

References

1. Baylin SB, Herman JG (2000). DNA hypermethylation in tumorigenesis: epigenetics joins genetics. *Trends in Genetics* **16**, 168–74.
2. Jones PA (1996). DNA methylation errors and cancer. *Cancer Research* **56**, 2463–7.
3. Jones PA, Laird PW (1999). Cancer epigenetics comes of age. *Nature Genetics* **21**, 163–7.
4. Timp W, Feinberg AP (2013). Cancer as a dysregulated epigenome allowing cellular growth advantage at the expense of the host. *Nature Reviews Cancer* **13**, 497–510.
5. Jones PA, Takai D (2001). The role of DNA methylation in mammalian epigenetics. *Science* **293**, 1068–70.
6. Takai D, Jones PA (2002). Comprehensive analysis of CpG islands in human chromosomes 21 and 22. *Proceedings of the National Academy of Sciences of the United States of America* **99**, 3740–5.
7. Jones PA (2012). Functions of DNA methylation: islands, start sites, gene bodies and beyond. *Nature Reviews Genetics* **13**, 484–92.
8. Hanahan D, Weinberg RA (2011). Hallmarks of cancer: the next generation. *Cell* **144**, 646–74.
9. Baylin SB, Jones PA (2011). A decade of exploring the cancer epigenome – biological and translational implications. *Nature Reviews Cancer* **11**, 726–34.
10. Sandoval J, Esteller M (2012). Cancer epigenomics: beyond genomics. *Current Opinion in Genetics & Development* **22**, 50–5.
11. Baylin SB (2012). The cancer epigenome: its origins, contributions to tumorigenesis, and translational implications. *Proceedings of the American Thoracic Society* **9**, 64–5.
12. Lister R, Pelizzola M, Kida YS, *et al.* (2011). Hotspots of aberrant epigenomic reprogramming in human induced pluripotent stem cells. *Nature* **471**, 68–73.
13. Lettini AA, Guidoboni M, Fonsatti E, *et al.* (2007). Epigenetic remodeling of DNA in cancer. *Histology and Histopathology* **22**, 1413–24.
14. Okano M, Bell DW, Haber DA, *et al.* (1999). DNA methyltransferases Dnmt3a and Dnmt3b are essential for de novo methylation and mammalian development. *Cell* **99**, 247–57.
15. Mizuno S, Chijiwa T, Okamura T *et al.* (2001). Expression of DNA methyltransferases DNMT1, 3A, and 3B in normal hematopoiesis and in acute and chronic myelogenous leukemia. *Blood* **97**, 1172–9.
16. Robertson KD (2001). DNA methylation, methyltransferases, and cancer. *Oncogene* **20**, 3139–55.
17. Goll MG, Kirpekar F, Maggert KA, *et al.* (2006). Methylation of tRNAAsp by the DNA methyltransferase homolog Dnmt2. *Science* **311**, 395–8.
18. Delpu Y, Cordelier P, Cho WC, *et al.* (2013). DNA methylation and cancer diagnosis. *International Journal of Molecular Sciences* **14**, 15029–58.
19. Baylin SB. Jones PA (2011). A decade of exploring the cancer epigenome–biological and translational implications. *Nature Reviews Cancer* **11**, 726–34.
20. Tsai HC, Baylin SB (2011). Cancer epigenetics: linking basic biology to clinical medicine. *Cell Research* **21**, 502–17.
21. Vinson C, Chatterjee R (2012). CG methylation. *Epigenomics* **4**, 655–63.
22. Herman JG, Baylin SB (2003). Gene silencing in cancer in association with promoter hypermethylation. *New England Journal of Medicine* **349**, 2042–54.
23. Ma Y, Wang X, Jin H (2013). Methylated DNA and microRNA in Body Fluids as Biomarkers for Cancer Detection. *International Journal of Molecular Sciences* **14**, 10307–31.
24. Lahtz C and Pfeifer GP (2011). Epigenetic changes of DNA repair genes in cancer. *Journal of Molecular Cell Biology* **3**, 51–8.
25. Nagy E, Gajjar KB, Patel II, *et al.* (2014). MGMT promoter hypermethylation and K-RAS, PTEN and TP53 mutations in tamoxifen-exposed and non-exposed endometrial cancer cases. *British Journal of Cancer.* doi: 10.1038/bjc.2014.263. [Epub ahead of print]
26. Pease M, Ling C, Mack WJ, *et al.* (2013). The role of epigenetic modification in tumorigenesis and progression of pituitary adenomas: a systematic review of the literature. *PLoS One* **8**, e82619.
27. Surana R, Sikka S, Cai W, *et al.* (2014). Secreted frizzled related proteins: Implications in cancers. *Biochimica et Biophysica Acta* **1845**, 53–65.
28. Xu LL, Shi Y, Petrovics G, *et al.* (2003). PMEPA1, an androgen-regulated NEDD4-binding protein, exhibits cell growth inhibitory function and decreased expression during prostate cancer progression. *Cancer Research* **63**, 4299–304.
29. Richter E, Masuda K, Cook C, *et al.* (2007). A role for DNA methylation in regulating the growth suppressor PMEPA1 gene in prostate cancer. *Epigenetics* **2**, 100–9.

30. Sharad S, Ravindranath L, Haffner MC, *et al.* (2014). Methylation of the PMEPA1 gene, a negative regulator of the androgen receptor in prostate cancer. *Epigenetics* **9**, 918–27.

31. Saito Y, Liang G, Egger G, *et al.* (2006). Specific activation of microRNA-127 with downregulation of the proto-oncogene BCL6 by chromatin-modifying drugs in human cancer cells. *Cancer Cell* **9**, 435–43.

32. Brueckner B, Stresemann C, Kuner R, *et al.* (2007). The human let-7a-3 locus contains an epigenetically regulated microRNA gene with oncogenic function. *Cancer Research* **67**, 1419–23.

33. Lujambio A, Ropero S, Ballestar E, *et al.* (2007). Genetic unmasking of an epigenetically silenced microRNA in human cancer cells. *Cancer Research* **67**, 1424–9.

34. Bandres E, Agirre X, Bitarte N, *et al.* (2009). Epigenetic regulation of microRNA expression in colorectal cancer. *International Journal of Cancer* **125**, 2737–43.

35. Fabbri M, Garzon R, Cimmino A, *et al.* (2007). MicroRNA-29 family reverts aberrant methylation in lung cancer by targeting DNA methyltransferases 3A and 3B. *Proceedings of the National Academy of Sciences of the United States of America* **104**, 15805–10.

36. Ng EK, Tsang WP, Ng SS, *et al.* (2009). MicroRNA-143 targets DNA methyltransferases 3A in colorectal cancer. *British Journal of Cancer* **101**, 699–706.

37. Fukushige S, Horii A (2013). DNA methylation in cancer: a gene silencing mechanism and the clinical potential of its biomarkers. *Tohoku Journal of Experimental Medicine* **229**, 173–85.

38. Suzuki H, Maruyama R, Yamamoto E, *et al.* (2013). Epigenetic alteration and microRNA dysregulation in cancer. *Frontiers in Genetics* **4**, 258.

39. Aryee MJ, Liu W, Engelmann JC, *et al.* (2013). DNA methylation alterations exhibit intraindividual *stability and interindividual heterogeneity in prostate cancer metastases*. *Science Translational Medicine* **5**, 169.

40. Esteller M (2008). Epigenetics in cancer. *New England Journal of Medicine* **358**, 1148–59.

41. Nogueira da Costa A, Herceg Z (2012). Detection of cancer-specific epigenomic changes in biofluids: powerful tools in biomarker discovery and application. *Molecular Oncology* **6**, 704–15.

42. Srivastava S (2013). The early detection research network: 10-year outlook. *Clinical Chemistry* **59**, 60–7.

43. Feng Z, Kagan J, Pepe M, *et al.* (2013). The Early Detection Research Network's Specimen reference sets: paving the way for rapid evaluation of potential biomarkers. *Clinical Chemistry* **59**, 68–74.

44. Moncada V, Srivastava S. (2008). Biomarkers in oncology research and treatment: early detection research network: a collaborative approach. *Biomarkers in Medicine* **2**, 181–95.

45. Imperiale TF, Ransohoff DF, Itzkowitz SH, *et al.* (2014). Multitarget stool DNA testing for colorectal-cancer screening. *New England Journal of Medicine* **370**, 1287–97.

46. Song BP, Jain S, Lin SY, *et al.* (2012). Detection of hypermethylated vimentin in urine of patients with colorectal cancer. *Journal of Molecular Diagnostics* **14**, 112–9.

47. Markowitz SD, Bertagnolli MM (2009). Molecular origins of cancer: Molecular basis of colorectal cancer. *New England Journal of Medicine* **361**, 2449–60.

48. Su SF, de Castro Abreu AL, Chihara Y, *et al.* (2014). A panel of three markers hyper- and hypomethylated in urine sediments accurately predicts bladder cancer recurrence. *Clinical Cancer Research* **20**, 1978–89.

49. Van Neste L, Bigley J, Toll A, *et al.* (2012). A tissue biopsy-based epigenetic multiplex PCR assay for prostate cancer detection. *BMC Urology* **12**, 6.

50. Narayan G, Arias-Pulido H, Koul S, *et al.* (2003). Frequent promoter methylation of CDH1, DAPK, RARB, and HIC1 genes in carcinoma of cervix uteri: its relationship to clinical outcome. *Molecular Cancer* **13**(2), 24.

51. Brock MV, Hooker CM, Ota-Machida E, *et al.* (2008). DNA methylation markers and early recurrence in stage I lung cancer. *New England Journal of Medicine* **358**, 1118–28

52. Azad N, Zahnow CA, Rudin CM, *et al.* (2013). The future of epigenetic therapy in solid tumours—lessons from the past. *Nature Reviews Clinical Oncology* **10**, 256–66.

53. Belinsky SA, Liechty KC, Gentry FD, *et al.* (2006). Promoter hypermethylation of multiple genes in sputum precedes lung cancer incidence in a high-risk cohort. *Cancer Research* **66**, 3338–44.

54. Glockner SC, Dhir M, Yi JM, *et al.* (2009). Methylation of TFPI2 in stool DNA: a potential novel biomarker for the detection of colorectal cancer. *Cancer Research* **69**, 4691–9.

55. Tomizawa Y, Kohno T, Kondo H, *et al.* (2002). Clinicopathological significance of epigenetic inactivation of RASSF1A at 3p21.3 in stage I lung adenocarcinoma. *Clinical Cancer Research* **8**, 2362–8.

56. Hesson LB, Cooper WN, Latif F (2007). The role of RASSF1A methylation in cancer. *Disease Markers* **23**, 73–87.

57. Figueroa ME, Lugthart S, Li Y, *et al.* (2010). DNA methylation signatures identify biologically distinct subtypes in acute myeloid leukemia. *Cancer Cell* **17**, 13–27.

58. Seligson DB, Horvath S, Shi T, *et al.* (2005). Global histone modification patterns predict risk of prostate cancer recurrence. *Nature* **435**, 1262–6.

59. Seligson DB, Horvath S, McBrian MA, *et al.* (2009). Global levels of histone modifications predict prognosis in different cancers. *American Journal of Pathology* **174**, 1619–28.

60. Manuyakorn A, Paulus R, Farrell J, *et al.* (2010). Cellular histone modification patterns predict prognosis and treatment response in resectable pancreatic adenocarcinoma: results from RTOG 9704. *Journal of Clinical Oncology* **28**, 1358–65.

61. Elsheikh SE, Green AR, Rakha EA, *et al.* (2009). Global histone modifications in breast cancer correlate with tumor phenotypes, prognostic factors, and patient outcome. *Cancer Research* **69**, 3802–9.

62. Warren D, Xiong W, Bunker AM, *et al.* (2011). Septin 9 methylated DNA is a sensitive and specific blood test for colorectal cancer. *BMC Medicine* **9**, 133.

63. Ahlquist DA, Zou H, Domanico M, *et al.* (2012). Next-generation stool DNA test accurately detects colorectal cancer and large adenomas. *Gastroenterology* **142**, 248–56.

64. Plumb JA, Strathdee G, Sludden J, *et al.* (2000). Reversal of drug resistance in human tumor xenografts by 2′-deoxy-5-azacytidine-induced demethylation of the hMLH1 gene promoter. *Cancer Research* **60**, 6039–44.

65. Strathdee G, MacKean MJ, Illand M, *et al.* (1999). A role for methylation of the hMLH1 promoter in loss of hMLH1 expression and drug resistance in ovarian cancer. *Oncogene* **18**, 2335–41.

66. Soengas MS, Capodieci P, Polsky D, *et al.* (2001). Inactivation of the apoptosis effector Apaf-1 in malignant melanoma. *Nature* **409**, 207–11.

67. Jia L, Srinivasula SM, Liu FT, *et al.* (2001). Apaf-1 protein deficiency confers resistance to cytochrome c-dependent apoptosis in human leukemic cells. *Blood* **98**, 414–21.

68. Silverman LR, Demakos EP, Peterson BL, *et al.* (2002). Randomized controlled trial of azacitidine in patients with the myelodysplastic syndrome: a study of the cancer and leukemia group B. *Journal of Clinical Oncology* **20**, 2429–40.

69. Issa JP, Garcia-Manero G, Giles FJ, *et al.* (2004). Phase 1 study of low-dose prolonged exposure schedules of the hypomethylating agent 5-aza-2′-deoxycytidine (decitabine) in hematopoietic malignancies. *Blood* **103**, 1635–40.

70. Kaminskas E, Farrell A, Abraham S, *et al.* (2005). Approval summary: azacitidine for treatment of myelodysplastic syndrome subtypes. *Clinical Cancer Research* **11**, 3604–8.

71. Kantarjian H, Issa JP, Rosenfeld CS, *et al.* (2006). Decitabine improves patient outcomes in myelodysplastic syndromes: results of a phase III randomized study. *Cancer* **106**, 1794–803.

72. Cashen AF, Schiller GJ, O'Donnell MR, DiPersio JF (2010). Multicenter, phase II study of decitabine for the first-line treatment of older patients with acute myeloid leukemia. *Journal of Clinical Oncology* **28**, 556–61.

73. Whittaker SJ, Demierre MF, Kim EJ, *et al.* (2010). Final results from a multicenter, international, pivotal study of romidepsin in refractory cutaneous T-cell lymphoma. *Journal of Clinical Oncology* **28**, 4485–91.

74. Rangwala S, Zhang C, Duvic M (2012). HDAC inhibitors for the treatment of cutaneous T-cell lymphomas. *Future Medicinal Chemistry* **4**, 471–86.

75. Saulnier Sholler G, Currier EA, Dutta A, Slavik MA, Illenye SA, Mendonca MCF, Dragon J, Roberts SS, Bond JP (2013). PCI-24781 (abexinostat), a novel histone deacetylase inhibitor, induces reactive oxygen species-dependent apoptosis and is synergistic with bortezomib in neuroblastoma. *Journal of Cancer Therapeutics and Research* **2**, 21.

76. Daigle SR, Olhava EJ, Therkelsen CA, *et al.* (2011). Selective killing of mixed lineage leukemia cells by a potent small-molecule DOT1L inhibitor. *Cancer Cell* **20**, 53–65.

77. Filippakopoulos P, Qi J, Picaud S, *et al.* (2010). Selective inhibition of BET bromodomains. *Nature* **468**, 1067–73.

78. Nicodeme E, Jeffrey KL, Schaefer U, *et al.* (2010). Suppression of inflammation by a synthetic histone mimic. *Nature* **468**, 1119–23.

79. Delmore JE, Issa GC, Lemieux ME, *et al.* (2011). BET bromodomain inhibition as a therapeutic strategy to target c-Myc. *Cell* **146**, 904–17.

80. Schnekenburgera M, Dicatoa M, Diedericc M (2014). Epigenetic modulators from "The Big Blue": A treasure to fight against cancer. *Cancer Letters* S0304-3835(14)00309-7. doi: 10.1016/j.canlet.2014.06.005. [Epub ahead of print]

CHAPTER 3

MicroRNA Biomarkers for Early Detection of Cancer

Wendy Wang,[1] Matthew R Young,[1] and Sudhir Srivastava[2]

[1]Cancer Biomarkers Research Group, Division of Cancer Prevention, National Cancer Institute, National Institutes of Health, Rockville, MD, USA

[2]Cancer Biomarkers Research Group, Division of Cancer Prevention, National Cancer Institute, National Institutes of Health, Bethesda, MD, USA

Introduction

Detecting cancer correctly at an early stage has dramatically increased the success of treatment, thereby decreasing the mortality caused by the disease. Cancer screening aims to detect cancer early, prior to symptoms or progression beyond a treatable stage. Biomarkers are measurable indicators of disease, and have the potential to be used as early indicators of cancer. While tremendous effort has been made to identify early cancer biomarkers, few molecular biomarkers for cancer have been approved by the Food and Drug Administration (FDA) for clinical diagnosis. Clearly, discovering novel molecular biomarkers is still urgently needed in order to detect early occurrence of carcinogenesis at molecular levels; to predict the aggressiveness of pre-cancerous lesions; and to incorporate this information into existing screening tools.

Non-coding RNAs (ncRNAs), particularly, microRNAs (miRNAs) belong to a new category of molecule markers that have only recently been identified as functionally important RNAs. Noncoding RNAs have been linked to the etiology of diseases, particularly cancer. This article will briefly review the history of miRNA discovery, types of ncRNAs, miRNAs' mechanisms of action, and the potential for using miRNAs for early detection, diagnosis, and prediction of progression.

MicroRNA discovery and non-coding RNA types

Ribonucleic acids (RNAs) include both messenger RNAs (mRNAs), which encode protein sequences, and non-coding RNAs (ncRNAs), which are gene transcripts but do not code for proteins. Historically, ncRNAs were not studied extensively, compared to protein-coding RNAs, because of the functions of ncRNAs were not properly recognized. In 1993, an activity for miRNAs was first discovered by Victor Ambros and his colleagues during a study of heterochronic gene lin-4 in *Caenorhabditis elegans* [1]. Since this initial finding, the number of studies that show evidence that miRNAs regulate gene expression, mRNA degradation, translation, cell proliferation, cancer initiation, and progression has increased rapidly.

MicroRNAs are 19–22 nucleotides (NTs) that bind to a complementary sequence on mRNAs and negatively regulate their expression. There are about 30 424 known miRNAs from 206 species, with about 2555 unique mature human miRNAs [2, 3]. Even though miRNAs are the most widely studied and characterized among all types of ncRNAs, with rapidly increasing knowledge of the functions of miRNAs, other types of ncRNAs have also been discovered in the human genome and have been studied for their functions.

Biomarkers in Cancer Screening and Early Detection, First Edition. Edited by Sudhir Srivastava.
© 2017 John Wiley & Sons, Inc. Published 2017 by John Wiley & Sons, Inc.

Piwi-interacting RNAs (piRNAs) are small ncRNAs with a length of 26–31 NTs. piRNAs regulate gene expression, translation and post-translational modification through forming a complex with P-element induced wimpy testis (piwi) proteins [4]. Even though most piRNAs are processed in the nucleus and cytoplasm, piRNAs have been detected in human mitochondria cancer cells [5].

Endogenous small interfering RNAs (endo-siRNAs) are small ncRNAs with a length of 20–24 NTs, which regulate target gene expression by forming a complex with genomic sequences to silence gene expression [6]. Decreased endo-siRNAs quantity in breast cancer epigenetically repress the expression of long interspersed nuclear element 1 (LINE-1) retrotransposons [7, 8].

Transfer RNA-derived RNA fragments (tRFs) are small RNAs derived from processing precursor or mature transfer-RNAs (tRNAs) that contain 5′ leader and 3′ trailer sequences. Three groups of tRFs have been mapped by genome-wide analysis. The tRF-1 series, which includes tRF1001, 1002, and 1003, are located between the 3′ end of the mature tRNA and the 3′ end of pre-tRNAs. The tRF-3 series mapped to the 3′ terminal region of mature tRNAs. Conversely, the tRF-5 series are derived from the 5′ end of mature tRNAs [9, 10]. These tRFs regulate cell proliferation through interacting with cancer susceptibility genes, such as in human bladder carcinoma and B cell lymphoma [11].

Long non-coding RNAs (lncRNAs) are RNA sequences with lengths greater than 200 NTs. The transcription of lncRNAs is similar to that of mRNAs, in that they are transcribed as single stranded RNAs, capped and polyadenylated. Based on the locations of the lncRNA with regard to protein-coding genes, several subtypes of lncRNAs have been characterized. Long intergenic ncRNAs (lincRNAs) are located between two protein coding genes. Sense lincRNAs reside within introns of a coding gene on the sense strand and antisense lincRNAs are transcripts that overlap with exons of protein-coding genes on the opposite strand [12, 13]. Recent studies indicate that lncRNAs can regulate cancer initiation and development, providing the potential for using them as cancer biomarkers [14–17].

MicroRNA biogenesis and mechanism of action

The common process of generating mature miRNAs occurs in both the nucleus and cytoplasm. In the nucleus, genes encoding miRNAs are transcribed, capped and polyadenylated by RNA polymerase II to generate double-strand primary-miRNAs (pri-miRNAs) with 500–3000 NTs [18]. The pri-miRNAs are cleaved by the RNAse III enzyme Drosha and its cofactor, double-stranded RNA [dsRNA)-binding protein DGCR (8DiGeorge syndrome critical region gene 8), into 60–120 NTs stem-loop precursor miRNAs (pre-miRNAs) [19, 20]. The pre-miRNAs are then transported to cytoplasm by Exportin 5 (XPO5) [21], and further processed by Dicer (a double-stranded RNA-specific endoribonuclease) to a 19–22-base RNA duplex [22, 23].

The duplex miRNA associates with Argonaute (Ago) proteins to form the RNA-induced silencing complex (RISC) [24, 25]. The guide strand of the miRNA duplex remains bound with Ago, while the passenger strand is degraded. The miRNA-Ago complexes are targeted to mRNAs, where the miRNA seed sequences determine binding specificity, accelerating degradation of the mRNA and reducing translation [26, 27]. Two major mechanisms are involved in the negative regulation of mRNAs expression by the complex of miRNA-RISC; one causes degradation of the target mRNA when the complementary miRNA binds to the mRNA's open reading frame (ORF); the other suppresses mRNA translation if the seed sequence of the miRNA binds the mRNA 3′ untranslated region (UTR) [28].

MicroRNAs act as oncogenes and tumor suppressor genes

More than 60% of all human genes can be regulated by miRNAs, including oncogenes and tumor suppressor genes [29]. Dysregulation of the interactions of miRNAs with oncogenes and tumor suppressor genes often occurs in early tumorigenesis, suggesting that variations in these miRNAs could be indicators of stages of cancer [28, 30–32].

By suppressing translation of oncogenes, miRNAs function as tumor suppressor genes. Lethal-7 (let-7) is an early example of miRNAs that have tumor suppressor activity [33]. The let-7 family interacts with the human KRAS oncogene, through binding to its 3′-UTR, to repress the expression of the gene. Dysregulation of let-7 miRNA expression in some human lung tumors causes increased expression of the KRAS oncogene, while overexpression of let-7 has been shown to inhibit cell proliferation by inhibiting KRAS expression [34, 35].

Other examples of miRNAs that have tumor suppressor activity include miR-34a and miR-608, which target several oncogenes including EGFR, Bcl-xL, B-Myb, and E2F1, to inhibit cell proliferation and glioblastoma growth [36–38], while miR-15a and miR-16-1 repress expression of proto-oncogene Bcl-2 (B-cell lymphoma 2) [39, 40]. Both miR-15a and miR-16-1 have been lost or downregulated in the majority of cases of chronic lymphocytic leukemia (CLL), the most common adult human leukemia [41–43]. miR-1 and miR-206 suppress expression of the proto-oncogene of mesenchymal-epithelial transition factor (c-MET) in several types of cancer including rhabdomyosarcoma [44–47].

In contrast, some miRNAs have the characteristics of oncogenes, in that they repress expression of tumor suppressor genes and promote cell proliferation; therefore, these miRNAs are called oncomiRs. The miRNA cluster, miR-17-92, encodes six miRNAs that are highly expressed in several cancers, such as lung cancers and anaplastic thyroid cancer (ATC) cells. The miR-17-92 cluster has been characterized as an oncomiR that suppresses the tumor suppressor PTEN (phosphatase and tensin homolog) [48, 49]. When miRNA-155 expression was upregulated in a panel of glioma cells, expression of the tumor suppressor FOXO3a (forkhead box O3) was significantly downregulated [50]. Moreover, miR-494 and miR-22 downregulate PTEN expression in malignant transformed cells [51, 52].

Thrombospondins (TSPs) are a multigene family of five secreted glycoproteins involved in the regulation of cell proliferation, adhesion, and migration. Expression of TSP-1, which acts as a tumor suppressor gene in colorectal cancer, is negatively regulated by miR-17-92 [53, 54]. These oncomiRs have the potential to serve as targets for diagnosis, chemoprevention, and treatment, because the inhi-

bition of the expression of oncomiRs could result in upregulation of repressed tumor suppressor genes [28, 40]. In addition, oncomiRs have potential as molecular markers for cancer early diagnosis and risk prediction.

Many miRNAs can function as both tumor suppressor genes and oncogenes. For example, as a tumor suppressor gene, miR-125b, which inhibits cell proliferation and cell-cycle progression in normal tissue, is downregulated in ovarian, thyroid, breast and oral squamous cell carcinomas [55, 56]. Conversely, as an oncomiR, miR-125b inhibits apoptosis in neuroblastoma cells and promotes cell proliferation and invasion in prostate cancer cells [57, 58].

MicroRNAs in cancer detection and prediction

MicroRNAs as risk indicators

MicroRNA markers have the potential to be used as molecular risk indicators for all types of cancer, especially for those tumors that may be rare or which lack standard screening and detection tools for the early events of cancer development. Triple negative breast cancer (TNBC), which is negative for estrogen receptor (ER), progesterone receptor (PR) and Her2/neu, accounts for 15–20% of all breast cancers. TNBC is the most deadly subtype of BC, and occurs most often in young women.

Screening mammograms are either not done or do not work well in young women. Currently, there is no method for accurate early detection of TNBC, so it is necessary to develop effective tools for early detection of TNBC. miRNAs have been studied in combination with oncogene variants in detecting TNBC. The KRAS oncogene is associated with TNBC risk in premenopausal women. Let-7 miRNA binds to the 3′-untranslated region of KRAS to suppress expression. Dysregulation of let-7 binding to the KRAS leads to increased expression of KRAS and initiation of TNBC. The combination of miRNA markers and the oncogene variant has been suggested as a new detection tool for TNBC [59, 60].

Glioma is a rare central nervous system cancer that affects only about 3.7 males and 2.6 females per 100 000 people, but it has a high mortality rate, with a median survival of only 12–15 months. Glioma, which can be divided into grades I to IV, is rarely detected in the early, possibly treatable grades I or II. Early detection should reduce mortality. The initial pilot study, in a small cohort with 33 glioma patients and 33 normal controls, showed that serum miR-125b was associated with all grades of glioma, with a sensitivity and specificity of 78% and 75% respectively [61]. Because glioma is a rare cancer, it is necessary to have international collaboration to collect large samples for validating miRNA markers for the detection of glioma.

MicroRNAs for detecting cancer and improving standard diagnostic tools

Multiple miRNAs have been identified that are associated with various types of cancer, including lung, colon, pancreatic, breast, prostate, brain, and liver cancer. Therefore, these miRNAs have a high potential as biomarkers that could be used to enhance the current standard tests of cancer diagnosis.

Colonoscopy is the current gold standard for early detection of colorectal cancer (CRC). However, it has been difficult in medical practice to use colonoscopy for regular screening, because it is costly, requires unpleasant bowel prep and is invasive. miRNA biomarkers have the potential to be used for developing noninvasive methods to identify patients needing initial screening, as well as to increase sensitivity and specificity. For developing noninvasive diagnostic tests, convenient samples, such as peripheral blood, serum, urine, and stool could be used. A number of miRNAs that are associated with CRC have been discovered, including miR-409, miR-7, and miR-93, which have been validated in independent sets of plasma samples. A panel of these miRNAs was shown to detect all stages of CRC, with 82% sensitivity and 89% specificity [62]. Further validation is necessary prior to use of these miRNAs in the clinic.

The gold standard screening technique for breast cancer is still mammography, although the sensitivity and specificity of this test is about 80–90% and 88–90%. Therefore, some breast cancers could potentially be missed by mammography. In addition, even though individuals with benign breast diseases (BBDs), such as ductal epithelial hyperplasia (DEH), atypical ductal hyperplasia (ADH) and ductal carcinoma *in situ* (DCIS) have a 4–5 fold

increased risk of developing breast cancer, it is still not predictable which individuals with BBDs will progress to invasive breast cancer.

A number of miRNAs have been identified that have the potential for use as biomarkers for early detection. One study showed that miR-21 and miR-191 were upregulated in breast cancer tissues, while miR-125b was downregulated. This study suggested that a combined expression profile of the ratio of 2 miRNAs could be used as a biomarker to discriminate between breast cancer and non-tumor tissue [63].

For lung cancer, the most common method for its detection involves incorporating imaging-based screening techniques – in particular, the use of low-dose helical computed tomography (LDCT; also referred as spiral CT), which could decrease lung cancer associated mortality by 20%. However, the false positive rate is high, with uncertainty as to whether the detected nodules are benign or malignant tumors. MicroRNAs have the potential to increase the accuracy of classification of spiral CT detected nodules.

To discover miRNAs for biomarkers of lung cancer that might distinguish malignant and normal tissue, profiles of more than 800–1000 human miRNAs were generated between paired malignancy, such as non-small cell lung cancer (NSCLC) and normal lung tissues. These miRNAs were then validated using easily accessible biofluids, such as sputum, collected from large populations. A number of miRNAs, including miR-21, miR-31, and miR-210, were identified to be able to distinguish between malignancy and indeterminate solitary pulmonary nodules (ISPN) with higher than 80% sensitivity and specificity [64,65].

MicroRNAs in body fluids

Detection of miRNAs in serum was first reported for patients with diffuse B-Cell lymphoma, where an increase in miR-21 levels was associated with relapse free survival [66]. These authors acknowledged that miR-21 is usually associated with a poor prognosis. Circulating miRNAs from solid tumors were first detected in mice transplanted with prostate cancer xenografts [67]. In the same studies, miR-141, a miRNA expressed in prostate cancer cells, was detected in serum from patients with prostate cancer. By showing that circulating miRNAs are protected from endogenous RNase, and are remarkably stable in the blood, these researchers established that detection of tumor-derived miRNAs in bodily fluids could be useful for non-invasive blood-based detection of cancer. Since this initial report, the number of studies reporting circulating tumor-associated miRNAs as potential biomarkers of cancers has been steadily increasing [68]. In addition, miRNAs have been detected, or are likely present, in other biofluids. These include urine, pancreatic juices, cyst fluids, saliva and sputum, tears, breast milk, bronchial lavage, colostrum, seminal, amniotic, pleural, peritoneal, and cerebrospinal fluids [69, 70].

Extracellular MicroRNAs as biomarkers of early detection

The detection of extracellular miRNAs in various biofluids has led to numerous studies that have evaluated whether miRNAs in body fluids have diagnostic and prognostic value [69]. For example, miRNA expression patterns in plasma have been used to discriminate patients with non-small cell lung cancer (NSCLC) from healthy controls [71, 72]. From sputum, Xing *et al.* [73] were able to distinguish lung squamous cell carcinoma (SCC) patients from normal healthy patients, using a panel of miRNAs which included miR-205, miR-210 and miR-708. Expression of miR-126 and miR-152 in urine can predict the presence of bladder cancer [74]. Circulating miRNAs detected in plasma or serum have been reported for lung, breast, prostate, colorectal, and gastric cancers, as well as for hepatocellular carcinoma. Panels of circulating miRNA detected in these cancers could be used as diagnostic and prognostic indicators [69].

As the number of studies detecting and validating extracellular miRNA increases, so does the possibility that screens will be developed that use extracellular miRNAs for early detection of cancers. However, more work is required prior to using circulating miRNA in the clinics. One problem is that miRNA signatures reported from over 154 studies lack concordance, and no single diagnostic signature emerges among various groups [75]. There is also a lack of correlation between levels of miRNA detected in extracellular fluids and the expression of these miRNA in cancer tissues.

Another problem is that circulating miRNAs can come from sources other than tumor cells. The levels of circulating miRNAs can be affected by other, non-cancer conditions, such as infection, hypoxia, diet and exercise [76]. In addition to miRNA from tumor cells or other tissues, circulating blood cells can interfere with the determination of a miRNA signature to predict cancer. The concentration of miRNAs in contaminating cells are several-fold higher than circulating miRNAs from tumors, so these signals must be accounted for when generating a diagnostic markers. Finally, the methods used to isolate, purify and detect extracellular miRNAs varies between labs, which can lead to a lack of concordance between labs and an inability to validate studies reported by other labs [75].

While there are a number of papers reporting extracellular miRNAs as potential biomarkers for early detection, more studies are needed in order to move these markers to the clinic. First, because it is not clear of the origins of circulating miRNAs, it is important to determine the source of the miRNA, and to establish well-characterized panels of miRNA that are specific to each tumor type. Second, the panels of miRNA need to differentiated patients with cancer from healthy patients or patients with unrelated disease. Third, detailed reproducible methods for detecting tumor-specific miRNA in body fluids need to be developed. Finally, large prospective clinical trials are needed to validate the use of circulating miRNA as biomarkers for early detection.

MicroRNAs in combination with other genomic and clinical indicators

Genomic variants of miRNA targets affect the normal processes by which miRNA regulate gene expression, cell proliferation, and cancer initiation. Molecular markers have been explored by combining genomic variations, particularly oncogene variants with microRNA variations of both mature and pri-miRNAs. Acute lymphoblastic leukemia (ALL) is the most common cancer in childhood. However, there is no reliable screening test for detecting ALL. Genetic variants of Has-miR-196a2 were found to be associated with increased risk of childhood ALL [77]. Similarly, a homozygous C>T single nucleotide polymorphism (SNP) in the pri-miR-16-1 was identified in chronic lymphocytic leukemia (CLL) patients [41] and a Has-mir-499 polymorphism, where genotypes of TC, TT, and CC, were found to be associated with esophageal cancer in Chinese populations [78].

MicroRNAs have been integrated with other clinical factors to predict prognostic outcome. miRNA-21 was identified as an additional indicator to predict unfavorable outcomes when combined with other clinical parameters, such as age, gender, T-category (a measure of the distance that a tumor has grown into the wall of the intestine and nearby areas), perforation, and vascular invasion [79–81]. Further validation studies of miRNA-21 in large, properly designed experiments with reproducible microRNA measurement methods, are needed to recommend the use of miR-21 to predict prognosis.

New development of miRNA research

While most studies on miRNA monitor the change in levels of the total quantity of miRNAs as molecular markers for early detection, recent developments in miRNA research include fractionation and isolation of carriers of miRNA to study the distribution of miRNAs. One such technology uses an asymmetrical flow field flow fractionation (AF4)-based method to fractionate different types of miRNA carriers [82]. The carriers being used include exosomes, which are membrane-bound miRNA containing particles excreted from cells, miRNA-bound proteins like Argonaute (AGO) 2 and GW182, and high-density lipoprotein particles (HDL). The carriers are fractionated based on the property of the carrier and the miRNA being isolated and quantified.

MicroRNA reproducibility and validation for cancer detection

As with all types of molecular markers, reproducibility is a major issue in using microRNAs for early detection of cancer. Inconsistent results existing in different experiments can be caused by various reasons, such as experimental design, sample preparation, handling, storage, and variations in standard operating procedures (SOPs). Increasing reproducibility needs to be emphasized in

discovering and validating miRNA molecular markers. Prior to using microRNAs as cancer biomarkers for early detection in the clinic, it will be critical to know whether these markers have been tested and validated in a large population. To enable circulating miRNAs-based biomarkers to be useful in clinical diagnosis, many of the problems encountered in biomarker research must be addressed.

Biological relevance

The biological relevance of miRNA as a diagnostic tool has to be determined. Circulating miRNA signatures should match the miRNA signature of the tumor, and the tumor miRNA signature should have biological relevance to the type of tumor. The miRNA signature also needs to correlate with the pathology. Biomarker levels should be proportional to the degree of severity of pathology. The role of miRNAs in other tumors or tissues also needs to be determined. Relative miRNA signatures that are associated with the tumor's biology should result in markers with higher sensitivity and specificity, while changes in non-relative miRNA signatures could reflect non-related or secondary disease states and increase the false positive or false negative rate.

Analytical variability

Pre-analytical variability needs to be minimized. Minimal and predictable pre-analytical variability is preferred. Currently, there are no universally implemented SOPs for the collection, preparation, and extraction of samples for miRNA analysis. Differences in specimen type (tissue, whole blood, plasma, or serum), and how the miRNAs are collected (centrifugation and small RNA enrichment), can have a profound effect on miRNA concentrations. Furthermore, miRNA content in both plasma and serum can be influenced by cell remnant contamination from erythrocytes, leukocytes, or platelets. Biological variance, which has been largely neglected, could be an extremely important variable that may affect the clinical utility of miRNAs.

Analytical standards

A set of standards that can be incorporated into isolation and detection techniques need to be generated. Detection and quantification of miRNAs should be robust, rapid, simple, accurate, reproducible and inexpensive. miRNA detection currently falls short of all of these prerequisites. There is often a low correlation of results obtained from different platforms, or even from the same platform using reagents from different vendors. Standardization of these assays is especially challenging for circulating miRNA, where the concentration of miRNA is small.

Data normalization, an often underestimated aspect of data processing, is crucially important and is a major concern in obtaining accurate results. Because the sequence and the platform used for detection of the miRNA can affect the efficiency of detection, a normalizer is needed to adjust the raw data to render it comparable between samples. However, the lack of agreement on a putative normalizer or "housekeeping miRNA" is preventing proper analysis of circulating miRNA. The lack of standardization and implementation of normalization methods is especially challenging. Some of the discrepant results between miRNA studies may be due, in part, to the application of different normalization methods.

Downregulation or loss of miRNA expression needs to be accurately quantified. A major determinant of the early stages of cancer is the dysregulation of miRNAs that negatively regulate oncogenes. In terms of measurement, an increase in expression of miRNA is preferable to a decrease in expression, because of the ease in quantification in relation to a non-pathological condition. However, in cancer tissue, the expression of miRNAs with tumor suppressing potential is mostly repressed. Studies are needed to determine if the decrease in miRNA expression can be considered for diagnostic use. Also needed is the level of circulating miRNA in healthy individuals for base line comparison.

To enable miRNAs-based biomarkers to be useful in clinical diagnosis, the reproducibility and performance should be clearly examined. First, with the use of a universal set of standards, the data must be reproducible in the lab and later validated in other labs. In addition, clinical validation studies are required, with relatively large sample sizes and sufficient quantity of specimens, based on study design and biomarker assay. To fulfill the validation requirement and produce sustained results, collaborations among scientists and clinicians are essential.

Summary

The ultimate expectation of miRNAs as novel biomarkers is to enhance the ability to manage the patient optimally. Despite considerable efforts to demonstrate that miRNAs have a high potential to be used for the early detection of cancer and improving standard diagnosis tools, many challenges remain. First, in order to clearly identify miRNA biomarkers for diagnostics and prognostics, definitive miRNA signatures for all cancers need to be identified, with large profiling studies. Second, all the targets of the miRNAs involved in cancer need to be identified. This will help to ensure the accuracy of any diagnosis inferred from changes in a miRNA biomarkers, and will reduce the possibility of false positives.

Currently, there still remains significant inconsistency in the isolation and detection of extracellular miRNAs, so it is necessary to increase reproducibility during miRNA research. In addition, for achieving the purpose of using miRNAs as cancer detection markers, accurate measurement of miRNAs in bodily fluid must be developed, and clinical validation is critically important. Enhancement of international and national collaborations among scientists, clinicians and technologic experts for systematically evaluating the usefulness of miRNAs for cancer risk assessment, detection and prevention should help in achieving this goal.

Only after these concerns have been addressed can we ask if miRNA biomarkers will significantly improve the diagnostic workup, and eventually lead to a positive targeted clinical outcome when compared to already current diagnostic standards.

References

1. Lee RC, Feinbaum RL, Ambros V (1993). The *C. elegans* heterochronic gene lin-4 encodes small RNAs with antisense complementarity to lin-14. *Cell* **75**, 843–54.
2. Kozomara A, Griffiths-Jones S (2014). miRBase: annotating high confidence microRNAs using deep sequencing data. *Nucleic Acids Research* **42**, 25.
3. Wang X (2008). miRDB: a microRNA target prediction and functional annotation database with a wiki interface. *RNA* **14**, 1012–7.

4. Tian Y, Simanshu DK, Ma JB, Patel DJ (2011). Structural basis for piRNA 2′-O-methylated 3′-end recognition by Piwi PAZ (Piwi/Argonaute/Zwille) domains. *Proceedings of the National Academy of Sciences of the United States of America* **108**, 903–10.

5. Kwon C, Tak H, Rho M, Chang HR, Kim YH, Kim KT, *et al.* (2014). Detection of PIWI and piRNAs in the mitochondria of mammalian cancer cells. *Biochemical and Biophysical Research Communications* **446**, 218–23.

6. Okamura K, Lai EC (2008). Endogenous small interfering RNAs in animals. *Nature Reviews Molecular Cell Biology* **9**, 673–8.

7. Chan WL, Yuo CY, Yang WK, Hung SY, Chang YS, Chiu CC, *et al.* (2013). Transcribed pseudogene psiPPM1K generates endogenous siRNA to suppress oncogenic cell growth in hepatocellular carcinoma. *Nucleic Acids Research* **41**, 3734–47.

8. Chen L, Dahlstrom JE, Lee SH, Rangasamy D (2012). Naturally occurring endo-siRNA silences LINE-1 retrotransposons in human cells through DNA methylation. *Epigenetics* **7**, 758–71.

9. Lee YS, Shibata Y, Malhotra A, Dutta A (2009). A novel class of small RNAs: tRNA-derived RNA fragments (tRFs). *Genes & Development* **23**, 2639–49.

10. Martens-Uzunova ES, Olvedy M, Jenster G (2013). Beyond microRNA – novel RNAs derived from small non-coding RNA and their implication in cancer. *Cancer Letters* **340**, 201–11.

11. Zhao H, Bojanowski K, Ingber DE, Panigrahy D, Pepper MS, Montesano R, *et al.* (1999). New role for tRNA and its fragment purified from human urinary bladder carcinoma conditioned medium: inhibition of endothelial cell growth. *Journal of Cellular Biochemistry* **76**, 109–17.

12. Derrien T, Johnson R, Bussotti G, Tanzer A, Djebali S, Tilgner H, *et al.* (2012). The GENCODE v7 catalog of human long noncoding RNAs: analysis of their gene structure, evolution, and expression. *Genome Research* **22**, 1775–89.

13. Marques AC, Ponting CP (2014). Intergenic lncRNAs and the evolution of gene expression. *Current Opinion in Genetics & Development* **27**, 48–53.

14. Li CH, Chen Y (2013). Targeting long non-coding RNAs in cancers: progress and prospects. *International Journal of Biochemistry & Cell Biology* **45**, 1895–910.

15. Wang L, Fu D, Qiu Y, Xing X, Xu F, Han C, *et al.* (2014). Genome-wide screening and identification of long non-coding RNAs and their interaction with protein coding RNAs in bladder urothelial cell carcinoma. *Cancer Letters* **349**, 77–86.

16. Cao W, Wu W, Shi F, Chen X, Wu L, Yang K, *et al.* (2013). Integrated analysis of long noncoding RNA and coding RNA expression in esophageal squamous cell carcinoma. *International Journal of Genomics* **480534**, 7.

17. Yu G, Yao W, Wang J, Ma X, Xiao W, Li H, *et al.* (2012). LncRNAs expression signatures of renal clear cell carcinoma revealed by microarray. *PLoS One* **7**, 6.

18. Lee Y, Kim M, Han J, Yeom KH, Lee S, Baek SH, *et al.* (2004). MicroRNA genes are transcribed by RNA polymerase II. *The EMBO Journal* **23**, 4051–60.

19. Han J, Lee Y, Yeom KH, Kim YK, Jin H, Kim VN (2004). The Drosha-DGCR8 complex in primary microRNA processing. *Genes & Development* **18**, 3016–27.

20. Yeom KH, Lee Y, Han J, Suh MR, Kim VN (2006). Characterization of DGCR8/Pasha, the essential cofactor for Drosha in primary miRNA processing. *Nucleic Acids Research* **34**, 4622–9.

21. Kim VN (2004). MicroRNA precursors in motion: exportin-5 mediates their nuclear export. *Trends in Cell Biology* **14**, 156–9.

22. Hutvagner G, McLachlan J, Pasquinelli AE, Balint E, Tuschl T, Zamore PD (2001). A cellular function for the RNA-interference enzyme Dicer in the maturation of the let-7 small temporal RNA. *Science* **293**, 834–8.

23. Ketting RF, Fischer SE, Bernstein E, Sijen T, Hannon GJ, Plasterk RH (2001). Dicer functions in RNA interference and in synthesis of small RNA involved in developmental timing in C. elegans. *Genes & Development* **15**, 2654–9.

24. Khvorova A, Reynolds A, Jayasena SD (2003). Functional siRNAs and miRNAs exhibit strand bias. *Cell* **115**, 209–16.

25. Schwarz DS, Hutvagner G, Du T, Xu Z, Aronin N, Zamore PD (2003). Asymmetry in the assembly of the RNAi enzyme complex. *Cell* **115**, 199–208.

26. Bartel DP (2009). MicroRNAs: target recognition and regulatory functions. *Cell* **136**, 215–33.

27. Djuranovic S, Nahvi A, Green R (2011). A parsimonious model for gene regulation by miRNAs. *Science* **331**, 550–3.

28. Esquela-Kerscher A, Slack FJ (2006). Oncomirs – microRNAs with a role in cancer. *Nature Reviews Cancer* **6**, 259–69.

29. Friedman RC, Farh KK, Burge CB, Bartel DP (2009). Most mammalian mRNAs are conserved targets of microRNAs. *Genome Research* **19**, 92–105.

30. He L, Thomson JM, Hemann MT, Hernando-Monge E, Mu D, Goodson S, *et al.* (2005). A microRNA polycistron as a potential human oncogene. *Nature* **435**, 828–33.

31. Song MS, Rossi JJ (2014). The anti-miR21 antagomir, a therapeutic tool for colorectal cancer, has a potential synergistic effect by perturbing an angiogenesis-associated miR30. *Frontiers in Genetics* **4**.

32. Couzin J (2005). Cancer biology. A new cancer player takes the stage. *Science* **310**(5749), 766–7.

33. Reinhart BJ, Slack FJ, Basson M, Pasquinelli AE, Bettinger JC, Rougvie AE, *et al.* (2000). The 21-nucleotide

let-7 RNA regulates developmental timing in *Caenorhabditis elegans*. *Nature* **403**, 901–6.

34. Johnson CD, Esquela-Kerscher A, Stefani G, Byrom M, Kelnar K, Ovcharenko D, et al. (2007). The let-7 microRNA represses cell proliferation pathways in human cells. *Cancer Research* **67**, 7713–22.

35. Johnson SM, Grosshans H, Shingara J, Byrom M, Jarvis R, Cheng A, et al. (2005). RAS is regulated by the let-7 microRNA family. *Cell* **120**, 635–47.

36. Zhang KL, Zhou X, Han L, Chen LY, Chen LC, Shi ZD, et al. (2014). MicroRNA-566 activates EGFR signaling and its inhibition sensitizes glioblastoma cells to nimotuzumab. *Molecular Cancer* **13**, 1476–4598.

37. Li Y, Tan W, Neo TW, Aung MO, Wasser S, Lim SG, et al. (2009). Role of the miR-106b-25 microRNA cluster in hepatocellular carcinoma. *Cancer Science* **100**, 1234–42.

38. Zauli G, Voltan R, di Iasio MG, Bosco R, Melloni E, Sana ME, et al. (2011). miR-34a induces the downregulation of both E2F1 and B-Myb oncogenes in leukemic cells. *Clinical Cancer Research* **17**, 2712–24.

39. Tagawa H, Ikeda S, Sawada K (2013). Role of microRNA in the pathogenesis of malignant lymphoma. *Cancer Science* **104**, 801–9.

40. Lee YS, Dutta A (2006). MicroRNAs: small but potent oncogenes or tumor suppressors. *Current Opinion in Investigational Drugs* **7**, 560–4.

41. Calin GA, Ferracin M, Cimmino A, Di Leva G, Shimizu M, Wojcik SE, et al. (2005). A MicroRNA signature associated with prognosis and progression in chronic lymphocytic leukemia. *New England Journal of Medicine* **353**, 1793–801.

42. Hanlon K, Rudin CE, Harries LW (2009). Investigating the targets of MIR-15a and MIR-16-1 in patients with chronic lymphocytic leukemia (CLL). *PLoS One* **4**, 0007169.

43. Cimmino A, Calin GA, Fabbri M, Iorio MV, Ferracin M, Shimizu M, et al. (2005). miR-15 and miR-16 induce apoptosis by targeting BCL2. *Proceedings of the National Academy of Sciences of the United States of America* **102**, 13944–9.

44. Mishra PJ, Merlino G (2009). MicroRNA reexpression as differentiation therapy in cancer. *Journal of Clinical Investigation* **119**, 2119–23.

45. Yan D, Dong Xda E, Chen X, Wang L, Lu C, Wang J, et al. (2009). MicroRNA-1/206 targets c-Met and inhibits rhabdomyosarcoma development. *Journal of Biological Chemistry* **284**, 29596–604.

46. Ahmad A, Sarkar SH, Bitar B, Ali S, Aboukameel A, Sethi S, et al. (2012). Garcinol regulates EMT and Wnt signaling pathways in vitro and in vivo, leading to anticancer activity against breast cancer cells. *Molecular Cancer Therapeutics* **11**, 2193–201.

47. Taulli R, Bersani F, Foglizzo V, Linari A, Vigna E, Ladanyi M, et al. (2009). The muscle-specific microRNA miR-206 blocks human rhabdomyosarcoma growth in xenotransplanted mice by promoting myogenic differentiation. *Journal of Clinical Investigation* **119**, 2366–78.

48. Mu P, Han YC, Betel D, Yao E, Squatrito M, Ogrodowski P, et al. (2009). Genetic dissection of the miR-17~92 cluster of microRNAs in Myc-induced B-cell lymphomas. *Genes & Development* **23**, 2806–11.

49. Olive V, Bennett MJ, Walker JC, Ma C, Jiang I, Cordon-Cardo C, et al. (2009). miR-19 is a key oncogenic component of mir-17-92. *Genes & Development* **23**, 2839–49.

50. Ling N, Gu J, Lei Z, Li M, Zhao J, Zhang HT, et al. (2013). microRNA-155 regulates cell proliferation and invasion by targeting FOXO3a in glioma. *Oncology Reports* **30**, 2111–8.

51. Bar N, Dikstein R (2010). miR-22 forms a regulatory loop in PTEN/AKT pathway and modulates signaling kinetics. *PLoS One* **5**, 0010859.

52. Liu L, Jiang Y, Zhang H, Greenlee AR, Han Z (2010). Overexpressed miR-494 down-regulates PTEN gene expression in cells transformed by anti-benzo(a)pyrene-trans-7,8-dihydrodiol-9,10-epoxide. *Life Sciences* **86**, 192–8.

53. Zhou L, Qi RQ, Liu M, Xu YP, Li G, Weiland M, et al. (2014). microRNA miR-17-92 cluster is highly expressed in epidermal Langerhans cells but not required for its development. *Genes & Immunity* **15**, 57–61.

54. Mogilyansky E, Rigoutsos I (2013). The miR-17/92 cluster: a comprehensive update on its genomics, genetics, functions and increasingly important and numerous roles in health and disease. *Cell Death & Differentiation* **20**, 1603–14.

55. Nam EJ, Yoon H, Kim SW, Kim H, Kim YT, Kim JH, et al. (2008). MicroRNA expression profiles in serous ovarian carcinoma. *Clinical Cancer Research* **14**, 2690–5.

56. Visone R, Pallante P, Vecchione A, Cirombella R, Ferracin M, Ferraro A, et al. (2007). Specific microRNAs are downregulated in human thyroid anaplastic carcinomas. *Oncogene* **26**, 7590–5.

57. Le MT, Teh C, Shyh-Chang N, Xie H, Zhou B, Korzh V, et al. (2009). MicroRNA-125b is a novel negative regulator of p53. *Genes & Development* **23**, 862–76.

58. Ozen M, Creighton CJ, Ozdemir M, Ittmann M (2008). Widespread deregulation of microRNA expression in human prostate cancer. *Oncogene* **27**, 1788–93.

59. Paranjape T, Heneghan H, Lindner R, Keane FK, Hoffman A, Hollestelle A, et al. (2011). A 3′-untranslated region KRAS variant and triple-negative breast cancer: a case-control and genetic analysis. *The Lancet Oncology* **12**, 377–86.

60. Kundu ST, Nallur S, Paranjape T, Boeke M, Weidhaas JB, Slack FJ (2012). KRAS alleles: the LCS6 3′UTR

variant and KRAS coding sequence mutations in the NCI-60 panel. *Cell Cycle* **11**, 361–6.

61. Wei X, Chen D, Lv T, Li G, Qu S (2014). Serum MicroRNA-125b as a Potential Biomarker for Glioma Diagnosis. *Molecular Neurobiology* **23**, 23.

62. Wang S, Xiang J, Li Z, Lu S, Hu J, Gao X, *et al.* (2015). A plasma microRNA panel for early detection of colorectal cancer. *International Journal of Cancer* **136**, 152–61.

63. Mar-Aguilar F, Luna-Aguirre CM, Moreno-Rocha JC, Araiza-Chavez J, Trevino V, Rodriguez-Padilla C, *et al.* (2013). Differential expression of miR-21, miR-125b and miR-191 in breast cancer tissue. *Asia-Pacific Journal of Clinical Oncology* **9**, 53–9.

64. Xing L, Su J, Guarnera MA, Zhang H, Cai L, Zhou R, *et al.* (2015). Sputum microRNA Biomarkers for Identifying Lung Cancer in Indeterminate Solitary Pulmonary Nodules. *Clinical Cancer Research* **21**, 484–9.

65. Liloglou T, Bediaga NG, Brown BR, Field JK, Davies MP (2014). Epigenetic biomarkers in lung cancer. *Cancer Letters* **342**, 200–12.

66. Lawrie CH, Gal S, Dunlop HM, Pushkaran B, Liggins AP, Pulford K, *et al.* (2008). Detection of elevated levels of tumour-associated microRNAs in serum of patients with diffuse large B-cell lymphoma. *British Journal of Haematology* **141**, 672–5.

67. Mitchell PS, Parkin RK, Kroh EM, Fritz BR, Wyman SK, Pogosova-Agadjanyan EL, *et al.* (2008). Circulating microRNAs as stable blood-based markers for cancer detection. *Proceedings of the National Academy of Sciences of the United States of America* **105**, 10513–8.

68. Cortez MA, Bueso-Ramos C, Ferdin J, Lopez-Berestein G, Sood AK, Calin GA (2011). MicroRNAs in body fluids – the mix of hormones and biomarkers. *Nature Reviews Clinical Oncology* **8**, 467–77.

69. Shen J, Stass SA, Jiang F (2013). MicroRNAs as potential biomarkers in human solid tumors. *Cancer Letters* **329**, 125–36.

70. Wang J, Zhang KY, Liu SM, Sen S (2014). Tumor-associated circulating microRNAs as biomarkers of cancer. *Molecules* **19**, 1912–38.

71. Shen J, Todd NW, Zhang H, Yu L, Lingxiao X, Mei Y, *et al.* (2011). Plasma microRNAs as potential biomarkers for non-small-cell lung cancer. *Laboratory Investigation* **91**, 579–87.

72. Shen J, Liu Z, Todd NW, Zhang H, Liao J, Yu L, *et al.* (2011). Diagnosis of lung cancer in individuals with solitary pulmonary nodules by plasma microRNA biomarkers. *BMC Cancer* **11**, 1471–2407.

73. Xing L, Todd NW, Yu L, Fang H, Jiang F (2010). Early detection of squamous cell lung cancer in sputum by a panel of microRNA markers. *Modern Pathology* **23**, 1157–64.

74. Hanke M, Hoefig K, Merz H, Feller AC, Kausch I, Jocham D, *et al.* (2010). A robust methodology to study urine microRNA as tumor marker: microRNA-126 and microRNA-182 are related to urinary bladder cancer. *Urologic Oncology* **28**, 655–61.

75. Jarry J, Schadendorf D, Greenwood C, Spatz A, van Kempen LC (2014). The validity of circulating microRNAs in oncology: five years of challenges and contradictions. *Molecular Oncology* **8**, 819–29.

76. Wang J, Wang Q, Liu H, Hu B, Zhou W, Cheng Y (2010). MicroRNA expression and its implication for the diagnosis and therapeutic strategies of gastric cancer. *Cancer Letters* **297**, 137–43.

77. Tong N, Xu B, Shi D, Du M, Li X, Sheng X, *et al.* (2014). Hsa-miR-196a2 polymorphism increases the risk of acute lymphoblastic leukemia in Chinese children. *Mutation Research/Fundamental and Molecular Mechanisms of Mutagenesis* **759**, 16–21.

78. Chen C, Yang S, Chaugai S, Wang Y, Wang D (2014). Meta-analysis of Hsa-mir-499 polymorphism (rs3746444) for cancer risk: evidence from 31 case-control studies. *BMC Medical Genetics* **15**, 126.

79. Hansen TF, Kjaer-Frifeldt S, Christensen RD, Morgenthaler S, Blondal T, Lindebjerg J, *et al.* (2014). Redefining high-risk patients with stage II colon cancer by risk index and microRNA-21: results from a population-based cohort. *British Journal of Cancer* **111**, 1285–92.

80. Kjaer-Frifeldt S, Hansen TF, Nielsen BS, Joergensen S, Lindebjerg J, Soerensen FB, *et al.* (2012). The prognostic importance of miR-21 in stage II colon cancer: a population-based study. *British Journal of Cancer* **107**, 1169–74.

81. Nielsen BS, Jorgensen S, Fog JU, Sokilde R, Christensen IJ, Hansen U, *et al.* (2011). High levels of microRNA-21 in the stroma of colorectal cancers predict short disease-free survival in stage II colon cancer patients. *Clinical & Experimental Metastasis* **28**, 27–38.

82. Ashby J, Flack K, Jimenez LA, Duan Y, Khatib AK, Somlo G, *et al.* (2014). Distribution profiling of circulating microRNAs in serum. *Analytical Chemistry* **86**, 9343–9.

CHAPTER 4

Inflammation and Cancer

Pamela L Beatty,[1] Sandra Cascio,[1,2] and Olivera J Finn[1]

[1] Department of Immunology, University of Pittsburgh School of Medicine, PA, USA
[2] Fondazione RiMED, Palermo, Italy

Background

Research into the prevention, treatment and causes of cancer has revealed that certain types of inflammation of various etiologies and afflicting various tissues can increase the risk for cancer development in those tissues. Initial support for this came from epidemiological studies which showed that reduction of inflammation, through the use of aspirin or non-steroidal anti-inflammatory drugs (NSAIDs), reduced the incidence of many cancers, including colorectal, esophageal, pancreatic, stomach, lung, brain, and prostate [1,2].

An association between inflammation and cancer is not a new observation, having already been first described in the 19th century by Virchow, who noted a cellular infiltrate in solid tumors [3]. He hypothesized that this phenomenon represented an attempt by the host to eliminate the tumor cells. Numerous studies since have shown that cellular infiltrate is a characteristic of most solid tumors. A positive correlation has been found between the presence in the tumor microenvironment of T cells expressing markers of Th1 type and memory T cells, and lower incidence of tumor recurrence [4]. In addition, the density and location of immune cells within tumors is a better predictor of patient survival than other methods used to stage cancer and predict its course [4].

Clinical studies have demonstrated that high density of intratumoral CD8+ T cells is also associated with improved disease outcome in breast, ovarian, bladder, colorectal and lung cancer [5–9].

However, not all immune cells in the tumor microenvironment contribute to tumor elimination. Tumor-promoting attributes have been assigned to a variety of cells of the innate immune system, but cells of the immune system are not solely responsible for tumor-promoting inflammation. They play a role through a complex interplay with other cell types in the tumor microenvironment, such as fibroblasts, endothelial and epithelial cells and tumor cells. This interplay results in the induction of transcriptional programs and production of soluble mediators that, together, foster an inflammatory environment conducive to tumor growth.

Introduction: inflammation

Key features of cancer-promoting inflammation include infiltration of macrophages and neutrophils that generate reactive oxygen species (ROS) and reactive nitrogen species (RNS) which, in the presence of repeated tissue damage, induce mutations in the DNA and RNA and profound changes in the structure of lipids, glycans and proteins. Activated macrophages also release inflammatory cytokines, including tumor necrosis factor-α (TNF-α), that stimulate ROS production in neighboring cells and perpetuate tumor-promoting inflammation. Furthermore, TNF-α activates NF-κB, a key transcription factor that is involved in the inflammatory pathway and is constitutively activated in most cancers [10]. Extracellular proteases, such as the matrix

Biomarkers in Cancer Screening and Early Detection, First Edition. Edited by Sudhir Srivastava.
© 2017 John Wiley & Sons, Inc. Published 2017 by John Wiley & Sons, Inc.

metalloproteinases (MMPs), cytokines, such as interleukin-6 (IL-6) and interleukin-8 (IL-8), and signal transducer and activator of transcription-3 (STAT3) are activated in most cancers, promoting cell growth, angiogenesis and survival. Their specific roles will be described in more detail later in the chapter.

Tumorigenesis is a multistage process comprising initiation, promotion and progression. Tumor initiation is governed by cumulative genetic and epigenetic changes, triggered by mutations in proto-oncogenes and/or tumor suppressor genes. Initiated (premalignant) cells can persist in tissues for years, where they encounter various promotion stimuli and acquire specific characteristics known as "hallmarks of cancer" that enable tumor growth and metastasis. Inflammation has recently emerged as an enabling factor in cancer development, and

the susceptibility of tumors to the promoting influence of inflammation has been recognized as a new important hallmark of cancer [11].

Inflammation is the body's response to infection (e.g. bacterial, viral and parasitic) or tissue damage. An acute inflammatory response is normally a self-limiting process and, once the infection is cleared and/or the damaged tissue is repaired, the inflammation resolves and tissue returns to the homeostatic state. Chronic inflammation, however, is characterized by the failure to eliminate the initiating factors and/or failure of the host defense mechanisms to resolve the inflammatory response. The types of inflammation that are associated with an increased risk for cancer development and the inflammatory signals differ depending on the nature of the initial insult (illustrated in Figure 4.1).

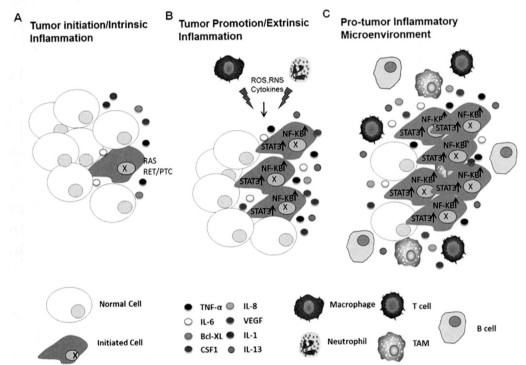

Figure 4.1 Co-evolution of cancer and its inflammatory microenvironment. **A**. Oncogenic mutations (e.g. Ras, RET/PTC) or other initiators of malignant transformation change the transcriptional program of initiated cells, including *de novo* transcription of inflammatory cytokines (intrinsic inflammation). **B**. These cytokines attract the cells of the innate immune system (e.g. macrophages and neutrophils), which produce their own cytokines and other inflammatory molecules (ROS, RNS) (extrinsic inflammation) that promote tumor development and tumor cell survival. **C**. The growing tumor attracts many cells of the immune system, creating a pro-tumor inflammatory microenvironment. Tumor-specific T cells and B cells are also present, but their function is compromised by the immunosuppressive effect of the tumor microenvironment. For a color version of this figure please see color plate section.

It is known that cancer and inflammation are connected by two pathways: *intrinsic pathway* and *extrinsic pathway* [12]. In the intrinsic pathway, genetic alterations and epigenetic mutations in somatic cells lead to transformation, and also enable those cells to elicit an inflammatory response that promotes malignant transformation. Activation of different classes of oncogenes induces the expression of tumor-promoting inflammatory cytokines and chemokines, creating an inflammatory microenvironment.

A well-known example of the intrinsic pathway is inflammatory hepatocellular adenoma, a benign liver tumor, characterized by an inflammatory infiltrate caused by a constitutively activated STAT3 pathway in the absence of ligand, due to a mutation in the binding site for IL-6 [13]. Similarly, chromosomal rearrangement of the genes encoding protein tyrosine kinase (*RET/PET*) or *Ras* family are frequent early events in papillary thyroid cancer or myeloma and pancreatic cancer, respectively. It has been shown that they induce the production of cytokines, enzymes and chemokines such as CSFs, IL-1 and COX-2 involved in the pro-tumor inflammatory pathways [14].

Infection-induced inflammation

Cancers that result from a known infection account for 17.8% of the global cancer burden [15]. Although some pathogens can directly induce cell transformation (e.g. human papillomavirus-inducing cervical cancer), the majority contribute to carcinogenesis by inducing a chronic inflammatory microenvironment. Infection-induced inflammation starts with the recognition by the innate immune system of pathogen-associated patterns (PAMPs) through pattern-recognition receptors (PRRs) on macrophages, neutrophils, mast cells and dendritic cells. The toll-like receptors (TLRs) are the predominant PPRs, and engagement of PAMPs with TLRs trigger signaling pathways, with the resultant release of cytokines and chemokines that activate and recruit lymphocytes.

Some of the strongest links between the cancer causing infection and pro-tumor inflammation can be made in hepatocellular carcinoma (HCC) caused by hepatitis B virus (HBV) and/or hepatitis C virus (HCV) infections [16], and gastric carcinomas caused by *Helicobacter pylori* (*H. pylori*) [17].

Both HBV and HCV establish persistent infection by blocking the initial innate immune response, or skewing it towards the Type 2 that promotes tissue repair instead of pathogen elimination. HBV alters Toll-like receptor (TLR) signaling, which severely impairs the innate immune response [18]. Inhibition of TLR signaling in antigen-presenting dendritic cells (DCs) leads to impaired Th1 response, with decreased IL-2, TNF-α and IFN-γ production [19]. The core protein of HCV has been shown to induce overproduction of ROS in the liver. HCV infection has also been shown to result in a skewed liver cytokine profile. Increased levels of IFN-a appear to polarize natural killer (NK) cells toward hyper-cytolytic activity without an increase in IFN-g, and this has been proposed as a mechanism of liver damage without virus clearance [20].

In *H. pylori* infection, activated neutrophils and macrophages, as well as increased levels of IL-8, are found in the gastric mucosa of infected individuals. Cellular damage is thought to be the result of production of oxygen metabolites, leading to DNA injury [21]. Individuals infected with strains containing cytotoxin-associated gene A (CagA) have an even higher incidence of developing cancer than individuals infected with strains without CagA. CagA has been shown to increase STAT3 in gastritis, intestinal metaplasia and stomach cancer, where it translocates to the nucleus and upregulates transcription of various genes involved in growth and proliferation [22].

Inflammation in sterile tissue injury

Inflammation in the absence of infection is referred to as "sterile inflammation". This type can occur when there is tissue damage accompanied by new or increased expression of damage-associated molecules high-mobility group box 1 (HMGB-1), heat shock proteins (HSPs), ATP and uric acid, released into the extracellular environment by the dying cells, or increased levels of molecules released by extracellular matrix (such as hyaluronan and heparin sulfate) [23]. All these tissue-injury related molecules are referred to collectively as damage-associated molecular patterns (DAMPs). In sterile inflammation, DAMPs are recognized by the TLRs of infiltrating macrophages and neutrophils, leading to the activation of pro-inflammatory pathways and release of histamines, cytokines and lipid mediators required to promote tissue repair (but, in the case of cancer, beneficial to its growth).

Examples of sterile inflammation promoting cancer development include pancreatitis leading to pancreatic cancer, lung inflammation progressing to mesothelioma, Barrett's Esophagus (BE) converting to esophageal cancer, and endometriosis giving rise to ovarian cancer (24-28]. Epidemiological studies have most recently associated obesity, another sterile inflammatory condition, with an increased risk of a wide range of cancers [29]. The initial injury that causes acute pancreatitis is usually sterile (e.g. alcohol consumption and gallstones), resulting in acinar cell necrosis and influx of monocytes and neutrophils. Recurrent acute pancreatitis can lead to chronic pancreatitis, which is a risk factor for the development of pancreatic ductal carcinoma (PDA) [28]. In the absence of resolution, there is a shift in the apoptosis-necrosis balance of acinar cell death in favor of necrosis [24]. This results in high levels of ROS perpetuating inflammation and DNA damage.

Lung inflammation is a hallmark of inhaled asbestos or silica particles, and asbestos fibers are associated with the development of malignant mesotheliomas [25]. Bronchial epithelial cells and macrophages are in constant contact with the inhaled particulates, and initiate and sustain lung inflammation [30]. Phagocytosis of asbestos particles leads to high production of ROS [25, 30]. Barrett's esophagus (BE) represents the only identified precursor lesion, and the most important risk factor for esophageal adenocarcinoma [27]. BE is the result of healing from esophageal mucosal injury, due to gastroesophagel reflux disease (GERD). Chronic mucosal injury induces production of ROS, and the bile salts can induce degradation of p53.

Tumor-promoting inflammatory cells

Cancer cells comprise 30% or less of the cells in a solid tumor mass, and the remaining mass is known as tumor stroma [31]. Stroma includes the extracellular matrix (ECM) (e.g. proteoglycans, hyaluronic acid and fibrous proteins), various soluble factors (chemokines and cytokines), and stromal cells (e.g. mesenchymal and immune cells)

[31]. Two key cell populations that drive inflammation are macrophages and neutrophils. Resident tissue macrophages are important sensors of, and responders to danger in the host tissues, and they also constitute a major cell population in the tumor microenvironment. Macrophages display incredible plasticity, and their function can be anti- or pro-tumorigenic, depending on the signals they receive from the tumor or the rest of tumor stroma during the transition from early preneoplasia to advanced tumor stages.

Classical, so-called Type 1 macrophages (M1), develop in the presence of IFNg and TNFa, and they produce increased superoxide anion, oxygen and nitrogen radicals, and secrete high levels of pro-inflammatory cytokines such as IL-12. M1 macrophages are tumoricidal, and they drive the polarization and recruitment of Th1 cells. High production of TNFa, ROS and RNS by macrophages, on the other hand, has been shown to support neoplastic transformation. In mammary tumors, macrophages have been shown to facilitate tumor cell intravasation, an important step in tumor cell dissemination and metastasis [32].

Type 2 macrophages (M2) develop in the presence of IL-4 and IL-13. They have impaired antigen-presenting capabilities, produce IL-10, downregulate IL-12 and secrete components of the extracellular matrix that cause tissue fibrosis. M2 macrophages are associated with tissue remodeling, and they support tumor promotion through the release of pro-angiogenic factors such as IL-8 and VEGF [33]. In addition to being bad presenters of antigen and, thus, ineffective at inducing adaptive immunity, they actively suppress anti-tumor T cells by releasing prostaglandins, IL-10 and TGFb.

Neutrophils are the first line of defense against microbial pathogens, due to their immediate ability to generate proteases and ROS. Their activation is important in the regulation of innate and adaptive immunity. Neutrophils can also be polarized toward a tumor-promoting Type 2 (N2), or tumor-inhibiting Type 1 (N1) [34]. Neutrophils contain an intracellular pool of VEGF that they release in response to various cytokines (TNF, IFN-γ, IL-4, IL-10 and IL-13), and contribute to tumor promotion by stimulating angiogenesis [35]. They also release enzymes that disrupt the basal membrane, thus facilitating extravasation of cancer cells [36].

Myeloid-derived suppressor cells (MDSCs) are a heterogenous population of myeloid progenitor cells and immature myeloid cells. MDSCs are found in many pathological conditions, and can regulate immune responses to infections, acute and chronic inflammation, traumatic stress, sepsis and organ transplants. MDSCs contribute to tumor promotion in part by driving angiogenesis, but their major effect is on inhibiting T cell activation [37]. In a mouse model of pancreatic ductal carcinoma (PDA), increased numbers of MDSCs in the pancreas was strongly correlated with the absence of $CD8^+$ T cells, even very early in the development of pancreatic intraepithelial neoplasia (PanIN) lesions [38].

Tumor-promoting inflammatory cytokines and chemokines

Through downstream effectors, some cytokines and chemokines promote anti-tumor immunity (e.g. IL-2, IFN-γ, TRAIL), while others can enhance tumor progression (e.g. TNF-α, IL-6, IL-17, IL-23, IL-11) and invasion and metastasis (e.g. IL-8, IL-6). Production of pro-inflammatory cytokines by stromal cells and immune/inflammatory cells, such as T cells and macrophages, activates transcription factors in pre-malignant cells, including NF-kB, AP-1 and STAT3, with a tumor-promoting effect. Pro-inflammatory cytokines are also produced by cancer cells which, in turn, enhances the recruitment of inflammatory cells into the tumor-site with a consequent overexpression of pro-inflammatory cytokines. Other molecules that work via autocrine and paracrine mechanisms are the pro-angiogenic factors VEGF, HIF-α, IL-8 and angiopetin2. In order to increase in size, tumors require blood supply. Hypoxia in the tumor microenvironment promotes angiogenesis and increases the probability of metastasis. Like cytokines and chemokines, these pro-angiogenic factors are released both by tumor cells and stromal and inflammatory cells.

IL-6, IL-8 and TNF-α are the major mediators of inflammation-driven tumorigenesis. They activate the key transcription factors in tumor-associated inflammation, NF-kB and STAT3, impacting different stages of tumorigenesis. IL-6 is a multifunctional cytokine that regulates both innate and adaptive immunity [39, 40]. It is involved in the regulation of the acute phase response by inducing the differentiation of monocytes to macrophages, resistance of T cells to apoptosis and Th2 cytokine production. IL-6 is also involved in chronic inflammation, inducing Th17 effector cells and inhibiting the differentiation of regulatory T cells (Treg). Expression of IL-6 is regulated by several transcription factors, such as NF-kB, CAAT/enhancer-binding protein beta (C/EBPbeta) or activator protein 1 (AP-1).

IL-6 is produced by various cell types, including monocytes, macrophages, fibroblasts, keratinocytes, endothelial cells, B cells, T cells, and also several tumor types. IL-6 can interact with both membrane-bound and soluble forms of its receptor, IL-6R, triggering signaling via dimerization of gp130, and leading to the activation of the JAK/STAT3 pathway, phosphorylation of the mitogen-activated protein kinases (MAPK) and Akt pathway. It also promotes epithelial-to-mesenchymal transition (EMT), a crucial process in tumor invasiveness and metastasis, which converts an adherent epithelial cell to a migratory cell that can invade through the extracellular matrix. As is the case with many inflammatory mediators, in addition to a pro-inflammatory activity, IL-6 has also been reported to play a role in terminating inflammation through STAT3-mediated signaling pathways [40]. Because of the importance of dysregulated IL-6 production and signaling in chronic inflammatory diseases, auto-immunity and cancer, IL-6 is the subject of translational research as a promising therapeutic target [41].

IL-8 is produced by various types of tumors, such as lung, breast, colon, prostate and gastric cancers, malignant melanoma and others. Its increased expression has been associated with advanced stages of tumor, and it has been used to differentiate between benign and malignant disease. It is produced in response to IL-1 and TNF-α, which activate NF-kB, AP-1 and SP1 signaling pathways. IL-8 produced by the tumor is important for the activation and chemotaxis of neutrophils in the tumor microenvironment. In contrast to IL-6 and TNF-α, whose effects may be both pro- and anti-tumor, IL-8 is a pro-tumor chemokine and a strong inducer of tumor proliferation, angiogenesis and metastasis [39].

TNF-α is involved in the regulation of embryonic development, sleep-wake cycle, lymph node follicle and germinal center formation, as well as in host defense against bacterial and viral infection. TNF-α is another pleiotropic cytokine that plays a dual role in tumorigenesis. A high level of TNF-α can destroy tumor vasculature and induce necrosis, thereby providing an anti-tumor function. On the other hand, at low levels, TNF-α can be a key intermediary in the process of cancer-associated chronic inflammation. Its overexpression is frequently detected in human breast, bladder, colorectal, prostate, ovarian and renal cancers, as well as in leukemia [3].

The pro-inflammatory role of TNF-α has been documented in all the steps involved in tumorigenesis. It contributes to tumor initiation by stimulation of genotoxic RNS and ROS species, and to tumor promotion by inducing angiogenesis, impairment of immunosurveillance through T-cell suppression, and inhibition of the cytotoxic activity of activated macrophages. Although macrophages are the major source of TNF-α, it can also be made by a variety of other cells, including fibroblasts, astrocytes, and tumor cells.

The molecular mechanisms behind TNF's actions have been extensively investigated. The binding of TNF-α to its receptor (TNFR1) activates several adaptor proteins, such as the TNFR-associated factor containing death domains (TRADD) which, in turn, recruits TNFR-associated factors (TRAFs), as well as the cellular inhibitor of apoptosis proteins 1 and 2 (c-IAP1/2), to form the TNF receptor signaling complex (TNF-RSC). This TNF-dependent signaling cascade regulates many pathways, including NF-kB, c-Jun N-terminal Kinase (JNK), MAPK, and the nuclear transcriptional factor AP1 [42].

Molecular pathways and networks that regulate tumor promoting inflammation

Two major nuclear transcription factors that regulate transcriptional activity of pro-inflammatory and pro-angiogenic factors, both in cancer cells and inflammatory cells, are NF-kB and STAT3. They are aberrantly expressed in most tumors, lymphoid or solid, and are responsible for responding to the signals from the tumor microenvironment and enhancing survival and progression of neoplastic cells.

The NF-κB family of molecules is composed of RelA (p65), c-Rel, RelB, p50 (NF-κB1) and p52 (NF-κB2). These proteins form homodimers and heterodimers, interact with IκBs and bind DNA. NF-κB complexes reside predominantly in the cytoplasm, in an inactive form bound to the IκB family of proteins. Exposure to pro-inflammatory cytokines, such as TNF-α and IL-1, or mutations of upstream components of IKK–NF-κB signaling pathways [10], activate NF-κB pathway in cancer cells. Upon activation, IκBα is phosphorylated and polyubiquitinated by the IKK complex. Then, NF-κB forms a dimer, predominantly RelA-p50, translocates to the nucleus, and interacts with the DNA at specific motifs known as kB sites [43]. NF-κB-binding sites have been found in the promoter genes encoding cytokines, chemokines, adhesion molecules, inhibitor of apoptosis, and enzymes that produce secondary inflammatory mediators (for a complete list of molecules and genes related to NF-κB regulation, see www.nf-kb.org).

The NF-κB pathway is active in both the cancer cells and the inflammatory cells in the tumor microenvironment, and it is involved in cancer initiation, promotion and progression. In cells that are destined to be converted to malignant cells after TNF-α and IL-1 activation, NF-kB upregulates genes that create resistance to apoptotic cell death and DNA damage, such as BCL-X, BFL1, SOD2, resulting in the survival and proliferation of tumorigenic cells. NF-κB activation in cancer cells can also lead to upregulation of chemokines that initiate and maintain the tumor microenvironment through the recruitment of the immune response and inflammatory cells. One interesting example is the activation of the NF-kB pathway through an overexpression of a tumor mucin MUC1 [44]. Upon TNF-α activation, NF-kB p65 associates with the tumor-specific form of the mucin MUC1, characterized by short O-glycans typical of tumor-type glycosylation, and translocates to the nucleus, where it binds to the kB consensus sites of IL-6 and TNF-α, increasing their transcription.

Activation of NF-κB and pro-inflammatory cytokine expression are constitutive not only in cancer cells, but also in cancer-associated fibroblasts (CAFs) [45], which drive neovascularization and tumor growth. Tumor progression is also facilitated by the production of colony-stimulating factor 1 (CSF1) and IL-6 by tumor-associated macrophages (TAMs) that inhibit DC maturation. There is also evidence that NF-κB is important for macrophage recruitment and maintenance of their immunosuppressive phenotype. Inhibition of IKKb activity in TAMs converts them from the tumor-polarized M2 phenotype to the M1 cytotoxic phenotype, driving tumor regression [46]. Although NF-kB activation is mostly known to stimulate tumor progression and to have anti-apoptotic influence, there is evidences to indicate that it can also have an inhibitory effect on onco-genesis, and can promote apoptosis in response to chemotherapeutic agents [47].

STAT3 is a convergent point for a number of oncogenic signaling pathways, and controls intra-cellular signal transduction of several pro-inflammatory cytokines and growth factors. As discussed above, IL-6 is one of the main inducers of STAT3 phosphorylation, through the activation of gp130-associated proteins Janus kinase (Jak). Phosphorylated STAT3 forms stable homodimers, translocates to the nucleus and binds the DNA. STAT3 recognizes an 8- to 10-base pair inverted repeat DNA element, with a consensus sequence of 5-TT(N)AA-3, and activates transcription of several genes, among them VEGF, IL-10, Bcl-xL, Cyclin D1, p21 and c-Myc [48].

In normal cells, activation of STAT3 is a transient and tightly controlled process, critical for transmission of cytokine-induced proliferation and differentiation signals. Elevated expression of STAT3 and its constitutive activation is a recurrent finding in HCC, leukemias, lymphomas, multiple myelomas, prostate, gastric, breast, lung, and head and neck cancer [49]. Chronic inflammatory conditions that drive carcinogenesis can also be attributed to altered STAT3 signaling. Studies in mice have demonstrated that an increase in STAT3 signaling leads to inflammation-associated gastric tumorigenesis [50].

Similar to the NF-kB pathway, constitutive activation of STAT3 is involved in many cellular processes, including cell growth, survival, metastasis, angiogenesis, and immune suppression. STAT3, indeed, plays a major role in tumor initiation and development. For example, it is required for oncogenic transformation by v-Src, and several studies reported that inhibition of STAT3 expression suppressed the transformed phenotype and tumor progression. IL-6/STAT3 signaling participates in initiation and promotion of tumor through upregulation of genes encoding apoptosis inhibitors Bcl-2, Bcl-xL, survivin, Mcl-1 and XIAP. It is also involved in the control of cell cycle progression, by regulating the expression of c-myc and Cyclin D1, which can associate with cdk4 or cdk6 and control progression from G1 to S phase. Thus, STAT3, by regulating the transcription of key proteins of the cell cycle, contributes to malignant progression [48].

It has also been proposed that STAT3 leads to tumor progression by negatively regulating immunosurveillance. Experiments in tumor-bearing mice with Stat3$^{-/-}$ hematopoietic cells revealed an enhanced function of dendritic cells, T cells, natural killer (NK) cells and neutrophils [51]. Thus STAT3 activation pathway is an important contributor to inflammation-induced cancers, making it an attractive target for treating and/or preventing cancer. Because IL-6 has been linked to constitutive or aberrant activation of STAT3 in various cancers, molecules that inhibit IL-6 or IL-6R may be good targets for inhibition of STAT3-mediated tumorigenesis. Interrupting STAT-3 signaling with selective inhibitors would not only have a direct antitumor effect, through growth suppression and apoptosis induction, but could also activate innate and adaptive anti-tumor immunity. There are multiple strategies that can be taken to design inhibitors of STAT3 signaling. Some involve pharmacologic inhibitors of upstream STAT3 activators, such as IL-6R, while others may rely on identifying small molecules that directly target STAT3 proteins and disrupt their function [48].

Tumor-associated antigens and inflammation

During the process of carcinogenesis, cancer cells express tumor antigens derived from genetic alterations and epigenetic dysregulation of normal molecules, which can then be recognized as abnormal by the immune system. Molecules such as CEA, MUC1 and NY-ESO-1, originally identified as tumor associated antigens, have been shown to induce innate inflammatory responses that inhibit an effective anti-tumor T cell response [28, 52, 53]. The C-type lectin DC-SIGN that is expressed on immature DCs can bind CEA released by tumor cells, resulting in the inhibition of DC antigen-presenting function, and thus preventing genera-tion of anti-tumor T cell responses [53].

Tumor antigen MUC1 has been shown to be chemotactic for immature DCs which, fol-lowing the encounter with MUC1 on tumors, fail to make IL-12 and to promote an effective Th1 anti-tumor response [52]. Inhibition of Th1 immune responses, and failure to eliminate can-cer cells, leads to a persistent chronic inflamma-tory environment that fosters continued tumor growth. Premalignant lesions of many cancers have now been identified, and many abnormal self antigens/tumor-associated antigens, expressed on the fully mature tumor cells, have also been found on premalignant cells [54, 55]. Thus, even at these early stages of tumor development, the immune response can be skewed toward promoting prema-lignant cell growth, and progression to fully malig-nant cells.

Transition from normal to cancerous tissue is often associated with alterations in posttransla-tional modifications of cellular proteins, which can change the biological properties and function of many molecules. Several studies indicate that aber-rant glycosylation accompanies oncogenic trans-formation and that, in turn, impacts tumor cell functions and promotes metastasis [56].

Some well-characterized tumor-specific carbo-hydrates are Tn (GalNAc-ser Thr), sialyl Tn (sTn), Thomsen-Friedenrech disaccharide (TF) and sialy-lated Lewis (S-LeX) antigens. These abnormal gly-cans are found in the serum of cancer patients, as well as on the surface of tumor cells, and are associated with poor prognosis. Their pattern of expression is useful for diagnosis, prognosis and monitoring of disease progression, and has been exploited to develop experimental therapies and immunization approaches to cancer treatment [57–59]. Glycan analysis of serum glycoproteins pro-vides a useful biomarker for the presence of ovar-ian and pancreatic tumors, and may also reflect the host response to the disease processes. An alter-native approach is to detect aberrant glycosyla-tion with small molecules such as peptides, capable of binding specific glycan epitopes on tumor cells [60].

One of the well-known glycoprotein antigens on human adenocarcinomas that is modified with abnormal glycans is MUC1. Aberrantly glycosy-lated MUC1 on the surface of tumor cells alters their interaction with other tumor cells or the sur-rounding stromal cells. Hypoglycosylated MUC1 attracts immature DCs to the tumor site, leading to a Th2-mediated response implicated in support-ing tumor metastasis and progression [52]. On the other hand, underglycosylation of tumor MUC1 also allows processing and presentation by antigen-presenting cells (APC) of otherwise cryptic normal peptide epitopes to the immune system, leading to an induction of tumor-specific immunity [61, 62].

Recent studies propose that pro-inflammatory signaling can affect both protein expression and glycosylation. Pro-inflammatory stimuli such as oxidative stress, and cytokines such as IFN-γ, IL-6 and TNF-α, regulate the expression and glycosyla-tion of several mucins, MUC1, MUC4, MUC5 and MUC16 in ovarian, breast and pancreatic tumor cells [18, 63, 64]. Hypoglycosylated MUC1 has been shown to interact with the promoter region of sev-eral pro-inflammatory cytokines, enhancing their transcriptional activity [44] and, thus, creating a positive feedback loop, leading to the establishment of pro-tumor chronic inflammation at the tumor site.

Disease-associated antigens in immunosurveillance of cancer and inflammation

The "cancer immunosurveillance" hypothesis orig-inally proposed in the 1950s stated that the immune system can detect the presence of early can-cer and can destroy it before it becomes clini-cal disease. This hypothesis was recently revised to better reflect dynamic interactions between the tumor, the tumor microenvironment and the immune system that can result in tumor elimina-tion, tumor/host equilibrium or tumor escape [65]. Adaptive immune responses against abnormally expressed molecules on tumors are important for successful tumor elimination. Tumor-associated antigens (TAAs) are abnormally expressed on both cancer cells and their precursor lesions, and can elicit adaptive immunity. Abnormal expression of these same molecules, as well as spontaneous immune responses against them, have also been found during other inflammatory but nonmalignant events, such as infections and sterile acute inflammations. Thus, molecules previously considered TAAs are more broadly associated with multiple diseases, and are better referred to as disease associated antigens (DAAs).

Memory responses against some of these antigens have been associated with a reduced risk for certain cancers. Examples include tumor antigens cyclin B1 and MUC1. Cyclin B1 is transiently expressed in the G2/M phase of the cell cycle in normal cells, but it is constitutively expressed in the cytoplasm of certain tumor cells. Antibodies and memory T cells specific for cyclin B1 have been found in healthy individuals with no history of cancer [66]. It has been shown that infection of human fibroblasts with Varicella Zoster virus or human Cytomegalovirus induces overexpression of cyclin B1 in the cytoplasm of infected cells similar to its abnormal expression found in tumor cells [67, 68]. MUC1, which is highly glycosylated and expressed at low levels on apical surfaces of ductal epithelial cells of several organs [62], is overexpressed and hypoglycosylated in the majority of adenocarcinomas and their precursor lesions. This abnormal, hypoglycosylated form of MUC1 has also been found in non-malignant inflammatory conditions that are associated with epithelial injury, such as breast mastitis, endometriosis, pancreatitis, colon polyps and IBD [26, 69–72], where it can lead to the development of anti-MUC1 immunity. This is the case with the aberrant expression of MUC1 in the salivary gland during mumps infection in humans [73] and, more recently, it has been shown in a mouse model of influenza infection [74].

Epidemiological studies have demonstrated that inflammatory events promote anti-MUC1 immunity and correlate with a significant reduction of cancer risk [75]. This suggests that, instead of focusing on identifying and targeting tumor associated antigens, research efforts should be focused on molecules that are abnormally expressed as a result of disease, and capable of further driving the disease. The type of an immune response generated against DAAs may be a defining determinant in the balance between tumor-promoting inflammation

and anti-tumor inflammation. Therapeutic modalities, such as vaccines that can elicit or strengthen adaptive immunity against DAAs, may tip the balance at the disease site, including in the cancer microenvironment, towards an acute inflammation carried out predominantly by the adaptive immunity and resulting in the disease elimination. Pre-existing immunity to one or more DAAs could be a biomarker of prognostic significance following cancer diagnosis.

Preventing tumor-promoting inflammation by eliciting DAA specific immunity: example from inflammatory bowel disease (IBD) promoting colitis associated colon cancer (CACC)

The tumor-promoting role of inflammation is exemplified in patients with inflammatory bowel disease who are at an increased risk of colitis-associated colon cancer (CACC). Several mouse models of IBD have been studied, the two most common being the IL-10$^{-/-}$ mouse that develops spontaneous IBD and dextran sodium sulfate (DSS)-induced IBD. In IL-10$^{-/-}$ mice, the lack of IL-10 causes an exaggerated immune response to intestinal microflora, leading to chronic inflammation. On the C57Bl/6 background, these mice develop colitis between 3–6 months of age, characterized by inflammatory cell infiltration, goblet cell depletion, crypt abscess formation and epithelial hyperplasia [76]. In the DSS-induced colitis model, DSS treatment causes loss of epithelial barrier integrity, resulting in colitis.

Both models have been used to evaluate the role of particular genes or the immune system in the pathogenesis of IBD. Unlike in human disease, neither mouse model develops CACC spontaneously. This is most likely because both models lack the human molecule MUC1 that, in human IBD, might play an important role in promoting inflammation and tumor development. To explore the importance of MUC1 promoted inflammation in IBD and progression to colon cancer, IL10$^{-/-}$ mice were crossed with MUC1-Tg mice. Mice transgenic for human MUC1 (MUC1-Tg) express MUC1 under its endogenous promoter [77]. These mice develop normally and express human MUC1 in the same tissue distribution seen in humans. When induced to develop cancer, their tumors overexpress the same hypoglycosylated form of MUC1 seen in human disease.

Using the MUC1⁺IL-10⁻/⁻ mouse model, it was shown that *de novo* expression of abnormally glycosylated MUC1 on affected colonocytes resulted in worse inflammation and in increased cancer development, compared with IL-10⁻/⁻ mice. A predominant neutrophil infiltrate was found in the colon of mice with IBD, and the majority of these mice developed colon tumors [70, 78]. These mice also had increased MDSCs in their spleens [78]. The same results were obtained in DSS-induced colitis in MUC1-Tg mice [57].

To determine if the tumor-promoting microenvironment driven by MUC1 expression could be prevented by strengthening adaptive immunity specific for aberrant MUC1 as both a DAA in IBD and a TAA in CAAC, mice were vaccinated prior to the onset of IBD with a tumor form of MUC1. In both models, vaccination resulted in less severe colonic inflammation, and prevention of progression to dysplasia and cancer [57, 78]. MUC1-specific T cells replaced the neutrophilic inflammation in the colon, and there was no increase of MDSCs in the spleen. Immunohistology revealed that abnormal MUC1-expressing cells were eliminated, halting the cycle of inflammation and preventing tumor development.

This work showed that DAAs, represented by MUC1, that are abnormally expressed in chronically inflamed tissues, and the cancers that arise from those tissues, are most likely playing a role in exacerbating inflammation and driving tumor-promotion. It also showed that these molecules could serve as therapeutic targets to halt chronic inflammation and reduce cancer risk. Evidence of a strong adaptive immune memory for several important and common TAAs that are also DAAs could serve as a biomarker for a reduced risk of development of chronic inflammatory diseases and cancer.

References

1. Hawk ET, Levin B (2005). Colorectal cancer prevention. *Journal of Clinical Oncology* **23**(2), 378–91.
2. Rothwell PM, Fowkes FG, Belch JF, Ogawa H, Warlow CP, Meade TW (2011). Effect of daily aspirin on long-term risk of death due to cancer: analysis of individual patient data from randomised trials. *The Lancet* **377**(9759), 31–41.
3. Balkwill F, Mantovani A (2001). Inflammation and cancer: back to Virchow? *The Lancet* **357**(9255), 539–45.
4. Galon J, Costes A, Sanchez-Cabo F, Kirilovsky A, Mlecnik B, Lagorce-Pages C, et al. (2006). Type, density, and location of immune cells within human colorectal tumors predict clinical outcome. *Science* **313**(5795), 1960–4.
5. Al-Shibli KI, Donnem T, Al-Saad S, Persson M, Bremnes RM, Busund LT (2008). Prognostic effect of epithelial and stromal lymphocyte infiltration in non-small cell lung cancer. *Clinical Cancer Research* **14**(16), 5220–7.
6. Camus M, Tosolini M, Mlecnik B, Pages F, Kirilovsky A, Berger A, et al. (2009). Coordination of intratumoral immune reaction and human colorectal cancer recurrence. *Cancer Research* **69**(6), 2685–93.
7. Mahmoud SM, Paish EC, Powe DG, Macmillan RD, Grainge MJ, Lee AH, et al. (2011). Tumor-infiltrating CD8+ lymphocytes predict clinical outcome in breast cancer. *Journal of Clinical Oncology* **29**(15), 1949–55.
8. Sharma P, Shen Y, Wen S, Yamada S, Jungbluth AA, Gnjatic S, et al. (2007). CD8 tumor-infiltrating lymphocytes are predictive of survival in muscle-invasive urothelial carcinoma. *Proceedings of the National Academy of Sciences of the United States of America* **104**(10), 3967–72.
9. Zhang L, Conejo-Garcia JR, Katsaros D, Gimotty PA, Massobrio M, Regnani G, et al. (2003). Intratumoral T cells, recurrence, and survival in epithelial ovarian cancer. *New England Journal of Medicine* **348**(3), 203–13.
10. Ben-Neriah Y, Karin M (2011). Inflammation meets cancer, with NF-kappaB as the matchmaker. *Nature Immunology* **12**(8), 715–23.
11. Hanahan D, Weinberg RA (2011). Hallmarks of cancer: the next generation. *Cell* **144**(5), 646–74.
12. Mantovani A, Allavena P, Sica A, Balkwill F (2008). Cancer-related inflammation. *Nature* **454**(7203), 436–44.
13. Rebouissou S, Amessou M, Couchy G, Poussin K, Imbeaud S, Pilati C, et al. (2009). Frequent in-frame somatic deletions activate gp130 in inflammatory hepatocellular tumours. *Nature* **457**(7226), 200–4.
14. Borrello MG, Alberti L, Fischer A, Degl'innocenti D, Ferrario C, Gariboldi M, et al. (2005). Induction of a proinflammatory program in normal human thyrocytes by the RET/PTC1 *Oncogene Proceedings of the National Academy of Sciences of the United States of America* **102**(41), 14825–30.
15. Parkin DM (2006). The global health burden of infection-associated cancers in the year 2002. *International Journal of Cancer* **118**(12), 3030–44.

16. Arzumanyan A, Reis HM, Feitelson MA (2013). Pathogenic mechanisms in HBV- and HCV-associated hepatocellular carcinoma. *Nature Reviews Cancer* **13**(2), 123–35.

17. Peek RM, Jr., Crabtree JE (2006). Helicobacter infection and gastric neoplasia. *Journal of Pathology* **208**(2), 233–48.

18. Wu J, Meng Z, Jiang M, Pei R, Trippler M, Broering R, *et al.* (2009). Hepatitis B virus suppresses toll-like receptor-mediated innate immune responses in murine parenchymal and nonparenchymal liver cells. *Hepatology* **49**(4), 1132–40.

19. Beckebaum S, Cicinnati VR, Zhang X, Ferencik S, Frilling A, Grosse-Wilde H, *et al.* (2003). Hepatitis B virus-induced defect of monocyte-derived dendritic cells leads to impaired T helper type 1 response *in vitro*: mechanisms for viral immune escape. *Immunology* **109**(4), 487–95.

20. Zhang Z, Zhang S, Zou Z, Shi J, Zhao J, Fan R, *et al.* (2011). Hypercytolytic activity of hepatic natural killer cells correlates with liver injury in chronic hepatitis B patients. *Hepatology* **53**(1), 73–85.

21. Ernst PB, Gold BD (2000). The disease spectrum of *Helicobacter pylori*: the immunopathogenesis of gastroduodenal ulcer and gastric cancer. *Annual Review of Microbiology* **54**, 615–40.

22. Bronte-Tinkew DM, Terebiznik M, Franco A, Ang M, Ahn D, Mimuro H, *et al.* (2009). Helicobacter pylori cytotoxin-associated gene A activates the signal transducer and activator of transcription 3 pathway in vitro and in vivo. *Cancer Research* **69**(2), 632–9.

23. Chen GY, Nunez G (2010). Sterile inflammation: sensing and reacting to damage. *Nature Reviews Immunology* **10**(12), 826–37.

24. Hoque R, Malik AF, Gorelick F, Mehal WZ (2012). Sterile inflammatory response in acute pancreatitis. *Pancreas. Apr;***41**(3), 353–7.

25. Mossman BT, Churg A (1998). Mechanisms in the pathogenesis of asbestosis and silicosis. *American Journal of Respiratory and Critical Care Medicine* **157**(5 Pt 1), 1666–80.

26. Vlad AM, Diaconu I, Gantt KR (2006). MUC1 in endometriosis and ovarian cancer. *Immunologic Research* **36**(1–3), 229–36.

27. Wiseman EF, Ang YS (2011). Risk factors for neoplastic progression in Barrett's esophagus. *World Journal of Gastroenterology* **17**(32), 3672–83.

28. Zheng L, Xue J, Jaffee EM, Habtezion A (2013). Role of immune cells and immune-based therapies in pancreatitis and pancreatic ductal adenocarcinoma. *Gastroenterology* **144**(6), 1230–40.

29. Calle EE, Kaaks R (2004). Overweight, obesity and cancer: epidemiological evidence and proposed mechanisms. *Nature Reviews Cancer* **4**(8), 579–91.

30. Dostert C, Petrilli V, Van Bruggen R, Steele C, Mossman BT, Tschopp J (2008). Innate immune activation through Nalp3 inflammasome sensing of asbestos and silica. *Science* **320**(5876), 674–7.

31. Becker JC, Andersen MH, Schrama D, Thor Straten P (2013). Immune-suppressive properties of the tumor microenvironment. *Cancer Immunology, Immunotherapy* **62**(7), 1137–48.

32. Wyckoff JB, Wang Y, Lin EY, Li JF, Goswami S, Stanley ER, *et al.* (2007). Direct visualization of macrophage-assisted tumor cell intravasation in mammary tumors. *Cancer Research* **67**(6), 2649–56.

33. Lin EY, Li JF, Gnatovskiy L, Deng Y, Zhu L, Grzesik DA, *et al.* (2006). Macrophages regulate the angiogenic switch in a mouse model of breast cancer. *Cancer Research* **66**(23), 11238–46.

34. Fridlender ZG, Sun J, Kim S, Kapoor V, Cheng G, Ling L, *et al.* (2009). Polarization of tumor-associated neutrophil phenotype by TGF-beta: "N1" versus "N2" TAN. *Cancer Cell* **16**(3), 183–94.

35. Scapini P, Calzetti F, Cassatella MA. (1999). On the detection of neutrophil-derived vascular endothelial growth factor (VEGF). *Journal of Immunological Methods* **232**(1–2), 121–9.

36. Huh SJ, Liang S, Sharma A, Dong C, Robertson GP. (2010). Transiently entrapped circulating tumor cells interact with neutrophils to facilitate lung metastasis development. *Cancer Research* **70**(14), 6071–82.

37. Ostrand-Rosenberg S, Sinha P, Beury DW, Clements VK. (2012). Cross-talk between myeloid-derived suppressor cells (MDSC), macrophages, and dendritic cells enhances tumor-induced immune suppression. *Seminars in Cancer Biology* **22**(4), 275–81.

38. Clark CE, Hingorani SR, Mick R, Combs C, Tuveson DA, Vonderheide RH. (2007). Dynamics of the immune reaction to pancreatic cancer from inception to invasion. *Cancer Research* **67**(19), 9518–27.

39. Culig Z (2011). Cytokine disbalance in common human cancers. *Biochimica et Biophysica Acta* **1813**(2), 308–14.

40. Scheller J, Chalaris A, Schmidt-Arras D, Rose-John S. (2011). The pro- and anti-inflammatory properties of the cytokine interleukin-6. *Biochimica et Biophysica Acta* **1813**(5), 878–88.

41. Shinriki S, Jono H, Ota K, Ueda M, Kudo M, Ota T, *et al.* (2009). Humanized anti-interleukin-6 receptor antibody suppresses tumor angiogenesis and in vivo growth of human oral squamous cell carcinoma. *Clinical Cancer Research* **15**(17), 5426–34.

42. Chu WM (2013). Tumor necrosis factor. *Cancer Letters* **328**(2), 222–5.

43. Hoffmann A, Baltimore D (2006). Circuitry of nuclear factor kappaB signaling. *Immunological Reviews* **210**, 171–86.

44. Cascio S, Zhang L, Finn OJ (2011). MUC1 protein expression in tumor cells regulates transcription of proinflammatory cytokines by forming a complex with nuclear factor-kappaB p65 and binding to cytokine promoters: importance of extracellular domain. *Journal of Biological Chemistry* **286**(49), 42248–56.

45. Erez N, Truitt M, Olson P, Arron ST, Hanahan D (2010). Cancer-Associated Fibroblasts Are Activated in Incipient Neoplasia to Orchestrate Tumor-Promoting Inflammation in an NF-kappaB-Dependent Manner. *Cancer Cell* **17**(2), 135–47.

46. Hagemann T, Lawrence T, McNeish I, Charles KA, Kulbe H, Thompson RG, *et al.* (2008). "Re-educating" tumor-associated macrophages by targeting NF-kappaB. *Journal of Experimental Medicine* **205**(6), 1261–8.

47. Baldwin AS (2001). Control of oncogenesis and cancer therapy resistance by the transcription factor NF-kappaB. *Journal of Clinical Investigation* **107**(3), 241–6.

48. Bowman T, Garcia R, Turkson J, Jove R (2000). STATs in oncogenesis. *Oncogene* **19**(21), 2474–88.

49. Song JI, Grandis JR (2000). STAT signaling in head and neck cancer. *Oncogene* **19**(21), 2489–95.

50. Ernst M, Najdovska M, Grail D, Lundgren-May T, Buchert M, Tye H, *et al.* (2008). STAT3 and STAT1 mediate IL-11-dependent and inflammation-associated gastric tumorigenesis in gp130 receptor mutant mice. *Journal of Clinical Investigation* **118**(5), 1727–38.

51. Kortylewski M, Kujawski M, Wang T, Wei S, Zhang S, Pilon-Thomas S, *et al.* (2005). Inhibiting Stat3 signaling in the hematopoietic system elicits multicomponent antitumor immunity. *Nature Medicine* **11**(12), 1314–21.

52. Carlos CA, Dong HF, Howard OM, Oppenheim JJ, Hanisch FG, Finn OJ (2005). Human tumor antigen MUC1 is chemotactic for immature dendritic cells and elicits maturation but does not promote Th1 type immunity. *Journal of Immunology* **175**(3), 1628–35.

53. van Gisbergen KP, Aarnoudse CA, Meijer GA, Geijtenbeek TB, van Kooyk Y (2005). Dendritic cells recognize tumor-specific glycosylation of carcinoembryonic antigen on colorectal cancer cells through dendritic cell-specific intercellular adhesion molecule-3-grabbing nonintegrin. *Cancer Research* **65**(13), 5935–44.

54. Dhodapkar MV (2005). Harnessing host immune responses to preneoplasia: promise and challenges. *Cancer Immunology, Immunotherapy* **54**(5), 409–13.

55. Finn OJ (2003). Premalignant lesions as targets for cancer vaccines. *Journal of Experimental Medicine* **198**(11), 1623–6.

56. Hakomori S (2002). Glycosylation defining cancer malignancy: new wine in an old bottle. *Proceedings of the National Academy of Sciences of the United States of America* **99**(16), 10231–3.

57. Beatty P, Ranganathan S, Finn OJ (2012). Prevention of colitis-associated colon cancer using a vaccine to target abnormal expression of the MUC1 tumor antigen. *Oncoimmunology* **1**(3), 263–70.

58. Hollingsworth MA, Swanson BJ (2004). Mucins in cancer: protection and control of the cell surface. *Nature Reviews Cancer* **4**(1), 45–60.

59. Kimura T, McKolanis JR, Dzubinski LA, Islam K, Potter DM, Salazar AM, *et al.* (2013). MUC1 vaccine for individuals with advanced adenoma of the colon: a cancer immunoprevention feasibility study. *Cancer Prevention Research (Philadelphia)* **6**(1), 18–26.

60. Moore A, Medarova Z, Potthast A, Dai G (2004). *In vivo* targeting of underglycosylated MUC-1 tumor antigen using a multimodal imaging probe. *Cancer Research* **64**(5), 1821–7.

61. Ryan SO, Vlad AM, Islam K, Gariepy J, Finn OJ (2009). Tumor-associated MUC1 glycopeptide epitopes are not subject to self-tolerance and improve responses to MUC1 peptide epitopes in MUC1 transgenic mice. *Biological Chemistry* **390**(7), 611–8.

62. Vlad AM, Kettel JC, Alajez NM, Carlos CA, Finn OJ (2004). MUC1 immunobiology: from discovery to clinical applications. *Advances in Immunology* **82**, 249–93.

63. Andrianifahanana M, Moniaux N, Batra SK (2006). Regulation of mucin expression: mechanistic aspects and implications for cancer and inflammatory diseases. *Biochimica et Biophysica Acta* **1765**(2), 189–222.

64. Choi S, Park YS, Koga T, Treloar A, Kim KC (2011). TNF-alpha is a key regulator of MUC1, an anti-inflammatory molecule, during airway Pseudomonas aeruginosa infection. *American Journal of Respiratory Cell and Molecular Biology* **44**(2), 255–60.

65. Dunn GP, Old LJ, Schreiber RD (2004). The three Es of cancer immunoediting. *Annual Review of Immunology* **22**, 329–60.

66. Vella LA, Yu M, Fuhrmann SR, El-Amine M, Epperson DE, Finn OJ (2009). Healthy individuals have T-cell and antibody responses to the tumor antigen cyclin B1 that when elicited in mice protect from cancer. *Proceedings of the National Academy of Sciences of the United States of America* **106**(33), 14010–5.

67. Leisenfelder SA, Moffat JF (2006). Varicella-zoster virus infection of human foreskin fibroblast cells results in atypical cyclin expression and cyclin-dependent kinase activity. *Journal of Virology* **80**(11), 5577–87.

68. Sanchez V, McElroy AK, Spector DH (2003). Mechanisms governing maintenance of Cdk1/cyclin B1 kinase activity in cells infected with human cytomegalovirus. *Journal of Virology* **77**(24), 13214–24.

69. Ajioka Y, Watanabe H, Jass JR (1997). MUC1 and MUC2 mucins in flat and polypoid colorectal adenomas. *Journal of Clinical Pathology* **50**(5), 417–21.

70. Beatty PL, Plevy SE, Sepulveda AR, Finn OJ (2007). Cutting edge: transgenic expression of human MUC1 in IL-10-/- mice accelerates inflammatory bowel disease and progression to colon cancer. *Journal of Immunology* **179**(2), 735–9.

71. Ho SB, Ewing SL, Montgomery CK, Kim YS (1996). Altered mucin core peptide immunoreactivity in the colon polyp-carcinoma sequence. *Oncology Research* **8**(2), 53–61.

72. Kadayakkara DK, Beatty PL, Turner MS, Janjic JM, Ahrens ET, Finn OJ (2010). Inflammation driven by overexpression of the hypoglycosylated abnormal mucin 1 (MUC1) links inflammatory bowel disease and pancreatitis. *Pancreas* **39**(4), 510–5.

73. Cramer DW, Vitonis AF, Pinheiro SP, McKolanis JR, Fichorova RN, Brown KE, *et al.* (2010). Mumps and ovarian cancer: modern interpretation of an historic association. *Cancer Causes and Control* **21**(8), 1193–201.

74. Iheagwara UK (2013). MUC-1 as a therapeutic target in cancer: programming the immune system through childhood infections. In: *Cancer Immunology and Immunotherapy*. Oxford: Oxford University Press.

75. Cramer DW, Titus-Ernstoff L, McKolanis JR, Welch WR, Vitonis AF, Berkowitz RS, *et al.* (2005). Conditions associated with antibodies against the tumor-associated antigen MUC1 and their relationship to risk for ovarian cancer. *Cancer Epidemiology, Biomarkers & Prevention* **14**(5), 1125–31.

76. Berg DJ, Davidson N, Kuhn R, Muller W, Menon S, Holland G, *et al.* (1996). Enterocolitis and colon cancer in interleukin-10-deficient mice are associated with aberrant cytokine production and CD4(+) TH1-like responses. *Journal of Clinical Investigation* **98**(4), 1010–20.

77. Rowse GJ, Tempero RM, VanLith ML, Hollingsworth MA, Gendler SJ (1998). Tolerance and immunity to MUC1 in a human MUC1 transgenic murine model. *Cancer Research* **58**(2), 315–21.

78. Beatty PL, Narayanan S, Gariepy J, Ranganathan S, Finn OJ (2010). Vaccine against MUC1 antigen expressed in inflammatory bowel disease and cancer lessens colonic inflammation and prevents progression to colitis-associated colon cancer. *Cancer Prevention Research (Philadelphia)* **3**(4), 438–46.

CHAPTER 5

Exosomes: A Valuable Biomedical Tool in Biomarker Discovery and Development

Jocelyn Lee,[1] Sharmistha Ghosh,[1] and Sudhir Srivastava[2]

[1]Cancer Biomarkers Research Group, Division of Cancer Prevention, National Cancer Institute, Rockville, MD, USA

[2]Cancer Biomarkers Research Group, Division of Cancer Prevention, National Cancer Institute, National Institutes of Health, Bethesda, MD, USA

Introduction

Bodily fluids are attractive sources of a range of analytes for diagnostic work-ups. Serum, plasma, urine and cervical fluid are examples of commonly used biofluids in clinical laboratories, and remain the "workhorse" in the diagnosis and prognosis of many cancers. The trafficking of biological analytes (e.g., proteins, metabolites, nucleotides) across the cell membrane is part of any normal cell homeostasis. In a vesicular transport mechanism, the analytes are transported across the cell membrane via microparticles or small extracellular vesicles (exosomes). In pathological states, such as cancer, the circulating exosomal analytes may mirror the altered state (e.g., over- or underexpressed key proteins and microRNAs) of the cell of origin and, therefore, can be of substantial diagnostic value [1,2].

Over the past decade, a number of studies have implicated exosomes in major tumor-related pathways, such as hypoxia-driven epithelial-to-mesenchymal transition, cancer stemness, angiogenesis, malignant formation, metastasis and drug resistance [3–7]. This chapter highlights the advancements in exosome research, with particular focus on the potential use of exosomes as a source of enriched biomarkers (e.g., RNA and protein biomarkers), and their clinical utilization as a non-invasive biomedical tool for diagnostic purposes.

Biogenesis and characterization of exosomes

Extracellular vesicles are membrane-bound particles, which include exosomes (30–100 nm), shedding microvesicles or microparticles (100–1000 nm), and apoptotic blebs (1000–5000 nm) [8]. Although many studies use the terms "microvesicles" and "exosomes" interchangeably, these vesicles do not just represent a continuum of size of the same vesicular entity, and can be categorized according to their biogenesis, biophysical properties, surface markers, and function [9–12]. However, a clear distinction between the different types is lacking.

Exosomes, the exocytosed vesicles of endosomal origin, are characterized as spherical or cup-shaped nanovesicles that constitutively express specific isoforms of tetraspanins (CD63, CD9, CD81, and CD82) on the cell surface [13–16]. The biogenesis, secretion, and function of exosomes in normal

Biomarkers in Cancer Screening and Early Detection, First Edition. Edited by Sudhir Srivastava.
© 2017 John Wiley & Sons, Inc. Published 2017 by John Wiley & Sons, Inc.

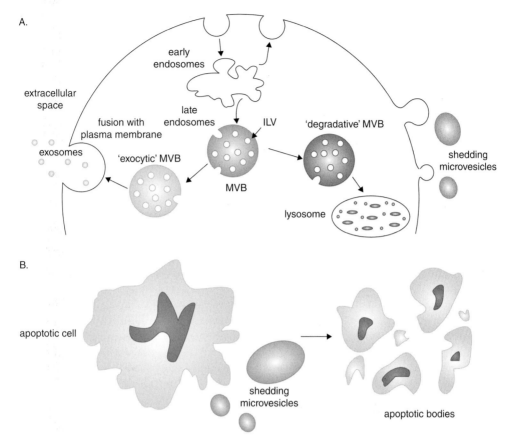

Figure 5.1 Schematic representation of biogenesis of extracellular vesicles. **A.** Release of exosomes and shedding microvesicles. Cytosolic components are trapped within intraluminal vesicles (ILVs) formed by invagination of endosomal membranes and contained within larger multivesicular bodies (MVBs). MVBs can release the ILVs into the extracellular space upon exocytic fusion with the plasma membrane (the released vesicles are defined as exosomes), or may be targeted for ubiquitination-dependent lysomal degradation. The role of the endosomal sorting complex responsible for transport (ESCRT) machinery in exosome biogenesis is unclear. There is support for both an ESCRT-dependent and an ESCRT-independent mechanism [19–22]. New studies may provide insights into the mechanisms governing MVB trafficking to the plasma membrane [23, 24]. Currently, it is not known whether there are MVB-independent mechanisms of exosome formation. The shedding microvesicles are formed directly by blebbing of the plasma membrane. **B.** Apoptotic bodies are vesicles with nuclear and cytoplasmic contents of apoptotic or dying cells. *Source:* Mathivanan 2010 [8]. Reproduced with permission of Elsevier. For a color version of this figure please see color plate section.

cells and during disease development have all been extensively studied [17]. Exosomes, which are actively secreted by almost all cell types (e.g., neural, epithelial, muscle, and stem cells) [9, 12], function as an intermediate compartment between the plasma membrane, where endocytosis of extracellular molecules takes place, and lysosomes, where these molecules are degraded [18], as shown in Figure 5.1 (Courtesy of [08]).

In multicellular organisms, localized or systemic cell-cell communication is vital for many cellular processes including growth, migration, differenti- ation, and apoptosis. Besides being involved in the removal of cellular waste, unwanted molecules, and the efflux of drugs [25, 26], exosomes are vehicles that transport molecules such as nucleotides (DNA, coding and non-coding RNAs), lipids, glycans, and proteins to adjacent cells or to distant sites via circulation. The range of proposed functions are extensive, including both autocrine (intracellular communication) and paracrine (intercellular communication) signaling [27] for normal physiological processes, or to modify a variety of cellular processes [28–31].

Because exosomes are composed of a lipid bilayer and contain transmembrane proteins, they can influence several cellular processes, including membrane trafficking, angiogenesis, cell proliferation, tumor-cell invasion, antigen presentation, and can even elicit immune responses [12, 31]. Exosomes were originally described, by two parallel publications in 1983, as vesicles transporting the transferrin receptor in reticulocytes [32, 33]. However, the utility of exosomes for clinical use did not gain much attention until it was discovered that they have the ability both to modulate the immune system [34,35] and to transfer genetic material [36].

Based on decades of data, exosomes are characterized by their size, extracellular membrane components, and the cell surface markers mentioned earlier [13–16]. However, despite substantial advancements, sufficient knowledge of the regulatory mechanism of exosome trafficking, sorting of biomolecules, targeting to recipient cells, and an understanding of the physiological relevance are lacking.

Importantly, there is evidence that some molecular components of exosomes can correctly identify the origin of cancer tissue [37], which is an important feature for their utilization as cancer biomarkers. Because exosomes are also released into bodily fluids (e.g., saliva, blood, urine, pleural effusion, semen) [9, 12], they have strong potential to serve as an excellent non-invasive source of pathognomonic indicators of a multitude of diseases.

Diagnostic potential of exosomal RNA

In 2007, the presence of mRNA, and other small RNAs such as microRNAs (miRNAs), encapsulated in the exosomes of mast cells was discovered, and these RNAs were named "exosomal shuttle RNA" (esRNA) [36]. Microarray analysis of the target cells revealed the presence of several novel mRNAs which were not present in the cytoplasm of the donor cells. Although, at the time, a definitive distinction between microvesicles and exosomes could not be made, a study found that purified exosomes contained functional miRNAs and small RNAs, but detected only small amounts of mRNA [38]. In addition, it was found that a proportion of the mRNA present in the exosomes could be translated into proteins in target cells, suggesting that

exosomes can facilitate the transfer of genetic information [36]. Although most circulating miRNAs are not encapsulated in vesicles, it has been shown that there may be specific targeting of some RNAs into released exosomes [39–42].

Although the functions of miRNAs and their influence on cancer development and progression are just being uncovered, it appears that miRNAs play a much greater role than expected [43, 44]. Several miRNAs with high expression levels in cancer tissues have been reported as suitable diagnostic or prognostic biomarkers [1]. Unlike exosomal mRNAs, miRNAs can reportedly identify cancer tissue origin [37]. Exosomes are thought to be the vehicle to protect and deliver these RNAs to target cells in which they modulate signaling cascades [27]. Due to the heterogeneity of the techniques used to isolate exosomes and other microvesicles, it is not clear how RNAs are sequestered in the exosomes. Understanding the mechanisms of RNA targeting to exosomes, and determining whether there are distinct targeting consensus sequences or common targeting components such as RNA-binding proteins, will allow a better understanding of the function and purpose of RNA delivery to secreted vesicles.

Although previous work has been centered on the comparison of RNA sequences in vesicles primarily isolated from normal and cultured cancer cell lines, lately the analysis of exosomes from the biological fluids of cancer patients has attracted much interest. Despite substantial advancement in highly sensitive technologies, the identification of low abundance biomarkers in biofluids remains a challenge, particularly in the early stages of cancer. A few years ago, a study reported that glioblastoma patients could be diagnosed and identified by analyzing the exosomal miRNA profile in their serum [41]. Another study reported that miR-141, an miRNA expressed in prostate cancer, can distinguish patients with prostate cancer from healthy controls [45, 46]. Further research, including independent validation of the reported markers in case-control and prospective studies, are needed.

Diagnostic potential of exosomal proteins

Over the past decade, extensive analysis and cataloging of the proteomic profiles of exosomes have shed new light on their molecular components, as well as their diagnostic potential as cancer biomarkers. New technologies, including improvements in mass spectrometric analysis and methods of exosomal purification and isolation, have fostered extensive proteomic analyses of exosomes and other microvesicles [2, 28].

As stated previously, exosomes are often characterized and isolated based on their expression of members of the tetraspanin protein superfamily, including CD63, CD9, CD81, and CD82 [13–16]. Exosomes not only contain a conserved group of proteins, but also express a subset of proteins that are tissue- or cell-type specific. These proteins include the cytoskeletal proteins actin and tubulin, in combination with cell-signaling proteins such as a diverse group of kinases, heterotrimeric G proteins, members of the RAS oncogene family, and heat shock proteins such as HSP-70 and HSP-90 [2, 28, 47, 48].

Exosomes are also enriched in matrix proteins, intracellular adhesion molecules and immunological proteins, including, but not limited to, $\alpha_v\beta_3$ integrin, Alix, phosphatidylserine, CD80, CD86, CD96, Rab-5b, and major histocompatibility complex (MHC) class I and MHC class II [48, 49]. Metabolic enzymes, such as peroxidases, pyruvate and lipid kinases and enolase-1, have also been detected in exosomes [50]. It has been reported that exosomal proteins remain functionally active throughout transportation and delivery to their new location [27]. The intracellular components and cell surface markers can initiate signaling cascades, influencing a range of cellular functions in the recipient cells. Several studies have revealed that the exosomal protein signatures may be tumor-specific as well, lending support to the idea that these proteins may have functional roles in tumor growth and development, and may also serve as potentially useful biomarkers for early detection, diagnosis and prognosis of cancers [51–53].

Role in immune regulation and tumor development

Exosomes, once considered to be cellular debris or artifacts [54], have recently been extensively studied because of their possible role in immune modulation as well as in tumor growth and progression [55–59]. Evidence suggests that exosomes do not contain a random array of intracellular proteins, but a specific set of protein classes or groups shuttled from the plasma membrane, the endocytic pathway and the cytosol, and also very limited amounts of proteins from other intracellular organelles, including the nucleus, endoplasmic reticulum, and Golgi apparatus which, ultimately, may influence their role in disease progression [17, 18]. It has also been reported that oncogenes can spread/circulate via exosomes and microvesicles secreted by tumor cells [60].

Since exosomes were initially characterized as mediators of antigen presentation in immune cells, there is a vast amount of information on the immunological effects of exosomes [61]. Although they have been found to be involved in intracellular communication and signaling during normal immune functioning, altering normal immune system function is one of the major mechanisms by which exosomes can affect cancer development [61]. When exosomes are released from tumor cells, they can induce T-cell activation, alter T-cell immunity, and stimulate inflammation which, subsequently, can affect cancer initiation and progression [62, 63].

Exosomes are also thought to change the cellular microenvironment through the transportation of viral components, such as Epstein-Barr virus (EBV) latent membrane protein 1 (LMP1), which is involved in the development of many cancers [64], including Burkitt's lymphoma, Hodgkin's disease, nasopharyngeal carcinoma (NPC), and gastric cancer [65]. In support of this, it has been found that exosomes released from NPC cells contain latent EBV-LMP1 [66]. These exosomes could activate certain signaling pathways, such as the ERK and AKT pathways, which play essential roles in cell proliferation, cell survival, angiogenesis, and metastasis [66, 67]. Due to their small size, it is thought that exosomes are able to access the lymphatic system and, thereby, elicit effects on tumor progression and possibly metastasis through unknown signaling mechanisms [61]. A number of studies have demonstrated that exosomes play important roles in cancer development, and have potential as biomarkers for various cancer types, including lung, breast, ovarian, and prostate cancer [68–72].

Exosomes from tumor cells

There have been several key publications recently that have examined the release of exosomes by tumor cells. Tumor cells release a specific subtype of exosomes into the interstitial space, or directly into lymphatic system, and thus are referred to as tumor-derived (TD) exosomes [54]. Exosomes and their components have been found to have both immunoactivating (tumor-suppressing) and immunosuppressing (tumor-promoting) effects [61]. Exosomes secreted by tumor cells have been found to carry antigens from the secreting tumors, and can be captured and used to present tumor antigens by dendritic cells. In addition, exosomes also carry immunosuppressive molecules and interact with normal cells, which can reduce immune surveillance and, ultimately, reduce the number of antigen-presenting cells (APCs) and inactivate T-cells or natural killer cells [54, 73, 74]. In contrast, exosomes also promote the differentiation of regulatory T-cells or myeloid cells [54, 75, 76].

The balance of these tumor-promoting and tumor-suppressing activities is not completely understood, although it is believed by some groups that tumor cell-secreted exosomes further support tumor growth by stimulating angiogenesis or cell migration from the metastatic niche. Although chemotaxis is believed to be involved in the migration of exosomes to these metastatic niches, the mechanism of this movement is not completely understood. Through intracellular signaling and activation, TD exosomes elicit growth, evasion, and metastasis of malignant cells to tumor nodes or other metastatic locations. They are also thought to participate in a feedback loop within the metastatic niche, facilitating the progression, growth, and eventual metastasis of the cancer. There is also emerging evidence that exosomes and their components may be instrumental in establishing and maintaining these metastatic locations, and also may be involved in the subsistence of neoplastic cells at these locations.

Because of their vascularity, there is evidence that more malignant tumors may release a greater amount of exosomes into circulation compared with non-malignant tissue, and may have increased access to the vascular system, potentially increasing the signal-to-noise ratio of cancer biomarkers that

may be used for the early detection and screening of cancer. In addition to their role in genetic transfer, exosomes may play an important role in chemoresistance, because of their involvement in removal of cellular waste and the efflux of drugs. TD exosomes are molecularly distinct from non-cancer derived exosomes and those released from other diseased cells.

Recent developments in utilization of exosomes as biomarkers for cancer

Several recent studies have demonstrated that circulating levels of exosomes and/or their molecular contents may have promise as biomarkers for early detection and screening for certain types of cancers that currently have no effective screening methods (see Table 5.1). In one study, to develop non-invasive methods for melanoma screening and follow-up care, the investigators analyzed exosomes isolated from plasma that expressed the proteins CD63 and caveolin-1 from melanoma patients and controls. Results demonstrated that exosomal CD63 and caveolin-1 levels in melanoma patients were significantly higher than those in control patients [77]. In another study, to develop non-invasive biomarkers for ovarian cancer screening, exosomes were isolated from the blood of ovarian cancer patients and controls. Results showed that ovarian cancer patients significantly expressed claudin-4-containing exosomes, compared with control patients [78].

The United States Preventive Services Task Force (USPSTF) has recommended against prostate-specific antigen (PSA)-based testing to screen for prostate cancer since 2012 [79]. There is an urgent need for sensitive, specific and accurate biomarkers to improve screening, diagnosis and prognosis of prostate cancer. Based on this existing need, there is great interest in deciphering the role of exosomes and their involvement in prostate cancer initiation, progression, and metastasis.

Several studies have examined the proteomic content and the structural components of exosomes in prostate cancer patient samples and cultured cell lines. Clinical prostate cancer samples have been shown to express cancer biomarkers such as CD9, CD81, and Annexin A2, as well as a

Table 5.1 Selected exosome-derived biomarkers differentially expressed during cancer.

Cancer type	mRNA marker	Source	Reference
Colorectal	CDK8, RAD21	Cell lines	[99]
Glioblastoma	EGFRvIII	Serum	[41]

Cancer type	miRNA marker	Source	Reference
Prostate	107, 130b, 141, 181, 181a-2, 2110, 301a, 326, 331-3p, 375, 432, 484, 574-3p, 625, 200b	Plasma, urine	[100]
NSCLC	1, 25, 30d, 223, 486, 499	Serum	[101, 102]
Lymphoma	21, 155, 210	Serum	[103]
Melanoma	15b, 182	Melanomas, cell lines	[104, 105]
Breast	155	Serum	[106]
Ovarian	21, 92	Serum	[107]
Colorectal	17-3p, 92	Serum	[108]
Glioblastoma	21	Serum	[41]
Laryngeal squamous cell carcinoma (LSCC)	21	Serum	[109]

Cancer type	ncRNA marker	Source	Reference
Prostate	PCA3	Urine	[110]
Bladder	MALAT1, HOTAIR	Urine, cell lines	[111]
Laryngeal squamous cell carcinoma (LSCC)	HOTAIR	Serum	[109]

Cancer type	Protein marker	Source	Reference
Ovarian	L1CAM, CD24, CD63, ADAM10, EpCAM, EMMPRIN, TGFB1, MAGE3/6, Claudin-4	Plasma, ascites, serum	[78, 112–115]
Glioblastoma	EGFRvIII, EGFR, EGFRvII, PDPN, IDH1	Serum	[41, 116]
Melanoma	CD63, Caveolin1	Plasma	[77]
Oral	FasL	Serum	[117]
Gastric	HER-2/neu, CCR6	Plasma	[118]
Breast	CA-15-3/MUC-1, CEA	Plasma	[119]
Prostate	TMPRSS2:ERG, PSA, PTEN, Annexin A3	Urine	[86, 120]
Bladder	EDIL-3	Urine	[111]

prostate cancer-specific biomarker, FOLH1/PMSA [80–82]. FOLH1/PSMA has been correlated with poorly differentiated, metastatic, hormone-refractory prostate cancers, and is associated with PSA recurrence [82–84]. Interestingly, exosomes containing PTEN, a negative regulator of PI3K signaling associated with more aggressive prostate disease, have been correlated with prostate cancer diagnosis [85, 86].

In addition, androgen receptor (AR), which is key to the normal development and maintenance of the prostate, and instrumental in the development and progression of prostate cancer [87], has also been examined in regards to exosome biology and signaling [88]. Exosomal populations from

AR-positive (VCaP, C4-2, LNCaP, and RWPE-1) and AR-negative cultured cells (DU145 and PC3) were determined to contain distinct proteins that may be used to determine AR-related prognosis and targeted therapies in prostate cancer patients [88].

In a recent report on developing plasma exosome biomarkers for early detection and progression of prostate cancer, patients with low-grade/localized prostate cancer, pre-inflammatory benign prostatic hyperplasia (BPH), recurrent prostate cancer, and healthy control subjects were recruited and studied. It was observed that the levels of exosomal survivin in plasma from patients with early-stage prostate cancer (Gleason score ≤ 6) were significantly higher than in those with BPH or in controls. There was also no significant observable difference in exosomal survivin levels between controls and BPH patients [89]. In addition, exosomal survivin levels were higher in patients that had relapsed during or after chemotherapy, compared with controls.

Recently, a study examined the potential for the quantity of TD exosomes to be used as a screening biomarker for colorectal cancer by quantifying exosomes from the plasma of colorectal cancer (CRC) patients using flow cytometry. It was found that the quantity of exosomes in CRC patients was significantly higher than in healthy controls. Among the CRC patients, higher levels of circulating TD exosomes were also correlated with poorly differentiated tumors and shorter overall survival [90]. In another study, the circulating levels of tumor exosomes, exosomal small RNAs, and specific exosomal miRNAs were evaluated in patients with and without lung adenocarcinoma. A significant difference in total exosome and exosomal miRNA levels was observed between lung cancer patients and controls. Importantly, similar levels of circulating exosomal miRNA and TD miRNA were observed in adenocarcinoma patients, suggesting that circulating exosomal miRNAs might be useful as a screening test for lung adenocarcinoma [91].

Although the results from these studies are promising, none of them have examined exosomes in preneoplasias or their usefulness in predicting progression from preneoplasia to cancer. Based on the cancer site-specific exosome and exosome component association, TD exosomes may have uses in early detection, risk assessment, diagnosis, and prognosis of certain cancers, as well as uses in evaluating surrogate endpoints. Further research is needed to confirm these findings and to validate the use of exosomes and their components as biomarkers of cancer initiation and progression.

Challenges in exosome utilization

One of the major challenges emerging in the field of exosome utilization for clinical use is the lack of robust and reproducible methods for the isolation of a pure vesicular population [92]. There is a lack of clear consensus for an optimal method of isolation of pure exosomal population that is devoid of

contamination with similarly sized microvesicles of different origins. This is a major hurdle for the utilization of exosomes and their components for clinical use and early detection and screening of cancer [92].

In addition to population heterogeneity, many proteins and other biomolecules may bind/associate nonspecifically to the exosomal surface, and confound the analysis of exosomal composition. In the traditional methods, exosomes are purified preferably by a combination of differential centrifugation and ultracentrifugation, filtration, concentration, and immmunocapture using beads. The ultrafiltration is performed using a 100–220 nm filter, followed by a $100\,000 \times g$ ultracentrifugation in a sucrose gradient to pellet exosomes. These methods allow for the removal of cellular debris and larger microvesicles while concentrating exosomes. High-performance liquid chromatography (HPLC)-based protocols can potentially allow highly pure exosomes to be obtained, although the methodology has limitations [93]. Exosome purification kits are commercially available, although the isolation technology needs further improvement, as kits have been reported to isolate non-exosomal contaminants in some cases.

A recent study that conducted a comprehensive evaluation of a few methods of exosome isolation including ultracentrifugation, OptiPrep^{TM} density-based separation, and immunoaffinity capture using anti-EpCAM coated magnetic beads, found immunoaffinity capture to be the most effective method [92]. Although comprehensive, it has been suggested that the serial isolation steps do not allow complete recovery of the secreted exosomes at any given time. In addition, it was presumed that only a fraction of secreted exosomes may be captured during purification, because they are reabsorbed by cells through phagocytosis.

At this time, because of their small size, visualization by electron microscopy is the only accepted method for the assessment of the purity of the exosomal population [12]. Exosomes appear as spherical or cup-shaped bilayered membrane-bound vesicles in electron micrographs [12]. Some speculate that the cup shape may be formed due to membrane shrinkage during the fixation procedure [94]. New methods, using western blot analysis and florescence-activated cell sorting (FACS) to assess the purity and components of exosome preparation, are currently being developed [54].

It is currently unknown whether the amounts of exosomes and their components that could be used for early detection and screening of cancer correspond to physiological levels secreted by tumor cells, or if information can be extrapolated from these levels to gain insight into the tumor stage or prognosis [54]. There is also a lack of understanding of how the differences in composition and size of the different microvesicle populations relate to their functional features. Ultimately, new technologies and approaches should focus not only on isolating pure exosomal populations, but on whether these populations accurately reflect the tumors from which they are derived.

Challenges in exosome-based diagnostics

The isolation and analysis of pure exosomes and their cargo remains a challenge. Challenges in purifying and analyzing exosomes include setting up high-performance, high-throughput, large-scale purification methods with minimum manual labor, and addressing the inter-laboratory variability in methodology and purity standards by establishing standardized protocols.

Although the presence of extracellular vesicles has been known for decades, techniques have been able to distinguish exosomes from microvesicles and apoptotic bodies only recently [8, 11, 95]. In order to explore the contents and the physiological roles of exosomes, it is important to use technology and procedures that are able to avoid cross-contamination with other microvesicles and non-vesicular components from the surrounding environment, and assess their presence, size and purity, prior to progressing to extensive molecular profiling for global mRNAs, miRNAs, or proteins in search of biomarkers.

The utility of extracellular vesicles as disease biomarkers, and their potential as therapeutic agents, have gained substantial interest in recent years [69, 96]. However, the fundamental question that remains to be answered satisfactorily is, how pure are the vesicle preparations? Estimating the purity of samples remains difficult, with inconsistent approaches across diverse studies.

Another major challenge with the isolation of exosome and utilization as a diagnostic tool is a challenging source material, such as serum, urine or cancer-related effusions [97].

The purity of exosome is of critical importance to demonstrate that a given biomarker or analyte is associated with vesicles, and not with co-isolated contaminants. There are several current approaches that attempt to address this. For example, an examination of samples by electron microscopy can give an indication of vesicular morphology, and can reveal the presence of larger non-vesicular particulates. However, although informative, this approach cannot measure the amount of soluble factors contaminating the sample [97]. The other practical problem is the routine use of electron microscopes, which are extremely expensive and may not be accessible to many research groups.

Being able to estimate and compare sample purity in a general, simple, and quantitative manner is not only useful for clinical use, but is equally important as a tool for inter- and intra-group comparisons, to monitor the quality of preparations across various laboratories, or more broadly as an approach to aid in establishing standards as to what is an acceptable pure exosome sample. This aspect is of particular importance in the context of exosome utilization as a diagnostic/therapeutic tool. Several companies are also investing in developing exosome-based diagnostics, and promising results may be obtained from such collective efforts.

Conclusion

Exosomes, and perhaps other EVs, may have great potential for the development of non-invasive markers for early detection of various cancers due to their unique properties, including their stability in biological fluids and their potential to be isolated efficiently [98]. Work in several different laboratories has centered on the analysis of exosomes and their components isolated from normal and cancer cell lines, and isolation from biological fluids of cancer patients is ongoing, However, more research, including case-control and prospective studies, needs to be conducted in order to develop new biomarkers for early detection, diagnosis and prognosis. In addition, exosomes, as well as the molecules contained in exosomes, may have potential to be multiplexed with other molecular markers or screening modalities (e.g., imaging) to develop integrated molecular tools for the early detection of cancer. The development of biologically-relevant sensitive biomarker-based assays that accurately detect cancer at an early stage will increase the effectiveness of intervention strategies.

References

1. Iorio MV, Croce CM (2012). MicroRNA dysregulation in cancer: diagnostics, monitoring and therapeutics. A comprehensive review. *EMBO Molecular Medicine* **4**, 143–59.

2. Simpson RJ, Lim JW, Moritz RL, Mathivanan S (2009). Exosomes: proteomic insights and diagnostic potential. *Expert Review of Proteomics* **6**, 267–83.

3. Azmi AS, Bao B, Sarkar FH (2013). Exosomes in cancer development, metastasis, and drug resistance: a comprehensive review. *Cancer and Metastasis Reviews* **32**, 623–42.

4. El Andaloussi S, Maeger I, Breakefield XO, Wood MJA (2013). Extracellular vesicles: biology and emerging therapeutic opportunities. *Nature Reviews Drug Discovery* **12**, 348–358.

5. Martins VR, Dias MS, Hainaut P (2013). Tumor-cell-derived microvesicles as carriers of molecular information in cancer. *Current Opinion in Oncology* **25**, 66–75.

6. Simona F, Laura S, Simona T, Riccardo A (2013). Contribution of proteomics to understanding the role of tumor-derived exosomes in cancer progression: State of the art and new perspectives. *Proteomics* **13**, 1581–1594.

7. Taylor DD, Gercel-Taylor C (2005). Tumour-derived exosomes and their role in cancer-associated T-cell signalling defects. *British Journal of Cancer* **92**, 305–11.

8. Mathivanan S, Ji H, Simpson RJ (2010). Exosomes: extracellular organelles important in intercellular communication. *Journal of Proteomics* **73**, 1907–20.

9. Keller S, Sanderson MP, Stoeck A, Altevogt P (2006). Exosomes: from biogenesis and secretion to biological function. *Immunology Letters* **107**, 102–8.

10. Simpson RJ, Jensen SS, Lim JW (2008). Proteomic profiling of exosomes: current perspectives. *Proteomics* **8**, 4083–99.

11. Thery C, Ostrowski M, Segura E (2009). Membrane vesicles as conveyors of immune responses. *Nature Reviews Immunology* **9**, 581–93.

12. van der Pol E, Boing AN, Harrison P, Sturk A, Nieuwland R (2012). Classification, functions, and clinical relevance of extracellular vesicles. *Pharmacological Reviews* **64**, 676–705.

13. Conde-Vancells J, Rodriguez-Suarez E, Embade N, Gil D, Matthiesen R, Valle M, Elortza F, Lu SC, Mato JM, Falcon-Perez JM (2008). Characterization and comprehensive proteome profiling of exosomes secreted by hepatocytes. *Journal of Proteome Research* **7**, 5157–66.

14. Escola JM, Kleijmeer MJ, Stoorvogel W, Griffith JM, Yoshie O, Geuze HJ (1998). Selective enrichment of tetraspan proteins on the internal vesicles of multivesicular endosomes and on exosomes secreted by human B-lymphocytes. *Journal of Biological Chemistry* **273**, 20121–7.

15. Jorgensen M, Baek R, Pedersen S, Sondergaard EK, Kristensen SR, Varming K (2013). Extracellular Vesicle (EV). Array: microarray capturing of exosomes and other extracellular vesicles for multiplexed phenotyping. *Journal of Extracellular Vesicles* **2**.

16. Stoorvogel W, Kleijmeer MJ, Geuze HJ, Raposo G (2002). The biogenesis and functions of exosomes. *Traffic* **3**, 321–30.

17. Staals, RH, Pruijn GJ (2010). The human exosome and disease. *Advances in Experimental Medicine and Biology* **702**, 132–42.

18. Vlassov AV, Magdaleno S, Setterquist R, Conrad R (2012). Exosomes: current knowledge of their composition, biological functions, and diagnostic and therapeutic potentials. *Biochimica et Biophysica Acta* **1820**, 940–8.

19. Geminard C, De Gassart A, Blanc L, Vidal M (2004). Degradation of AP2 during reticulocyte maturation enhances binding of hsc70 and Alix to a common site on TFR for sorting into exosomes. *Traffic* **5**, 181–93.

20. Theos AC, Truschel ST, Tenza D, Hurbain I, Harper DC, Berson JF, Thomas PC, Raposo G, Marks MS (2006). A lumenal domain-dependent pathway for sorting to intralumenal vesicles of multivesicular endosomes involved in organelle morphogenesis. *Developmental Cell* **10**, 343–54.

21. Hurley JH (2008). ESCRT complexes and the biogenesis of multivesicular bodies. *Current Opinion in Cell Biology* **20**, 4–11.

22. Babst M (2006). A close-up of the ESCRTs. *Developmental Cell* **10**, 547–8.

23. Williams RL, Urbe S (2007). The emerging shape of the ESCRT machinery. *Nature Reviews Molecular Cell Biology* **8**, 355–68.

24. Tamai K, Tanaka N, Nakano T, Kakazu E, Kondo Y, Inoue J, Shiina M, Fukushima K, Hoshino T, Sano K, Ueno Y, Shimosegawa T, Sugamura K (2010). Exosome secretion of dendritic cells is regulated by Hrs, an ESCRT-0 protein. *Biochemical and Biophysical Research Communications* **399**, 384–90.

25. Shedden K, Xie XT, Chandaroy P, Chang YT, Rosania GR (2003). Expulsion of small molecules in vesicles shed by cancer cells: association with gene expression and chemosensitivity profiles. *Cancer Research* **63**, 4331–7.

26. Safaei R, Larson BJ, Cheng TC, Gibson MA, Otani S, Naerdemann W, Howell SB (2005). Abnormal lysosomal trafficking and enhanced exosomal export of cisplatin in drug-resistant human ovarian carcinoma cells. *Molecular Cancer Therapeutics* **4**, 1595–604.

27. Schorey JS, Bhatnagar S (2008). Exosome function: from tumor immunology to pathogen biology. *Traffic* **9**, 871–81.

28. Mathivanan S, Fahner CJ, Reid GE, Simpson RJ (2012). ExoCarta 2012: database of exosomal proteins, RNA and lipids. *Nucleic Acids Research* **40**, D1241–4.

29. Breakefield XO, Frederickson RM, Simpson RJ (2011). Gesicles: Microvesicle "cookies" for transient information transfer between cells. *Molecular Therapy* **19**, 1574–6.

30. Lee TH, D'Asti E, Magnus N, Al-Nedawi K, Meehan B, Rak J (2011). Microvesicles as mediators of intercellular communication in cancer – the emerging science of cellular 'debris'. *Seminars in Immunopathology* **33**, 455–67.

31. Li XB, Zhang ZR, Schluesener HJ, Xu SQ (2006). Role of exosomes in immune regulation. *Journal of Cellular and Molecular Medicine* **10**, 364–75.

32. Harding C, Stahl P (1983). Transferrin recycling in reticulocytes: pH and iron are important determinants of ligand binding and processing. *Biochemical and Biophysical Research Communications* **113**, 650–8.

33. Pan BT, Johnstone RM (1983). Fate of the transferrin receptor during maturation of sheep reticulocytes in vitro: selective externalization of the receptor. *Cell* **33**, 967–78.

34. Andre F, Andersen M, Wolfers J, Lozier A, Raposo G, Serra V, Ruegg C, Flament C, Angevin E, Amigorena S, Zitvogel L (2001). Exosomes in cancer immunotherapy: preclinical data. *Advances in Experimental Medicine and Biology* **495**, 349–54.

35. Chaput N, Taieb J, Schartz NE, Andre F, Angevin E, Zitvogel L (2004). Exosome-based immunotherapy. *Cancer Immunology, Immunotherapy* **53**, 234–9.

36. Valadi H, Ekstrom K, Bossios A, Sjostrand M, Lee JJ, Lotvall JO (2007). Exosome-mediated transfer of mRNAs and microRNAs is a novel mechanism of genetic exchange between cells. *Nature Cell Biology* **9**, 654–9.

37. Rosenfeld N, Aharonov R, Meiri E, Rosenwald S, Spector Y, Zepeniuk M, Benjamin H, Shabes N, Tabak S, Levy A, Lebanony D, Goren Y, Silberschein E, Targan N, Ben-Ari A, Gilad S, Sion-Vardy N, Tobar A, Feinmesser M, Kharenko O, Nativ O, Nass D, Perelman M, Yosepovich A, Shalmon B, Polak-Charcon S, Fridman E, Avniel A, Bentwich I, Bentwich Z, Cohen D, Chajut A, Barshack I (2008). MicroRNAs accurately identify cancer tissue origin. *Nature Biotechnology* **26**, 462–9.

38. Zomer A, Vendrig T, Hopmans ES, van Eijndhoven M, Middeldorp JM, Pegtel DM (2010). Exosomes: Fit to deliver small RNA. *Communicative & Integrative Biology* **3**, 447–50.

39. Bellingham SA, Coleman BM, Hill AF (2012). Small RNA deep sequencing reveals a distinct miRNA signature released in exosomes from prion-infected neuronal cells. *Nucleic Acids Research* **40**, 10937–49.

40. Taylor DD, Gercel-Taylor C (2008). MicroRNA signatures of tumor-derived exosomes as diagnostic biomarkers of ovarian cancer. *Gynecologic Oncology* **110**, 13–21.

41. Skog J, Wurdinger T, van Rijn S, Meijer DH, Gainche L, Sena-Esteves M, Curry WT, Jr, Carter BS, Krichevsky AM, Breakefield XO (2008). Glioblastoma microvesicles transport RNA and proteins that promote tumour growth and provide diagnostic biomarkers. *Nature Cell Biology* **10**, 1470–6.

42. Michael A, Bajracharya SD, Yuen PS, Zhou H, Star RA, Illei GG, Alevizos I (2010). Exosomes from human saliva as a source of microRNA biomarkers. *Oral Diseases* **16**, 34–8.

43. Sassen S, Miska EA, Caldas C (2008). MicroRNA: implications for cancer. *Virchows Archiv* **452**, 1–10.

44. Jansson MD, Lund AH (2012). MicroRNA and cancer. *Molecular Oncology* **6**, 590–610.

45. Gilad S, Meiri E, Yogev Y, Benjamin S, Lebanony D, Yerushalmi N, Benjamin H, Kushnir M, Cholakh H, Melamed N, Bentwich Z, Hod M, Goren Y, Chajut A (2008). Serum microRNAs are promising novel biomarkers. *PLoS One* **3**, e3148.

46. Mitchell, PS, Parkin RK, Kroh EM, Fritz BR, Wyman SK, Pogosova-Agadjanyan EL, Peterson A, Noteboom, J. O'Briant KC, Allen A, Lin DW, Urban N, Drescher CW, Knudsen BS, Stirewalt DL, Gentleman R, Vessella RL, Nelson PS, Martin DB, Tewari M (2008). Circulating microRNAs as stable blood-based markers for cancer detection. *Proceedings of the National Academy of Sciences of the United States of America* **105**, 10513–8.

47. Raposo G, Stoorvogel W (2013). Extracellular vesicles: exosomes, microvesicles, and friends. *Journal of Cell Biology* **200**, 373–83.

48. Gastpar R, Gehrmann M, Bausero MA, Asea A, Gross C, Schroeder JA, Multhoff G (2005). Heat shock protein 70 surface-positive tumor exosomes stimulate migratory and cytolytic activity of natural killer cells. *Cancer Research* **65**, 5238–47.

49. Segura E, Amigorena S, Thery C (2005). Mature dendritic cells secrete exosomes with strong ability to induce antigen-specific effector immune responses. *Blood Cells, Molecules and Diseases* **35**, 89–93.

50. Hegmans JP, Bard MP, Hemmes A, Luider TM, Kleijmeer MJ, Prins JB, Zitvogel L, Burgers SA, Hoogsteden HC, Lambrecht BN (2004). Proteomic analysis of exosomes secreted by human mesothelioma cells. *American Journal of Pathology* **164**, 1807–15.

51. Duijvesz D, Burnum-Johnson KE, Gritsenko MA, Hoogland AM, Vredenbregt-van den Berg MS, Willemsen R, Luider T, Pasa-Tolic L, Jenster G (2013). Proteomic profiling of exosomes leads to the identification of novel biomarkers for prostate cancer. *PLoS One* **8**, e82589.

52. Nicholas J (2013). A new diagnostic tool with the potential to predict tumor metastasis. *Journal of the National Cancer Institute* **105**, 371–2.

53. Peinado H, Aleckovic M, Lavotshkin S, Matei I, Costa-Silva B, Moreno-Bueno G, Hergueta-Redondo M, Williams C, Garcia-Santos G, Ghajar C, Nitadori-Hoshino A, Hoffman C, Badal K, Garcia BA, Callahan MK, Yuan J, Martins VR, Skog J, Kaplan RN, Brady MS, Wolchok JD, Chapman PB, Kang Y, Bromberg J, Lyden D (2012). Melanoma exosomes educate bone marrow progenitor cells toward a pro-metastatic phenotype through MET. *Nature Medicine* **18**, 883–91.

54. Zhang HG, Grizzle WE (2014). Exosomes: a novel pathway of local and distant intercellular communication that facilitates the growth and metastasis of neoplastic lesions. *American Journal of Pathology* **184**, 28–41.

55. Alderton GK (2012). Metastasis. Exosomes drive premetastatic niche formation. *Nature Reviews Cancer* **12**, 447.

56. Fang DY, King HW, Li JY, Gleadle JM (2012). Exosomes and the Kidney: Blaming the Messenger. *Nephrology (Carlton)* **18**(1):1–10.

57. Aung T, Chapuy B, Vogel D, Wenzel D, Oppermann M, Lahmann M, Weinhage T, Menck K, Hupfeld T, Koch R, Trumper L, Wulf GG (2011). Exosomal evasion of humoral immunotherapy in aggressive B-cell lymphoma modulated by ATP-binding cassette transporter A3. *Proceedings of the National Academy of Sciences of the United States of America* **108**, 15336–41.

58. Kharaziha P, Ceder S, Li Q, Panaretakis T (2012). Tumor cell-derived exosomes: A message in a bottle. *Biochimica et Biophysica Acta* **1826**, 103–11.

59. Taylor DD, Gercel-Taylor C (2011). Exosomes/microvesicles: mediators of cancer-associated immunosuppressive microenvironments. *Seminars in Immunopathology* **33**, 441–54.

60. Al-Nedawi K, Meehan B, Micallef J, Lhotak V, May L, Guha A, Rak J (2008). Intercellular transfer of the oncogenic receptor EGFRvIII by microvesicles derived from tumour cells. *Nature Cell Biology* **10**, 619–24.

61. Zhang HG, Grizzle WE (2011). Exosomes and cancer: a newly described pathway of immune suppression. *Clinical Cancer Research* **17**, 959–64.

62. Chaput N, Thery C (2011). Exosomes: immune properties and potential clinical implementations. *Seminars in Immunopathology* **33**, 419–40.

63. Filipazzi P, Burdek M, Villa A, Rivoltini L, Huber V (2012). Recent advances on the role of tumor exosomes in immunosuppression and disease progression. *Seminars in Cancer Biology* **22**, 342–9.

64. Keryer-Bibens C, Pioche-Durieu C, Villemant C, Souquere S, Nishi N, Hirashima M, Middeldorp J, Busson P (2006). Exosomes released by EBV-infected nasopharyngeal carcinoma cells convey the viral latent membrane protein 1 and the immunomodulatory protein galectin 9. *BMC Cancer* **6**, 283.

65. Nanbo A, Kawanishi E, Yoshida R, Yoshiyama H (2013). Exosomes derived from Epstein-Barr virus-infected cells are internalized via caveola-dependent endocytosis and promote phenotypic modulation in target cells. *Journal of Virology* **87**, 10334–47.

66. Meckes D.G, Jr, Shair KH, Marquitz AR, Kung CP, Edwards RH, Raab-Traub N (2010). Human tumor virus utilizes exosomes for intercellular communication. *Proceedings of the National Academy of Sciences of the United States of America* **107**, 20370–5.

67. Bose S, Chandran S, Mirocha JM, Bose N (2006). The Akt pathway in human breast cancer: a tissue-array-based analysis. *Modern Pathology* **19**, 238–45.

68. Arscott WT, Camphausen KA (2011). Analysis of urinary exosomes to identify new markers of non-small-cell lung cancer. *Biomarkers in Medicine* **5**, 822.

69. Duijvesz D, Luider T, Bangma CH, Jenster G (2011). Exosomes as biomarker treasure chests for prostate cancer. *European Urology* **59**, 823–31.

70. Friel AM, Corcoran C, Crown J, O'Driscoll L (2010). Relevance of circulating tumor cells, extracellular nucleic acids, and exosomes in breast cancer. *Breast Cancer Research and Treatment* **123**, 613–25.

71. Peng P, Yan Y, Keng S (2011). Exosomes in the ascites of ovarian cancer patients: origin and effects on antitumor immunity. *Oncology Reports* **25**, 749–62.

72. Roberson CD, Atay S, Gercel-Taylor C, Taylor DD (2010). Tumor-derived exosomes as mediators of disease and potential diagnostic biomarkers. *Cancer Biomarkers* **8**, 281–91.

73. Thery C, Duban L, Segura E, Veron P, Lantz O, Amigorena S (2002). Indirect activation of naive CD4+ T cells by dendritic cell-derived exosomes. *Nature Immunology* **3**, 1156–62.

74. Vincent-Schneider H, Stumptner-Cuvelette P, Lankar D, Pain S, Raposo G, Benaroch P, Bonnerot C (2002). Exosomes bearing HLA-DR1 molecules need dendritic cells to efficiently stimulate specific T cells. *International Immunology* **14**, 713–22.

75. Xiang X, Poliakov A, Liu C, Liu Y, Deng ZB, Wang J, Cheng Z, Shah SV, Wang GJ, Zhang L, Grizzle WE, Mobley J, Zhang HG (2009). Induction of myeloid-derived suppressor cells by tumor exosomes. *International Journal of Cancer* **124**, 2621–33.

76. Liu C, Yu S, Kappes J, Wang J, Grizzle WE, Zinn KR, Zhang HG (2007). Expansion of spleen myeloid suppressor cells represses NK cell cytotoxicity in tumor-bearing host. *Blood* **109**, 4336–42.

77. Logozzi M, De Milito A, Lugini L, Borghi M, Calabro L, Spada M, Perdicchio M, Marino ML, Federici C, Iessi E, Brambilla D, Venturi G, Lozupone F, Santinami M, Huber V, Maio M, Rivoltini L, Fais S (2009). High levels of exosomes expressing CD63 and caveolin-1 in plasma of melanoma patients. *PLoS One* **4**, e5219.

78. Li J, Sherman-Baust CA, Tsai-Turton M, Bristow RE, Roden RB, Morin PJ. (2009). Claudin-containing exosomes in the peripheral circulation of women with ovarian cancer. *BMC Cancer* **9**, 244.

79. Andriole GL, Crawford ED, Grubb RL, 3rd, Buys SS, Chia D, Church TR, Fouad MN, Isaacs C, Kvale PA, Reding DJ, Weissfeld JL, Yokochi LA, O'Brien B, Ragard LR, Clapp JD, Rathmell JM, Riley TL, Hsing AW, Izmirlian G, Pinsky PF, Kramer BS, Miller AB, Gohagan JK, Prorok PC, Team PP (2012). Prostate cancer screening in the randomized Prostate, Lung, Colorectal, and Ovarian Cancer Screening Trial: mortality results after 13 years of follow-up. *Journal of the National Cancer Institute* **104**, 125–32.

80. Gonzalez-Begne M, Lu B, Han X, Hagen FK, Hand AR, Melvin JE, Yates JR (2009). Proteomic analysis of human parotid gland exosomes by multidimensional protein identification technology (MudPIT). *Journal of Proteome Research* **8**, 1304–14.

81. Gonzalez-Begne M, Lu B, Liao L, Xu T, Bedi G, Melvin JE, Yates JR, 3rd (2011). Characterization of the human submandibular/sublingual saliva glycoproteome using lectin affinity chromatography coupled to multidimensional protein identification technology. *Journal of Proteome Research* **10**, 5031–46.

82. Soekmadji C, Russell PJ, Nelson CC (2013). Exosomes in prostate cancer: putting together the pieces of a puzzle. *Cancers (Basel)* **5**, 1522–44.

83. Perner S, Hofer MD, Kim R, Shah RB, Li H, Moller P, Hautmann RE, Gschwend JE, Kuefer R, Rubin MA (2007). Prostate-specific membrane antigen expression as a predictor of prostate cancer progression. *Human Pathology* **38**, 696–701.

84. Wright GL, Jr, Haley C, Beckett ML, Schellhammer PF (1995). Expression of prostate-specific membrane antigen in normal, benign, and malignant prostate tissues. *Urologic Oncology* **1**, 18–28.

85. Phin S, Moore MW, Cotter PD (2013). Genomic Rearrangements of in Prostate Cancer. *Frontiers in Oncology* **3**, 240.

86. Gabriel K, Ingram A, Austin R, Kapoor A, Tang D, Majeed F, Qureshi T, Al-Nedawi K (2013). Regulation of the tumor suppressor PTEN through exosomes: a diagnostic potential for prostate cancer. *PLoS One* **8**, e70047.

87. Heinlein, CA, Chang C (2004). Androgen receptor in prostate cancer. *Endocrine Reviews* **25**, 276–308.

88. Trajkovic K, Hsu C, Chiantia S, Rajendran L, Wenzel D, Wieland F, Schwille P, Brugger B, Simons M (2008). Ceramide triggers budding of exosome vesicles into multivesicular endosomes. *Science* **319**, 1244–7.

89. Khan S, Jutzy JM, Valenzuela MM, Turay D, Aspe JR, Ashok A, Mirshahidi S, Mercola D, Lilly MB, Wall NR (2012). Plasma-derived exosomal survivin, a plausible biomarker for early detection of prostate cancer. *PLoS One* **7**, e46737.

90. Silva J, Garcia V, Rodriguez M, Compte M, Cisneros E, Veguillas, P. Garcia JM, Dominguez G, Campos-Martin Y, Cuevas J, Pena C, Herrera M, Diaz R, Mohammed N, Bonilla F (2012). Analysis of exosome release and its prognostic value in human colorectal cancer. *Genes Chromosomes Cancer* **51**, 409–18.

91. Rabinowits G, Gercel-Taylor C, Day JM, Taylor DD, Kloecker GH (2009). Exosomal microRNA: a diagnostic marker for lung cancer. *Clinical Lung Cancer* **10**, 42–6.

92. Tauro BJ, Greening DW, Mathias RA, Ji H, Mathivanan S, Scott AM, Simpson RJ (2012). Comparison of ultracentrifugation, density gradient separation, and immunoaffinity capture methods for isolating human colon cancer cell line LIM1863-derived exosomes. *Methods* **56**, 293–304.

93. Lai RC, Arslan F, Lee MM, Sze NS, Choo A, Chen TS, Salto-Tellez, M. Timmers L, Lee CN, El Oakley RM, Pasterkamp G, de Kleijn DP, Lim SK (2010). Exosome secreted by MSC reduces myocardial ischemia/ reperfusion injury. *Stem Cell Research* **4**, 214–22.

94. Cicero AL, Raposo G (2013). *Emerging Concepts of Tumor Exosome-Mediated Cell-Cell Communication.* Springer.

95. Beyer C, Pisetsky DS (2010). The role of microparticles in the pathogenesis of rheumatic diseases. *Nature Reviews Rheumatology* **6**, 21–9.

96. Alvarez-Erviti L, Seow Y, Yin H, Betts C, Lakhal S, Wood MJ (2011). Delivery of siRNA to the mouse brain

by systemic injection of targeted exosomes. *Nature Biotechnology* **29**, 341–5.

97. Webber J, Clayton A (2013). How pure are your vesicles? *Journal of Extracellular Vesicles* **2**. doi: 10.3402/jev.v2i0.19861.

98. Henderson MC, Azorsa DO. (2012). The genomic and proteomic content of cancer cell-derived exosomes. *Frontiers in Oncology* **2**, 38.

99. Hong BS, Cho JH, Kim H, Choi EJ, Rho S, Kim J, Kim JH, Choi DS, Kim YK, Hwang D, Gho YS (2009). Colorectal cancer cell-derived microvesicles are enriched in cell cycle-related mRNAs that promote proliferation of endothelial cells. *BMC Genomics* **10**, 556.

100. Bryant RJ, Pawlowski T, Catto JW, Marsden G, Vessella RL, Rhees B, Kuslich C, Visakorpi T, Hamdy FC (2012). Changes in circulating microRNA levels associated with prostate cancer. *British Journal of Cancer* **106**, 768–74.

101. Hu Z, Chen X, Zhao Y, Tian T, Jin G, Shu Y, Chen Y, Xu L, Zen K, Zhang C, Shen H (2010). Serum microRNA signatures identified in a genome-wide serum microRNA expression profiling predict survival of non-small-cell lung cancer. *Journal of Clinical Oncology* **28**, 1721–6.

102. Chen X, Ba Y, Ma L, Cai X, Yin Y, Wang K, Guo J, Zhang Y, Chen J, Guo X, Li Q, Li X, Wang W, Zhang Y, Wang J, Jiang X, Xiang Y, Xu C, Zheng P, Zhang J, Li R, Zhang H, Shang X, Gong T, Ning G, Wang J, Zen K, Zhang J, Zhang CY (2008). Characterization of microRNAs in serum: a novel class of biomarkers for diagnosis of cancer and other diseases. *Cell Research* **18**, 997–1006.

103. Lawrie CH, Gal S, Dunlop HM, Pushkaran B, Liggins AP, Pulford K, Banham AH, Pezzella F, Boultwood J, Wainscoat JS, Hatton CS, Harris AL (2008). Detection of elevated levels of tumour-associated microRNAs in serum of patients with diffuse large B-cell lymphoma. *British Journal of Haematology* **141**, 672–5.

104. Satzger I, Mattern, A. Kuettler U, Weinspach D, Niebuhr M, Kapp A, Gutzmer R (2012). microRNA-21 is upregulated in malignant melanoma and influences apoptosis of melanocytic cells. *Experimental Dermatology* **21**, 509–14.

105. Segura MF, Hanniford D, Menendez S, Reavie L, Zou X, Alvarez-Diaz S, Zakrzewski J, Blochin, E. Rose A, Bogunovic D, Polsky D, Wei J, Lee P, Belitskaya-Levy I, Bhardwaj N, Osman I, Hernando E (2009). Aberrant miR-182 expression promotes melanoma metastasis by repressing FOXO3 and microphthalmia-associated transcription factor. *Proceedings of the National Academy of Sciences of the United States of America* **106**, 1814–9.

106. Zhu W, Qin W, Atasoy U, Sauter ER (2009). Circulating microRNAs in breast cancer and healthy subjects. *BMC Research Notes* **2**, 89.

107. Resnick, KE, Alder H, Hagan JP, Richardson DL, Croce CM, Cohn DE. (2009). The detection of differentially expressed microRNAs from the serum of ovarian cancer patients using a novel real-time PCR platform. *Gynecologic Oncology* **112**, 55–9.

108. Ng EK, Chong WW, Jin H, Lam EK, Shin VY, Yu J, Poon TC, Ng SS, Sung JJ (2009). Differential expression of microRNAs in plasma of patients with colorectal cancer: a potential marker for colorectal cancer screening. *Gut* **58**, 1375–81.

109. Wang J, Zhou Y, Lu J, Sun Y, Xiao H, Liu M, Tian L (2014). Combined detection of serum exosomal miR-21 and HOTAIR as diagnostic and prognostic biomarkers for laryngeal squamous cell carcinoma. *Medical Oncology* **31**, 148.

110. Dijkstra S, Birker IL, Smit FP, Leyten GH, de Reijke TM, van Oort IM, Mulders PF, Jannink SA, Schalken JA (2014). Prostate cancer biomarker profiles in urinary sediments and exosomes. *Journal of Urology* **191**, 1132–8.

111. Beckham CJ, Olsen J, Yin PN, Wu CH, Ting HJ, Hagen FK, Scosyrev E, Messing EM, Lee YF (2014). Bladder Cancer Exosomes Contain EDIL-3/Del1 and Facilitate Cancer Progression. *Journal of Urology* **192**, 583–92.

112. Keller S, Konig AK, Marme F, Runz S, Wolterink S, Koensgen D, Mustea A, Sehouli J, Altevogt P (2009). Systemic presence and tumor-growth promoting effect of ovarian carcinoma released exosomes. *Cancer Letters* **278**, 73–81.

113. Szajnik M, Derbis M, Lach M, Patalas P, Michalak M, Drzewiecka H, Szpurek D, Nowakowski A, Spaczynski M, Baranowski W, Whiteside TL (2013). Exosomes in Plasma of Patients with Ovarian Carcinoma: Potential Biomarkers of Tumor Progression and Response to Therapy. *Gynecology & Obstetrics (Sunnyvale)* Suppl 4, 3.

114. Rank A, Liebhardt S, Zwirner J, Burges A, Nieuwland R, Toth B (2012). Circulating microparticles in patients with benign and malignant ovarian tumors. *Anticancer Research* **32**, 2009–14.

115. Rupp AK, Rupp C, Keller S, Brase JC, Ehehalt R, Fogel M, Moldenhauer G, Marme F, Sultmann H, Altevogt P (2011). Loss of EpCAM expression in breast cancer derived serum exosomes: role of proteolytic cleavage. *Gynecologic Oncology* **122**, 437–46.

116. Shao H, Chung J, Balaj L, Charest A, Bigner DD, Carter BS, Hochberg FH, Breakefield XO, Weissleder R, Lee H (2012). Protein typing of circulating microvesicles

allows real-time monitoring of glioblastoma therapy. *Nature Medicine* **18**, 1835–40.

117. Kim JW, Wieckowski E, Taylor DD, Reichert TE, Watkins S, Whiteside TL (2005). Fas ligand-positive membranous vesicles isolated from sera of patients with oral cancer induce apoptosis of activated T lymphocytes. *Clinical Cancer Research* **11**, 1010–20.

118. Baran J, Baj-Krzyworzeka M, Weglarczyk K, Szatanek R, Zembala M, Barbasz J, Czupryna A, Szczepanik A, Zembala M (2010). Circulating tumour-derived microvesicles in plasma of gastric cancer patients. *Cancer Immunology, Immunotherapy* **59**, 841–50.

119. Toth B, Nieuwland R, Liebhardt S, Ditsch N, Steinig K, Stieber P, Rank A, Gohring P, Thaler CJ, Friese K, Bauerfeind I (2008). Circulating microparticles in breast cancer patients: a comparative analysis with established biomarkers. *Anticancer Research* **28**, 1107–12

120. Nilsson J, Skog J, Nordstrand A, Baranov V, Mincheva-Nilsson L, Breakefield XO, Widmark A (2009). Prostate cancer-derived urine exosomes: a novel approach to biomarkers for prostate cancer. *British Journal of Cancer* **100**, 1603–7.

CHAPTER 6

Epithelial-to-Mesenchymal Transition (EMT): Clinical Implications

Elisa C Woodhouse and Suresh Mohla

Tumor Biology and Metastasis Branch, Division of Cancer Biology, National Cancer Institute, National Institutes of Health, Bethesda, MD, USA

Biology of epithelial-to-mesenchymal transition (EMT)

Epithelial-mesenchymal transition is a process in which epithelial cells acquire a less-differentiated mesenchymal phenotype. During EMT, epithelial cells lose their attachments to neighboring cells as well as apico-basal polarity, and gain migratory properties. The gain of mesenchymal markers (e.g. N-cadherin, vimentin, fibronectin) and loss of epithelial markers (e.g. E-cadherin, cytokeratins) accompany these phenotypic changes [1].

EMT was first described by Elizabeth Hay, who observed the formation of the primitive streak in chick development, a process that involves the conversion of epithelial cells to mesenchymal cells [2]. The loss of cell polarity and intercellular junctions disrupt the basement membrane, allowing cells to penetrate the extracellular matrix-rich compartment [3]. The reverse process, mesenchymal-epithelial transition (MET), allows phenotypic plasticity as cells can move from one state to the other [4].

EMT has since been found to occur in a range of biological contexts and was recently classified into three types:

1 developmental EMT
2 fibrosis and wound healing EMT
3 EMT in cancer [5,6].

Type 1 EMT is associated with implantation, embryogenesis, and organ development, whereas Type 2 EMT takes place in the context of tissue regeneration and organ fibrosis and is largely inflammation-driven. Type 3, or carcinoma EMT, is associated with cancer progression and metastasis and is the focus of this chapter.

Evidence points to EMT as a key event in the progression to a malignant phenotype [7]. Cancer cells expressing mesenchymal markers have been observed most often at the invasive front of tumors [8], leading to the suggestion that cells undergoing EMT enhance tumor invasion. In addition, EMT is also associated with expanded stem-like and tumor initiation properties. A direct link between EMT and a cancer stem cell (CSC) phenotype was first demonstrated by the finding that EMT induction resulted in the acquisition of mesenchymal traits and the expression of stem cell markers ($CD44^{high}/CD24^{low}$) – mammary epithelial cells that have undergone EMT have an enhanced ability to form mammospheres, a property associated with mammary epithelial stem cells. Moreover, stem-like cells isolated from mouse or human mammary glands, or mammary carcinomas, express EMT markers [9].

Although EMT has generally been regarded as a late event in cancer progression, it is now understood that EMT (and tumor dissemination) can

---

Biomarkers in Cancer Screening and Early Detection, First Edition. Edited by Sudhir Srivastava.
© 2017 John Wiley & Sons, Inc. Published 2017 by John Wiley & Sons, Inc.

occur quite early in tumorigenesis [10]. In a mouse model of pancreatic cancer, pancreatic epithelial cells were found to enter the circulation very early, even before a primary tumor is detectable. This behavior is associated with EMT, since the circulating pancreatic epithelial cells maintain a mesenchymal phenotype and exhibit stem cell properties. Interestingly, inflammation, a common occurrence in pancreatic cancers, promotes the EMT process, thereby enhancing tumor progression [10].

EMT: effects on cells and tissues

The EMT process involves numerous changes in the cell [5], including the activation of specific transcription factors, changes in expression and reorganization of cytoskeleton proteins, and production of ECM-degrading proteins. There has been skepticism regarding the existence of EMT *in vivo*, due to a lack of evidence at secondary metastatic sites. The transient nature and reversibility of this process are likely to confound the observation of EMT in tissues. Furthermore, carcinoma cells that have undergone EMT may be difficult to distinguish from mesenchymal fibroblasts [11].

The occurrence of EMT *in vivo* was first shown through lineage tracing of epithelial and stromal cells in a Myc-induced breast cancer model. Stromal fibroblasts were demonstrated to be of epithelial origin (since the epithelial cells were genetically marked), being devoid of cytokeratins and E-cadherin but enriched with mesenchymal markers such as vimentin and fibronectin [12]. There are reports of detection of stem cells and EMT in human tissues, as shown recently with breast cancer [11]. Further investigation of EMT in patient samples will be important for the development of predictive or prognostic tests related to EMT markers.

Downregulation of E-cadherin is a key event in EMT, and the relationship between E-cadherin loss and EMT has been established in many systems [1, 5, 13]. Many oncogenes can induce EMT by suppressing E-cadherin expression, or via loss of the E-cadherin gene. It is possible to reverse the mesenchymal phenotype in cells that have undergone EMT by expressing E-cadherin (full length, or the cytoplasmic portion that binds β-catenin) [5]. During EMT, the loss of E-cadherin results in relocalization of β-catenin from the cytoplasm to the nucleus, where it forms part of the Tcf/LEF

complex [5]. The presence of E-cadherin, and the resulting cytoplasmic sequestration of β-catenin, are important for the epithelial phenotype, as they function to maintain cell-cell adhesion via adherens junctions, to coordinate cellular organization, and to transmit information from the extracellular microenvironment to the cells [14]. E-cadherin expression is maintained in most differentiated tumors (including breast, colon, head and neck, liver, lung, prostate and skin). However, an inverse correlation exists between E-cadherin levels and tumor grade/differentiation or survival [13], and E-cadherin loss in breast cancer has been shown to correlate with increased metastasis [15].

The induction of the mesenchymal/stem cell state of carcinoma cells, and its functional consequences (viz., EMT/stemness imparts a more aggressive phenotype), has been delineated by a number of investigators. EMT induction and its maintenance is controlled by three signaling pathways – TGFβ, and Wnt canonical and non-canonical signaling. These pathways first induce EMT, then perpetuate the mesenchymal state in an autocrine manner [16]. Also, EMT enhances filopodia-like protrusions in carcinoma cells through blockade of cofilin-mediated actin filament severing, resulting in stable filopodia. The stable filopodia contribute to the tumor initiating capabilities to carcinoma cells [17].

Induction of EMT: contribution of the tumor microenvironment

EMT in carcinoma cells can be initiated by a number of intra- and extra-cellular signals such as growth factors, inflammatory cytokines, oncogenes, and enhanced NF-κB signaling [1]. Hypoxia (one of the most common features of a majority of carcinomas), and the resulting increase in hypoxia-inducible factor-1, can promote EMT in cancer cells by promoting expression of Twist [18], or by activating urokinase receptor (uPAR) signaling. Following hypoxia, re-oxygenation of carcinoma cells results in decreased uPAR expression levels, and a reversal of EMT to mesenchymal-to-epithelial transition [19]. EMT/cancer stem cells (CSCs) and hypoxia markers have been shown to co-localize within tumors, supporting the notion that hypoxia promotes EMT. In fact, studies show that CSCs are the cells that acquire high migratory potential in response to hypoxia and are, therefore, responsible for invasion and metastasis [20].

Like hypoxia, autophagy is considered to be an important mediator in cancer progression. The precise role of autophagy in tumor progression is an active area of investigation. However, autophagy has been shown to induce EMT in some cancers, such as hepatocellular carcinoma; the shift from epithelial to mesenchymal markers is accompanied by increased expression of matrix metalloproteinase-9 and increased invasiveness [21].

It is increasingly appreciated that factors produced by the tumor microenvironment can exert effects on tumor cells that influence cancer progression, including the induction of EMT. TGFβ is a potent inducer of EMT, and is a major regulator of this process [22]. During EMT induction, TGFβ signaling ultimately regulates the expression and activity of several EMT transcription factors, including Snail1, Slug, Zeb1/2, Twist 1/2, Six family of homeobox (Six 1), and Forkhead (FOXC2), as well as members of the High Mobility Group Proteins (HMG2a), which enhance transcription factor binding [23].

Stromal cells in tumors and their role in EMT induction

It is now accepted that tumor cells and the associated stroma have dynamic and reciprocal interactions throughout the cancer continuum (from initiation-progression-metastasis, to resistance and recurrence). Stromal cells include fibroblasts, adipocytes, endothelial cells, and myeloid and lymphoid immune cells. Essentially, all stromal cells have been shown to induce EMT in carcinoma cells via secretion of growth factors, inflammatory cytokines, or proteases.

Macrophages

Among the stromal cells, tumor-associated macrophages occupy a central role. Macrophages constitute the largest fraction of the leukocyte population. Once they are associated with tumor cells (tumor-associated macrophages, or TAMs), they can induce inflammation, angiogenesis, intra- and extra-vasation, tumor growth, progression and EMT, via production of growth factors and inflammatory cytokines. They can also modulate

the tumor microenvironment through the expression of proteases (e.g., matrix metallo-proteinases, cathepsins, and urokinase plasminogen activator), lysyl oxidases and SPARC [24].

It is unlikely that the majority of pro-tumoral functions belong to one population of TAMs. For clinical approaches to succeed, these various populations of TAMs in the tumor microenvironment must first be properly identified and characterized. However, the plasticity of macrophages during tumor evolution makes accurate characterization a challenging task [25]. Indeed, using the macrophage transcriptome, a recent paper identified both distinct and universally associated genes with mature tissue resident macrophages, but the results also showed the extreme diversity of macrophages [26].

Recently, the Pollard laboratory has made substantial contributions to the understanding of the role of tumor-associated macrophages in cancer progression. Their results suggest that macrophage diversity enhances tumor progression and metastasis [27], and provide further elaboration of macrophage heterogeneity, based on the various roles that macrophages play in specialized organs such as brain, bone and heart and vasculature, as well as a variety of functions they modulate, such as angiogenesis, metabolism, adipogenesis and immunity. Specifically during cancer progression, macrophages exhibit unique activation profiles that regulate cancer invasion, migration, progression and metastasis, as well as EMT in carcinoma cells [24].

There is, thus, an increasing clinical interest to delete or silence the pro-tumorigenic and immunosuppressive TAMs from the tumor microenvironment. Targeting cells in the microenvironment that induce EMT could be a means to disrupt this process via the suppression of tumor migration and invasion. Several approaches have been used to ablate TAMs or to inhibit their tumor-promoting functions in mouse models of cancer. One strategy used is CSF-1R inhibition, which depletes macrophages and reduces tumor volume in several xenograft models [28, 29].

Recent studies show that a new CSF-1R inhibitor (BLZ945) blocks malignant progression, regresses established gliomas, and markedly enhances survival in a transgenic mouse model of proneural glioblastoma *multiforme* (GBM). Moreover, multiple proneural GBM human xenografts responded similarly to CSF-1R inhibition, underscoring the therapeutic relevance of these findings. Surprisingly, it was found that TAMs in all models were specifically protected from CSF-1R inhibitor-induced death. This contrasted with the observed depletion of microglia in the normal brain and the depletion of macrophages in other tissues, consistent with previous reports [28, 29]. These results suggest that glioma-supplied factors (e.g., IGFγ and GM-SCF) facilitate TAM survival in the presence of BLZ945, whereas neighboring microglia outside of the tumor mass are not exposed to these protective signals and are, thus, depleted. However, the surviving TAMs are now converted to immunocompetent and cytotoxic macrophages, resulting in the regression of established GBMs [30].

CD8T cells

Other immune cells can also induce EMT. For example, CD8T cells have been found to play a role in immunoediting and the promotion of EMT [31]. Immunoediting [32], describes the process by which the immune system has both host protective and tumor-promoting functions. Immunoediting is divided into three phases: elimination (involving extrinsic tumor suppression), equilibrium (involving tumor dormancy and editing), and escape (involving tumor growth promotion).

CD8T cells were required for outgrowth of mesenchymal variants in a MMTV-Neu model of mammary carcinoma, suggesting local induction of EMT. The resulting carcinoma cells with EMT were also enriched with stem cell markers (CD44^{high}/CD24^{low}) and formed mammospheres *in vitro*, as well as tumor formation *in vivo*, suggesting that EMT may be one mechanism underlying immunoediting in cancer [31]. In a recent study, neutrophils have also been shown to promote EMT in carcinoma cells [33].

Carcinoma-associated fibroblasts and endothelial cells

Carcinoma-associated fibroblasts (CAFs) are frequently present in the stroma and have been shown to promote tumor progression. In differentiation into CAFs, resident fibroblasts establish two autocrine signaling loops, mediated by TGF-β and stromal cell-derived factor-1 (SDF-1) [34]. The CAFs acquire a tumor-promoting activity, possibly via promotion of EMT by TGF-β produced in the tumor microenvironment [35].

Endothelial cells are also potent inducers of EMT, inducing a shift from E-cadherin to N-cadherin expression and causing increased migratory properties in carcinoma cells and the acquisition of stem cell-like properties. In clinical samples, tumor cells near the vasculature have had little or no E-cadherin expression, suggesting that cells in these areas undergo EMT [36].

Epithelial-to-mesenchymal transition regulators

Transcription factors

A complex system of regulatory networks define EMT during cancer initiation and progression [37]. Downregulation of E-cadherin, one of the central hallmarks of EMT, occurs during the tumor progression process via transcriptional repression [13]. While many transcriptional repressors target the CDH1 (E-cadherin) gene, EMT is primarily controlled by three transcription factor families that downregulate E-cadherin by transcriptional repression: the Snail (Snail and Slug) and ZEB families (ZEB1/ZEB2), and Twist [1]. In addition to E-cadherin down regulation, they also regulate other epithelial markers and induce mesenchymal genes [22].

Snail, a zinc-finger containing transcriptional repressor, strongly binds to two E-boxes near the transcriptional start site of E-cadherin [13]. Snail and Slug (also known as Snail2) have both been detected at sites of EMT in vertebrates [13]. Furthermore, Snail is expressed in high grade human breast carcinoma tissues and lymph node positive tumors [13], and Snail overexpression predicts decreased relapse-free survival [38]. Twist1, a basic helix-loop-helix transcription factor, can bind the Slug promoter region, which induces Slug transcription and promotes EMT [1]. Like Snail and Slug, ZEB1 and ZEB2 are zinc-finger-containing transcription factors that promote EMT through binding E-cadherin E-boxes and repressing transcription. In addition to repression of epithelial genes (e.g., E-cadherin, plakophilin-2, ZO-3), ZEB transcription factors also activate expression of

MMP family members, particularly MMP2, which further promotes the invasive phenotype [1].

MicroRNAs

MicroRNAs (miRs) are important post-transcriptional regulators of EMT that suppress their targets through mRNA destabilization and translational inhibition [22]. Individual miRs are often capable of targeting multiple mRNAs, and it is also possible for a single RNA to be regulated by multiple miRs that target distinct sequences. For example, miR-200a, miR-200b, miR-200c, miR-141 and miR-429 all target ZEB1 and ZEB2. The expression of these miRs is reduced in EMT, increasing the levels of ZEB1 and ZEB2 [22]. Interestingly, a negative feedback loop exists between ZEB1/2 and the miR200 family members, as ZEB1 and ZEB2 also repress the miR200s [1]. The Snail transcription factor is also regulated by microRNAs (miR-29b and miR-30). However, regulation of EMT by microRNAs is not restricted to direct targeting of transcriptional factors. For example, the let-7 miR targets HMGA2, a chromatin-binding protein that regulates TGF-β-induced responses via activation of Snail and Twist [22].

Concerted efforts are also being made to determine whether microRNAs can be used as therapeutic agents in cancer patients. For example, miR-34a has recently been reported as a potential therapeutic agent for lung cancer patients [39]. miR34a, one of 27 miRs downregulated by ZEB1, has been shown to decrease tumor cell invasion and metastasis, and its overexpression inhibits TGF-β-induced invasion of lung cancer cells, even in the presence of other upregulated mesenchymal markers. miR34a elicits its effects via downregulation of *Arhgap1 gene*, a critical mediator of cell invasion that encodes a RHO GTPase-activating protein [39].

Further elucidation of ZEB1-induced regulation of miRs has recently been reported by the Weinberg lab, where it was found that a critical factor in the responsiveness of breast cancer cells to EMT signals is the chromatin conformation of the promoter of the gene encoding ZEB1, a key regulator of the EMT program. The researchers made the seminal observation that explains as to why basal, but not luminal, breast cancer cells show propensity to become stem-like, and they attributed this to a difference in ZEB1 gene expression. The promoter of the ZEB1 gene in luminal cancer cells was in a "repressed" chromatin configuration, but in basal cells it was in a "bivalent poised" state (containing chromatin marks of both repressive and activated chromatin), allowing it to be activated by microenvironmental signals, such as TGF-β [40].

One of the key growth factors that regulate EMT in carcinoma cells is TGF-β. Several excellent reviews have been written on this topic, and a few are cited here [5, 23, 41]. Using a mathematical model for the core regulatory network controlling TGF-β-induced EMT, it was recently demonstrated that EMT is a sequential two-step program – epithelial cells first transit to partial EMT, and then to the mesenchymal state. The extent of the process is dependent on the strength and duration of TGF-β stimulation. The SNAIL1/miR-34 double negative feedback loop is responsible for a reversible switch that regulates the initiation of EMT, while the ZEB/miR-200 feedback loop is accountable for an irreversible switch that controls the establishment of the mesenchymal state. The second switch is made irreversible through an autocrine TGF-β-miR-200 feedback loop [42].

Mesenchymal-to-epithelial transition (MET)

While EMT is associated with the invasive migratory phenotype and helps in tumor dissemination, the reverse process, mesenchymal-to-epithelial transition, or MET, has been shown to be important in colonization of disseminated tumor cells in many cancers, including breast cancer [43]. Mesenchymal-to-epithelial transition is a reversible process by which mesenchymal cells transdifferentiate to epithelial cells with cell-cell junctions and adherens complexes [23]. MET results in the transformation of motile, nonpolarized mesenchymal cells into nonmotile, polarized epithelial cells [44]. During MET, there is a decrease in mesenchymal markers such as N-cadherin and vimentin, while epithelial markers such as E-cadherin increase. EMT-inducing transcription factors can directly inhibit proliferation, so tumor cells must undergo MET in order to revert to the epithelial state and proliferate at the metastatic site [1]. While EMT allows dissemination of tumor cells from the primary tumor, MET is needed to drive proliferation of the disseminated cancer cell and formation of the secondary tumor [23].

Both EMT and MET are recognized as critical events that can determine the extent of carcinoma metastasis. For example, using bladder cancer lines with differing degrees of epithelial characteristic showed differential metastatic efficacy – when injected intracardially, the cancer cell lines that had acquired more epithelial characteristics were more metastatic, compared with less epithelial-like cells. However, if injected orthotopically, the more epithelial lines produced fewer lung metastases, compared with cell lines that had both epithelial and mesenchymal markers, showing the importance of EMT in allowing escape from the primary tumor [45].

A more complete understanding of the MET process is still developing. MET can be induced by various mechanisms, including E-cadherin overexpression, FGF Receptor 2 isoform switching, EGFR inhibition, and knock-down of plasminogen-activator-1 [46]. A novel MET-inducing function was recently discovered for two transcription factors – OVOL1 and OVOL2. The MET function of these transcription factors occurs through a regulatory feedback loop with ZEB1 and the regulation of mRNA splicing by inducing Epithelial Splicing Regulation Protein 1 (ESRP1). Expression of OVOL1 and 2 in mesenchymal prostate cancer cells decreases the invasive potential and migratory properties of the cells, and reduces the metastatic potential of mesenchymal cells in a murine tumor model of prostate cancer [47].

Accumulating evidence from experimental studies supports a direct role of MET on carcinoma metastasis, suggesting that targeting the MET process at distant sites of metastasis may offer opportunities to inhibit metastatic tumor formation [44].

As EMT is linked to therapeutic resistance, inducing MET may allow increased efficacy of cancer therapeutics; the induction of epithelial phenotypes has been shown to increase sensitivity of ovarian cancer cells to carboplatin treatment [48].

EMT: clinical implications

Circulating tumor cells (CTCs) in the blood are increasingly recognized for their usefulness for disease monitoring or for their potential role in influencing therapeutic approaches [49]. Analysis of CTCs to determine the properties of the cells can yield valuable information regarding the disease state. EMT has been clearly linked to the cancer stem cell phenotype and tumor dissemination in pre-clinical models, and its clinical relevance is now being investigated. Measuring EMT transcription factors in CTCs in patients with metastatic breast cancer showed the presence of multiple EMT transcription factors such as Twist1 and Snail1. Patients whose CTCs were enriched with EMT transcription factors had a shorter progression-free and overall survival, compared with patients lacking the EMT transcription factor signature in their CTCs [50].

In breast cancer patients, characterization of EMT status in CTCs shows that primary tumor cells rarely express both epithelial and mesenchymal markers (except for a few EMT-positive cells at the leading edge of the invasive carcinomas such as in breast cancer), but mesenchymal cells were highly enriched in CTCs [51]. Serial monitoring of patients has found a link between mesenchymal CTCs and disease progression. Interestingly, mesenchymal cells tend to be present in multi-cellular clusters, many of which carry attached platelets. Earlier work showed that CTCs, when attached to the platelets (which are known to be TGF-β rich), can undergo EMT [52]. Thus, the TGF-β signature observed in the mesenchymal CTC clusters strongly suggests that platelet-enriched TGF-β promotes EMT in the circulating carcinoma cells.

Similarly, EMT-related gene signatures in metastatic prostate cancer have also been revealed by single cell analysis of CTCs. Although expression patterns are heterogeneous for individual CTCs, genes that promote EMT, including IGF1, IGF2, EGFR, FoxP3, and TGF-β3 are expressed in these cells, while another subset of EMT-related genes (PTPRN2, ALDH1, ESR2, and WNT5A) are expressed more frequently in CTCs of castration-resistant prostate cancer [53]. Thus, evidence is emerging that EMT in carcinomas can occur *in situ*, mostly at the leading/invasive edge of tumors, where the tumor cells are in close proximity to stromal cells, but also in CTCs when they are attached to platelets. The presence of EMT in CTCs, and their correlation with therapeutic response, suggest that CTCs can be used as a surrogate biomarker for monitoring therapeutic responses.

EMT and chemoresistance

EMT has been linked to chemoresistance in many cancer types. EMT association with the resistant phenotype has been reported for classical chemotherapeutic agents such as taxol, platinum-containing drugs, and vinca alkaloids, as well as targeted therapies such as EGFR or HER-2 inhibitors [54]. Although multiple resistance mechanisms appear to be involved in resistance to trastuzumab, a HER-2 targeting antibody, evidence indicates that EMT (which leads to a basal phenotype) is one mechanism by which HER-2+ luminal breast cancer cells escape from trastuzumab treatment [55].

An emerging concept to explain the genotoxic therapy-induced resistance was shown to be mediated through cell non-autonomous effects elicited by the tumor microenvironment [56]. Treatment-associated DNA damage responses in benign cells comprising the tumor microenvironment promote therapy resistance and subsequent tumor progression in prostate cancer patients. A recent study provided *in vivo* evidence of chemotherapy-induced alterations in prostate cancer tumor stroma that include the expression of a diverse spectrum of secreted cytokines and growth factors. Among these, *WNT16B* is activated in fibroblasts through NF-κB, and promotes an epithelial-to-mesenchymal transition (EMT) in neoplastic prostate epithelium through paracrine signaling. Furthermore, WNT16B, acting in a cell nonautonomous manner, promotes the survival of cancer cells after cytotoxic therapy. Given that treatment can induce changes in the tumor microenvironment that affect cancer cells, approaches that target constituents of the tumor microenvironment, in conjunction with conventional cancer therapeutics, may enhance treatment responses [56].

Cancer therapeutics can also have an effect on inhibition of EMT. Sorafenib, a VEGF inhibitor with activity against RAF kinase, is active against hepatocellular carcinoma or HCC, and this drug was found to inhibit HGF-induced EMT via inhibition of MAPK signaling and SNAI1 expression in HCC. These results may provide insights into the anti-EMT effects of tyrosine kinase inhibitors [57].

Inhibition of EMT

Given the contribution of EMT to tumor progression, metastasis, and chemoresistance, targeting EMT could be an important therapeutic approach for cancer patients. Some natural EMT inhibitors exist and their mechanisms of action have recently become better understood. For example, curcumin, a phenolic compound extracted from *Zingiberaceae turmeric*, has been known to have anti-inflammatory and anti-tumor properties. Recent studies indicate that curcumin can inhibit TGF-β-induced EMT in pancreatic cells, and this response is associated with decreased proliferation, increased apoptosis, decreased mesenchymal markers, and increased expression of E-cadherin. Curcumin also affects invasion and migration of TGF-β-treated pancreatic cancer cells [58].

Another natural inhibitor of EMT, pterostilbene, a component of blueberries, has also been proposed to have anti-tumor properties. The effects of pterostilbene treatment on breast cancer cells caused cells to overcome M2 TAM-induced enrichment of CD44$^+$/CD24$^-$ CSCs. Pterostilbene modulates EMT pathways, suppressing NF-βB, Twist1, and vimentin and increasing levels of E-cadherin [59].

Cinnamomi cortex extract, one of ten herbal components of Juzentaihoto (a Japanese traditional medicine) also inhibits TGF-β-induced EMT. The active component in *Cinnamomi cortex* that inhibits EMT, identified as procyanidin C1, could potentially be useful in the development of inhibitors of metastasis [60].

Caffeic acid phenethyl ester (CAPE), a bee propolis component with known anti-oxidant properties [61,62], inhibits EMT of human pancreatic cells [63]. CAPE treatment suppresses tumor growth and, interestingly, attenuates expression of vimentin and Twist 2, but does not reduce Smad 2/3, Snail1, and Zeb expression levels [63].

Downregulation of CMTM8, a chemokine-like MARVEL transmembrane domain-containing protein with tumor suppressor-like activities, induces EMT phenotypes via interfering with c-MET/ERK signaling in some tumor types cell types. Being a novel EMT regulator, CMTM8 may be useful as a therapeutic target for cancer with hyperactivated c-MET/ERK signaling [64].

It has recently been shown that a subset of SCLC patients have activation of the Met receptor by HGF, resulting in EMT and chemoresistance, and treatment with the Met inhibitor Crizotinib sensitizes cells to standard SCLC chemotherapy (etoposide) [65].

Given the potential therapeutic benefits of EMT inhibitors, there is a need to identify additional EMT-blocking drugs. Recently, global gene expression data, generated from cell lines treated with various drugs to identify compounds with negative correlations to EMT gene profiles, identified rapamycin as a novel inhibitor of TGF-β signaling-blocking EMT and the associated migratory/invasive phenotype [66]. A novel EMT inhibitor-screening assay, where cell growth and migration were evaluated simultaneously via time course imaging, found that targeting ALK5, MEK, and SRC block tumor growth factor-induced EMT, providing a foundation for improving the therapeutic value of recently developed compounds to target advanced stage carcinoma [67].

Summary

The transition of epithelial carcinoma cells to mesenchymal phenotype confers migratory, invasive, and stem-like properties. A more complete understanding of EMT in tumor progression and chemoresistance may provide novel therapeutic strategies. A variety of growth factors and inflammatory molecules secreted by cancer cells or the tumor microenvironment (including fibroblasts, immune cells and endothelial cells) can induce EMT, and continue to have an impact during response to treatment. Now that technologies are available to analyze epithelial and mesenchymal markers in CTCs, EMT status may serve as a surrogate marker to monitor therapeutic response. In addition to standard chemotherapy, the identification of patients who might benefit from EMT inhibition may also be possible.

Acknowledgements

The authors gratefully acknowledge Dr. Dinah Singer of NCI for her many helpful suggestions and review of this chapter.

References

1. Zheng H, Kang Y (2013). Multilayer control of the EMT master regulators. *Oncogene* **33**(14), 1755–63. doi: 10.1038/onc.2013.128.
2. Trelstad RL, Hay ED, Revel JD (1967). Cell contact during early morphogenesis in the chick embryo. *Developmental Biology* **16**, 78–107.
3. Lim J, Thiery JP (2012). Epithelial-mesenchymal transitions: insights from development. *Development* **139**, 3471–86.
4. Nieto MA (2013). Epithelial plasticity: a common theme in embryonic and cancer cells. *Science* **342**(6159), 1234850. doi: 10.1126/science.1234850.
5. Kalluri R, Weinberg RA (2009). The basics of epithelial-mesenchymal transition. *Journal of Clinical Investigation* **119**, 1420–8.
6. Zeisberg M, Neilson EG (2009). Biomarkers for epithelial-mesenchymal transition. *Journal of Clinical Investigation* **119**, 1429–37.
7. Savagner P, Yamada KM, Thiery JP (1997). The zinc-finger protein slug causes desmosome dissociation, an initial and necessary step for growth factor-induced epithelial-mesenchymal transition. *Journal of Cell Biology* **137**(6), 1403–19.
8. Yang J, Weinberg RA (2008). Epithelial-mesenchymal transition: at the crossroads of development and tumor metastasis. *Developmental Cell* **14**, 818–29.
9. Mani SA, Guo W, Liao MJ, *et al.* (2008). The epithelial-mesenchymal transition generated cells with properties of stem cells. *Cell* **133**, 704–15.
10. Rhim AD, Mirek ET, Aiello NM, *et al.* (2012). EMT and dissemination precede pancreatic tumor formation. *Cell* **148**, 349–61.
11. Anwar TE, Kleer CG (2013). Tissue-based identification of stem cells and epithelial-to-mesenchymal transition in breast cancer. *Human Pathology* **44**, 1457–64.
12. Trimboli AJ, Fukino K, de Bruin A, *et al.* (2008). Direct evidence for epithelial-mesenchymal transitions in breast cancer. *Cancer Research* **68**, 937–45.
13. Thiery JP (2002). Epithelial-mesenchymal transitions in tumor progression. *Nature Reviews Cancer* **2**, 442–54.
14. Nistico P, Bissell MJ, Radisky DC (2012). Epithelial-mesenchymal transition: General principles and pathological relevance with special emphasis on the role of matrix metalloproteinases. *Cold Spring Harbor Perspectives in Biology* **4**, a011908.
15. Oka H, Shiozaki H, Kobayashi K, *et al.* (1993). Expression of E-cadherin cell adhesion molecules in human breast cancer tissues and its relationship to metastasis. *Cancer Research* **53**, 1696–701.
16. Scheel C, Eaton EN, Li S H-J, *et al.* (2011). Paracrine and autocrine signals induce and maintain mesenchymal and stem cell states in the breast. *Cell* **145**, 926–40.

17. Shibue T, Brooks MW, Weinberg RA (2013). An integrin-linked machinery of cytoskeletal regulation that enables experimental tumor initiation and metastatic colonization. *Cancer Cell* 24, 481–98.

18. Yang MH, Wu MZ, Chiou SH, *et al.* (2008). Direct regulation of TWIST by HIF-α promotes metastasis. *Nature Cell Biology* 10, 295–305.

19. Jo MJ, Lester RD, Montel V, *et al.* (2009). Reversibility of epithelial-mesenchymal transition (EMT) induced in breast cancer cells by activation of urokinase receptor-dependent cell signaling. *Journal of Biological Chemistry* 284, 22825–33.

20. Salnikov AV, Liu L, Platen M, *et al.* (2012). Hypoxia induces EMT in low and highly aggressive pancreatic tumor cells but only cells with cancer stem cell characteristics acquire pronounced migratory potential. *PLoS One* 7, e4639. doi: 10.1371.

21. Li J, Yang B, Zhou Q, *et al.* (2013). Autophagy promotes hepatocellular carcinoma cell invasion through activation of epithelial-mesenchymal transition. *Carcinogenesis* 34, 1343–51. doi: 10.1093/carcin/bgt063.

22. Lamouille S, Subramanyam D, Blelloch R, *et al.* (2013). Regulation of epithelial-mesenchymal and mesenchymal-epithelial transitions by microRNAs. *Current Opinion in Cell Biology* 25, 200–7.

23. Morrison CD, Parvani JG, Schiemann WP (2013). The relevance of the TGF-β paradox to EMT-MET programs. *Cancer Letters* 341(1), 30–40. doi: 10.1016/j.canlet.2013.02.048.

24. Wynn T, Chawla A, Pollard JW (2013). Macrophage biology in development, homeostasis and disease. *Nature* 496, 445–55.

25. Quatromoni JG, Eruslanov E (2012). Tumor-associated macrophages: function, phenotype, and link to prognosis in human lung cancer. *American Journal of Translational Research* 4, 376–89.

26. Gautier EL, Shay T, Miller J, *et al.* (2012). Gene expression profiles and transcriptional regulatory pathways that underlie the identity and diversity of mouse tissue macrophages *Nature Immunology* 13, 1118–28.

27. Qian BZ, Pollard JW (2010). Macrophage diversity enhances tumor progression and metastasis *Cell* 141, 39–51.

28. Manthey CL, Johnson DL, Illig CR, *et al.* (2009). JNJ-28312141, a novel orally active colony-stimulating factor-1 receptor/FMS-related receptor tyrosine kinase-3 receptor tyrosine kinase inhibitor with potential utility in solid tumors, bone metastases, and acute myeloid leukemia. *Molecular Cancer Therapeutics* 8, 3151–61.

29. Patel S, Player MR (2009). Colony-stimulating factor-1 receptor inhibitors for the treatment of cancer and inflammatory disease. *Current Topics in Medicinal Chemistry* 9, 599–10.

30. Pyonteck SM, Akkari L, Schuhmacher AL, *et al.* (2013). CSF-1R inhibition alters macrophage polarization and blocks glioma progression. *Nature Medicine* 19, 1264–72.

31. Reiman JM, Knutson KL, Radisky DC (2010). Immune promotion of epithelial-mesenchymal transition and generation of breast cancer stem cells. *Cancer Research* 70, 3005–8.

32. Schreiber RD, Old LJ, Smyth MJ (2011). Cancer immunoediting: Integrating immunity's roles in cancer suppression and promotion. *Science* 331, 1565–70.

33. Große-Steffen T, Giese T, Giese N, *et al.* (2012). Epithelial-to-mesenchymal transition in pancreatic ductal adenocarcinoma and pancreatic tumor cell lines: The role of neutrophils and neutrophil-derived elastase. *Clinical and Developmental Immunology* 2012, article ID 720768, 12 pages. doi: 10.1155/2012/720768.

34. Kojima Y, Acar A, Eaton EN, *et al.* (2010). Autocrine TGF-β and stromal cell-derived factor-1 (SDF-1) signaling drives the evolution of tumor promoting mammary stromal myofibroblasts. *PNAS* 107, 20009–14.

35. Biddle A, Mackenzie IC (2012). Cancer stem cells and EMT in carcinoma. *Cancer and Metastasis Reviews* 31, 285–93.

36. Sigurdsson V, Hilmarsdottir B, Sigmundsdottir H, *et al.* (2011). Endothelial induced EMT in breast epithelial cells with stem cell properties. *PLoS One* 6(9), e23833. doi: 10.1371/journal.pone.00238333.

37. De Craene B, Berx G (2013). Regulatory networks defining EMT during cancer initiation and progression. *Nature Reviews Cancer* 13, 97–110. doi: 10.1038/nrc3447.

38. Moody SE, Perez D, Pan TC, *et al.* (2005). The transcriptional repressor Snail promotes mammary tumor recurrence. *Cancer Cell* 8, 197–209.

39. Ahn YH, Gibbons DL, Chakravarti D, *et al.* (2012). ZEB1 drives prometastatic actin cytoskeletal remodeling by downregulating miR-34a expression. *Journal of Clinical Investigation* 122, 3170–83. doi: 10.1172/JCI63608.

40. Chaffer CL, Marjanovic ND, Lee T, *et al.* (2013). Poised chromatin at the ZEB1 Promoter enables breast cancer cell plasticity and enhances tumorigenicity. *Cell* 154, 61–74.

41. Heldin CH, Vanlandewijck M, Moustakas A (2012). Regulation of EMT by TGFβ in cancer. *FEBS Letters* 586, 1959–70.

42. Tian XJ, Zhang H, Xing J (2013). Coupled reversible and irreversible bistable switches underlying TGFβ-induced epithelial to mesenchymal transition. *Biophysical Journal* 105, 1079–89.

43. Gunasinghe NP, Wells A, Thompson EW, *et al.* (2012). Mesenchymal-epithelial transition (MET) as a mechanism for metastatic colonisation in breast cancer. *Cancer and Metastasis Reviews* 31, 469–78.

44. Yao, D, Dai C, Peng S (2011). Mechanism of the mesenchymal–epithelial transition and its relationship with metastatic tumor formation. *Molecular Cancer Research* **9**, 1608–20.

45. Chaffer CL, Brennan JP, Blick T, *et al.* (2006). Mesenchymal-to-epithelial transition facilitates bladder cancer metastasis: Role of fibroblast growth factor receptor-2. *Cancer Research* **66**, 11271–8.

46. Lupu-Meiri M, Geras-Raaka E, Lupu R, *et al.* (2012). Knock-down of plasminogen-activator inhibitor-1 enhances expression of E-cadherin and promotes epithelial differentiation of human pancreatic adeno-carcinoma cells. *Journal of Cellular Physiology* **227**, 3621–8.

47. Roca H, Hernandez J, Weidner S, *et al.* (2013). Transcription factors OVOL1 and OVOL2 induce the mesenchymal to epithelial transition in human cancer. *PLoS One* **8**(10), e76773. doi: 10.1371/journal.pone.0076773.

48. Yew K-H, Crow J, Hirst J, *et al.* (2013). Epimorphin-induced MET sensitizes ovarian cancer cells to platinum. *PLoS One* **8**(9), e72637. doi: 10.1371/journal.pone.0072637.

49. Kang Y, Pantel K (2013). Tumor cell dissemination: Emerging biological insights from animal models and cancer patients. *Cancer Cell* **23**, 573–80.

50. Mego M, Gao H, Lee BN, *et al.* (2012). Prognostic value of EMT-circulating tumor cells in metastatic breast cancer patients undergoing high-dose chemotherapy with autologous hematopoietic stem cell transplantation. *Journal of Cancer* **3**, 369–80. doi: 10.7150/jca.5111.

51. Yu M, Bardia A, Wittner BS, *et al.* (2013). Circulating breast tumor cells exhibit dynamic changes in epithelial and mesenchymal composition. *Science* **339**, 580–4.

52. Labelle M, Begum S, Hynes RO (2011). Direct signaling between platelets and cancer cells induces an epithelial-mesenchymal-like transition and promotes metastasis. *Cancer Cell* **20**, 576–90.

53. Chen C-L, Mahalingam D, Osmulski P, *et al.* (2013). Single-cell analysis of circulating tumor cells identifies cumulative expression patterns of EMT-related genes in metastatic prostate cancer. *The Prostate* **73**, 813–26.

54. Foroni C, Broggini M, Generali D, *et al.* (2012). Epithlial-mesenchymal transition and breast cancer: Role, molecular mechanisms and clinical impact. *Cancer Treatment Reviews* **38**, 689–697.

55. Lesniack D, Sabri S, Xu Y, *et al.* (2013). Spontaneous epithelial-mesenchymal transition and resistance to HER-2-targetd therapies in HER-2-positive luminal breast cancer. *PLoS One* **8**, e71987. doi: 10.1371/journal.pone.0071987.

56. Sun Y, Campisi J, Higano C, *et al.* (2012). Treatment-induced damage to the tumor microenvironment promotes prostate cancer therapy resistance through WNT16B. *Nature Medicine* **18**, 1359–68.

57. Nagai T, Arao T, Furuta K, *et al.* (2011). Sorafenib inhibits the hepatocyte growth factor-mediated epithelial mesenchymal transition in hepatocellular carcinoma. *Molecular Cancer Therapeutics* **10**, 169–177.

58. Sun XD, Liu XE, Huang DS (2013). Curcumin reverses the epithelial-mesenchymal transition of pancreatic cancer cells by inhibiting the Hedgehog signaling pathway. *Oncology Reports* **29**, 2401–7. doi: 10.3892/or.2013.2385.

59. Mak KK, Wu AT, Lee WH, *et al.* (2013). Pyerostilbene, a bioactive component of blueberries, suppresses the generation of breast cancer stem cells within tumor microenvironment and metastasis via modulating NF-KB/microRNA 448 circuit. *Molecular Nutrition & Food Research* **57**, 1123–34. doi: 10.1002/mnfr.201200549.

60. Kin R, Kato S, Kaneto N, *et al.* (2013). Procyanidin C1 from Cinnamomi Cortex inhibits TGF-β-induced epithelial-to-mesenchymal transition in the A549 lung cancer cell line. *International Journal of Oncology* **43**, 1901–6. doi: 10.3892/ijo.2013.2139.

61. Russo A, Longo R, Vanella A (2002). Antioxidant activity of propolis: role of caffeic acid phenethyl ester and galangin. *Fitoterapia* **73**, S21–9.

62. Sudina GF, Mirzoeva OK, Pushkareva MA, *et al.* (1993). Caffeic acid phenethyl ester as a lipoxygenase inhibitor with antioxidant properties. *FEBS Letters* **329**, 21–4.

63. Chen MJ, Shih SC, Wang HY (2013). Caffeic Acid phenethyl ester inhibits epithelial-mesenchymal transition of human pancreatic cancer cells. *Evidence-Based Complementary and Alternative Medicine* **2013**, 270906. doi: 10.1155/2013/270906.

64. Zhang W, Mendoza MC, Pei X, *et al.* (2012). Downregulation of CMTM8 induces epithelial-to-mesenchymal transition-like changes via c-MET/extracellular signal-regulated kinase (ERK) signaling. *Journal of Biological Chemistry* **287**, 118450–8.

65. Canadas I, Rojo F, Taus A, *et al.* (2013). Targeting epithelial to mesenchymal transition with Met inhibitors reverts chemoresistance in small cell lung cancer. *Clinical Cancer Research* **20**(4), 938–50.

66. Reka AK, Kuick R, Kurapati H, *et al.* (2011). Identifying inhibitors of epithelial-mesenchymal transition by connectivity map-based systems approach. *Journal of Thoracic Oncology* **6**, 1784–92. doi: 10.1097/JTO.0b013e31822adfb0.

67. Chua KN, Sim WJ, Racine V, *et al.* (2012). A cell-based small molecule screening method for identifying inhibitors of epithelial-mesenchymal transition in carcinoma. *PLoS One* **7**(3), e33183. doi: 10.1371/journal.pone.0033183.

PART II

State-of-the-Science in Organ-Specific Biomarker Research

CHAPTER 7

Breast Cancer

Benjamin A Katchman,[1] Christos Patriotis,[2] and Karen S Anderson[1]

[1]Center for Personalized Diagnostics, Biodesign Institute, Arizona State University, Tempe, AZ, USA
[2]Cancer Biomarkers Research Group, Division of Cancer Prevention, National Cancer Institute, National Institutes of Health, Bethesda, MD, USA

Introduction

Breast cancer is one of the most frequently diagnosed cancers among women, with over 200 000 new cases of invasive breast cancer and over 60 000 cases of *in situ* breast cancer diagnosed each year [1]. Since 1990, there has been a steady decrease in breast cancer deaths attributed to progress in early detection, treatment and reduced disease incidence. The five-year survival rate of locoregional cancers is now over 80%. However, those who present with distant metastases have five-year survival rates of only 23%, and extremely low ten-year survival rates.

Currently, the primary screening tool for early detection is mammography, which has an 80-90% sensitivity, with a low specificity of detection [1]. Blood- and tissue-based biomarkers have the potential to increase the detection of invasive cancers, especially for rapidly proliferative cancers that are not as frequently detected by mammography. These biomarkers may also aid in the detection of cancers arising within dense breast tissue, where mammography is less effective. Mammographic screening is also associated with the overdiagnosis of benign breast disease. The presence of atypia with benign breast disease is associated with a 3–5 fold increased risk of subsequent breast cancer [1]. Identifying the biomarkers associated with the higher risk benign breast disease and *in situ*

carcinomas could significantly improve targeted screening. The rapid development of these molecular markers have the potential to shift the field from population-based screening to risk-stratified targeted screening, which both decreases the consequences of false discovery and improves early breast cancer detection.

Genomic biomarkers of risk

Breast cancer is a heterogeneous disease that exhibits hereditary (5–10% of cases) as well as sporadic (90–95% of cases) tumor development [2, 3]. Familial linkage studies (Table 7.1) have identified high-penetrance genes that are strong predictors of breast cancer over a woman's lifetime (BRCA1, BRCA2, PTEN, and TP53) [4]. The combination of heritable and population-based approaches has identified genes involved in DNA repair (CHEK2, ATM, BRIP, and PALB2) that are associated with moderate risk [5]. In total, these known genes account for 25% of the familial cases [4]. These results suggest that the majority of familial risk in breast cancer is due to the involvement of multiple low-penetrance susceptibility alleles that have a multiplicative effect in determining overall risk.

Genome-wide association studies (GWAS) provide a powerful tool to identify the lower penetrance alleles that cannot be detected by genetic linkage studies. Recent GWAS in breast cancer have

Biomarkers in Cancer Screening and Early Detection, First Edition. Edited by Sudhir Srivastava.
© 2017 John Wiley & Sons, Inc. Published 2017 by John Wiley & Sons, Inc.

Table 7.1 Genome-wide association studies.

High penetrance, low frequency	Low penetrance, low frequency	Low penetrance, high frequency	
BRCA1	CHEK2	FGFR2	SLC4A7
BRCA2	ATM	TNRC9	COX11
p53	PALB2	LSP1	
PTEN	BRIP1	MAP3K1	

revealed single nucleotide polymorphisms (SNPs) in five novel genes (TNRC9, FGFR2, MAP3K1, H19, and lymphocyte-specific protein 1 (LSP1)) associated with increased susceptibility (Table 7.1). Allelic variants associated with breast cancer risk have recently been discovered that are involved in the regulation of the cell cycle, apoptosis, metabolism, and mitochondrial functions [2]. The identification of susceptible loci associated with disease detection and prognosis may lead to an improved understanding of the biological mechanisms contributing to breast cancer.

Breast cancer development

The development of breast tissue biomarkers has been focused on molecular changes that identify at-risk individuals for additional screening. Discovery of these biomarkers have resulted from analysis of the development of normal breast tissue and the breast microenvironment. The breast is composed of a branching system of ducts that begin at the nipple and terminate in the many terminal ductal lobular units (TDLU) [6, 7]. The ductal system consists of two cell layers – a luminal epithelial layer, surrounded by myoepithelial cells. The surrounding microenvironment is composed of extracellular matrix (ECM) and numerous stromal cell types, including fibroblasts, adipocytes, endothelial and immune cells, which function in mammary duct formation.

The normal development of the mammary gland depends on cooperation between these multiple cell types to form a complex network. The cell-cell and cell-microenvironment interactions have dramatic effects on mammary epithelial cells contributing to normal development of branching milk ducts and lactation, as well as neoplastic development and metastatic progression. There are several proposed models of breast cancer initiation, malignant progression and metastasis, such as sporadic clonal evolution [6, 8], the cancer stem cell [9], and the seed and soil model [10]. Overall, there is no inclusive model that describes breast cancer progression, and significant data supports each of these proposed models which incorporate tumor initiation, heterogeneity and the invasive and metastatic progression of breast cancer.

Benign breast disease

Benign breast disease (BBD) accounts for the majority (90%) of referrals to breast clinics, and it comprises a heterogeneous population of proliferative cells, with or without atypia. BBD is associated with an increased risk of subsequent breast cancer, based on degree of proliferation and atypia. Molecularly, a subset of BBD may be non-obligate precursors for *in situ* and invasive disease [11]. Compared to the general population, women with non-proliferative lesions, which account for 70% of biopsies, do not have an elevated risk of breast cancer [12]. Women diagnosed with a proliferative disease without atypia (30%) have a relative risk of 1.3–1.9 of developing breast cancer. BBD with atypia (4%) increases the relative risk to 3.9–13.0 [12, 13].

Ductal carcinoma *in situ* (DCIS)

Pre-invasive breast cancer, confined to the ductal-lobular network, falls into two histological categories – ductal and lobular types [6, 7], which are distinguished by cell morphology. The ductal subtype comprises 80% of all diagnosed pre-invasive and invasive breast cancers [7]. Recent advances in tissue micro-dissection, high-throughput genomic analysis, and proteomic technologies, have provided new insights into the pre-invasive stages of breast cancer progression [6, 7]. Comparative genomic hybridization (CGH) and serial analysis of gene expression (SAGE) have been used to identify loss of 16q in low-grade DCIS, whereas intermediate-grade DCIS had a higher frequency of 1q gain and 11q loss [14]. High-grade DCIS has increasing and complex genomic alterations, loss of 8p, 11q, 13q, and 14q, and gains in 1q, 5p, 8p, and 17q [15]. Together, this data supports a direct relationship between DCIS and invasive ductal carcinoma (IDC).

A.

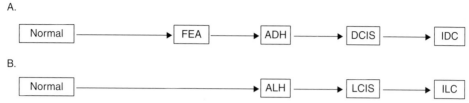

B.

Figure 7.1 Pathological models of breast cancer progression. **A.** The classic model of breast cancer progression of the ductal type proposes that neoplastic evolution initiates in normal epithelium (normal), progresses to flat epithelial atypia (FEA), advances to atypical ductal hyperplasia (ADH), evolves to ductal carcinoma *in situ* (DCIS) and culminates as invasive ductal carcinoma (IDC). Immunohistochemical, genomic and transcriptomic data strongly support the evidence of a continuum from FEA to ADH, DCIS and IDC, indicating FEA as the potential non-obligate precursor of ADH. **B.** The model of lobular neoplasia proposes a multi-step progression, from normal epithelium to atypical lobular hyperplasia, lobular carcinoma *in situ* (LCIS) and invasive lobular carcinoma (ILC). For a more detailed explanation please refer to [6, 7].

The development of the majority of DCIS consists of a well-recognized linear progression from flat epithelial atypia (FEA) to atypical ductal hyperplasia (ADH) to DCIS (Figure 7.1). Flat epithelial atypia (FEA) has been classified as a precursor to ADH and low-grade DCIS. By immunohistochemistry (IHC), FEA is similar in profile to ADH and low-grade DCIS (weak positivity for ER, PR, and CK19; negative for HER2) and, genetically, it overlaps with low-grade DCIS [16].

Pathological, clinical, and epidemiological data support the role of atypical ductal hyperplasia (ADH) as a precursor to low-grade DCIS [6, 7]. DCIS is also characterized by degrees of architectural atypia, and is further sub-classified into low-, intermediate-, and high-grade [6, 7]. There is such strong morphological and molecular overlap between ADH and DCIS that it has led some researchers to question the classification as distinct pathological entities. Patients with DCIS have excellent clinical outcomes with surgical excision and radiation, but have a 3.4–8.6 fold higher risk of developing a second breast cancer [13]. DCIS is further characterized by the loss of the myoepithelial cell layer and basement membrane degradation, by staining with SMA, calponin and CD10 [17].

Lobular carcinoma *in situ* (LCIS)

The lobular subtype represents 10–15% of all diagnosed breast cancers, [1, 6, 7, 18] (Figure 7.1). LCIS is molecularly characterized by weak Ki-67, negative p53, low erb-B2, and loss of E-cadherin. CGH-based studies have identified recurrent loss of 16q in classic ILC, ALH and LCIS, supporting an evolutionary link between these lesions and a common pathway of progression. The pleomorphic variant of LCIS (PLCIS) is associated with higher proliferation rates, p53 overexpression and occasional ER and PR negativity. At this time, little is known about biomarkers associated with the risk of subsequent invasive cancer after a diagnosis of LCIS (reviewed in [6, 7]).

Blood-based biomarkers for early detection

Current clinical practice

Significant advances in breast cancer treatment have been made over the past two decades. The identification of somatic mutations, copy number variants, and pathway alterations have led to rapid translational clinical trials of targeted therapeutics, especially for higher-grade cancers with increased recurrence rates. In contrast, few significant advances have resulted in clinical impact on early breast cancer detection. Current screening is still based on mammography, with concurrent MRI reserved for patients at high risk of breast cancer development, such as BRCA1 and BRCA2 mutation carriers [19]. There are no blood-based biomarkers in clinical use for the early detection or monitoring of early-stage breast cancer. Existing biomarkers, such as CEA, CA27.29, and CA15-3, are used routinely for monitoring patients with metastatic disease, but have insufficient sensitivity for detection of early breast cancer [20].

Molecular profiling of serum or plasma has been used to discover many potential biomarkers for early detection, monitoring disease response to treatment, prognosis, and detection of recurrent disease of breast cancers. These biomarkers include protein markers, autoantibodies, glycans, circulating tumor cells (CTCs), exosomes, cell-free DNA, and microRNA (miR) (Table 7.2). The majority of these studies are small, pilot studies using single-institution retrospective biorepositories, which remain to be rigorously evaluated using blinded, multi-institutional sample

Table 7.2 Circulating Tumor Markers.

Circulating biomarkers			
Protein biomarkers			
Name of biomarker	Material		Reference
RS/DJ-1	Autoantibody/protein		[75]
p53	Autoantibody/protein		[76]
HSP60	Autoantibody/protein		[77]
HSP90	Autoantibody/protein		[78]
Mucin-related proteins (MUC1)	Autoantibody/protein		[79]
28 Antigen panel	Autoantibody/protein		[29]
7 Antigen panel	Autoantibody/protein		[30]
29 Antigen panel	Autoantibody/protein		[25]
CA15-3	Protein		[80]
HER-2/neu	Protein		[81]
miRNA as diagnostic/prognostic biomarkers			
Name of biomarker	Potential role		Reference
miR-195	Increased in breast cancer patients.		[45]
let-7a, miR-10b, and miR-21	Distinguish nodal and ER status.		[45]
miR-10b, miR-34a, miR-141, and miR-155	Distinguish healthy controls from primary and metastatic breast cancer.		[46]
miR-202	Identify patients with early stage breast cancer.		[82]
miR-148b, miR-376c, miR-409-3p, and miR-801	Identify patients with early stage breast cancer.		[47]
miR-125b	Predict chemoresistance of breast cancer.		[83]
miR-221	Predict sensitivity to neoadjuvent therapy.		[84]
miR-425, let-7d, let-7c, and miR-589	Identify early stage breast cancer from healthy controls.		[48]
Circulating tumor cell detection techniques			
Assay system	Enrichment	Detection	Reference
CellSearch system	Immunomagnetic beads: EpCAM.	ICC (Immunocytochemistry): Pos. CK-8, -18, -19. Neg. CD45.	[85]
MACS technology/dynal magnetic beads	CD45+ cell depletion.	ICC: Pan-CK positive	[86]
EPISPOT assay	Ficoll density gradient: CD45+ cell depletion.	Viable epithelial cells secreting: CK-19, MUC1, and cathepsin D.	[87]
AdnaTest	Immunomagnetic beads: MUC1 and EpCAM.	RT-PCR: positive for at least one marker (MUC1, HER2, or EpCAM mRNA)	[88]
Screen cell	Micropore filtration	ICC: epithelial markers (CK and EpCAM) or mesenchymal markers	[89]
ISET	8 μm pore filters	ICC: epithelial markers (CK and EpCAM) or mesenchymal markers	[90]

Table 7.2 *(Continued)*

Molecular characterization of CTCs in breast cancer		
Expressed markers in CTCs	*Analytical method*	*Reference*
CK-19, hMAM (human MAM), HER2	Multimarker RT-PCR	[91]
CK-19, HER2, MAGE-A3, hMAM, TWIST-1	Liquid bead array	[92]
CK-19	qRT-PCR	[93]
ER/PR	RT-PCR	[88]

Cell-free DNA as diagnostic and prognostic biomarkers			
Expressed markers in cfDNA	*Analytical method*	*Findings*	*Reference*
HER2 amplification	quantitative (q) PCR	Demonstrated the amplified HER2 in cfDNA of breast cancer patients who are disease free.	[94]
Copy number variation (CNV) and loss of heterozygosity (LOH)	Genome-wide SNP 6.0 arrays	Using SNP/CNV analysis of cfDNA to distinguish breast cancer and healthy controls during follow-up. Results indicate cancer dormancy.	[42]
APC and GSTP1 methylation	Methylation-specific qPCR	Methylated APC and GSTP1 associate with CTC and more aggressive tumors.	[95]
APC, RASSF1A and DAP-kinase promoter hypermethylation	Methylation-specific PCR	Serum DNA contained hypermethylation in pre-invasive and early-stage breast cancer.	[96]
ESR1 and 14-3-3-σ methylation	Methylation-specific qPCR	Potential use as biomarkers.	[97]
β-globin quantification; GSTP1 promoter hypermethylation; RASSF1A and ATM methylation	qPCR; methylation-specific qPCR	cfDNA is able to distinguish cancer patients from disease-free individuals.	[98]
BRCA1 hypermethylation	Methylation-specific qPCR	BRCA1 methylation correlates with response to neoadjuvent therapy.	[99]
LOH and microsatellite instability (MSI)	PCR	Chromosomes 10, 16, and 17 contains frequent genomic aberrations in cfDNA.	[100]
LOH and MSI	PCR	LOH and MSI identified in plasma DNA and reflected in the primary tumor.	[101]
LOH and TP53 mutation	PCR	cfDNA in plasma has potential as a prognostic marker of disease-free survival.	[102]

collections. The recent development of clinical pipelines for large-scale phase II and phase III clinical validation studies should facilitate moving these biomarkers forward into clinical practice.

Protein biomarkers

Advances in mass spectrometry and proteomic technologies have led to a resurgence of interest in serum- or plasma-based protein biomarkers for the early detection of breast cancer (reviewed in [21,22]). The use of liquid chromatography coupled with mass spectrometry (LC-MS/MS) to directly analyze the proteins or peptides contained in serum or plasma offers numerous advantages over the traditional enzyme-linked immunosorbent assay (ELISA). Unlike ELISA, MS can be used for unbiased discovery of differential protein/peptide content in case and control plasma.

Multiple reaction monitoring (MRM), combined with stable isotope standards and capture by antipeptide antibodies (SISCAPA), have been developed to enrich low-abundance peptides from complex mixtures such as trypsin-digested serum or plasma. This enhances identification of underrepresented peptides [23]. MS is also used to detect post-translational modifications, such as glycosylation patterns, that could be early indicators of disease progression [21].

Custom ELISA microarrays were used to evaluate 23 selected candidate biomarkers in plasma samples from newly diagnosed women and compared with benign controls [24]. Of these, ten analytes were significantly elevated in at least one of four breast cancer subtypes, including RANTES, which was consistently elevated in all four subtypes. Two distinct biomarker panels were identified based on tumor subtype ER+/HER2- (PDGF, RANTES, and VEGF; AUC = 0.82) and for ER+/HER2+ (RANTES, PDGF, VEGF, and TNFα; AUC = 0.88). A pilot study to identify biomarkers of triple negative breast cancer (TNBC) detected 29 novel antigens (TNBC) [25] from an array of more than 1,000 antibodies.

The challenge of tumor heterogeneity

The biologic heterogeneity of breast cancer impacts the research design of biomarker discovery. Early biomarker discovery studies used unselected samples from many breast cancer subtypes, resulting in under-representation of hormone receptor negative cancers. Since protein expression varies between cancer subtypes, it is expected that the composition of shed proteins from cancer cells into the bloodstream will be highly subtype-specific, while biomarkers of the inflammatory or

stromal response may be less dependent on tumor subtype. Mathematical modeling results in different recommended strategies for biomarker discovery in the setting of homogeneous vs. heterogeneous disease [26]. As a result, most investigators now focus discovery on defined tumor subtypes.

Autoantibodies

Autoantibodies (AAb) are another potential type of blood-based biomarkers that are elicited against aberrantly expressed native proteins, as well as mutated proteins. These AAb include p53, heat shock protein 60 (HSP60), HSP90, NY-ESO-1, and mucin related antigens [27–29]. Improvements in protein microarray, reversed-phase protein display, and phage display technology have resulted in the identification of panels of AAb as potential biomarkers for breast cancer (reviewed in [27,28]). In contrast to protein antigens, AAb are highly stable proteins that may amplify *in vivo* protein signals.

As with protein biomarkers, individual AAb generally have low clinical sensitivity (< 20% of patients), but panels of AAb have been identified that improve the clinical sensitivity of the detection of breast cancer. Custom protein microarrays have been used to screen 5000 candidate tumor antigens with sera from patients with early stage breast cancer [29]. A 28-AAb classifier was identified with a sensitivity of 80.8% and a specificity of 61.6% (AUC = 0.756). Similarly, a panel of seven autoantigens (p53, c-myc, NY-ESO-1, BRCA1, BRCA2, HER2, and MUC1) had a sensitivity of 64% at a specificity of 85% for breast cancer detection [30]. AAb against p53, c-myc, and MUC1 have been detected up to 27 months before cancer was diagnosed by mammography. Both protein and AAb biomarkers remain to be validated in blinded, controlled studies.

Glycosylation

Altered protein glycosylation is a common feature of tumor cells, including N-glycans, O-glycans, glycoproteins, glycolipids, and glycosaminoglycans [31]. The most widely used serum markers for monitoring metastatic breast cancer, CA15-3 and CA27.29, detect the soluble forms of the mucin MUC1, which is heavily glycosylated [31].

The alteration of glycoproteins is a critical event in early cancer development and progression, although the functional consequences of these alterations are not yet well understood [31]. N-glycome analysis of whole serum has revealed alterations in sialylation (sLe^x) and fucosylation that correlates with metastatic breast cancer [32, 33]. Glycans containing alteration of sLe^x epitopes have been detected in circulating tumor cells [32]. Lectin affinity-based glycan enrichment, followed by nanospray ionization mass spectrometry (NSI-MS/MS), has been used to identify L-PHA-enriched glycoproteins in breast tumor tissue [34], and 30 proteins with elevated branched glycosylation were detected, including periostin. Glycosylphosphatidylinositol (GPI)-anchored proteins include many known tumor antigens, such as CEA, mesothelin, prostate-specific stem cell antigen, and urokinase plasminogen activator receptor [35, 36]. Of the GPI-anchored proteins, FERMT3 and FLNA have been specifically detected in plasma of breast cancer patients.

Exosomes

Exosomes are 40–100 nm vesicles secreted by a wide range of mammalian cell types [37]. They consist of a lipid bilayer membrane surrounding a small cytosol, and are devoid of cellular organelles, but they contain various molecular components of their cell of origin, including proteins and nucleic acids (DNA, mRNA, miRNA). Most exosomes contain an evolutionary-conserved common set of proteins (reviewed in [37, 38]). Exosome proteomes of different cell origins include a common set of membrane and cytosolic proteins, and specific subsets of proteins, likely correlated to cell-type associated functions.

The prevalence and clinical relevance of tumor exosomes in blood and urine from breast cancer patients are beginning to be evaluated [39]. Tumor exosomes may function to manipulate the metastatic cascade through angiogenesis, stromal remodeling, signal transduction interference by growth factor/receptor transfer, chemoresistance, and genetic intercellular exchange through the expression and transfer of a number of proteins (TGFB, MMP-14, MMP-1, Hsp90a, and HER ligands) [39]. Both the presence, and the specific content, of tumor exosomes may provide useful biomarkers for cancer detection.

Circulating tumor cells (CTC)

CTCs are cancer cells that disseminate to secondary sites via the peripheral blood, and are associated with decreased progression-free survival [22]. CTCs originate from primary tumors and from metastatic lesions, and may acquire features of invasiveness and migration. The accurate identification and further molecular profiling of CTCs remains a tremendous technical challenge [40], as they occur at a very low yield, present in blood at one per million hematological cells. Therefore, there is a need to enrich CTCs, based on physical and/or biological properties that discriminate CTCs from normal hematopoietic cells present in the blood.

Antibodies targeting epithelial cell adhesion molecule (EpCAM), or tumor associated antigens such as cytokeratin (CK)19, CK18, mucin-1 (MUC1), carcinoembryonic antigen (CEA) and mammaglobin have been used to detect CTCs [40], and PCR is used to amplify the nucleic acids in CTCs (and exosomes). CellSearch^{TM} (Veridex LLC, NJ, USA) is the first automated, standardized and FDA approved system to detect and quantify CTCs in the peripheral blood of metastatic breast cancer patients. The system performs automated immunomagnetic EpCAM-based enrichment of CTCs, followed by IHC of cytokeratins. The epithelial cells are differentiated from leukocytes using fluorescently labeled antileukocytes (CD45) and antiepithelial (CK8, -18, and -19) specific monoclonal antibodies. Proteins isolated from CTCs include HER2/neu, EGFR, PI3Kα/Akt and topoisomerase 2 (TOP2A) [40]. At this time, the primary use of CTCs is the identification of molecular alterations that correlate with alterations in tumor sites (primary and metastatic), providing a potential alternative to tissue biopsy.

Cell-free DNA

Apoptotic and necrotic cells of the primary tumor can release DNA into the bloodstream, which can be measured as cell-free DNA (cfDNA). cfDNA can also be detected in exosomes, or in combination with CTCs. The concentration of circulating cfDNA is higher in cancer patients, compared with healthy individuals [22, 41]. Since cfDNA circulates in the form of nucleosomes, both genetic and epigenetic alterations can be measured, including DNA methylation patterns and changes in chromatin histone proteins [41].

cfDNA are potential biomarkers for the metastatic spread of solid tumors [42]. However, there are no established standards, normalization procedures, DNA concentration or reference standards available for assay standardization [22]. Targeted mutation analyses in the peripheral blood have been limited by the rare content of mutated cfDNA within wild-type sequences from hematopoietic cells. Still, the direct correlation of cfDNA with tumor genomic alterations makes these attractive candidate biomarkers for detection.

microRNA

MicroRNAs (miRNA or miR) are a class of evolutionary conserved non-coding RNA molecules, 17–25 nt in length, which function as negative regulators of gene expression by directing specific mRNA cleavage or translational inhibition [43, 44]. miRNAs are more stable than mRNA in the peripheral blood, as well as in formalin-fixed tissue [43]. Tissue miRNA profiles have been used to classify human cancers [22].

Circulating miRNA, either free miRNA or CTC/exosome-associated miRNAs, are potential biomarkers for breast cancer detection. Elevated miR-195 levels have been detected in breast cancer patient plasma (sensitivity of 88% at a specificity of 91% [45]), and miRNA signatures have been detected in serum [46–48]. Overall, these are highly promising and stable biomarkers with emerging biologic relevance. However, isolation and quantitation of miRNAs by quantitative reverse-transcriptase PCR remains a technical challenge, including the lack of standardized endogenous controls and sample preparation procedures, as well as robust clinical-grade assays.

Prognostic tissue biomarkers of BBD and DCIS

Improvements in mammographic and clinical screening of breast cancer have led to a marked increase in the diagnosis of BBD and DCIS. A critical unmet need in breast cancer management today is the discovery of tissue biomarkers that

will identify patients who present with atypia or DCIS/LCIS, and who are at high risk of developing IBC. In a retrospective study, Hartmann and colleagues identified all women ($n = 9,087$) who received a diagnosis of benign breast disease at the Mayo Clinic between 1967 and 1991 with a median follow-up of 15 years [13]. Of the women in this cohort, 67% had non-proliferative lesions, 30% had proliferative lesions without atypia, and 4% had atypical ductal hyperplasia. A total of 707 women subsequently developed invasive breast cancer, with an overall risk of 1.56; the relative risk of progression from non-proliferative disease was 1.27, from proliferative disease (without atypia) 1.88, and from atypical ductal hyperplasia 4.24. The most important risk factor associated with risk of invasive disease was family history.

Over the past two decades, molecular biomarkers have been identified in breast tissues of non-invasive lesions that predict the subsequent diagnosis of invasive cancer. In the case of DCIS, such studies have confirmed the existence of distinct molecular subtypes although, at present, it is not clear whether these parallel the distinct molecular subtypes present in invasive cancer [49]. Similar studies have also led to the identification of mRNAs, miRNAs, proteins and differentially methylated gene promoter sequences, which may be useful as markers for the assessment of risk of progression from BBD or DCIS/LCIS to IBC (Figure 7.2).

Poola and colleagues have shown that the elevated protein expression of MMP1, HYAL-1 and CEACAM-6 in benign hyperplastic lesions of the breast can predict, with high sensitivity (0.80–0.98) and specificity (0.76–0.89), the subsequent development of IBC [50]. Similarly, Gauthier and colleagues reported a number of tissue markers, including p16, Ki-67, and COX-2, whose combined elevated expression is associated with high risk for subsequent tumor events in women diagnosed with DCIS. This set of markers together also define a basal-like subset of IBC and, hence, their combined elevated expression could be utilized as a prognostic marker to stratify women diagnosed with DCIS that are more likely to benefit from more aggressive therapy [51] (Table 7.3).

More recently, Genomic Health announced the development of Oncotype DX® Breast Cancer Test

Figure 7.2 Candidate risk biomarkers for progression from benign breast disease/ductal carcinoma *in situ* to invasive breast carcinoma. Red indicates proteomic and genomic markers of benign breast disease; blue indicates proteomic and genomic markers of ductal carcinoma in situ. This figure is courtesy of Andrew K. Godwin. For a color version of this figure please see color plate section.

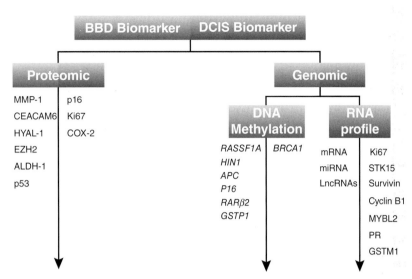

for DCIS (DCIS Score™ Gene Selection). This test is based on the elevated tissue expression of genes associated with cell proliferation, including Ki-67, STK15, Survivin, Cyclin B1 and MYBL2, as well as the expression of hormone receptor group genes, including PR and GSTM1 [20] (Table 7.4).

Prognostic biomarkers of invasive carcinoma

For decades, the clinical subtypes of breast cancer have been defined by IHC of estrogen receptor (ER), progesterone receptor (PR) and HER2/neu (ERBB2), which are routinely used in clinical laboratories to classify tumors and determine treatment options [18, 52]. The hormone-receptor positive subtype (80%, ER$^+$/PR$^+$), has the most favorable prognosis and response to targeted endocrine therapy [18, 53]. Fewer than 1% of breast cancers are PR$^+$/ER$^-$, as the expression of PR is strongly dependent on ER expression. The hormone-receptor negative subtype (ER$^-$/PR$^-$) are typically higher grade lesions, and have higher recurrence and mortality rates [53]. The HER2/neu$^+$ subset (15%) have an increased response to HER2-targeted therapies [18, 53].

Table 7.3 Tissue-based biomarkers.

Tissue-based biomarkers			
miRNA as diagnostic biomarkers			
Name of biomarker	*Technology used for discovery*	*Material*	*References*
miR-10b, miR-34a, and miR155	Tissue – qRT-PCR	RNA	[46]
29 miRNA signature	Tissue – qRT-PCR	RNA	[66]
9 miRNA signature	Tissue – qRT-PCR	RNA	[67]
miRNA as prognostic biomarkers			
Name of biomarker	*Technology used for discovery*	*Material*	*References*
miR-195 and let-7a	Tissue – qRT-PCR	RNA	[45], [66]
miR-335 and miR-126	Tissue – qRT-PCR	RNA	[68]
miR-10b, miR-34a, and miR155	Tissue – qRT-PCR	RNA	[46], [103], [104]
Protein as prognostic markers			
Name of biomarker		*Material*	*Reference*
MMP-1, HYAL-1, and CEACAM-6		Tissue	
p16, Ki-67, and COX-2		Tissue	[551]

Table 7.4 Multigene parameters in breast cancer.

Gene signatures	Number of genes assessed	Application	Reference
MammaPrint	70	Prognostic for recurrence within 5 years in all ER+ and node-positive patients.	Agendia Inc. [71]
Oncotype DX	21	Risk of distant recurrence in ER+ patients. Predictive of chemotherapy benefit.	Genomic Health, Inc. [72]
Genomic-grade Index	97	Predictive of relapse in endocrine therapy treated ER+ patients.	[73]
Molecular Grade Index	5	Predictive of overall survival in ER+ patients.	[73]
Rotterdam Signature	76	Prognostic for distant metastasis within 5 years.	[74]

In addition to these classic tissue biomarkers, high Ki67 is frequently used as a prognostic biomarker of poor overall survival. Ki67 is a nuclear non-histone protein that is universally expressed by proliferating cells and detected by IHC [54]. High Ki67 has been shown to distinguish between Luminal A and B [54]. Additional protein biomarkers, such as p53 and urokinase plasminogen activator/plasminogen activator inhibitor-1, are under evaluation as predictive markers [52]. Overall, current protein biomarkers are insufficient to predict responses to emerging targeted therapies and to provide sufficient prognostic accuracy to aid in adjuvant chemotherapy treatment decisions. There is a need for broader, more predictive biomarker panels [18].

Recent advances in multiparametric gene analysis have led to several gene expression signatures for clinical prognosis and prediction of response to chemotherapeutics. Oncotype DX® was developed to improve prediction of the risk of distant recurrence in patients with ER+ early breast cancer receiving tamoxifen. The test uses RT-PCR from FFPE tissue to quantitate the expression of 16 genes with known significance in breast cancer, and five reference genes. The resulting recurrence score is a continuous measurement of risk, but patients can be stratified into three groups: low, intermediate, and high risk of distant metastasis. The RS has been shown to be predictive of distant recurrence independent of age and tumor size as well as of overall survival. Similarly, MammaPrint was developed as a prognostic and predictive 70-gene signature using frozen tissue samples [55]. Both Mammaprint and Oncotype DX® have been independently validated

with node-positive and node-negative disease [56, 57] (Table 7.4).

Potential clinical applications of biomarkers for breast cancer

Improving risk assessment of healthy populations

Large, population-based epidemiologic studies have led to the identification of numerous risk factors of breast cancer. The highest risk populations with strong family histories and/or known genomic alterations in BRCA1, BRCA2, PTEN, and TP53 represent a minority (5–10%) of breast cancers, and these alterations lead to intensive targeted screening pathways with physical exams, mammography, MRIs, and/or prophylactic mastectomies and oophorectomies [19, 58]. The few SNPs identified through GWAS studies have a much lower estimated contribution to overall breast cancer risk, and may be insufficiently prognostic for targeted screening [2, 59].

Additional clinical risk factors include gender, age, early menarche, late menopause, and delayed pregnancy [60]. These risk factors primarily impact lifetime estrogen exposure. Environmental exposures, such as ionizing chest wall irradiation, have clear mechanisms of carcinogenesis, but the combined impact of chemical environmental exposures (such as endocrine-disruptors) remains unknown. Other factors associated with increased breast cancer risk, such as weight gain during menopause, alcohol intake, benign breast disease, and elevated mammographic breast density, increase risk through poorly understood molecular mechanisms

[61]. Dynamic risk-assessment tools are needed to rapidly integrate the known and emerging clinical, epidemiologic, and genomic risk factors to improved risk stratification for targeted screening and prevention clinical trials. Future studies, such as incorporating early random breast biopsies of healthy women, may lead to further epigenetic and proteomic biomarkers for risk stratification.

Complementing mammographic screening

Improving access to care
The establishment of routine annual or biannual mammographic screening for women over the age of 40 has increased the detection of DCIS and early-stage (< 2 cm) node-negative breast cancer, and has led to improved survival [1]. Lesions less than 0.5 cm in size remain largely undetectable [21]. Despite these successes, mammographic screening has many limitations. First, it is markedly lower in underserved, underinsured, and minority populations, including American Indian/Alaska Natives, those who do not have a high school degree, those with an annual household income ≤ $15 000, those with no health insurance, and those with no usual source of health care [62]. Even within insured populations, up to 25% of eligible women have not had mammograms within the previous four years [56].

It is estimated that a 5% increase in mammography use could prevent 560 deaths annually in the US [63]. With improving microfluidic technologies, point-of-care devices for blood-based biomarker measurements may become highly cost-effective and accessible for rapid population screening. These have the potential to complement screening mammography to improve population coverage.

Increased detection of missed cancers
Even within populations undergoing routine screening, mammography has an estimated sensitivity, ranging from 98% in women with fatty breast parenchyma, to 36% in women with dense breasts [64]. The sensitivity of mammography for the detection of invasive cancers is limited in the setting of high breast density, which also confers a four-fold increased risk of breast cancer. The population of women with extremely dense breasts, in particular, would likely benefit from complementary

tissue- and blood-based biomarkers for early detection, as well as risk assessment tools to select patients for cost-effective MRI screening [64].

Increased detection of interval cancers
Recent multi-institutional clinical trials, such as ISPY-1 and ISPY-2, have targeted patients diagnosed with large, high-grade cancers for neoadjuvant chemotherapy. The majority of patients with high-grade cancers enrolled in ISPY-1 were diagnosed by clinical palpation, not screening mammography, as these cancers often present in the intervals between routine mammographic screening [65]. Rapidly proliferative, high-grade cancers can develop to clinically detectable cancers within months, limiting the clinical effectiveness of annual mammography for detection of these cancers. The low prevalence of these cancers within the general population prohibits more frequent mammography. Blood-based biomarkers, in particular, may be useful as more frequent screening tools for higher-risk populations.

Limiting overdiagnosis and improving prognosis of benign breast disease and DCIS
The majority of abnormal mammograms are not associated with cancer, leading to unnecessary biopsies and the overdiagnosis of benign breast disease [19]. Additional patients are diagnosed with low-grade DCIS of unclear clinical significance, and current trials of post-excision watchful waiting of these lesions in selected populations are ongoing. The surgical, economic, and emotional impact of the overdiagnosis of BBD and DCIS is significant. Tissue-based biomarkers that stratify risk after a diagnosis of BBD or DCIS would have significant impact on the follow-up and clinical management of these patients.

Summary

The rapidly-evolving field of biomarker science has led to the discovery of hundreds of blood-based and tissue-based biomarkers for the early detection and risk assessment of breast cancer. Moving these biomarkers into clinical use requires rigorous and systematic validation in the setting of intended use. Development of tissue and blood repositories with relevant controls, standardized collections that minimize pre-analytical variables, assay and clinical lab standardization, as well as accurate annotation of clinical outcomes and co-variates, is necessary to evaluate these biomarkers. Clinical trial pipelines, designed to assess both tissue and blood biomarkers for breast cancer detection and screening, are under way. These integrated efforts require the coordinated efforts of basic scientists, biomarker researchers, clinicians, biostatisticians, industry, and patient advocates. If successful, these biomarkers have the potential to impact survival and quality of life for women undergoing breast cancer screening.

Conflict of interest

Dr. Anderson has served as a consultant and scientific advisory board member for Provista Dx.

References

1. American Cancer Society (2013). *Cancer Facts and Figures 2013*. Atlanta: American Cancer Society.
2. Cancer Genome Atlas N (2012). Comprehensive molecular portraits of human breast tumours. *Nature* **490**(7418), 61–70.
3. Polyak K (2011). Heterogeneity in breast cancer. *Journal of Clinical Investigation* **121**(10):3786–8.
4. Thompson D, Easton D (2004). The genetic epidemiology of breast cancer genes. *Journal of Mammary Gland Biology and Neoplasia* **9**(3), 221–36.
5. Hollestelle A, Wasielewski M, Martens JW, Schutte M (2010). Discovering moderate-risk breast cancer susceptibility genes. *Current Opinion in Genetics & Development* **20**(3), 268–76.
6. Bombonati A, Sgroi DC (2011). The molecular pathology of breast cancer progression. *Journal of Pathology* **223**(2), 307–17.
7. Sgroi DC (2010). Preinvasive breast cancer. *Annual Review of Pathology* **5**, 193–221.
8. Shackleton M, Quintana E, Fearon ER, Morrison SJ (2009). Heterogeneity in cancer: cancer stem cells versus clonal evolution. *Cell* **138**(5), 822–9.
9. Cole K, Tabernero M, Anderson KS (2010). Biologic characteristics of premalignant breast disease. *Cancer Biomarkers* **9**(1–6), 177–92.
10. Langley RR, Fidler IJ (2011). The seed and soil hypothesis revisited – the role of tumor-stroma interactions in metastasis to different organs. *International Journal of Cancer* **128**(11), 2527–35.
11. Datta S, Davies EL (2013). Benign breast disease. *Surgery (Oxford)* **31**(1), 22–6.
12. Guray M, Sahin AA (2006). Benign breast diseases: classification, diagnosis, and management. *The Oncologist* **11**(5), 435–49.
13. Hartmann LC, Sellers TA, Frost MH, Lingle WL, Degnim AC, Ghosh K, *et al.* (2005). Benign breast disease and the risk of breast cancer. *New England Journal of Medicine* **353**(3), 229–37.
14. Buerger H, Otterbach F, Simon R, Poremba C, Diallo R, Decker T, *et al.* (1999). Comparative genomic hybridization of ductal carcinoma in situ of the breast-evidence of multiple genetic pathways. *Journal of Pathology* **187**(4), 396–402.
15. Yao J, Weremowicz S, Feng B, Gentleman RC, Marks JR, Gelman R, *et al.* (2006). Combined cDNA array comparative genomic hybridization and serial analysis of gene expression analysis of breast tumor progression. *Cancer Research* **66**(8), 4065–78.
16. Moinfar F (2009). Flat ductal intraepithelial neoplasia of the breast: a review of diagnostic criteria, differential diagnoses, molecular-genetic findings, and clinical relevance – it is time to appreciate the Azzopardi concept! *Archives of Pathology & Laboratory Medicine* **133**(6), 879–92.
17. Polyak K, Kalluri R (2010). The role of the microenvironment in mammary gland development and cancer. *Cold Spring Harbor Perspectives in Biology* **2**(11), a003244.
18. Cole KD, He HJ, Wang L (2013). Breast cancer biomarker measurements and standards. *Proteomics Clinical Applications* **7**(1–2), 17–29.
19. Warner E (2011). Breast-Cancer Screening. *New England Journal of Medicine* **365**(11), 1025–32.
20. Galanina N, Bossuyt V, Harris LN (2011). Molecular predictors of response to therapy for breast cancer. *Cancer Journal* **17**(2), 96–103.
21. Misek DE, Kim EH (2011). Protein biomarkers for the early detection of breast cancer. *International Journal of Proteomics* **2011**, 343582.
22. Guttery DS, Blighe K, Page K, Marchese SD, Hills A, Coombes RC, *et al.* (2013). Hide and seek: tell-tale signs of breast cancer lurking in the blood. *Cancer Metastasis Reviews* **32**(1–2), 289–302.
23. Kim JW, You J (2013). Protein target quantification decision tree. *International Journal of Proteomics* **2013**, 701247.
24. Gonzalez RM, Daly DS, Tan R, Marks JR, Zangar RC (2011). Plasma biomarker profiles differ depending on breast cancer subtype but RANTES is consistently increased. *Cancer epidemiology, Biomarkers & Prevention* **20**(7):1543–51.

25. Li CI, Mirus JE, Zhang Y, Ramirez AB, Ladd JJ, Prentice RL, et al. (2012). Discovery and preliminary confirmation of novel early detection biomarkers for triple-negative breast cancer using preclinical plasma samples from the Women's Health Initiative observational study. *Breast Cancer Research and Treatment* **135**(2), 611–8.

26. Wallstrom G, Anderson KS, LaBaer J (2013). Biomarker discovery for heterogeneous diseases. *Cancer Epidemiology, Biomarkers & Prevention* **22**(5), 747–55.

27. Tan HT, Low J, Lim SG, Chung MC (2009). Serum autoantibodies as biomarkers for early cancer detection. *FEBS Journal* **276**(23), 6880–904.

28. Anderson KS (2011). Multiplexed detection of antibodies using programmable bead arrays. *Methods in Molecular Biology* **723**, 227–38.

29. Anderson KS, Sibani S, Wallstrom G, Qiu J, Mendoza EA, Raphael J, et al. (2011). Protein microarray signature of autoantibody biomarkers for the early detection of breast cancer. *Journal of Proteome Research* **10**(1), 85–96.

30. Chapman C, Murray A, Chakrabarti J, Thorpe A, Woolston C, Sahin U, et al. (2007). Autoantibodies in breast cancer: their use as an aid to early diagnosis. *Annals of Oncology* **18**(5), 868–73.

31. Adamczyk B, Tharmalingam T, Rudd PM (2012). Glycans as cancer biomarkers. *Biochimica et Biophysica Acta* **1820**(9), 1347–53.

32. Kyselova Z, Mechref Y, Kang P, Goetz JA, Dobrolecki LE, Sledge GW, et al. (2008). Breast cancer diagnosis and prognosis through quantitative measurements of serum glycan profiles. *Clinical Chemistry* **54**(7), 1166–75.

33. Abbott KL, Lim JM, Wells L, Benigno BB, McDonald JF, Pierce M. (2010). Identification of candidate biomarkers with cancer-specific glycosylation in the tissue and serum of endometrioid ovarian cancer patients by glycoproteomic analysis. *Proteomics* **10**(3), 470–81.

34. Abbott KL, Aoki K, Lim JM, Porterfield M, Johnson R, O'Regan RM, et al. (2008). Targeted glycoproteomic identification of biomarkers for human breast carcinoma. *Journal of Proteome Research* **7**(4), 1470–80.

35. Zhao P, Nairn AV, Hester S, Moremen KW, O'Regan RM, Oprea G, et al. (2012). Proteomic identification of glycosylphosphatidylinositol anchor-dependent membrane proteins elevated in breast carcinoma. *Journal of Biological Chemistry* **287**(30), 25230–40.

36. Wu G, Guo Z, Chatterjee A, Huang X, Rubin E, Wu F, et al. (2006). Overexpression of glycosylphosphatidylinositol (GPI) transamidase subunits phosphatidylinositol glycan class T and/or GPI anchor attachment 1 induces tumorigenesis and contributes to invasion in human breast cancer. *Cancer Research* **66**(20), 9829–36.

37. Azmi AS, Bao B, Sarkar FH (2013). Exosomes in cancer development, metastasis, and drug resistance: a comprehensive review. *Cancer Metastasis Reviews* **32**(3–4), 623–42.

38. Vlassov AV, Magdaleno S, Setterquist R, Conrad R (2012). Exosomes: current knowledge of their composition, biological functions, and diagnostic and therapeutic potentials. *Biochimica et Biophysica Acta* **1820**(7), 940–8.

39. Hendrix A, Hume AN (2011). Exosome signaling in mammary gland development and cancer. *International Journal of Developmental Biology* **55**(7–9), 879–87.

40. Nadal R, Lorente JA, Rosell R, Serrano MJ (2013). Relevance of molecular characterization of circulating tumor cells in breast cancer in the era of targeted therapies. *Expert Review of Molecular Diagnostics* **13**(3), 295–307.

41. Alix-Panabieres C, Schwarzenbach H, Pantel K (2012). Circulating tumor cells and circulating tumor DNA. *Annual Review of Medicine* **63**, 199–215.

42. Shaw JA, Page K, Blighe K, Hava N, Guttery D, Ward B, et al. (2012). Genomic analysis of circulating cell-free DNA infers breast cancer dormancy. *Genome Research* **22**(2), 220–31.

43. Ferracin M, Veronese A, Negrini M (2010). Micromarkers: miRNAs in cancer diagnosis and prognosis. *Expert Review of Molecular Diagnostics* **10**(3), 297–308.

44. Shen J, Stass SA, Jiang F (2013). MicroRNAs as potential biomarkers in human solid tumors. *Cancer Letters* **329**(2), 125–36.

45. Heneghan HM, Miller N, Kelly R, Newell J, Kerin MJ (2010). Systemic miRNA-195 differentiates breast cancer from other malignancies and is a potential biomarker for detecting noninvasive and early stage disease. *The Oncologist* **15**(7), 673–82.

46. Roth C, Rack B, Muller V, Janni W, Pantel K, Schwarzenbach H (2010). Circulating microRNAs as blood-based markers for patients with primary and metastatic breast cancer. *Breast Cancer Research* **12**(6), R90.

47. Cuk K, Zucknick M, Heil J, Madhavan D, Schott S, Turchinovich A, et al. (2013). Circulating microRNAs in plasma as early detection markers for breast cancer. *International Journal of Cancer* **132**(7), 1602–12.

48. Zhao H, Shen J, Medico L, Wang D, Ambrosone CB, Liu S (2010). A pilot study of circulating miRNAs as potential biomarkers of early stage breast cancer. *PloS One* **5**(10), e13735.

49. Hannemann J, Velds A, Halfwerk JB, Kreike B, Peterse JL, van de Vijver MJ (2006). Classification of ductal

carcinoma in situ by gene expression profiling. *Breast Cancer Research* **8**(5), R61.

50. Poola I, Abraham J, Marshalleck JJ, Yue Q, Lokeshwar VB, Bonney G, *et al.* (2008). Molecular risk assessment for breast cancer development in patients with ductal hyperplasias. *Clinical Cancer Research* **14**(4), 1274–80.

51. Gauthier ML, Berman HK, Miller C, Kozakeiwicz K, Chew K, Moore D, *et al.* (2007). Abrogated response to cellular stress identifies DCIS associated with subsequent tumor events and defines basal-like breast tumors. *Cancer Cell* **12**(5), 479–91.

52. Danova M, Delfanti S, Manzoni M, Mariucci S (2011). Tissue and soluble biomarkers in breast cancer and their applications: ready to use? *Journal of the National Cancer Institute Monographs* **2011**(43), 75–8.

53. Chung L, Shibli S, Moore K, Elder EE, Boyle FM, Marsh DJ, *et al.* (2013). Tissue biomarkers of breast cancer and their association with conventional pathologic features. *British Journal of Cancer* **108**(2), 351–60.

54. Dowsett M, Nielsen TO, A'Hern R, Bartlett J, Coombes RC, Cuzick J, *et al.* (2011). Assessment of Ki67 in breast cancer: recommendations from the International Ki67 in Breast Cancer working group. *Journal of the National Cancer Institute* **103**(22), 1656–64.

55. van't Veer LJ, Dai H, van de Vijver MJ, He YD, Hart AA, Mao M, *et al.* (2002). Gene expression profiling predicts clinical outcome of breast cancer. *Nature* **415**(6871), 530–6.

56. Buyse M, Loi S, van't Veer L, Viale G, Delorenzi M, Glas AM, *et al.* (2006). Validation and clinical utility of a 70-gene prognostic signature for women with node-negative breast cancer. *Journal of the National Cancer Institute* **98**(17), 1183–92.

57. Albain KS, Barlow WE, Shak S, Hortobagyi GN, Livingston RB, Yeh IT, *et al.* (2010). Prognostic and predictive value of the 21-gene recurrence score assay in postmenopausal women with node-positive, oestrogen-receptor-positive breast cancer on chemotherapy: a retrospective analysis of a randomised trial. *The Lancet Oncology* **11**(1), 55–65.

58. Filippini SE, Vega A (2013). Breast cancer genes: beyond BRCA1 and BRCA2. *Frontiers in Bioscience* **18**, 1358–72.

59. Bayraktar S, Thompson PA, Yoo SY, Do KA, Sahin AA, Arun BK, *et al.* (2013). The relationship between eight GWAS-identified single-nucleotide polymorphisms and primary breast cancer outcomes. *The Oncologist* **18**(5), 493–500.

60. Evans DG, Howell A (2007). Breast cancer risk-assessment models. *Breast Cancer Research* **9**(5), 213.

61. Gemignani ML (2011). Breast cancer screening: why, when, and how many? *Clinical Obstetrics and Gynecology* **54**(1), 125–32.

62. Centers for Disease Control and Prevention (2012). Cancer screening – United States, 2010. *MMWR Morbidity and Mortality Weekly Report* **61**(3), 41–5.

63. Farley TA, Dalal MA, Mostashari F, Frieden TR (2010). Deaths preventable in the U.S. by improvements in use of clinical preventive services. *American Journal of Preventive Medicine* **38**(6), 600–9.

64. Drukteinis JS, Mooney BP, Flowers CI, Gatenby RA (2013). Beyond mammography: new frontiers in breast cancer screening. *American Journal of Medicine* **126**(6), 472–9.

65. Mukhtar RA, Yau C, Rosen M, Tandon VJ, The IST, Investigators A, *et al.* (2013). Clinically Meaningful Tumor Reduction Rates Vary by Prechemotherapy MRI Phenotype and Tumor Subtype in the I-SPY 1 TRIAL (CALGB 150007/150012; ACRIN 6657). *Annals of Surgical Oncology* **20**(12), 3823–30.

66. Iorio MV, Ferracin M, Liu CG, Veronese A, Spizzo R, Sabbioni S, *et al.* (2005). MicroRNA gene expression deregulation in human breast cancer. *Cancer Research* **65**(16), 7065–70.

67. Blenkiron C, Goldstein LD, Thorne NP, Spiteri I, Chin SF, Dunning MJ, *et al.* (2007). MicroRNA expression profiling of human breast cancer identifies new markers of tumor subtype. *Genome Biology* **8**(10), R214.

68. Tavazoie SF, Alarcon C, Oskarsson T, Padua D, Wang Q, Bos PD, *et al.* (2008). Endogenous human microRNAs that suppress breast cancer metastasis. *Nature* **451**(7175), 147–52.

69. Poola I, DeWitty RL, Marshalleck JJ, Bhatnagar R, Abraham J, Leffall LD (2005). Identification of MMP-1 as a putative breast cancer predictive marker by global gene expression analysis. *Nature Medicine* **11**(5), 481–3.

70. Poola I, Shokrani B, Bhatnagar R, DeWitty RL, Yue Q, Bonney G (2006). Expression of carcinoembryonic antigen cell adhesion molecule 6 oncoprotein in atypical ductal hyperplastic tissues is associated with the development of invasive breast cancer. *Clinical Cancer Research* **12**(15), 4773–83.

71. Knauer M, Mook S, Rutgers EJ, Bender RA, Hauptmann M, van de Vijver MJ, *et al.* (2010). The predictive value of the 70-gene signature for adjuvant chemotherapy in early breast cancer. *Breast Cancer Research and Treatment* **120**(3), 655–61.

72. Paik S, Shak S, Tang G, Kim C, Baker J, Cronin M, *et al.* (2004). A multigene assay to predict recurrence of tamoxifen-treated, node-negative breast cancer. *New England Journal of Medicine* **351**(27), 2817–26.

73. Metzger Filho O, Ignatiadis M, Sotiriou C (2011). Genomic Grade Index: An important tool for assessing breast cancer tumor grade and prognosis. *Critical Reviews in Oncology/Hematology* **77**(1), 20–9.

74. Wang Y, Klijn JG, Zhang Y, Sieuwerts AM, Look MP, Yang F, et al. (2005). Gene-expression profiles to predict distant metastasis of lymph-node-negative primary breast cancer. The Lancet 365(9460), 671–9.

75. Le Naour F, Misek DE, Krause MC, Deneux L, Giordano TJ, Scholl S, et al. (2001). Proteomics-based identification of RS/DJ-1 as a novel circulating tumor antigen in breast cancer. Clinical Cancer Research 7(11), 3328–35.

76. Kulic A, Sirotkovic-Skerlev M, Jelisavac-Cosic S, Herceg D, Kovac Z, Vrbanec D (2010). Anti-p53 antibodies in serum: relationship to tumor biology and prognosis of breast cancer patients. Medical Oncology 27(3), 887–93.

77. Desmetz C, Bascoul-Mollevi C, Rochaix P, Lamy PJ, Kramar A, Rouanet P, et al. (2009). Identification of a new panel of serum autoantibodies associated with the presence of in situ carcinoma of the breast in younger women. Clinical Cancer Research 15(14), 4733–41.

78. Conroy SE, Sasieni PD, Amin V, Wang DY, Smith P, Fentiman IS, et al. (1998). Antibodies to heat-shock protein 27 are associated with improved survival in patients with breast cancer. British Journal of Cancer 77(11), 1875–9.

79. von Mensdorff-Pouilly S, Petrakou E, Kenemans P, van Uffelen K, Verstraeten AA, Snijdewint FG, et al. 2000 (). Reactivity of natural and induced human antibodies to MUC1 mucin with MUC1 peptides and n-acetylgalactosamine (GalNAc) peptides. International Journal of Cancer 86(5), 702–12.

80. Duffy MJ, Evoy D, McDermott EW (2010). CA 15-3: uses and limitation as a biomarker for breast cancer. Clinica Chimica Acta 411(23–24), 1869–74.

81. Goodell V, Waisman J, Salazar LG, de la Rosa C, Link J, Coveler AL, et al. (2008). Level of HER-2/neu protein expression in breast cancer may affect the development of endogenous HER-2/neu-specific immunity. Molecular Cancer Therapeutics 7(3), 449–54.

82. Schrauder MG, Strick R, Schulz-Wendtland R, Strissel PL, Kahmann L, Loehberg CR, et al. (2012). Circulating micro-RNAs as potential blood-based markers for early stage breast cancer detection. PloS One 7(1), e29770.

83. Wang H, Tan G, Dong L, Cheng L, Li K, Wang Z, et al. (2012). Circulating MiR-125b as a marker predicting chemoresistance in breast cancer. PloS One 7(4), e34210.

84. Zhao G, Cai C, Yang T, Qiu X, Liao B, Li W, et al. (2013). MicroRNA-221 induces cell survival and cisplatin resistance through PI3K/Akt pathway in human osteosarcoma. PloS One 8(1), e53906.

85. Riethdorf S, Fritsche H, Muller V, Rau T, Schindlbeck C, Rack B, et al. (2007). Detection of circulating tumor cells in peripheral blood of patients with metastatic breast cancer: a validation study of the CellSearch system. Clinical Cancer Research 13(3), 920–8.

86. Gaforio JJ, Serrano MJ, Sanchez-Rovira P, Sirvent A, Delgado-Rodriguez M, Campos M, et al. (2003). Detection of breast cancer cells in the peripheral blood is positively correlated with estrogen-receptor status and predicts for poor prognosis. International Journal of Cancer 107(6), 984–90.

87. Alix-Panabieres C, Vendrell JP, Slijper M, Pelle O, Barbotte E, Mercier G, et al. (2009). Full-length cytokeratin-19 is released by human tumor cells: a potential role in metastatic progression of breast cancer. Breast Cancer Research 11(3), R39.

88. Fehm T, Hoffmann O, Aktas B, Becker S, Solomayer EF, Wallwiener D, et al. (2009). Detection and characterization of circulating tumor cells in blood of primary breast cancer patients by RT-PCR and comparison to status of bone marrow disseminated cells. Breast Cancer Research 11(4), R59.

89. Desitter I, Guerrouahen BS, Benali-Furet N, Wechsler J, Janne PA, Kuang Y, et al. (2011). A new device for rapid isolation by size and characterization of rare circulating tumor cells. AntiCancer Research 31(2), 427–41.

90. Pinzani P, Salvadori B, Simi L, Bianchi S, Distante V, Cataliotti L, et al. (2006). Isolation by size of epithelial tumor cells in peripheral blood of patients with breast cancer: correlation with real-time reverse transcriptase-polymerase chain reaction results and feasibility of molecular analysis by laser microdissection. Human Pathology 37(6), 711–8.

91. Ignatiadis M, Rothe F, Chaboteaux C, Durbecq V, Rouas G, Criscitiello C, et al. (2011). HER2-positive circulating tumor cells in breast cancer. PloS One 6(1), e15624.

92. Markou A, Strati A, Malamos N, Georgoulias V, Lianidou ES (). Molecular characterization of circulating tumor cells in breast cancer by a liquid bead array hybridization assay. Clinical Chemistry 57(3), 421–30.

93. Xenidis N, Ignatiadis M, Apostolaki S, Perraki M, Kalbakis K, Agelaki S, et al. (2009). Cytokeratin-19 mRNA-positive circulating tumor cells after adjuvant chemotherapy in patients with early breast cancer. Journal of Clinical Oncology 27(13), 2177–84.

94. Page K, Hava N, Ward B, Brown J, Guttery DS, Ruang-pratheep C, et al. (2011). Detection of HER2 amplification in circulating free DNA in patients with breast cancer. British Journal of Cancer 104(8), 1342–8.

95. Matuschek C, Bolke E, Lammering G, Gerber PA, Peiper M, Budach W, et al. (2010). Methylated APC and GSTP1 genes in serum DNA correlate with the presence of circulating blood tumor cells and are associated with a more aggressive and advanced breast cancer disease. European Journal of Medical Research 15, 277–86.

96. Dulaimi E, Hillinck J, Ibanez de Caceres I, Al-Saleem T, Cairns P (2004). Tumor suppressor gene promoter hypermethylation in serum of breast cancer patients. *Clinical Cancer Research* **10**(18 Pt 1), 6189–93.

97. Martinez-Galan J, Torres B, Del Moral R, Munoz-Gamez JA, Martin-Oliva D, Villalobos M, *et al.* (2008). Quantitative detection of methylated ESR1 and 14-3-3-sigma gene promoters in serum as candidate biomarkers for diagnosis of breast cancer and evaluation of treatment efficacy. *Cancer Biology & Therapy* **7**(6), 958–65.

98. Papadopoulou E, Davilas E, Sotiriou V, Georgakopoulos E, Georgakopoulou S, Koliopanos A, *et al.* (2006). Cell-free DNA and RNA in plasma as a new molecular marker for prostate and breast cancer. *Annals of the New York Academy of Sciences* **1075**, 235–43.

99. Sharma G, Mirza S, Parshad R, Gupta SD, Ralhan R (2012). DNA methylation of circulating DNA: a marker for monitoring efficacy of neoadjuvant chemotherapy in breast cancer patients. *Tumour Biology* **33**(6), 1837–43.

100. Schwarzenbach H, Muller V, Stahmann N, Pantel K (2004). Detection and characterization of circulating microsatellite-DNA in blood of patients with breast cancer. *Annals of the New York Academy of Sciences* **1022**, 25–32.

101. Shaw JA, Smith BM, Walsh T, Johnson S, Primrose L, Slade MJ, *et al.* (2000). Microsatellite alterations plasma DNA of primary breast cancer patients. *Clinical Cancer Research* **6**(3), 1119–24.

102. Silva JM, Gonzalez R, Dominguez G, Garcia JM, Espana P, Bonilla F (1999). TP53 gene mutations in plasma DNA of cancer patients. *Genes, Chromosomes & Cancer* **24**(2), 160–1.

103. Iorio MV, Casalini P, Tagliabue E, Menard S, Croce CM. (2008). MicroRNA profiling as a tool to understand prognosis, therapy response and resistance in breast cancer. *European Journal of Cancer* **44**(18), 2753–9.

104. Ma L, Teruya-Feldstein J, Weinberg RA (2007). Tumour invasion and metastasis initiated by microRNA-10b in breast cancer. *Nature* **449**(7163), 682–8.

CHAPTER 8

Ovarian Cancer

Christos Patriotis,[1] Archana Simmons,[2] Karen H Lu,[3] Robert C Bast, Jr,[2] and Steven J Skates[4]

[1]Cancer Biomarkers Research Group, Division of Cancer Prevention, National Cancer Institute, National Institutes of Health, Bethesda, MD, USA

[2]Department of Experimental Therapeutics, University of Texas MD Anderson Cancer Center, Houston, TX, USA

[3]Department of Gynecologic Oncology, University of Texas MD Anderson Cancer Center, Houston, TX, USA

[4]Massachusetts General Hospital and Harvard Medical School, Boston, MA, USA

Introduction

Recent morphologic and molecular genetic studies have shed light on our understanding of ovarian carcinogenesis in ways that have been quite unexpected and have challenged the conventional wisdom regarding their origin and development. Indeed, they have resulted in a paradigm shift that has important implications for research, and for radically changing our approaches to early detection, prevention, and treatment [1].

Origin of ovarian cancer

Ovarian surface

The traditional view of ovarian carcinogenesis has been that epithelial ovarian cancer originates from the ovarian surface mesothelial epithelium, or coelomic epithelium [1]. This epithelium undergoes metaplasia to müllerian epithelium which, morphologically, resembles the epithelia of the fallopian tube, endometrium, gastrointestinal tract, endocervix, and urinary bladder. Ovulation leads to trapping of this metaplastic mesothelium in the ovary, forming inclusion cysts and, under conditions of incessant ovulation and an ongoing repetitive wound-healing process, this leads to neoplastic epithelial ovarian cancer. This theory is based on the observation that surface epithelial inclusion cysts are often found in the ovary. Pothuri *et al.* showed, in a recent study, that TP53 mutations and BRCA LOH are often present in inclusion cysts in morphologically normal ovaries from BRCA mutation carriers [2]. However, precursor lesions were rarely found in the ovary. A recent study that followed women with inclusion cysts showed no increase in ovarian cancer in these women [3].

Secondary müllerian system

Another theory suggests that epithelial ovarian cancer originates from the "secondary müllerian system" [4]. This alternate theory proposes that tumors with a müllerian phenotype (serous, endometrioid) are derived from müllerian-type tissue, and not from the mesothelium. This tissue, such as glands of endometriosis, endosalpingiosis, and endocervicosis, and the rete ovarii, lines cysts located in the para-tubal and para-ovarian locations. These cysts, as well as endometriosis and any other müllerian tissue located outside of the müllerian system, are collectively referred to as the "secondary müllerian system" [5]. According to this theory, ovarian tumors develop in these cysts, enlarge and compress, and eventually obliterate

Biomarkers in Cancer Screening and Early Detection, First Edition. Edited by Sudhir Srivastava.
© 2017 John Wiley & Sons, Inc. Published 2017 by John Wiley & Sons, Inc.

normal ovarian tissue, resulting in an adnexal tumor that seems to have arisen from the ovary [1].

This theory is based on the observation that, morphologically, ovarian tumors of the serous, endometrioid, and clear cell subtypes resemble the müllerian epithelium, while the ovary itself is not of müllerian origin. However, precursor lesions resembling serous, endometrioid, and clear cell carcinomas have rarely, if ever, been reported in paratubal and para-ovarian cysts [1].

Fallopian tube

Most recently, it has been postulated that the majority of high-grade serous ovarian carcinomas arise from serous intraepithelial carcinoma of the fallopian tube, which then disseminates to the adjacent ovarian surface and the peritoneum. Data to support this theory are derived from the systematic characterization of salpingo-oophorectomy specimens removed prophylactically from women with inherited high risk for ovarian cancer (BRCA mutation carriers), where *in situ* and small early invasive tubal carcinomas were detected in the fimbriated end of the fallopian tube [1,6–12]. Further observations to support this theory include the recognition that serous tumor is morphologically indistinguishable from tubal intraepithelial carcinoma.

Serous tubal intraepithelial carcinoma (STIC) is the earliest morphologic manifestation of serous carcinoma, and is composed of secretory cells showing significant atypia, such as loss of nuclear polarity, prominent nucleoli, and increased nuclear to cytoplasmic ratio [13, 14]. The STIC lesion overexpresses p53 [14], is common (approximately 80%) in prophylactic salpingo-oophorectomy specimens from women with BRCA1/2 mutations [15], and is associated with 70% of sporadic (non-hereditary) advanced serous ovarian cancer [16]. In addition, PAX2/8, a müllerian marker and a transcription factor that is expressed in normal female genital track epithelium (fallopian tube, endometrium, endocervix), is expressed in high-grade serous tumors, but not in ovarian surface epithelium, while calretinin, a mesothelial marker, is expressed in ovarian surface epithelium. but not in high-grade serous carcinoma [17, 18]. Identical TP53 mutations exist in STIC lesions and concomitant ovarian serous carcinoma in some BRCA1/2 carriers, indicating clonal relationship [1].

Another tubal lesion, the P53 Signature, a possible precursor lesion that is characterized by intense P53 staining and TP53 mutations in a morphologically normal tubal epithelium, is found adjacent to STICs. However, mutations in the P53 signature are not always the same as in the STIC lesion [14, 19]. Finally, there is an improved survival of primary fallopian tube cancer, compared with ovarian cancer [20].

On the other hand, only 10–15% of epithelial ovarian cancers arise in patients with BRCA1 and BRCA2 germ line mutations, and a large fraction of high-grade serous cancers appears to grow from ovaries, rather than the fallopian tube, in patients with sporadic disease. While up to 80% of the 10–15% of high-grade serous ovarian cancers may well arise from the fallopian tube, this represents only 10% of all epithelial ovarian cancers. In addition, approximately 20% of high-grade serous carcinomas coat the ovary, rather than grow from it, and have been termed primary peritoneal carcinomas. Some of these may have grown from the peritoneum, but it is as likely that they could have arisen in the fallopian tube. Consequently, at least 30% of high-grade serous ovarian cancers may be of fallopian tube origin, but it is unlikely that all high-grade serous cancers come from the fallopian tube.

Endometriosis

Endometrioid and clear cell ovarian cancer are hypothesized to arise from endometrial tissue implanted on the ovary (endometriosis). This is supported by well-documented identification of transitional areas of endometriosis, ranging from benign to atypical, adjacent to ovarian cancer. In addition, epidemiological studies show that risk of ovarian cancer among women with endometriosis is higher, by 30 to 40%, than among women without endometriosis. Molecular genetic studies showed that many of the same genes (β-catenin, PTEN) are mutated both in endometrial cancers and in endometrioid ovarian cancers. A recent pooled analysis has shown that endometriosis is associated with higher risk of developing low-grade serous, endometrioid, and clear-cell ovarian cancer, but not with mucinous or high-grade serous ovarian cancer. [21] ARID1A mutations were found in 46% of clear cell carcinomas and 30% endometrial carcinomas, and none in high-grade serous tumors. [22].

Based on morphologic, molecular, genetic and epidemiological evidence, a fraction of high-grade serous ovarian cancers likely originates from fallopian tubes, while most, if not all, low-grade serous ovarian cancers arise from the ovarian surface epithelium. [1] Endometrioid and clear cell ovarian cancers arise from ectopic implants of the endometrium. [1] The cell origin of mucinous ovarian cancer is unclear.

Heterogeneity of epithelial ovarian cancer

Based on morphologic, molecular and genetic data, Kurman *et al.* proposed a dualistic model that categorizes various types of ovarian cancer into two groups – one group designated Type I, the other Type II [1]. Type I tumors include low-grade serous, low-grade endometrioid, clear cell, and mucinous carcinomas. In contrast to the clear-cut and distinctive morphologic differences among Type I tumors, the morphologic differences among Type II tumors are more subtle and, as a result, there is considerable overlap in the diagnosis of these tumors by different pathologists. Type II tumors exhibit papillary, glandular, and solid patterns, and are diagnosed as high-grade serous, high-grade endometrioid and undifferentiated carcinomas, depending on the dominant pattern; they also include carcinosarcomas. These Type II tumors represent 75% of all ovarian carcinomas, and are responsible for 90% of ovarian cancer deaths [23].

As a group, Type I tumors are genetically more stable than Type II tumors, and display specific mutations in different histologic cell types [1, 34]. For example, KRAS (19%), BRAF (38%), and/or ERBB2 mutations occur in approximately two-thirds of low-grade serous carcinomas, whereas TP53 mutations are rare in these tumors [25]. Low-grade endometrioid carcinomas have aberrations in the Wnt signaling pathway involving somatic mutations of CTNNB1 (encoding β-catenin), PTEN (20%), and PIK3CA [26]. PIK3CA leads to activation of the PI3K/AKT pathway, resulting in improved cell survival and invasion. Clear cell carcinoma is unique, in that it has a high percentage of PIK3CA (33%) mutations [24]. The HNF1β gene is upregulated in reactive or atypical endometriosis, as well as clear cell carcinomas associated with

endometriosis, and plays a major role in glucose-glycogen homeostasis [25, 27, 28]. Mucinous carcinomas have KRAS mutations in more than 50% of specimens, and HER2 gene amplification in 15–20% of specimens [1, 29, 30].

High-grade serous carcinoma, the prototypic Type II epithelial ovarian cancer, is characterized by very frequent TP53 mutations (in greater than 95% of cases) [31] and CCNE1 (encoding cyclin E1) amplification, but rarely the mutations that characterize most Type I tumors, such as KRAS, BRAF, ERBB2, PTEN, CTNNB1, and PIK3CA [1, 26]. When BRCA1 or BRCA2 is mutated, ovarian cancers are generally high-grade.

In summary, Type I tumors as a group are genetically more stable than Type II tumors, and display a distinctive pattern of mutations that occur in specific cell types (low-grade serous, low-grade endometrioid, clear cell and mucinous) [1]. In contrast, Type II tumors (high-grade serous, high-grade endometrioid, malignant mixed mesodermal tumors, and undifferentiated carcinomas) show greater morphologic and molecular homogeneity, are genetically unstable with frequent amplification and deletion, and have a very high frequency of TP53 mutations [1].

Early detection of ovarian cancer

In 2015, ovarian cancer was diagnosed in 21 290 women in the United States, and more than 14 000 died from this disease [60]. Effective early detection of ovarian cancer through regularly repeated screening tests may have a real impact on survival and, potentially, on mortality from the disease. A stochastic model of annual CA125 screening shifting diagnosis of ovarian cancer from late stage III/IV to early stage I/II could result in 3.4 years of life saved on average, per case of ovarian cancer, if survival of screen-detected early stage cases resembled survival of clinically detected early stage cases [32].

Epithelial ovarian cancer is detected through physical assessment and presence of symptoms, the use of the serum protein biomarker CA125, and imaging methods that include trans-vaginal sonography (TVS), magnetic resonance imaging (MRI) and positron emission tomography (PET). However, due to moderate sensitivity and specificity of all of these methods, and the low prevalence of the disease (1 in 2500 in postmenopausal women), resulting in unacceptably low expected positive predictive value (PPV), no screening of the general population is recommended [33, 34]. At the same time, given that 85–90% of ovarian cancer is sporadic in nature, with highest incidence in postmenopausal women with no other known strong risk factors, a successful screening program will have to target the general population in order to have a significant impact on the survival and mortality from the disease.

As described above, serous ovarian cancers are subdivided into two types, based on histopathology: Type I low-grade tumors, which represent approximately 10% of serous ovarian cancers and are usually detected at an early stage (I or II); and Type II – high-grade tumors, which are usually diagnosed at an advanced stage (III/IV). Type I and type II ovarian cancers differ by characteristic genetic aberrations. While type I mostly harbor K-Ras and B-Raf mutations, more than 95% of type II ovarian cancers carry a mutant TP53, and display significant heterogeneity with regard to chromosomal aberrations [35] which, for the most part as shown by the recent results from The Cancer Genome Atlas (TCGA) ovarian cancer project, represent amplification and deletion of diverse genetic loci [36, 37].

With most (> 75%) ovarian cancers detected in late stage with poor prognosis, yet excellent prognosis if detected in early stage, early detection holds the promise of having an impact on ovarian cancer mortality. For this to become a reality, tumors destined to be lethal must be detected and eliminated at a very early stage. The window of opportunity (i.e., the period before tumors become incurable) is most likely to be the time when aggressive tumors are still at the level of precursor lesions, carcinoma *in situ* (CIS), or Stage I/II cancer [38].

Challenges for early detection of ovarian cancer

Brown and Palmer performed a mathematical analysis of the size and stage of prophylactic bilateral salpingo-oophorectomy (PBSO) specimens obtained from women who carried mutations in the BRCA1 gene, taking into account the incidence and prevalence of serous ovarian cancers in BRCA1

mutation carriers, and the size of serous ovarian tumors at clinical diagnosis [39]. Based on their analysis, they concluded that the average period during which serous ovarian tumors in BRCA1 carriers are in an occult, early stage is 4.3 years, and the duration in stage III/IV prior to clinical diagnosis is approximately one year. While in early stage, more than 90% of the lesions had a diameter between 0.3 and 0.9 cm. Hence, to detect 50% of ovarian cancers in Stage I/II that would have progressed to Stage III/IV at clinical diagnosis, an annual screening program must be capable of detecting ovarian tumors with a diameter no greater than 1.3 cm.

Detection of 80% of ovarian cancers while in early stage would achieve a 50% reduction in ovarian cancer mortality. To achieve this level of sensitivity, the screening test must detect tumors with a diameter less than 0.4 cm. When detected clinically in stage I/II, serous ovarian cancers are typically 8 cm or more in diameter, and it is therefore clear that the required average tumor size to achieve 50% mortality reduction or better within the window of opportunity is > 200-fold smaller than the serous tumors that present clinically in early stage.

It is important, however, to note that this analysis pertains to Type II high grade serous ovarian cancers in genetically predisposed carriers of mutant BRCA1 genes. As many as 80% of these cancers may arise from the fimbriae of the fallopian tube, where there is no anatomic barrier to dissemination to the peritoneal cavity, permitting stage III disease to develop from very small cancers. Sporadic ovarian cancers that arise within cysts beneath the ovarian surface might well grow to larger size before metastasizing. This analysis does suggest, however, that caution is required in extrapolating the performance of biomarkers in patients at clinical diagnosis to their utility in early detection.

The minimally acceptable positive predictive value for a clinically useful ovarian cancer detection test, which would result in a surgical laparotomy, is > 10% (i.e., one or more ovarian cancers detected for every ten positive tests resulting in surgery). Given the low prevalence of ovarian cancer in the postmenopausal population ($\approx$ 1 in 2500), a sensitivity of > 75% for preclinical disease and a specificity of 99.6% are required. With only moderate sensitivity and/or specificity for currently available ovarian cancer biomarkers and imaging, one way to achieve a PPV > 10% is to utilize a multi-modal screening strategy [40]. For example, if the target is to identify one ovarian cancer in every five screen-indicated operations, a screening strategy should provide a 500-fold improvement, from an incidence of ovarian cancer of 1 in 2500, to a frequency of 1 in 5 at surgery.

Screening trials so far have shown that while transvaginal sonography (TVS) is not highly specific for ovarian cancer when used as a first line test, it can reduce the rate of false positive tests ten-fold among subjects with a positive CA125 test (absolute or longitudinal). Hence, a 500-fold increase in "incidence" could be achieved by a sequential bimodal test – a 50-fold improvement by a blood test, followed by a 10-fold improvement by TVS. To achieve a 50-fold improvement in "incidence", a blood test must have a false positive rate of at most 2% (1 in 50), which is equivalent to a specificity of at least 98%. This sets the minimum desired specificity of a blood test at 98% when sequentially combined with TVS as a screening strategy.

Two-stage screening strategies

While specificity for any blood biomarker can be set at 98%, the sensitivity for early stage pre-diagnostic disease remains a vital concern. To improve the sensitivity of an existing marker while maintaining the high specificity, retrospective analyses of CA125 data from ovarian cancer screening trials conducted in the 1980s and 1990s were undertaken. These analyses demonstrated that CA125 profiles over time differentiated subjects diagnosed with ovarian cancer from all other subjects. In ovarian cancer cases, CA125 increased exponentially over time while, in most other subjects, CA125 was relatively stable.

A method for interpreting serial CA125 values was developed which builds on the biological foundations that (ovarian) cancers have a doubling time and, therefore, exponential growth – likely reflected in the exponential CA125 rise – and that each woman has her own serum CA125 baseline [41,42]. The method calculates the probability, or risk, of having a change-point profile where CA125 rises exponentially from a baseline, as distinct from a flat profile where the CA125 is relatively stable. The probability of the profile having a change-point is interpreted as the risk of having ovarian cancer, and

the strategy that makes screening decisions on the basis of this risk is referred to as the risk of ovarian cancer algorithm (ROCA). This approach personalizes early detection for each woman, identifying her own baseline CA125, and thereby increasing sensitivity while maintaining the high specificity of 98%.

ROCA was investigated in a series of retrospective and prospective studies in the 1990s, culminating in the United Kingdom Collaborative Trial of Ovarian Cancer Screening (UKCTOCS) begun in 2001 [40]. This trial enrolled 200 000 normal-risk postmenopausal women, and screened half of the women annually for 11 years, with an additional three years of follow-up, while the other half were the control group. Half the screened women were randomized to a multi-modal screening group using ROCA followed by ultrasound, and the other half to annual trans-vaginal sonography screening as a first line test.

In the multimodal arm, CA125 was measured annually, ROCA calculated for each woman after every new CA125 value, and the women triaged with ROCA after every CA125 test into normal risk, intermediate risk, or elevated risk. If risk was normal, women returned for an annual test. If it was intermediate, women returned in three months for another CA125 test and were ROCA re-evaluated. If risk was elevated, subjects were referred to TVS screening. Screening and follow-up are completed, and preliminary results are encouraging. Specificity exceeds 99.6%, and no more than 3–4 operations will be required for each case of ovarian cancer detected.

ROCA detected 86% of ovarian cancers, with half of these cancers detected by ROCA earlier than would have been detected by a single threshold rule (> 35 U/mL) and the other half at the same time as a single threshold rule [43]. Final analyses of the effect of screening on ovarian cancer mortality were expected by the end of 2015.

Over the last 14 years, in parallel with UKC-TOCS, a smaller screening study has been conducted in the United States by the University of Texas MD Anderson Specialized Program of Research Excellence (SPORE) in Ovarian Cancer using the same two-stage multimodal screening arm of the UKCTOCS, in 5115 postmenopausal women at normal risk of developing ovarian cancer

(NROSS) [44]. Based on annual CA125 and ROCA analysis, less than 1% of women were referred for TVS each year, and less than 3% were referred over multiple years.

To date, 18 operations have been performed based on the ROCA algorithm, and 12 cases of ovarian cancer have been detected. Two were borderline and ten invasive, with nine of the 12 (75%) in stage I or II, compared to the 25% expected. While the numbers were small, several early stage cancers were discovered by a rise of CA125 within the normal range, suggesting that sensitivity can be improved, and the stage shifted with ROCA analysis and a two-stage strategy. Importantly, no more than three operations were required to detect each cancer, consistent with the high specificity observed in the UKCTOCS study. If the UKCTOCS shows a mortality advantage, screening should be feasible in the United States.

If a two-stage screening strategy is approved for early detection, point-of-service immunoassay tests that can assess finger-stick quantities of blood for ovarian cancer biomarkers may permit rapid screening of women in under 45 minutes, allowing prompt ROCA calculations and subsequent triage to TVS in the same visit, if necessary. A programmable bio-nano-chip (p-BNC), which is a miniaturized immunoanalyzer system with a credit-card-sized footprint, has been developed. This integrates automated sample metering, bubble and debris removal, reagent storage and waste disposal, all within the same platform, to permit point-of-service analysis. Utilizing this platform, miniaturized immunoassays have been developed for small volumes of blood (100 μL) for CA125 alone [45], and for CA125 multiplexed with HE4, CA 72-4 and MMP-7 [46], suitable for ovarian cancer applications in 43 minutes, with low detection limits and high analytical precision.

Enhancing the first stage of a two-stage screening strategy

Based on a simulated model with annual screening of women at average risk of ovarian cancer, using a parametric empirical Bayes (PEB) method to analyze rising CA125 and to prompt TVS, mortality from the disease could be reduced by $\approx$ 13% [47]. The PEB method interpreted serial CA125 levels by comparing the last CA125 value (log transformed) to the average of all previous (log) CA125 values. To reduce overall ovarian cancer mortality by at least 25% in a cost-effective manner, a first-line test must be identified that performs substantially better than PEB-CA125, and with a similar cost. As CA125 is expressed by only 80% of epithelial ovarian cancers, one approach is to develop a panel of blood biomarkers that complements CA125, to increase the proportion of ovarian cancers detected by CA125 and, ideally, to detect cancers earlier than with CA125.

In 2011, investigators of the Early Detection Research Network (EDRN), the Ovarian SPOREs and the Prostate, Lung, Colorectal and Ovarian (PLCO) Screening Trial published the results on the performance of 28 candidate ovarian cancer biomarkers tested in an EDRN-defined Phase III validation trial on PLCO serum samples [48]. The specimens from cases were the last pre-diagnostic sample collected, and the control samples were obtained from subjects without an ovarian cancer diagnosis at the end of the trial. These biomarkers were rated previously in a Phase II trial among a set of > 65 promising candidates, using clinical samples from 180 ovarian cancer cases and 660 benign controls assembled from four EDRN or Ovarian Cancer SPORE sites. Top performing biomarkers were CA125, HE4 (human epididymis protein), CA15-3, and CA72-4, with pre-diagnostic sensitivity ranging from 73% to 40% at 95% specificity. Biomarkers were tested individually as well as in panels. The conclusion was that no single biomarker or biomarker panel performed better than CA125 alone [49, 50].

From the mathematical models described above, and the extrapolation from larger tumors at diagnosis to presumably much smaller tumors six months or more prior to diagnosis, biomarker performance at diagnosis is expected to decrease, possibly substantially, in pre-diagnostic samples. In fact, most of the 28 biomarkers fail to have an appreciable sensitivity in pre-diagnostic samples. Possible explanations for the failure of most of these biomarkers tested at diagnosis, to detect ovarian cancer at an acceptable sensitivity and lead time in pre-diagnostic samples, are that the majority of them were identified and developed without taking into consideration the large histological heterogeneity of ovarian cancer as a disease, or using specimens from late stage disease, ascites or cystic fluids or cell lines [51]. While some of them may represent changes occurring late during the development of ovarian cancer, others may also be induced as a response of the individual to the disseminated cancer (i.e., acute phase reactants), as well as systematic differences in the conditions of sample collection. For example, samples from healthy controls are normally collected at regular gynecological check-up clinics, whereas cases are obtained before, during or after surgical procedure at the diagnostic surgery clinic.

To address this latter bias, samples from cases and controls from the same clinic, such as blood samples from women with pelvic masses prior to differential diagnosis (benign/malignant), are to be preferred, in order to evaluate biomarker performance at diagnosis, over case samples and control samples obtained from different clinics. Furthermore, samples to assess diagnostic performance should include samples from both late- and early-stage samples, to reduce the chance of identifying biomarkers arising only in late stage. Diagnostic performance is to be understood as an upper bound on, not as an estimate of, the performance in pre-diagnostic samples.

As was observed, most diagnostic biomarkers will fail as pre-diagnostic biomarkers, but the expectation is that a few of the diagnostic biomarkers will also prove to be present in earlier stages and will, therefore, be sensitive pre-diagnostic biomarkers with utility for early detection. Thus, the challenge is to test a large number of candidates, with strong validation in unbiased samples at diagnosis, in pre-diagnostic specimens, while consuming a minimum volume of a precious resource obtainable only from multi-year screening trials on a large cohort of subjects (10 000s or more).

Hori and Gambhir developed a mathematical model to describe biomarker kinetics relative to tumor growth from a single cancer cell, based on CA125 shedding data and ovarian tumor growth [52]. Based on their model, a tumor could reach a volume of 20.44 mm^3 and grow undetected for 10.1 years before currently available blood based assays could detect early cancer. Current blood-based markers were found to be 10^4-fold too low to provide a useful diagnostic role in the first decade of tumor growth. This limitation highlights the need

for highly sensitive methods, and/or biomarkers that detect smaller tumor volumes.

Autoantibodies to tumor-associated antigens could be induced by relatively small volumes of cancer early in the development of the disease. A variety of high-throughput strategies, including SEREX, phage display, high-density protein microarrays, serological proteome analysis and immunoaffinity purification, have sought to identify autoantibody biomarkers for ovarian cancer [53]. As virtually all high-grade serous cancers have mutations in TP53, anti-TP53 autoantibodies are of particular interest. With samples from UT MD Anderson Cancer Center, the NROSS trial, the Australia Ovarian Cancer Study Group (AOCSO) and the UKCTOCS, anti-TP53 autoantibodies have been found in 21–26% of ovarian cancer patients with similar fractions in early (I-II) and late (III-IV) stage disease) [54].

Using preclinical sera from the UKCTOCS study, anti-TP53 autoantibodies were elevated five (median) to 13.5 (mean) months prior to CA125 in patients detected with the ROCA algorithm, and 29 (median) to 33 (mean) months prior to clinical diagnosis in patients missed by CA125 and the ROCA algorithm. Of more than 110 candidates, this is the first biomarker to provide significant lead time over CA125. As anti-TP53 autoantibodies are only associated with 20–25% of ovarian cancers, the challenge remains to find a larger panel of autoantibodies or other biomarkers that would detect a larger fraction of ovarian cancers in advance of CA125. Utilizing the high-throughput methodologies described above, several researchers have sought to complement CA125 and anti-p53 autoantibodies with other suitable autoantibody biomarkers [55]. However, the utility of these promising autoantibody biomarkers remains to be validated in multiple preclinical specimens before their clinical utility and complementarity can be fully defined.

On the basis of the experience of the EDRN, and in the presence of the currently validated biomarkers for early detection of ovarian cancer, including CA125, HE4, CA15-3 and CA72-4, EDRN investigators have developed a number of criteria of acceptable values for sensitivity and specificity in the further development of a first-line biomarker test. The selection of 5–6 additional markers that complement CA125 and HE4, each with a pre-diagnostic sensitivity of at least 5% at a specificity of 98%, along with CA125 and HE4, could be candidates to form a panel that covers most ovarian cancer types, is presumed to be an achievable task [56]. Biomarkers of highest priority must be able to identify ovarian cancers that are not identified by CA125/HE4 and/or identify ovarian cancers earlier than CA125/HE4. Any biomarkers that are correlated in cases and, therefore, identify ovarian cancers that are being identified simultaneously by CA125, although not ideal, are a secondary priority. These would still contribute information on the presence of undetected tumors in situations where the longitudinal CA125 signal is weak to moderate, under the testable assumption that the variation of the new biomarkers and CA125 over time is uncorrelated in control subjects.

Investigators from six sites of the EDRN Breast/ Gynecology Collaborative group have launched a collaborative study to validate a set of more than 150 candidate biomarkers, which were identified during previous funding cycles of the Network. Considering that these biomarkers were identified via different approaches, and using diverse ovarian cancer-related samples, including tumor tissues, ascites and cystic fluids, and cell lines, many of them may be associated only with the very late stages in the development of ovarian cancers, and may not add any significant value to CA125. Hence, the EDRN has developed a process of prioritization of these biomarkers, based on *in silico* analysis of the differential expression of these markers at the RNA levels among ovarian cancer and healthy controls, on functional information as to whether they represent secreted or cell membrane-bound proteins, and on whether these biomarkers are present in blood, by employing multiple reaction monitoring (MR), a mass-spectrometry approach.

Following prioritization, high analytical sensitivity assays for the top 50 candidate biomarkers were developed by the EDRN Biomarker Laboratory (BRL) at Pacific Northwest National Laboratory (PNNL), using a multiplexed selective reaction monitoring-mass spectrometry approach. The PNNL assays identified 11 candidates for their ability to distinguish ovarian cancer cases from benign adnexal mass (BAM) controls at 98% specificity.

Multiplexed assays, using the MesoScale Discovery (MSD) platform, have been developed at the Johns Hopkins University EDRN BRL, for simultaneous measurement on small volume samples.

Any of the tested biomarkers that pass this criterion ($\geq$5% sensitivity at 98% specificity) will be re-tested in plasma from patients with benign and malignant pelvic masses at diagnosis, ranked by sensitivity at 98% specificity, and the top candidates further tested in a limited phase III validation study, using serial, pre-diagnostic samples obtained from the ROCA trial cohorts and from the Fox Chase Cancer Center biorepository. Finally, this evidence from a small number of biomarkers that potentially pass this last criterion will be presented to PLCO and/or UKCTOCS investigators, to request samples for a phase III retrospective longitudinal validation trial using pre-diagnostic serial samples.

Independently, efforts to identify and develop biomarkers for the early detection of ovarian cancers have also been undertaken using cervico-vaginal fluids (CVF). Based on the currently accepted assumption that high-grade serous ovarian cancers originate in the fimbriated portion of the fallopian tube, it is hypothesized that cells, DNA and proteins expressed by cells in precursor lesions, or in early stage neoplastic lesions, are shed directly into the mucous fluid discharge that ends up being collected during Pap tests, even before neoplastic lesions become vascularized.

Recently, a panel of genes that are commonly mutated in endometrial and ovarian cancers was used as a basis to identify mutations that are common in ovarian cancers, by employing sensitive massively parallel sequencing of DNA extracted from liquid Pap smear specimens [57]. The analysis led to the development of a panel of mutations in 12 genes, which could be tested simultaneously in a single liquid Pap smear specimen without previous knowledge of the tumor's genotype. DNA from 41% of ovarian cancers (nine of 22 samples tested) could be detected in a standard liquid-based Pap smear specimen obtained during routine pelvic examination. Whether this approach will detect early stage (I–II) cancer in a sporadic population remains to be determined. Perhaps the greatest potential would be in monitoring women with BRCA1 or BRCA2 mutations, prior to elective salpingo-oophorectomy.

Enhancing the second stage of two-stage screening

In addition to enhancing the initial stage of a two-stage screening strategy, there is substantial room for improvement in imaging during the second stage. TVS rarely images fallopian tubes and their fimbriae, and has limited resolution for small lesions. Efforts are underway to utilize nitrogen-filled albumin micro-bubbles that are FDA-approved for cardiovascular imaging to image the vasculature in pelvic masses [58]. While this approach clearly could improve specificity, how much it will augment sensitivity is uncertain.

Superconducting quantum interference detection (SQUID) has extraordinary sensitivity for measuring magnetic fields. Studies are underway to use ferritin nanoparticles coated with antibodies reactive with ovarian cancers to detect occult ovarian cancers using SQUID. In patients with rising biomarkers and negative TVS, a SQUID probe could be positioned over each ovary after injection of antibody-coated ferritin nanoparticles. When a magnetic pulse is passed through the region, free-floating nanoparticles do not affect its relaxation, whereas nanoparticles bound to ovarian cancer cells impede relaxation of a magnetic pulse. As few as 10^5 cancer cells can be detected with this technique [59]. If these observations can be confirmed and extended in ovarian cancers, sensitivity of the second phase in screening could be improved by more than an order of magnitude.

References

1. Kurman RJ, Shih Ie M (2010). The origin and pathogenesis of epithelial ovarian cancer: a proposed unifying theory. *American Journal of Surgical Pathology* **34**(3), 433–443.

2. Pothuri B, *et al.* (2010). Genetic analysis of the early natural history of epithelial ovarian carcinoma. *PLoS One* **5**(4), e10358.

3. Sharma A, *et al.* (2011). Assessing the malignant potential of ovarian inclusion cysts in postmenopausal women within the UK Collaborative Trial of Ovarian Cancer Screening (UKCTOCS): a prospective cohort study. *British Journal of Obstetrics and Gynaecology* **119**, 207–219.

4. Dubeau L (2008). The cell of origin of ovarian epithelial tumours. *The Lancet Oncology* **12**, 1191–1197.

5. Lauchlan SC (1972). The secondary Mullerian system. *Obstetrical & Gynecological Survey* **27**(3), 133–146.

6. Colgan TJ, *et al.* (2001). Occult carcinoma in prophylactic oophorectomy specimens: prevalence and association with BRCA germline mutation status. *American Journal of Surgical Pathology* **25**, 1283–1289.

7. Paley PJ, *et al.* (2001). Occult cancer of the fallopian tube in BRCA-1 germline mutation carriers at prophylactic oophorectomy: a case for recommending hysterectomy at surgical prophylaxis. *Gynecologic Oncology* **80**(2), 176–180.

8. Carcangiu ML, *et al.* (2004). Atypical epithelial proliferation in fallopian tubes in prophylactic salpingo-oophorectomy specimens from BRCA1 and BRCA2 germline mutation carriers. *International Journal of Gynecological Pathology* **23**(1), 35–40.

9. Finch, A, *et al.* (2006). Clinical and pathologic findings of prophylactic salpingo-oophorectomies in 159 BRCA1 and BRCA2 carriers. *Gynecologic Oncology* **100**, 58–64.

10. Medeiros F, *et al.* (2006). The tubal fimbria is a preferred site for early adenocarcinoma in women with familial ovarian cancer syndrome. *American Journal of Surgical Pathology* **30**, 230–236.

11. Callahan MJ, *et al.* (2007). Primary fallopian tube malignancies in BRCA-positive women undergoing surgery for ovarian cancer risk reduction. *Journal of Clinical Oncology* **25**, 3985–3990.

12. Shaw PA, *et al.* (2009). Candidate serous cancer precursors in fallopian tube epithelium of BRCA1/2 mutation carriers. *Modern Pathology* **22**, 1133–1138.

13. Jarboe E, *et al.* (2008). Serous carcinogenesis in the fallopian tube: a descriptive classification. *International Journal of Gynecological Pathology* **27**, 1–9.

14. Folkins, A. K, *et al.* (2009). Precursors to pelvic serous carcinoma and their clinical implications. *Gynecologic Oncology* **113**, 391–396.

15. Piek JM, *et al.* (2001). Dysplastic changes in prophylactically removed Fallopian tubes of women predisposed to developing ovarian cancer. *Journal of Pathology* **195**, 451–456.

16. Kindelberger DW, *et al.* (2007). Intraepithelial carcinoma of the fimbria and pelvic serous carcinoma: Evidence for a causal relationship. *American Journal of Surgical Pathology* **31**, 161–169.

17. Tong GX, *et al.* (2007). Expression of PAX2 in papillary serous carcinoma of the ovary: immunohistochemical evidence of fallopian tube or secondary Mullerian system origin? *Modern Pathology* **20**, 856–863.

18. Chen EY, *et al.* (2010). Secretory cell outgrowth, PAX2 and serous carcinogenesis in the Fallopian tube. *Journal of Pathology* **222**, 110–116.

19. Lee Y, *et al.* (2007). A candidate precursor to serous carcinoma that originates in the distal fallopian tube. *Journal of Pathology* **211**, 26–35.

20. Wethington SL, *et al.* (2008). Improved survival for fallopian tube cancer: a comparison of clinical

characteristics and outcome for primary fallopian tube and ovarian cancer. *Cancer* **113**, 3298–3306.

21. Pearce CL, *et al.* (2012). Association between endometriosis and risk of histological subtypes of ovarian cancer: a pooled analysis of case-control studies. *The Lancet Oncology* **13**(4), 385–394.

22. Wiegand KC, *et al.* (2010). ARID1A mutations in endometriosis-associated ovarian carcinomas. *New England Journal of Medicine* **363**(16), 1532–1543.

23. Guth U, Huang DJ, Bauer G, *et al.* (2007). Metastatic patterns at autopsy in patients with ovarian carcinoma. *Cancer* **110**, 1272–1280.

24. Kuo KT, *et al.* (2009). Analysis of DNA copy number alterations in ovarian serous tumors identifies new molecular genetic changes in low-grade and high-grade carcinomas. *Cancer Research* **69**, 4036–4042.

25. Lalwani N, *et al.* (2011). Histologic, molecular, and cytogenetic features of ovarian cancers: implications for diagnosis and treatment. *Radiographics* **31**, 625–646.

26. Cho KR, Shih Ie M (2010). Ovarian cancer. *Annual Review of Pathology* **4**, 287–313.

27. Gilks CB, Prat J (2009). Ovarian carcinoma pathology and genetics: recent advances. *Human Pathology* **40**, 1213–1223.

28. Kobayashi H, *et al.* (2009). The role of hepatocyte nuclear factor-1beta in the pathogenesis of clear cell carcinoma of the ovary. *International Journal of Gynecological Cancer* **19**, 471–479.

29. Mok SC, *et al.* (1993). Mutation of K-ras protooncogene in human ovarian epithelial tumors of borderline malignancy. *Cancer Research* **53**, 1489–1492.

30. Auner V, *et al.* (2009). KRAS mutation analysis in ovarian samples using a high sensitivity biochip assay. *BMC Cancer* **9**, 111.

31. Lalwani N, *et al.* (2011). Histologic, molecular, and cytogenetic features of ovarian cancers: implications for diagnosis and treatment. *Radiographics* **31**, 625–646.

32. Skates SJ, Singer D (1991). Quantifying the potential benefit of CA125 screening for ovarian cancer. *Journal of Clinical Epidemiology* **44**, 365–380

33. US Preventive Services Task Force (2005). Screening for ovarian cancer: recommendation statement. *American Family Physician* **71**, 759–762.

34. Brown DL, *et al.* (2010). ACR appropriateness criteria(c) ovarian cancer screening. *Ultrasound* **26**, 219–223.

35. Bast RC Jr, Hennessy B, Mills GB (2009). The Biology of Ovarian Cancer: New Opportunities for Translation. *Nature Reviews Cancer* **9**, 415–28.

36. Durinck S, Ho C, Wang NJ, *et al.* (2011). Temporal dissection of tumorigenesis in primary cancers. *Cancer Discovery* **1**(2), 137–143.

37. TCGA Network (2011). Integrated genomic analyses of ovarian carcinoma. *Nature* **474**, 609–615.

38. Nolen BM, Lokshin AE (2011). Screening for ovarian cancer: old tools, new lessons. *Cancer Biomarkers* **8**, 177–186.

39. Brown PO, Palmer C (2009). The preclinical natural history of serous ovarian cancer: defining the target for early detection. *PLoS Medicine* **6**(7), e1000114.

40. Menon U, Gentry-Maharaj A, *et al.* (2009). Sensitivity and specificity of multimodal and ultrasound screening for ovarian cancer, and stage distribution of detected cancers: results of the prevalence screen of the UK Collaborative Trial of Ovarian Cancer Screening (UKCTOCS). *The Lancet Oncology* **10**, 327–340.

41. Skates SJ, Xu FJ, Yu YH, *et al.* (1995). Toward an optimal algorithm for ovarian cancer screening with longitudinal tumor markers. *Cancer* **76**, 2004–2010.

42. Skates SJ, Jacobs IJ, Knapp RC (2001). Tumor markers in screening for ovarian cancer. *Methods in Molecular Medicine* **39**, 61–73.

43. Menon U, Ryan A, Gentry Maharaj A, *et al.* (2015). Risk algorithm using serial biomarker measurements doubles the number of screen-detected cancers compared with a single-threshold rule in the United Kingdom Collaborative Trial of Ovarian Cancer Screening. *Journal of Clinical Oncology* **33**, 2016–31.

44. Lu KH, Skates SJ, Hernandez MH, *et al.* (2013). A 2-stage ovarian cancer screening strategy using the Risk of Ovarian Cancer Algorithm (ROCA) identifies early-stage incident cancers and demonstrates high positive predictive value. *Cancer* **119**, 3454–619.

45. Raamanathan A, Simmons GW, Christodoulides N, Floriano PN, Furmaga WB, Lu KH, Bast RC Jr, McDevitt IT (2012). Programmable Bio-nano-chip system for serum CA125 quantification: Toward ovarian cancer diagnostics at point of care. *Cancer Prevention Research* **5**, 706–13.

46. Shadfan BH, Simmons AR, Simmons GW, *et al.* (2015). A multiplexable, microfluidic platform for the rapid quantitation of a biomarker panel for early ovarian cancer detection at the point-of-care. *Cancer Prevention Research* **8**, 37–48.

47. Drescher CW, Hawley S, *et al.* (2012). Impact of Screening Test Performance and Cost on Mortality Reduction and Cost-effectiveness of Multimodal Ovarian Cancer Screening. *Cancer Prevention Research* **5**, 1015–1024.

48. Pepe MS, *et al.* (2001). Phases of biomarker development for early detection of cancer. *Journal of the National Cancer Institute* **93**, 1054–1061.

49. Cramer DW, *et al.* (2011). Ovarian cancer biomarker performance in prostate, lung, colorectal, and ovarian cancer screening trial specimens. *Cancer Prevention Research* **4**, 365–374.

50. Zhu CS, *et al.* (2011). A framework for evaluating biomarkers for early detection: validation of biomarker

panels for ovarian cancer. *Cancer Prevention Research* **4**, 375–383.

51. Diamandis EP (2010). Cancer biomarkers: can we turn recent failures into success? *Journal of the National Cancer Institute* **102**, 1462–1467.

52. Hori SS, Gambhir SS (2011). Mathematical model identifies blood biomarker-based early cancer detection strategies and limitations. *Science Translational Medicine* **3**, 109

53. Martin K, Ricciardelli C, Hoffman P, *et al.* (2011). Exploring the immunoproteome for ovarian cancer biomarker discovery. *International Journal of Molecular Sciences* **12**, 410–28.

54. Yang WL, Simmons A, Lu Z, *et al.* (2015). TP53 autoantibody can detect CA125 screen negative ovarian cancer cases and can be elevated prior to CA125 in preclinical ovarian cancer. *Proceedings of the American Association for Cancer Research* **56**, (A#2838).

55. Chatterjee M, Tainsky MM (2010). Autoantibodies as biomarkers for ovarian cancer. *Cancer Biomarkers* **8**, 187–201.

56. Rodland KD, Maihle NJ (2011). Searching for a system: the quest for ovarian cancer biomarkers. *Cancer Biomarkers* **8**, 223–230.

57. Kinde I, Bettegowda C, Wang Y, *et al.* (2013). Evaluation of DNA from the Papanicolaou test to detect ovarian and endometrial cancers. *Science Translational Medicine* **5**, 167.

58. Willmann JK, Kimura RH, Deshpande N, *et al.* (2010). Targeted contrast-enhanced ultrasound imaging of tumor angiogenesis with contrast microbubbles conjugated to integrin-binding knottin peptides. *Journal of Nuclear Medicine* **51**, 433–40.

59. De Haro LP, Karaulanov T, Vreeland EC, *et al.* (2015). Targeted contrast-enhanced ultrasound imaging of tumor angiogenesis with contrast microbubbles conjugated to integrin-binding knottin peptides. *Biomedical Engineering/Biomedizinische Technik* **60**, 445–455.

60. Ferlay J, *et al.* (2008). Estimates of worldwide burden of cancer in 2008: GLOBOCAN 2008. *International Journal of Cancer* **127**, 2893–2917.

61. Howlader N, *et al.* (2012). *SEER Cancer Statistics Review, 1975–2009.* National Cancer Institute, Bethesda, MD.

62. Siegel RL, Miller KD, Jemel A (2015). Cancer Statistics 2015. *CA: A Cancer Journal for Clinicians* **65**, 5–29.

CHAPTER 9

Esophageal Cancer Biomarkers

Yanxin Luo,[1,2] Kishore Guda,[5] Sanford D Markowitz,[6]
Amitabh Chak,[7] Andrew M Kaz,[2,3,4] and William M Grady[2,4]

[1] Department of Colorectal Surgery, The Sixth Affiliated Hospital, Sun Yat-Sen University, Guangzhou, P.R. China

[2] Clinical Research Division, Fred Hutchinson Cancer Research Center, Seattle, WA, USA

[3] Research and Development Service, VA Puget Sound Health Care System, Seattle, WA, USA

[4] Department of Medicine, University of Washington School of Medicine, Seattle, WA, USA

[5] General Medical Sciences-Oncology, Case Western Reserve University, University Hospitals of Cleveland, Cleveland, OH, USA

[6] Oncology Division, Case Western Reserve University, University Hospitals of Cleveland, Cleveland, OH, USA

[7] Gastroenterology Division, Case Western Reserve University, University Hospitals of Cleveland, Cleveland, OH, USA

Introduction

Esophageal cancer, which is most commonly either esophageal squamous cell carcinoma (ESCC) or esophageal adenocarcinoma (EAC), is one of the most common causes of cancer-related death worldwide, especially in developing countries [1]. In contrast to the steadily decreasing incidence of the four most common malignancies (lung, colorectal, prostate and breast cancer), the incidence of esophageal cancer has been rapidly increasing globally in the past two decades [1,2]. Notably, not only the incidence rates, but also the histology types of esophageal cancer, vary by region [3]. ESCC is the predominant histological type of esophageal cancer worldwide, and is the most common type of esophageal cancer in developing Asian countries [4]. However, in some developed countries, such as Australia, the UK, the USA, and southern European countries, EAC is more common, and exceeds that of SCC [5].

Major risk factors for ESCC in the developing Asian countries include poor nutritional status, low intake of fruits and vegetables, and drinking very hot beverages. In developed countries, smoking and excessive alcohol consumption appear to be the most common risk factors, and are found in approximately 90% of all cases of ESCC. Risk factors for EAC include smoking, obesity, and chronic gastroesophageal reflux disease (GERD) [6]. Chronic GERD is thought to induce Barrett's esophagus (BE) – a metaplastic change of the esophageal mucosa that is associated with an increased risk of EAC [7]. Individuals with BE are estimated to have an approximate 30× increased risk for EAC, compared with the average population, and 0.3–0.5% of patients with BE are estimated to develop EAC each year [8,9].

With regards to the pathogenesis of ESCC, it is thought to develop from a hyperproliferative squamous epithelium that can progress to low, intermediate, and then high-grade dysplasia before evolving into invasive cancer. In contrast, most EAC originates in Barrett's esophagus (BE), a pre-malignant condition where the squamous epithelium of the tubular esophagus is replaced

Biomarkers in Cancer Screening and Early Detection, First Edition. Edited by Sudhir Srivastava.
© 2017 John Wiley & Sons, Inc. Published 2017 by John Wiley & Sons, Inc.

by specialized intestinal-type columnar epithelium. EAC appears to arise via a metaplasia-dysplasia-carcinoma sequence, whereby Barrett's metaplasia can progress to low-grade dysplasia, followed by indeterminate dysplasia, and then high-grade dysplasia, before becoming intramucosal carcinoma and, finally, invasive carcinoma [10, 11].

Despite advances in treatment, the overall five-year survival of esophageal cancers ranges from 15% to 25% [11], predominantly due to the fact that only ≈ 20% of cancers are localized at the time of diagnosis [12]. Esophageal cancer also appears to have a propensity to metastasize, even when the tumors are superficial [13]. Hence, the development of methods to improve the early detection of these cancers is believed to be important, in order to improve the outcomes of patients with esophageal cancer. Towards this goal, the molecular alterations underlying the initiation and progression of esophageal cancer have been under intense investigation over the past three decades, which has resulted in a deeper understanding of the molecular pathogenesis of ESCC and EAC and identification of potential molecular markers for esophageal cancer. The purpose of this review is to summarize our current understanding of candidate biomarkers for BE, EAC, and ESCC, and to discuss their use as early detection or diagnostic markers for estimating prognosis, and for predicting response to treatment. Finally, we will address some of the challenges that must be overcome in order to develop clinically useful esophageal cancer biomarkers.

Molecular alterations in pre-malignant and malignant disease of the esophagus

Most of our knowledge of gene mutations and epigenetic alterations in BE, EAC, and ESCC has been derived from studies of individual candidate genes. Our understanding of the molecular pathology of esophageal cancer has been recently accelerated by technologic advances in DNA sequencing (e.g., next-generation sequencing) and in array design technologies (e.g., HumanMethylation450 array (Illumina)). A comprehensive analysis of somatic mutations in EAC, using whole-exome sequencing and whole-genome sequencing, has been recently

performed [14]. The investigators analyzed 149 EAC tumor-normal matched fresh-frozen samples, and identified a series of significantly mutated genes, including "classical" tumor-driver genes, such as *TP53, CDKN2A, SMAD4, ARID1A* and *PIK3CA*, as well as new candidate driver genes, such as *SPG20, TLR4, ELMO1* and *DOCK2* among others.

In another whole-exome sequencing study of a smaller collection of BE, EAC, and ESCC cases, *NOTCH1* mutations were found in ESCC cases, but not EACs [15]. Chromosomal instability and copy number alterations have been found in BE, EAC and ESCC [16, 17]. Paulson *et al.* identified 9p loss encompassing the p16/CDKN2A locus in BE, high-grade dysplasia (HGD) and EAC cases and losses on chromosome 5q, 13q and 18q in HGD and EAC, and high-level amplification at ERBB2 on chromosome 17q in EAC [18].

In addition, a genome-wide association study completed recently has taken a step further and identified common variants that are associated with genetic susceptibility to BE [19]. These investigators carried out a genome-wide association study on Barrett's esophagus (1852 cases and 5172 controls in the discovery stage, and 5986 cases and 12 825 controls in the replication stage). and identified variants at two loci that associated with BE: chromosome 6p21, rs9257809 (odds ratio (OR) = 1.21, 95% confidence interval (CI) = 1.13–1.28), within the major histocompatibility complex locus, and chromosome 16q24, rs9936833 (OR = 1.14, 95% CI = 1.10–1.19), for which the closest protein-coding gene is *FOXF1*. They also found evidence that many common variants of small effect contribute to genetic susceptibility to BE, and that SNP alleles predisposing to obesity also increase risk for BE [19].

Epigenetic alterations, such as DNA hypermethylation in the promoter regions of genes, have also been identified in pre-neoplastic (Barrett's esophagus and dysplastic squamous epithelium) and neoplastic tissues (EAC and ESCC) in the esophagus [7, 20]. Hypermethylated genes identified include known tumor-suppressor genes, such as *APC, CDKN2A (p16INK4a), RUNX3, MGMT, CDH1,* and *SFRP* family members, among others [7]. A subset of the hypermethylated genes are silenced by the aberrant methylation, and play a role in driving the formation of EAC. Aberrant methylation of classic tumor suppressor genes such as *CDKN2A* and *MGMT* has been shown in the BE→EAC progression sequence, and has been shown to correlate with loss of mRNA and protein expression in the metaplasia-dysplasia-carcinoma sequence of Barrett's esophagus and ESCC [21,22]. These findings suggest that aberrant DNA methylation is one of the molecular mechanisms that mediates the development of esophageal cancer.

MicroRNAs are small noncoding RNA molecules of approximately 20 nucleotides that play important roles in diverse cellular processes associated with carcinogenesis. There have been a growing number of studies focused on the potential biological roles of microRNAs (miRNA/miR) in esophageal cancer development [23,24]. For example, several studies have shown overexpression of miR-192 during BE→EAC progression [20]. miR-192 is a downstream target of p53, and plays a tumor-suppressor role through cell-cycle arrest [25]. From a clinical perspective, an interesting finding is that altered miRNAs can be detected in the blood of patients with esophageal cancer [26], which suggests there may be readily accessible molecular markers for early detection, monitoring chemotherapeutic responsiveness, etc. [27].

A subset of the genetic and epigenetic alterations found in different steps of the progression of BE or dysplasia to esophageal cancer are believed to contribute to the pathogenesis of these cancers through deregulated protein expression. For example, the expression levels of Fhit and E-cadherin have been shown to be suppressed, and that of p53 is increased, in expression in advanced disease [28, 29]. These changes in protein expression are being assessed as possible cancer molecular markers, using a variety of different techniques [30,31].

Early detection markers for Barrett's esophagus (BE)

Genetic and epigenetic alterations occurring at the early stage of esophageal cancer development can be used as early detection biomarkers. Candidate early detection markers include somatic mutations, aberrantly methylated genes and overexpressed miRNAs, as well as deregulated proteins.

Somatic mutations

There is a rich literature based on studies that have assessed for somatic mutations in specific candidate genes. These studies have identified common mutations in *CDKN2A, APC, FANCD2, CTNNB1, DVL3, MLF1, ABCC5, BCL6, AGTR1* and others [32]. A more recent study used whole exome-sequencing identified novel somatic mutations in genes such as *SPG20, TLR4, ELMO1* and *DOCK2*, as well as mutations in well-known cancer-associated mutated genes, such as *TP53, CDKN2A, SMAD4, ARID1A* and *PIK3CA* in esophageal cancers [14]. The most frequent somatic mutations found in this study of 149 EACs were *TP53* (72%), *SYNE1* (25%), *CDKN2A* (12%), *DOCK2* (12%) and *CNTNAP5* (10%) [14]. It is not known when most of these mutations arise in the BE→EAC progression sequence, although at least one study suggested that many of these mutations arise in the BE step in this process [15].

Aberrantly methylated genes

Aberrant DNA methylation occurring in BE or LGD/HGD has also been demonstrated in studies published over the past two decades. For example, the tumor suppressor *CDKN2A/p16INK4a*, which blocks phosphorylation of Retinoblastoma (RB) and inhibits cell cycle progression, was one of the first genes shown to be aberrantly methylated in BE and EAC. Hypermethylation of this gene promoter, combined with loss of heterozygosity (LOH) of 9p21 (which contains the p16INK4a locus), leads to CDKN2A inactivation in some individuals with EAC, or BE with dysplasia [33].

In a study that evaluated the methylation frequency of a 20-gene panel in 104 tissue samples from 51 people, *CDKN2A* was found to be methylated in 15% of BE tissue samples, and was unmethylated in normal gastric and esophageal tissues [34]. Methylation of the *CDKN2A* promoter was also found to be associated with other established genetic biomarkers in BE, including 17p (p53) LOH and increased aneuploidy/tetraploidy which, together, are thought to promote the clonal expansion of BE at high risk of transformation and to drive the process of carcinogenesis [35]. Hypermethylation of *CDKN2A* appears to occur early in the metaplasia-dysplasia-carcinoma sequence, with various studies reporting promoter methylation in

15–66% of BE cases [33–37]. These studies suggest that methylated *CDKN2A* might be a useful marker in a noninvasive assay for the diagnosis of BE.

Eads *et al.* assessed additional candidate methylated genes beyond CDKN2A in BE, including *APC, ESR1,* and *CDH1* in six esophagectomy specimens, which contained both BE and EAC. They performed discrete methylation analyses of numerous regions of each resected sample, to create spatial methylation maps comprised of 107 sites per specimen. They found a high incidence of methylation of *ESR1, APC* and *CDKN2A* in BE, BE with dysplasia, and EAC, in a pattern suggesting clonal expansion of those cells that had acquired methylated alleles of these genes. In contrast, *CDH1* was unmethylated in almost all of the samples [42]. These studies suggest that aberrant methylation of these genes occurs in contiguous fields, possibly indicative of clonal expansion of a hypermethylated cell or group of cells. Similar patterns consistent with clonal expansion in BE have been reported in studies that focused on LOH or mutations of *APC, TP53,* and *CDKN2A* [43].

Of note, the incidence of DNA methylation of the genes *CDKN2A, APC, SOCS-3* and *CDH13* was evaluated in some studies with larger size of BE samples (>30 cases), as listed in Table 9.1 In all of these studies, the prevalence of gene methylation was increased in EAC and ESCC, as well as in BE and BE with dysplasia, compared with normal esophagus. Experiments in cell lines with the demethylating agent 5-aza-2'-deoxcytidine established the relationship between methylation of these genes and reduced mRNA expression levels. Of note, although all of these genes have potential to be used as diagnostic molecular markers for BE and/or EAC, none of them have been subjected to rigorous validation studies.

miRNA

MicroRNAs (miRNA/miR) are a class of small noncoding RNAs that are often abnormally expressed in cancer. Growing evidence supports their role as tumor promoters and tumor suppressors in a variety of cancers. Expression profiles of miRNAs have been used to characterize molecular subtypes of cancers, and as prognostic and predictive markers for certain cancers. With regard to their use as biomarkers, miRNAs have been shown to be exceptionally stable in various tissues and body fluids and, thus, can be detected and quantitated reliably, which is an essential feature of a biomarker. These findings strongly underscore the clinical utility of miRNAs as predictive and prognostic biomarkers.

Given the low progression rate and lack of reliable epidemiological or histological grading predictors of cancer risk in Barrett's patients, there is a critical need for developing evidence-based

Table 9.1 Candidate methylated gene biomarkers for the early detection of BE.

Gene	Method	Normal	BE	LGD	HGD	EAC	Ref.
CDKN2A	MSP		8/21 (38%)				[33]
(p16INK4a)	MethyLight	Gastric: 0/12 (0%); Esophageal: 0/31 (0%)	2/10 (20%)	2/9 (22%)		9/22 (41%)	[34]
	MSP	2/64 (3%)	14/93 (15%)			34/76 (45%)	[36]
	MSP		27/41 (66%)	21/45 (47%)	17/21 (81%)	65/107 (61%)	[35]
	MSP	0/17 (0%)	14/47 (30%)	9/27 (33%)	10/18 (56%)	22/41 (54%)	[37]
APC	MSP	0/17 (0%)	24/48 (50%)	14/28 (50%)	14/18 (78%)	20/32 (63%)	[37]
	MS-SSCA and MS-DBA	0/16 (0%)	11/11 (100%)			20/21 (95%)	[38]
TAC1	MSP	5/67 (7%)	38/60 (63%)	12/19 (63%)	11/21 (52%)	41/67 (61%)	[39]
MGMT	MethyLight	Gastric: 3/12 (25%); Esophageal: 17/31 (55%)	6/10 (60%)	8/9 (89%)		16/22 (73%)	[34]
	MSP	6/29 (21%)	24/27 (89%)	13/13 (100%)		37/47 (79%)	[22]
SOCS-3	MSP	0/20 (0%)	4/30 (13%)	6/27 (22%)	20/29 (69%)	14/19 (74%)	[40]
CDH13	MSP	0/66 (0%)	42/60 (70%)	15/19 (79%)	16/21 (76%)	51/67 (76%)	[41]

molecular biomarkers of risk in this disease model. Recently, a number of studies have demonstrated the potential of miRNAs as predictive biomarkers of cancer risk in BE. By employing high-throughput techniques, such as microarrays and next generation sequencing, a number of recent studies have identified candidate miRNAs as markers of malignant progression in Barrett's esophagus.

Using concurrent BE, dysplasia and esophageal adenocarcinoma, Maru and colleagues identified miR-196a as a potential marker that shows incremental increases in expression with each step of progression from normal esophagus to metaplasia to dysplasia and carcinoma [44]. A positive correlation of miR-196a expression with progression from intestinal metaplasia to adenocarcinoma was also reported by Luzna et al. [45]. Furthermore, in a five-year follow-up study, miR-196a, in addition to miR-192, -194, and -196b, showed differential expression in BE patients who progressed to cancer compared to those who did not progress to cancer [46], providing additional support for miR-196a as a potential marker of cancer risk.

Kan et al. reported a modest but progressive increase in expression of a different set of miRNAs, including miR-106b, -25, and -93, which are part of the miR-106b polycistron, in metaplasia and carcinoma in cultured cells and tissues. They proposed an oncogenic role for these miRNAs in driving esophageal tumor progression [47]. The upregulation of these oncomirs was further associated with genomic amplification and overexpression of the MCM7 locus on chromosome 7q22.1.23 [47].

In a pilot, phase 2, cross-sectional study, Bansal and colleagues compared miRNA expression signatures in metaplasia tissues from BE patients with or without dysplasia/cancer, and identified miR-15b, -203, and -21 as being discriminatory between BE patients with and without dysplasia/cancer, which suggested their potential utility for risk stratification [48]. Smith et al. showed decreased expression of miR-200 family members in esophageal adenocarcinomas when compared to Barrett's esophagus, and implicated their potential association with malignant progression [49]. On the other hand, Fassan et al. proposed a 5-miR signature, including let-7c, miR-203, -205, -192, and -215, as potential molecular biomarkers of neoplastic progression in BE, based on their significant alteration

in expression in a majority of metaplasia, dysplasia, and carcinoma lesions when compared with normal squamous tissues [50].

Recently, Leidner and colleagues comprehensively characterized miRNA alterations during progressive stages of esophageal adenocarcinoma [51]. Using next generation sequencing as an agnostic discovery platform, followed by quantitative real-time PCR validation, 26 miRNAs that are highly and frequently deregulated in esophageal adenocarcinomas when compared to paired normal esophageal squamous tissue were identified [51]. Their results showed that the majority of cancer-associated miRNAs are deregulated at the metaplasia stage, suggesting these miRs to be metaplasia-derived rather than markers of progression [51]. Two miRNAs, miR-31 and -31* however showed frequent downregulation only in high-grade dysplasia and cancer cases, suggesting association with transition from metaplasia to dysplasia, while another miRNA, miR-375, showed marked downregulation exclusively in cancer, suggesting its association with progression to invasive carcinoma [51]. These findings suggest miR-31 and -375 as potential markers of progression during early and late stages of tumorigenesis, respectively.

More recently, Wu et al., using a microarray approach, identified progressive alterations in expression of miR-21, -25, -223, -205, -203, let-7c, -133a, -301b, -618, and -23b from Barrett's esophagus to esophageal adenocarcinoma [24]. Similar to the findings from our study [51], Wu et al. identified miR-375 as a miRNA being downregulated exclusively in cancers, additionally supporting its role as a marker of cancer progression in Barrett's esophagus. Interestingly, several of the above miRNAs associated with progression have also been shown to be correlated with overall survival in cancer patients. For example, reduced expression of miR-375 in EAC has been associated with poor prognosis [52, 53], and miR-375 has been shown to have functional activity in suppressing growth of gastro-esophageal malignant cells [54, 55]. In addition, using global miRNA expression profiling or in situ hybridization, several miRNAs, including miR-143, -199a_3p, -199a_5p, -100, -99a, -16-2, -30e and -200a, have been shown to be associated with reduced overall survival in cancers [56].

Table 9.2 miRNAs as biomarkers for BE/EAC.

miRNAs	Result	Normal	BE	LGD	HGD	EAC	Ref.
Increased in BE/EAC							
miR-192	$P < 0.00001$		12	27		12	[45]
	1.7-fold	9	5		1	10	[60]
	6.34-fold	15	15	15	15	15	[50]
	ROC AUC = 0.61		24 (7 BE progressed to EAC; 17 not progressed)				[46]
miR-196a	ROC AUC = 0.80		24 (7 BE progressed to EAC; 17 not progressed)				[46]
	28.9 fold		11	11	11	11	[44]
	$P < 0.05$		12	27		12	[45]
miR-21	1.7-fold	100				100	[52]
	3.7-fold	9	5		1	10	[60]
	2.8-fold		7			9	[61]
miR-194	126-fold		7			9	[61]
	3.7-fold	9	5		1	10	[60]
	ROC AUC = 0.70		24 (7 BE progressed to EAC; 17 not progressed)				[46]
	3.5-fold	100				100	[52]
Decreased in BE/EAC							
miR-203	$P < 0.00001$		12	27		12	[45]
	3.0-fold	100				100	[52]
	6.67-fold	15	15	15	15	15	[50]
	1.49-fold	91		31	29	31	[57]
	17-fold		7			9	[61]
Let-7a	3.3-fold		22 (11 BE with dysplasia; 11 without dysplasia)				[48]
	1.75-fold	91		31	29	31	[57]
Let-7c	2.04-fold	15	15	15	15	15	[50]
	1.69-fold	91		31	29	31	[57]

Table 9.2 is a summary table of miRNAs in BE/EAC that have been shown to be over- or underexpressed in at least two independent studies. The expression of some of these candidate miRNAs, such as miR-192 and 196a, have been consistently found to be increased by many groups, while others, such as miR-143, are less consistent [20]. The Let-7 family member is consistently repressed in BE/EAC or BE with dysplasia, which is consistent with having a tumor suppressor function by suppressing KRAS [48, 50, 57].

Regarding the potential for miRNAs to be used as biomarkers, miRNA levels in serum or plasma have been assessed in patients with BE and/or EAC. Takeshita and colleagues conducted miRNA profiling on serum from patients with ESCC, and identified miR-1246 as a novel biomarker capable of detecting 71.3% of ESCC with a specificity of 73.9% [58]. In addition, they also demonstrated that miR-1246 was an independent risk factor for unfavorable survival (HR, 4.032; $P = 0.017$). Zhang and colleagues also carried out serum miRNA profiling of patients with ESCC. They identified a miRNA-panel with seven miRNAs (miR-10a, miR-22, miR-100, miR-148b, miR-223, miR-133a, and miR-127-3p) that can identify patients with early stage ESCC [59]. These findings highlight the potential of using the miRNAs as biomarkers for the non-invasive early detection of esophageal cancers.

Although significant progress has been made in characterizing miRNA alterations in BE and EAC, there are still substantial limitations in the existing data, including most notably the lack of a consensus miRNA signature of cancer risk across the different studies. This is likely a consequence of studies with small sample sizes, inherent variations among study populations, differing methods for detecting miR-NAs, and cellular heterogeneity in BE and EAC. In order to advance the field, large cohort studies, using uniform detection methods, are needed.

Protein biomarkers

In addition to nucleic acid-based biomarkers, there has been considerable effort to identify protein biomarkers for BE, esophageal dysplasia, ESCC and EAC. Several teams of investigators have used two-dimensional gel electrophoresis, coupled with mass spectrometry, to identify differentially expressed proteins during the esophageal cancer development [30]. For example, Pawar and colleagues used comparative proteomics on 10 ESCC, and matched normal samples and found 257 proteins that were differentially expressed in ESCC, compared with the normal samples. Some of these proteins were further confirmed by immunostaining on an independent collection of samples [30, 62]. Zhao and colleagues used comparative proteomics on the Barrett metaplasia and EAC, and found 38 differentially expressed proteins, which they verified by immunohistochemistry [31].

At this time, the majority of protein biomarkers have not progressed past phase II studies. One notable exception is TFF3, which has been shown to be an effective detection marker for BE by immunostaining of cytology samples obtained with the Cytosponge device (sensitivity of >93% for BE >2 cm in length) [63].

Biomarkers for predicting the risk of progression of BE to EAC

BE is associated with a 30× increased risk of EAC, which has led to the recommendation that patients with BE undergo regular endoscopic surveillance [9]. However, only 0.2% of people with Barrett's esophagus will progress to high-grade dysplasia or EAC each year, so a biomarker (or biomarker panel) that can more accurately risk stratify patients with BE would be of great clinical utility. Such a marker could potentially spare the great majority of individuals with a diagnosis of BE from the cost, inconvenience, and minimal risk of regular endoscopic surveillance. Being placed in a "low-risk" group

might also reduce the feelings of anxiety about developing EAC that have been shown to be associated with a diagnosis of BE [64].

The search for accurate risk stratification markers for BE is an area of intense investigation that has led to the identification of a number of promising risk biomarkers. None of these markers have proven adequate to be used in the clinical setting, although immunostaining assays for p53 and aneuploidy appear highly promising [9].

Another panel assay that has shown potential to identify BE at increased risk of transformation was assessed in a retrospective study that compared BE patients who progressed to HGD or EAC against those who did not. Hypermethylated CDKN2A (OR 1.74, 95% CI 1.33–2.20), RUNX3 (OR 1.80, 95% CI 1.08–2.81), and HPP1 (OR 1.77, 95% CI 1.06–2.81) were associated with an increased risk of progression. Age, BE segment length, and hypermethylation of other genes (TIMP3, APC, or CRBP1) were not found to be independent risk factors [36].

A follow-up study using these same epigenetic markers, in combination with three clinical parameters (gender, BE segment length (SL), and pathologic assessment), demonstrated this multi-parameter method could stratify BE patients into high, intermediate, and low risk for progression to HGD or EAC. However, it has not been adopted into routine clinical use to date [65]. In a later iteration of this approach, this risk assessment tool was expanded to include additional genes previously shown to be hypermethylated in BE and/or EAC, most of which have been described in the previous section, to generate an eight-marker risk-of-progression panel. In a retrospective analysis of 145 nonprogressors and 50 progressors, this panel predicted progression with a sensitivity of ≈ 50% when the specificity was set at 90% [66].

In addition to methylated gene biomarkers, there is evidence that microRNAs may be effective predictive markers for BE progressing to EAC. Revilla-Nuin and colleagues found that a series miRNAs (miR-192, 194, 196a, and 196b) were more highly expressed in BE samples from patients with progression to EAC, compared with those who did not progress to EAC [46]. As mentioned above, the let-7 family has also been found to be associated with progression of BE to EAC [24, 46]. However, none of these candidates have advanced to phase III or IV biomarker trials.

Biomarkers for prognosis and disease recurrence

Currently, tumor grade, stage, histological type, and residual disease following surgery are the most accurate prognostic factors for survival and disease recurrence in patients with esophageal cancer. Although these parameters are the best available prognostic markers, they are suboptimal for the accurate prediction of an individual's disease-free and overall survival [7]. In order to improve our ability to determine an individual's prognosis, recent research has focused on genetic and epigenetic changes in esophageal cancers, based on the premise that these alterations are responsible for the heterogenous clinical behavior of EAC and ESCC.

Brock *et al.* examined the methylation status of seven genes in 41 esophagectomy specimens containing EAC with matched normal tissue, and found increased methylation in the genes *APC*, E-cadherin (*CDH1*), *MGMT, ER, CDKN2A, DAPK*, and *TIMP3*. Individuals with >50% of their gene profile showing aberrant methylation had significantly reduced survival ($p = 0.04$) and earlier tumor recurrence ($p = 0.05$), compared with those individuals with <50% of their genes showing aberrant methylation. A positive methylation status was a better predictor of survival than either age or tumor stage [67]. Other methylated genes that have been associated with a poor prognosis in EAC include *NELL1* and *TAC1* [7].

With regards to the miRNAs, Komatsu and colleagues reported that patients with high miR-21 and low miR-375 concentrations in plasma had significantly worse prognosis (three-year survival rate: 48.4 and 83.1%, $p = 0.039$; $n = 50$) [68]. Decreased miR-375 expression in ESCC was found to associate with tumor metastasis and a poor prognosis in a large ($N = 300$) retrospective cohort study [69].

Protein biomarkers have also shown potential to be used as prognostic biomarkers for esophageal cancer. Kelly and colleagues identified three proteins (apolipoprotein A-I, serum amyloid A and transthyretin) in pre-treatment serum samples that associated with disease-free survival and overall survival in univariate and multivariate analysis [70]. Uemura and colleagues identified TGM3 as an unfavorable prognostic biomarker for esophageal cancer, and confirmed this observation in a validation set of samples. They found the five-year disease-specific survival rate was 64.5% and 32.1% for patients with TGM3-positive vs. TGM3-negative tumors, respectively [71].

Biomarkers to predict treatment response

Patients with advanced esophageal cancer often have recurrent cancer after curative surgical resection, which has led to the use of neoadjuvant and adjuvant chemoradiotherapy. However, many esophageal cancers fail to respond to these therapies. Thus, molecular markers that can predict sensitivity to specific chemotherapeutic agents or radiation therapy would dramatically enhance the treatment of these patients by allowing customization of the treatment regimens to maximize benefit, while limiting the toxicity associated with these therapies (Table 9.3).

One promising class of predictive markers is aberrantly methylated DNA damage repair genes (e.g. *MGMT, MLH1, BLM*), cell cycle checkpoint regulators (e.g. *CDKN2A, p14ARF*) and apoptosis regulating genes (e.g. *PTEN*). Methylation of these genes has the potential to affect treatment response by making the tumor cells vulnerable to the genotoxic effects of chemotherapy [72]. When chemoradiation responders ($N = 13$) and nonresponders ($N = 22$) with esophageal cancer were compared in one study, the number of methylated genes was found to be lower in responders (1.4 versus 2.4 genes per patient when the genes *CDKN2A, REPRIMO, p57, p73, RUNX3, CHFR, MGMT, TIMP3*, and *HPP1* were analyzed) [73]. With respect to individual genes, in this study, methylated *REPRIMO* was detected at significantly lower levels (and less frequently) in chemoradiotherapy responders versus nonresponders.

Sugimura and colleagues showed that let-7 expression in esophageal cancer may predict the response to cisplatin-based chemotherapy [74]. Odentha and colleagues compared the miRNA profiles between four responders and four nonresponders, and identified miR-192, miR-194

Table 9.3 Biomarkers to predict treatment response.

Samples	Size	Methodologies	Validation	Conclusion	Ref
Methylated loci/genes					
Tissue	35 patients (13 responders and 22 non-responders)	MSP	no	Reprimo methylation occurred at significantly lower levels and less frequently in chemoradioresponsive than in nonresponsive esophageal cancer patients	[73]
miRNAs					
Serum samples	64 patients (39 responders and 25 nonresponders)	qPCR	no	High expression of miR-200c was associated with shortened progression-free survival	[79]
Tissue samples	8 patients (4 major responder and 4 minor responders)	miRNA arrays	qPCR on 30 major responder and 50 minor responders	miR-192 and miR-194 in pretherapeutic biopsies are considered as indicators of major histopathologic regression	[75]
Tissue samples	19 patients (9 good responders and 10 poor responders)	miRNA arrays	qPCR on 37 samples and 29 sample using DNA repair gene study	high miR-31 expression were more likely to respond to the radiation	[76]
Tissue samples	cisplatin-resistant esophageal cancer cell lines compared with those parent cell lines	qPCR	74 patients in training set; 24 samples in validation set	low expression of let-7b and let-7c in pretreatment biopsies correlated significantly with poor response to chemotherapy	[74]
Proteins					
Serum samples	31 (16 poor response to neoadjuvant chemoradiation; 15 responders)	SELDI-TOF-MS	ELISA on the same set of samples	Pretreatment serum C4a and C3a levels were significantly higher in poor responders versus good responders	[48]
Tissue samples	20 (not sure of the number for chemotherapy responders and nonresponders)	2D/MS	34 samples (including the 20 samples used for proteomics experiments)	Low HSP27 expression was associated with no response to neoadjuvant chemotherapy	[78]

and miR-622 as the predictors for multimodality therapy response. Among these, miR-192 and miR-194 in pretherapeutic biopsies were validated in an independent collection of 80 samples. These microRNAs predicted major histopathologic regression [75]. Interestingly, certain miRNAs appear to modulate the sensitivity to radiation. For insistence, Lynam-Lennon and colleagues found that patients with esophageal cancers with high miR-31 expression were more likely to have a favorable response to radiation than those with low miR-31 expression [76].

There are also promising protein biomarkers that have been shown in phase II studies to predict tumor sensitivity to neoadjuvant therapy. This sort of studies had not only done *in vitro* cell line systems [77], but also in human serum or tissue samples. Langer and colleagues identified HSP27 as a marker for sensitivity to neoadjuvant chemotherapy [78]. Bansal and colleagues found that pretreatment serum C4a and C3a levels were significantly higher in poor responders versus good responders to the neoadjuvant chemoradiation [48].

Obstacles to the discovery of useful biomarkers for BE and esophageal cancer

The clinical application of methylated molecular biomarkers for both the diagnosis and prognosis of BE and esophageal cancer is hindered by the lack of adequate validation clinical trials (Phase 2–3 biomarker studies) [80]. A thorough review by Kaz *et al.* summarizes many of these issues, which are not unique to the field of esophageal cancer but are problematic for cancer biomarkers in general [7]. Most of the epigenetic biomarkers described in the current review are Phase 1–3 biomarkers, with only "any p16 lesion" (which includes hypermethylation, LOH, and sequencing of p16INK4a) having been assessed in a phase 4 study [81].

The primary barrier to developing clinically useful biomarkers is the lack of suitably large prospective clinical trials, which are hindered by the lack of sizeable esophageal tissue repositories that include complete clinical annotation. The design and implementation of large-scale trials will likely require multi-institutional cooperation and significant funding, in order to generate the cohorts needed to validate the promising biomarkers that have been identified to date.

Conclusions

In summary, there are increasing numbers of studies focusing on the biomarker development in esophageal cancers. Although many of these studies involve the analysis of relatively few patients, and are generally not prospective in nature, genetic and epigenetic alterations, as well as altered protein expression, appear to be associated with Barrett's esophagus and esophageal cancer and, thus, show considerable potential to be used as diagnostic biomarkers. Additionally, in some cases, these molecular alterations have been shown to be associated with clinical outcomes, including disease prognosis or response to treatment, which demonstrates the potential of these alterations to serve also as prognostic or predictive biomarkers.

More recently, genome-wide, microarray-based approaches have begun to uncover additional differences in the genetic and epigenetic levels between the normal esophagus, esophageal precursor lesions, and esophageal cancer. Further evaluation of these molecular changes between these groups, in the form of relatively large, prospective clinical trials, is needed in order to develop clinically useful biomarkers for the management of individuals with esophageal cancer or BE.

Acknowledgements

Grant support: Efforts on preparing this manuscript were supported by National Institutes of Health (NIH) National Cancer Institute (NCI) Program award P01CA77852; RO1CA115513, P30CA15704, UO1CA152756, U01CA086402, U54CA163060, U54CA143862, and P01CA077852 (WMG); Burroughs Wellcome Fund Translational Research Award for Clinician Scientist (WMG).

References

1. Jemal A, Bray F, Center MM, Ferlay J, Ward E, Forman D (2011). Global cancer statistics. *CA: A Cancer Journal for Clinicians* **61**(2), 69–90.

2. Ferlay J, Shin HR, Bray F, Forman D, Mathers C, Parkin DM (2010). Estimates of worldwide burden of cancer in 2008: GLOBOCAN 2008. *International Journal of Cancer* **127**(12), 2893–917.

3. Kamangar F, Dores GM, Anderson WF (2006). Patterns of cancer incidence, mortality, and prevalence across five continents: defining priorities to reduce cancer disparities in different geographic regions of the world. *Journal of Clinical Oncology* **24**(14), 2137–50.

4. Hongo M, Nagasaki Y, Shoji T (2009). Epidemiology of esophageal cancer: Orient to Occident. Effects of chronology, geography and ethnicity. *Journal of Gastroenterology and Hepatology* **24**(5), 729–35.

5. Pohl H, Welch HG (2005). The role of overdiagnosis and reclassification in the marked increase of esophageal adenocarcinoma incidence. *Journal of the National Cancer Institute* **97**(2), 142–6.

6. Paulson TG, Reid BJ (2004). Focus on Barrett's esophagus and esophageal adenocarcinoma. *Cancer Cell* **6**(1), 11–6.

7. Kaz AM, Grady WM (2012). Epigenetic biomarkers in esophageal cancer. *Cancer Letters* **342**(2), 193–9.

8. Moyes LH, Going JJ (2011). Still waiting for predictive biomarkers in Barrett's oesophagus. *Journal of Clinical Pathology* **64**(9), 742–50.

9. Fitzgerald RC, di Pietro M, Ragunath K, Ang Y, Kang JY, Watson P, *et al.* (2014). British Society of Gastroenterology guidelines on the diagnosis and management of Barrett's oesophagus. *Gut* **63**(1), 7–42.

10. Sharma P (2009). Clinical practice. Barrett's esophagus. *New England Journal of Medicine* **361**(26), 2548–56.

11. Pennathur A, Gibson MK, Jobe BA, Luketich JD (2013). Oesophageal carcinoma. *The Lancet* **381**(9864), 400–12.

12. Siegel R, Naishadham D, Jemal A (2012). Cancer statistics, 2012. *CA: A Cancer Journal for Clinicians* **62**(1), 10–29.

13. Pennathur A, Farkas A, Krasinskas AM, Ferson PF, Gooding WE, Gibson MK, *et al.* (2009). Esophagectomy for T1 esophageal cancer: outcomes in 100 patients and implications for endoscopic therapy. *Annals of Thoracic Surgery* **87**(4), 1048–54; discussion 54–5.

14. Dulak AM, Stojanov P, Peng S, Lawrence MS, Fox C, Stewart C, *et al.* (2013). Exome and whole-genome sequencing of esophageal adenocarcinoma identifies recurrent driver events and mutational complexity. *Nature Genetics* **45**(5), 478–86.

15. Agrawal N, Jiao Y, Bettegowda C, Hutfless SM, Wang Y, David S, *et al.* (2012). Comparative genomic analysis of esophageal adenocarcinoma and squamous cell carcinoma. *Cancer Discovery* **2**(10), 899–905.

16. Reid BJ (2010). Early events during neoplastic progression in Barrett's esophagus. *Cancer Biomarkers* **9**(1–6), 307–24.

17. Hu N, Wang C, Ng D, Clifford R, Yang HH, Tang ZZ, *et al.* (2009). Genomic characterization of esophageal squamous cell carcinoma from a high-risk population in China. *Cancer Research* **69**(14), 5908–17.

18. Paulson TG, Maley CC, Li X, Li H, Sanchez CA, Chao DL, *et al.* (2009). Chromosomal instability and copy number alterations in Barrett's esophagus and esophageal adenocarcinoma. *Clinical Cancer Research* **15**(10), 3305–14.

19. Su Z, Gay LJ, Strange A, Palles C, Band G, Whiteman DC, *et al.* (2012). Common variants at the MHC locus and at chromosome 16q24.1 predispose to Barrett's esophagus. *Nature Genetics* **44**(10), 1131–6.

20. Shah AK, Saunders NA, Barbour AP, Hill MM (2013). Early diagnostic biomarkers for esophageal adenocarcinoma – the current state of play. *Cancer Epidemiology, Biomarkers & Prevention* **22**(7), 1185–209.

21. Salam I, Hussain S, Mir MM, Dar NA, Abdullah S, Siddiqi MA, *et al.* (2009). Aberrant promoter methylation and reduced expression of p16 gene in esophageal squamous cell carcinoma from Kashmir valley: a high-risk area. *Molecular and Cellular Biochemistry* **332**(1–2), 51–8.

22. Kuester D, El-Rifai W, Peng D, Ruemmele P, Kroeckel I, Peters B, *et al.* (2009). Silencing of MGMT expression by promoter hypermethylation in the metaplasia-dysplasia-carcinoma sequence of Barrett's esophagus. *Cancer Letters* **275**(1), 117–26.

23. Song JH, Meltzer SJ (2012). MicroRNAs in pathogenesis, diagnosis, and treatment of gastroesophageal cancers. *Gastroenterology* **143**(1), 35–47 e2.

24. Wu X, Ajani JA, Gu J, Chang DW, Tan W, Hildebrandt MA, *et al.* (2013). MicroRNA expression signatures during malignant progression from Barrett's esophagus to esophageal adenocarcinoma. *Cancer Prevention Research (Philadelphia)* **6**(3), 196–205.

25. Braun CJ, Zhang X, Savelyeva I, Wolff S, Moll UM, Schepeler T, *et al.* (2008). p53-Responsive micrornas 192 and 215 are capable of inducing cell cycle arrest. *Cancer Research* **68**(24), 10094–104.

26. Komatsu S, Ichikawa D, Takeshita H, Tsujiura M, Morimura R, Nagata H, *et al.* (2011). Circulating microRNAs in plasma of patients with oesophageal squamous cell carcinoma. *British Journal of Cancer* **105**(1), 104–11.

27. Kurashige J, Kamohara H, Watanabe M, Tanaka Y, Kinoshita K, Saito S, *et al.* (2012). Serum microRNA-21 is a novel biomarker in patients with esophageal squamous cell carcinoma. *Journal of Surgical Oncology* **106**(2), 188–92.

28. Hayashi A, Yashima K, Takeda Y, Sasaki S, Kawaguchi K, Harada K, *et al.* (2012). Fhit, E-cadherin, p53, and activation-induced cytidine deaminase expression in endoscopically resected early stage esophageal squamous neoplasia. *Journal of Gastroenterology and Hepatology* **27**(11), 1752–8.

29. Chava S, Mohan V, Shetty PJ, Manolla ML, Vaidya S, Khan IA, *et al.* (2012). Immunohistochemical evaluation

of p53, FHIT, and IGF2 gene expression in esophageal cancer. *Diseases of the Esophagus* **25**(1), 81–7.

30. Qi YJ, Chao WX, Chiu JF (2012). An overview of esophageal squamous cell carcinoma proteomics. *Journal of Proteomics* **75**(11), 3129–37.

31. Zhao J, Chang AC, Li C, Shedden KA, Thomas DG, Misek DE, *et al.* (2007). Comparative proteomics analysis of Barrett metaplasia and esophageal adenocarcinoma using two-dimensional liquid mass mapping. *Molecular & Cellular Proteomics* **6**(6), 987–99.

32. Chen J, Guo L, Peiffer DA, Zhou L, Chan OT, Bibikova M, *et al.* (2008). Genomic profiling of 766 cancer-related genes in archived esophageal normal and carcinoma tissues. *International Journal of Cancer* **122**(10), 2249–54.

33. Wong DJ, Barrett MT, Stoger R, Emond MJ, Reid BJ (1997). p16INK4a promoter is hypermethylated at a high frequency in esophageal adenocarcinomas. *Cancer Research* **57**(13), 2619–22.

34. Eads CA, Lord RV, Wickramasinghe K, Long TI, Kurumboor SK, Bernstein L, *et al.* (2001). Epigenetic patterns in the progression of esophageal adenocarcinoma. *Cancer Research* **61**(8), 3410–8.

35. Wong DJ, Paulson TG, Prevo LJ, Galipeau PC, Longton G, Blount PL, *et al.* (2001). p16(INK4a) lesions are common, early abnormalities that undergo clonal expansion in Barrett's metaplastic epithelium. *Cancer Research* **61**(22), 8284–9.

36. Schulmann K, Sterian A, Berki A, Yin J, Sato F, Xu Y, *et al.* (2005). Inactivation of p16, RUNX3, and HPP1 occurs early in Barrett's-associated neoplastic progression and predicts progression risk. *Oncogene* **24**(25), 4138–48.

37. Wang JS, Guo M, Montgomery EA, Thompson RE, Cosby H, Hicks L, *et al.* (2009). DNA promoter hypermethylation of p16 and APC predicts neoplastic progression in Barrett's esophagus. *American Journal of Gastroenterology* **104**(9), 2153–60.

38. Clement G, Braunschweig R, Pasquier N, Bosman FT, Benhattar J (2006). Alterations of the Wnt signaling pathway during the neoplastic progression of Barrett's esophagus. *Oncogene* **25**(21), 3084–92.

39. Jin Z, Olaru A, Yang J, Sato F, Cheng Y, Kan T, *et al.* (2007). Hypermethylation of tachykinin-1 is a potential biomarker in human Esophageal cancer. *Clinical Cancer Research* **13**(21), 6293–300.

40. Tischoff I, Hengge UR, Vieth M, Ell C, Stolte M, Weber A, *et al.* (2007). Methylation of SOCS-3 and SOCS-1 in the carcinogenesis of Barrett's adenocarcinoma. *Gut* **56**(8), 1047–53.

41. Jin Z, Cheng YL, Olaru A, Kan T, Yang J, Paun B, *et al.* (2008). Promoter hypermethylation of CDH13 is a

common, early event in human esophageal adenocarcinogenesis and correlates with clinical risk factors. *International Journal of Cancer* **123**(10), 2331–6.

42. Eads CA, Lord RV, Kurumboor SK, Wickramasinghe K, Skinner ML, Long TI, *et al.* (2000). Fields of aberrant CpG island hypermethylation in Barrett's esophagus and associated adenocarcinoma. *Cancer Research* **60**(18), 5021–6.

43. Barrett MT, Sanchez CA, Prevo LJ, Wong DJ, Galipeau PC, Paulson TG, *et al.* (1999). Evolution of neoplastic cell lineages in Barrett oesophagus. *Nature Genetics* **22**(1), 106–9.

44. Maru DM, Singh RR, Hannah C, Albarracin CT, Li YX, Abraham R, *et al.* (2009). MicroRNA-196a Is a Potential Marker of Progression during Barrett's Metaplasia-Dysplasia-Invasive Adenocarcinoma Sequence in Esophagus. *American Journal of Pathology* **174**(5), 1940–8.

45. Luzna P, Gregar J, Uberall I, Radova L, Prochazka V, Ehrmann J, Jr. (2011). Changes of microRNAs-192, 196a and 203 correlate with Barrett's esophagus diagnosis and its progression compared to normal healthy individuals. *Diagnostic Pathology* **6**, 114.

46. Revilla-Nuin B, Parrilla P, Lozano JJ, de Haro LF, Ortiz A, Martinez C, *et al.* (2013). Predictive value of MicroRNAs in the progression of barrett esophagus to adenocarcinoma in a long-term follow-up study. *Annals of Surgery* **257**(5), 886–93.

47. Kan T, Meltzer SJ (2009). MicroRNAs in Barrett's esophagus and esophageal adenocarcinoma. *Current Opinion in Pharmacology* **9**(6), 727–32.

48. Bansal A, Lee IH, Hong X, Anand V, Mathur SC, Gaddam S, *et al.* (2011). Feasibility of mcroRNAs as biomarkers for Barrett's Esophagus progression: a pilot cross-sectional, phase 2 biomarker study. *American Journal of Gastroenterology* **106**(6), 1055–63.

49. Smith CM, Watson DI, Leong MP, Mayne GC, Michael MZ, Wijnhoven BP, *et al.* (2011). miR-200 family expression is downregulated upon neoplastic progression of Barrett's esophagus. *World Journal of Gastroenterology* **17**(8), 1036–44.

50. Fassan M, Volinia S, Palatini J, Pizzi M, Baffa R, De Bernard M, *et al.* (2011). MicroRNA expression profiling in human Barrett's carcinogenesis. *International Journal of Cancer* **129**(7), 1661–70.

51. Leidner RS, Ravi L, Leahy P, Chen Y, Bednarchik B, Streppel M, *et al.* (2012). The microRNAs, MiR-31 and MiR-375, as candidate markers in Barrett's esophageal carcinogenesis. *Genes, Chromosomes and Cancer* **51**(5), 473–9.

52. Mathe EA, Nguyen GH, Bowman ED, Zhao Y, Budhu A, Schetter AJ, *et al.* (2009). MicroRNA expression in

squamous cell carcinoma and adenocarcinoma of the esophagus: associations with survival. *Clinical Cancer Research* **15**(19), 6192–200.

53. Nguyen GH, Schetter AJ, Chou DB, Bowman ED, Zhao R, Hawkes JE, *et al.* (2010). Inflammatory and microRNA gene expression as prognostic classifier of Barrett's-associated esophageal adenocarcinoma. *Clinical Cancer Research* **16**(23), 5824–34.

54. Lin RJ, Xiao DW, Liao LD, Chen T, Xie ZF, Huang WZ, *et al.* (2012). MiR-142-3p as a potential prognostic biomarker for esophageal squamous cell carcinoma. *Journal of Surgical Oncology* **105**(2), 175–82.

55. Liu Z, Xiao B, Tang B, Li B, Li N, Zhu E, *et al.* (2010). Up-regulated microRNA-146a negatively modulate Helicobacter pylori-induced inflammatory response in human gastric epithelial cells. *Microbes and Infection* **12**(11), 854–63.

56. Abel AG, Brown WA, Smith A, Nottle P (2013). Spontaneous esophageal perforation leading to vertebral osteomyelitis and spinal cord compression. *Diseases of the Esophagus* **26**(3), 334–5.

57. Yang H, Gu J, Wang KK, Zhang W, Xing J, Chen Z, *et al.* (2009). MicroRNA expression signatures in Barrett's esophagus and esophageal adenocarcinoma. *Clinical Cancer Research* **15**(18), 5744–52.

58. Takeshita N, Hoshino I, Mori M, Akutsu Y, Hanari N, Yoneyama Y, *et al.* (2013). Serum microRNA expression profile: miR-1246 as a novel diagnostic and prognostic biomarker for oesophageal squamous cell carcinoma. *British Journal of Cancer* **108**(3), 644–52.

59. Zhang C, Wang C, Chen X, Yang C, Li K, Wang J, *et al.* (2010). Expression profile of microRNAs in serum: a fingerprint for esophageal squamous cell carcinoma. *Clinical Chemistry* **56**(12), 1871–9.

60. Feber A, Xi L, Luketich JD, Pennathur A, Landreneau RJ, Wu M, *et al.* (2008). MicroRNA expression profiles of esophageal cancer. *Journal of Thoracic and Cardiovascular Surgery* **135**(2), 255–60; discussion 60.

61. Wijnhoven BP, Hussey DJ, Watson DI, Tsykin A, Smith CM, Michael MZ, *et al.* (2010). MicroRNA profiling of Barrett's oesophagus and oesophageal adenocarcinoma. *British Journal of Surgery* **97**(6), 853–61.

62. Pawar H, Kashyap MK, Sahasrabuddhe NA, Renuse S, Harsha HC, Kumar P, *et al.* (2011). Quantitative tissue proteomics of esophageal squamous cell carcinoma for novel biomarker discovery. *Cancer Biology & Therapy* **12**(6), 510–22.

63. Kadri SR, Lao-Sirieix P, O'Donovan M, Debiram I, Das M, Blazeby JM, *et al.* (2010). Acceptability and accuracy of a non-endoscopic screening test for Barrett's oesophagus in primary care: cohort study. *BMJ* **341**, c4372.

64. Chiba T, Marusawa H, Ushijima T (2012). Inflammation-associated cancer development in digestive organs: mechanisms and roles for genetic and epigenetic modulation. *Gastroenterology* **143**(3), 550–63.

65. Sato F, Jin Z, Schulmann K, Wang J, Greenwald BD, Ito T, *et al.* (2008). Three-Tiered Risk Stratification Model to Predict Progression in Barrett's Esophagus Using Epigenetic and Clinical Features. *PLoS One* **3**(4).

66. Jin Z, Cheng Y, Gu W, Zheng Y, Sato F, Mori Y, *et al.* (2009). A multicenter, double-blinded validation study of methylation biomarkers for progression prediction in Barrett's esophagus. *Cancer Research* **69**(10), 4112–5.

67. Brock MV, Gou M, Akiyama Y, Muller A, Wu TT, Montgomery E, *et al.* (2003). Prognostic importance of promoter hypermethylation of multiple genes in esophageal adenocarcinoma. *Clinical Cancer Research* **9**(8), 2912–9.

68. Komatsu S, Ichikawa D, Takeshita H, Konishi H, Nagata H, Hirajima S, *et al.* (2012). Prognostic impact of circulating miR-21 and miR-375 in plasma of patients with esophageal squamous cell carcinoma. *Expert Opinion on Biological Therapy* **12** Suppl **1**, S53–9.

69. Li X, Galipeau PC, Paulson TG, Sanchez CA, Arnaudo J, Liu K, *et al.* (2013). Temporal and spatial evolution of somatic chromosomal alterations: A case-cohort study of Barrett's esophagus. *Cancer Prevention Research (Philadelphia)* **7**(1), 114–27.

70. Kelly P, Paulin F, Lamont D, Baker L, Clearly S, Exon D, *et al.* (2012). Pre-treatment plasma proteomic markers associated with survival in oesophageal cancer. *British Journal of Cancer* **106**(5), 955–61.

71. Uemura N, Nakanishi Y, Kato H, Saito S, Nagino M, Hirohashi S, *et al.* (2009). Transglutaminase 3 as a prognostic biomarker in esophageal cancer revealed by proteomics. *International Journal of Cancer* **124**(9), 2106–15.

72. Esteller M (2000). Epigenetic lesions causing genetic lesions in human cancer. promoter hypermethylation of DNA repair genes. *European Journal of Cancer* **36**(18), 2294–300.

73. Hamilton JP, Sato F, Greenwald BD, Suntharalingam M, Krasna MJ, Edelman MJ, *et al.* (2006). Promoter methylation and response to chemotherapy and radiation in esophageal cancer. *Clinical Gastroenterology and Hepatology* **4**(6), 701–8.

74. Sugimura K, Miyata H, Tanaka K, Hamano R, Takahashi T, Kurokawa Y, *et al.* (2012). Let-7 Expression Is a Significant Determinant of Response to Chemotherapy through the Regulation of IL-6/STAT3 Pathway in Esophageal Squamous Cell Carcinoma. *Clinical Cancer Research* **18**(18), 5144–53.

75. Odenthal M, Bollschweiler E, Grimminger PP, Schroder W, Brabender J, Drebber U, *et al.* (2013). MicroRNA profiling in locally advanced esophageal cancer

indicates a high potential of miR-192 in prediction of multimodality therapy response. *International Journal of Cancer* **133**(10), 2454–2463.

76. Lynam-Lennon N, Reynolds JV, Pidgeon GP, Maher SG (2011). Microrna-31 modulates tumour sensitivity to radiation in oesophageal cancer. *British Journal of Surgery* **98**, 23.

77. Wen J, Zheng B, Hu Y, Zhang X, Yang H, Li Y, *et al.* (2010). Comparative proteomic analysis of the esophageal squamous carcinoma cell line EC109 and its multi-drug resistant subline EC109/CDDP. *International Journal of Oncology* **36**(1), 265–74.

78. Langer R, Ott K, Specht K, Becker K, Lordick F, Burian M, *et al.* (2008). Protein expression profiling in esophageal adenocarcinoma patients indicates association of heat-shock protein 27 expression and chemotherapy response. *Clinical Cancer Research* **14**(24), 8279–87.

79. Tanaka K, Miyata H, Yamasaki M, Sugimura K, Takahashi T, Kurokawa Y, *et al.* (2013). Circulating miR-200c Levels Significantly Predict Response to Chemotherapy and Prognosis of Patients Undergoing Neoadjuvant Chemotherapy for Esophageal Cancer. *Annals of Surgical Oncology* **20**(Suppl 3), S607–15.

80. Pepe MS, Etzioni R, Feng Z, Potter JD, Thompson ML, Thornquist M, *et al.* (2001). Phases of biomarker development for early detection of cancer. *Journal of the National Cancer Institute* **93**(14), 1054–61.

81. Sullivan Pepe M, Etzioni R, Feng Z, Potter JD, Thompson ML, Thornquist M, *et al.* (2001). Phases of biomarker development for early detection of cancer. *Journal of the National Cancer Institute* **93**(14), 1054–61.

CHAPTER 10

Predictive Biomarkers for Therapy in Adenocarcinoma of the Upper Digestive Tract

Heath D Skinner,[1] Qiongrong Chen,[2] Elena Elimova,[2] Roopma Wadhwa,[2] Shumei Song,[2] and Jaffer A Ajani[2]

[1] Department of Radiation Oncology, The University of Texas MD Anderson Cancer Center, Houston, TX, USA

[2] Department of GI Medical Oncology, The University of Texas MD Anderson Cancer Center, Houston, TX, USA

Introduction

Adenocarcinoma of the upper digestive tract (UDT) (distal esophagus, gastro-esophageal junction (GEJ) and stomach) comprises a group of deadly malignancies, accounting for over 20 000 deaths annually [1]. Additionally, the incidence of these malignancies is on the rise in the West, most likely due to a combination of factors, including rising rates of obesity and increased incidence of gastro-esophageal reflux (GERD) [2, 3]. Although tumors in this region are becoming increasingly common, widespread screening is not often performed. Thus, many tumors present as locally advanced, with long-term survival ranging from 30–50% with the most aggressive therapy [4–6].

Currently, one of the key difficulties in the management of this disease is the lack of predictive biomarkers of response to either standard cytotoxic chemotherapy and radiotherapy, or targeted therapy. Thus, in the current chapter, we will discuss studies using several key biomarkers in predicting patient outcome and response to therapy, as well as the current obstacles to the clinical use of biomarkers in this context. We will then focus on studies examining panels of biomarkers to improve the ability to predict response. A discussion of the current state of targeted therapy and recent advances in tumor sequencing will follow. We will then conclude with possible future directions for biomarker development in adenocarcinoma of the upper digestive tract.

Importance of biomarkers in adenocarcinoma of the upper digestive tract (UDT)

As mentioned above, a majority of patients with adenocarcinoma of the UDT present with locally advanced disease. In early stage tumors, the most common form of therapy is surgical resection. However, with tumors invading a significant portion of the wall of the lumen or nodal involvement, multiple modalities of therapy are required. Typically, this will involve a combination of external beam radiotherapy and/or chemotherapy, delivered prior to or after surgery. Multi-modality therapy has been shown to improve patient outcome in multiple randomized trials [4, 7, 8]. However,

Biomarkers in Cancer Screening and Early Detection, First Edition. Edited by Sudhir Srivastava.
© 2017 John Wiley & Sons, Inc. Published 2017 by John Wiley & Sons, Inc.

despite these advances, the likelihood of survival following a diagnosis of UDT adenocarcinoma is poor. Additionally, multi-modality therapy has significant toxicities, with long-term decreases in UDT function and patient quality of life [9]. As such, the use of biomarkers in this field has several goals.

The first goal is to identify those patients sensitive to current treatment modalities, for whom treatment de-escalation can be considered. For example, approximately 20–30% of patients treated with neoadjuvant chemoradiation for adenocarcinoma of the UDT have a complete pathological response (pCR) following surgical resection [4, 10]. It is probable that these patients do not benefit from surgical resection. However, current methods of determining *a priori* the patients who will have a pCR – PET-CT and endoscopy – are not sufficiently reliable in this regard to definitively guide clinical decision-making [10–12]. Thus, the current clinical recommendation remains surgical resection in all medically operable patients.

However, if a biomarker or group of biomarkers were to exist to predict for response to chemotherapy or chemoradiation, these patients could be spared a very morbid surgical resection. Additionally, biomarkers for the patients with extreme resistance to current modalities of therapy are also needed. Knowing that a particular patient is highly resistant to chemotherapy and/or radiation may allow the patient to receive upfront surgery, sparing them from relatively greater toxicity of multi-modality therapy. Finally, the discovery of targetable biomarkers in adenocarcinoma of the UDT could allow for more personalized therapy of this malignancy, with the goal of improving survival.

Predictive biomarkers in UDT adenocarcinoma

Excision repair cross-complementing 1 (ERCC1)

Cisplatin and other platinum compounds lead to the formation of cross-linked DNA adducts, which is the primary mechanism by which these compounds exert their cytotoxic effects. These DNA lesions are primarily repaired by nucleotide excision repair, a complex process involving the recognition of damaged DNA strand, excision of the

DNA-adduct, and a "filling in" of the excised strand. One key protein in this process is ERCC1, which is necessary for the cleavage of the damaged DNA strand.

Multiple studies examining the association between low levels of ERCC1 expression and response to platinum-based chemotherapy have been performed. One of the first studies examining ERCC1 in this context examined pre-treatment biopsy specimens from 38 gastric adenocarcinoma patients treated with cisplatin and 5-flurouracil for expression of ERCC1, and correlated this marker with response [13]. In this study, low levels of ERCC expression were associated with higher response rates, as well as improved survival. Several retrospective and prospective studies have linked pre-treatment ERCC1 expression to the response to platinum-based chemotherapy, as well as to patient outcomes in UDT adenocarcinoma [14–18]. Additionally, poor responses to platinum-based chemoradiation have been observed in patients whose tumors have high ERCC1 expression levels [19–21]. However, this phenomenon is not universal, with at least two retrospective studies finding no association between ERCC1 expression and response to platinum-based chemotherapy in UDT adenocarcinoma [22, 23]. Thus, ERCC1 expression is not commonly used for clinical decision-making regarding the management of this disease.

NF-κB

Progression to frank invasive adenocarcinoma of the UDT is known to involve chronic inflammatory processes, mediated in large part by NF-κB [24]. This protein is highly expressed in adenocarcinoma of the UDT and has been linked to *in vitro* chemo and radioresistance [25]. These findings have led to multiple studies examining its role in predicting response to therapy. Izzo and colleagues examined pre-treatment NF-κB expression in 43 patients with UDT adenocarcinoma treated on a prospective protocol [26]. They noted that high levels of pre-treatment NF-κB expression correlated with poor response to docetaxel-based chemoradiation and poor survival outcomes. This finding has been confirmed by others.

Additionally, it has been shown that chemoradiation can lead to activation of NF-κB, and that this effect is associated with poor survival [28]. Others have noted that downregulation of NF-κB by chemoradiation is associated with improved therapeutic response [29]. This phenomenon appears to be directly predictive of response to chemoradiation, and not necessarily prognostic, as at least one group have linked NF-κB overexpression with improved prognosis in UDT adenocarcinoma in patients treated with surgery only [30].

TP53

The most commonly mutated gene in adenocarcinomas of the UDT is *TP53*, the gene encoding the p53 protein. p53 is one of the most well-studied proteins in the cancer cell, and is linked to a broad array of cellular functions, ranging from maintenance of genomic integrity, to cell motility, to apoptosis [31]. It is known that this transcription factor is activated by DNA damage and other stressors to activate apoptosis, and its mutation or absence can render cancer cells resistant to this form of cell death. Additionally, it has been shown that certain TP53 mutations can endow p53 with oncogenic "gain of function" attributes [32].

Because of the known relationship between p53 and apoptosis, multiple investigators have tried to link TP53 mutation and resistance to therapy in UDT adenocarcinoma. However the results of these studies have been mixed at best. While several studies have shown poor response to therapy and/or outcome in UDT tumors with high levels of p53 expression [33–36], others have shown no relationship between p53 and response [18, 37, 38]. This discordance could partially be explained by the common use of high p53 expression levels as a surrogate for mutation status. Many mutations in *TP53* lead to a lack of transcription of this gene and a p53-null cell. These mutations are not detected by protein expression, and may adversely affect the use of p53 expression as a predictive marker [39]. Additionally, as has been noted, some *TP53* mutations can lead to the transcription and translation of a p53 protein that has acquired some function not present in the wild type [32]. The resultant "gain of function" likely has relevance to therapeutic resistance [40], which further complicates a simple classification of tumors as mutant or wild type *TP53*.

Chemotherapy-associated metabolism genes

One of the most common chemotherapeutic agents used in UDT adenocarcinoma is 5-flurouracil (5-FU). This uracil analog is easily transported into the cancer cell, where it is converted by dihydropyrimidine dehydrogenase (DPD) into its active metabolite. Once activated, 5-FU inhibits thymidylate synthase (TS), preventing the formation of thymidylate and impairing DNA repair. Because of the multiple enzymatic steps involved in the function of 5-FU, it has been hypothesized that examination of the tumor expression of these enzymes may provide insight regarding response to 5-FU. Indeed, high TS expression has been shown to be associated with decreased therapeutic response, and poor outcome in UDT adenocarcinoma treated with 5-FU-based chemotherapy alone [15,17] or in combination with radiation [20, 41]. However, this observation is not universal, with at least one group showing no relationship between TS levels and outcome following treatment with a 5-FU-containing regimen [18].

Additionally, several other 5-FU-related enzymes, including DPD, orotate phosphoribosyltransferase (OPRT), methylenetetrahydrofolate reductase (MTHFR), and thymidine phosphorylase (TP) have all been examined in the context of predicting response to 5-FU-containing regimens [42–44]. Furthermore, both TP and TS are downregulated by treatment with 5-FU-containing regimens, with the downregulation of TP correlating with tumor response [44].

ATP-binding cassette transporters (ABC transporters)

One of the most well-studied mechanisms of chemotherapeutic resistance involves efflux of drug from the cell prior to reaching therapeutic concentration. This is accomplished via ABC transporters, which transport drug out of the cell in an ATP-dependent fashion [45]. Multiple proteins within the ABC superfamily have been associated with chemotherapeutic resistance. Specifically, both overexpression of Multidrug Resistance Protein 1 (p-glycoprotein, MDR-1) [46, 47] and multidrug resistance-associated protein-1 (MRP-1) [23] have been associated with poor response to chemotherapy in UDT adenocarcinoma. MDR-1 overexpression has been shown to be associated with poor response to concurrent chemoradiation in UDT adenocarcinoma [41]. Additionally, treatment with chemotherapy has been shown to downregulate the expression of MRP-1 in UDT adenocarcinoma [44]. However, conflicting data are present concerning MDR 1, with at least one study showing no relationship to tumor response following chemotherapy [23].

MicroRNA

MicroRNAs (miRNAs) are short, non-coding RNA sequences that are known to modulate gene expression at the transcriptional and post-transcriptional levels. These miRNAs bind to complementary mRNA within the cell, leading to the silencing of the gene in question. Thousands of these miRNAs are known, with many modulating a broad variety of cellular processes. Specifically, multiple miRNAs are overexpressed in adenocarcinomas of the UDT, leading to speculation that they may contribute to therapeutic resistance [48]. For example, miR-31 has been shown to be overexpressed in UDT adenocarcinoma with a "good response" to chemoradiation, an effect which can be recapitulated *in vitro* by the overexpression of miR-31 [49]. However, most studies in this context have examined only one, or a small group of miRNAs, in the context of sensitivity to therapy.

Using a more non-biased approach, Ko and colleagues examined tumor specimens from 25 patients treated with chemoradiation, and found several miRNAs differentially expressed between those patients with and without pCR, although a miRNA signature associated with pCR could not be found [50]. However, this and similar other studies have been limited by small numbers of patients as well as a lack of validation limit.

More recently, we examined over 700 miRNAs in esophageal adenocarcinoma, and developed a 4 miRNA signature predictive of response to chemoradiation in 40 esophageal adenocarcinoma patients [51]. This signature was then validated in a similarly treated cohort of 65 patients. In both groups of patients, pCR could be predicted with a high degree of accuracy, particularly when combined with clinical stage and grade. However, this signature requires further prospective validation before it allows for the generation of more sensitive prediction methods of response to therapy.

Germline alterations (single nucleotide polymorphisms (SNPs))

One significant difficulty in generating useful predictive markers of response in UDT adenocarcinoma is the requirement for tumor tissue. Obtaining sufficient pre-therapeutic tumor tissue for analysis is difficult and labor intensive, with tumor heterogeneity possibly skewing results [52]. Examination of post-therapy markers is usually unhelpful for determining response, as the treatment itself can certainly affect the expression of many candidate biomarkers. This has led to the examination of germline genetic alterations – usually single nucleotide polymorphisms or SNPs – as possible predictive biomarkers in UDT adenocarcinoma.

This approach has the benefit of being reasonably non-invasive (peripheral blood can be used), as well as cost-effective. Indeed, multiple groups have examined the relationship between therapeutic response and SNPs for a variety of genes [53–58]. Specifically, SNPs in Akt/mammalian target or rapamycin (mTOR) [53], X-ray repair cross-complementing protein 1 (XRCC1) [54], epidermal growth factor receptor (EGFR) [58], p53 [56, 57] and cyclin D1 [55] have all been associated with therapeutic response. However, one disadvantage of using SNPs for predicting therapeutic response is the requirement for a larger patient cohort and validation sets to make clinically useful conclusions. There is a high likelihood of finding significant association, since a large number of SNPs are available for analysis.

Biomarker signatures

Unfortunately, all individual biomarkers lack in high predictive power. This predictive power is necessary for any routine clinical use, but it is unlikely to be provided by any one biomarker gene or protein. Using several biomarkers in tandem to create a more predictive profile can surmount this difficulty. For example, this approach has been used effectively in breast cancer, with two biomarker panels in widespread clinical use to guide chemotherapeutic decision-making [59]. In UDT adenocarcinoma, several predictive and prognostic biomarker panels have been investigated (Table 10.1).

Ajani and colleagues have developed a three-protein expression panel to predict response to chemoradiation in esophageal adenocarcinoma

Table 10.1 Selected biomarker signatures in UDT adenocarcinoma.

Authors	Site/Stage	n	Treatment	Method	Signature	Outcome (s)	Comments
Ajani et al. [60]	Esophagus and GEJ/Locally advanced	Discovery: 60 Validation: 167	Neoadjuvant chemoradiation and surgical resection	IHC	NF-kB, Gli-1, and sonic hedgehog	Pathologic complete response (pCR): $\approx$ 80% (47/47 pts) in most favorable group and 0% (0/57) in least favorable group.	
Kim et al. [62]	Gastric/ Metastatic	Discovery: 96 Validation 1: 27 Validation 2: 40	CDDP & 5-FU	mRNA expression array	Myc, EGFR, FGFR2. Overexpression associated with poor outcome.	Median OS: low risk 7.4 mos., high risk 16.8 mos., $p = 0.047$	Signature not associated with survival in patients not treated with chemotherapy.
Ong et al. [61]	Esophagus and GEJ/All stages	Discovery: 374 Validation 1: 363 Validation 2: 314	Surgery	IHC	Overexpression: EGFR, TRIM44 Underexpression: SIRT2	Median survival for 0 (45 mos), 1 (18.2 mos), 2 (14 mos.), and 3 (7 mos.) dysregulated molecular markers ($p \leq 0.01$)	Prognostic, not predictive
Skinner et al. [51]	Esophagus and GEJ/Locally advanced	Discovery: 10 Model: 41 Validation: 61	Neoadjuvant chemoradiation and surgical resection	microRNA expression	4 miRNAs	Pathologic complete response (pCR): $\approx$ 80% in most favorable group and 10% in least favorable group.	Clinical stage and miRNA expression combined to improve predictive model

[60]. The authors examined the expression of two members of the Hedgehog signaling pathway, sonic hedgehog and Gli-1 and NFκB, via immunohisto-chemistry (IHC), with overexpression associated with therapeutic resistance. In patients defined by this signature as chemoradiation sensitive, the pCR rate was ≈ 80% in both the discovery and validation set, with a specificity of ≈ 95%. This signature has led to the first commercially available predictive biomarker panel in UDT adenocarci-noma – DecisionDx-EC. A separate panel of three protein (EGFR, tripartite motif-containing 44 (TRIM44) and sirtuin 2 (SIRT2), have been shown to be prognostic in patients treated with surgery alone for UDT adenocarcinoma, however it is unclear whether this panel is predictive of response to therapy [61].

Kim and colleagues examined mRNA expression in patients with metastatic gastric cancer, and iden-tified a three-gene panel to predict response to cis-platin and 5-FU [62]. Specifically, overexpression of Myc, EGFR and FGFR2, appear to be associated with both radiographic response to therapy, as well as overall survival, in this patient population. The same group identified a 72-gene panel that appears to be associated with acquired chemoresistance in gastric adenocarinoma [63]. Additionally, as men-tioned above, we have found a 4 miRNA expression profile that, combined with clinical stage and grade, is highly predictive of response to chemoradiation in esophageal adenocarcinoma [51].

Currently targeted biomarkers in UDT adenocarcinoma

At present, a limited number of markers have been evaluated for targeted therapy in UDT adenocarci-noma. Although none are currently used to direct standard first line therapy for this disease in the localized setting, many have a proven benefit in the metastatic setting, and are being evaluated in randomized trials. The optimum combination of targeted therapy, standard cytotoxic chemotherapy, and radiotherapy has yet to be determined.

Epidermal growth factor receptor (EGFR) and human epidermal growth factor receptor 2 (HER 2)

Both HER2 and EGFR are closely related tyrosine kinases located at the cell membrane, consisting of three domains. While EGFR has a number of known activating ligands, such as EGF and TGFα, HER 2 has no known activating ligand. These two proteins (as well as other members of this fam-ily) can homo- and heterodimerize, leading to the activation of a number of signaling cascades. Sev-eral agents targeting EGFR and/or HER2 have been used clinically, with the most dramatic example being significantly improved survival in HER2+ breast cancer with the addition of trastuzumab, a monoclonal antibody that inhibits Her2 mediated signaling [64].

In regards to UDT adenocarcinoma, studies regarding HER 2 overexpression are mixed. In one large study, HER 2 overexpression was associated with improved survival in patients treated with surgery alone [65]. However, additional studies have reported the opposite conclusion [66]. HER2 heterogeneity may also be a factor, with HER 2-positive UDT adenocarcinoma patients with sig-nificant heterogeneity having worse outcomes [67]. Regardless, Her2 positivity does not appear to affect response or outcome in patients treated with neoadjuvant chemotherapy [68] or chemoradiation [69]. However, because up to 20% of patients with UDT adenocarcinoma over-express Her2, target-ing this receptor has been, and continues to be, investigated.

Several phase I/II trials confirmed the safety of combining Her2 targeted therapy with either stan-dard cytotoxic chemotherapy or chemoradiation [70–72]. This culminated in the ToGA trial, a phase III randomized trial which showed a significant survival benefit of adding trastuzumab to cytotoxic chemotherapy in HER 2 positive UDT adenocar-cinoma (median survival 13.8 vs. 11 months) [73]. However, the question of the benefit of adding Her2 targeted therapy to chemoradiation remains.

EGFR targeting has also been examined in UDT adenocarcinoma. Although this approach has largely been found to be safe, multiple phase II and phase III randomized trials in this disease have found minimal benefit to this approach [74–77].

Vascular endothelial growth factor (VEGF)

VEGF, or more specifically VEGF-A, is one of the main drivers of tumor angiogenesis. This secreted protein was the first discovered member of the VEGF family of proteins, all derived from alternative mRNA splicing of the product of the VEGF gene. VEGF binds to one of a number of VEGF receptors (VEGFRs 1, 2 and 3), leading to the activation of multiple signaling cascades associated with angiogenesis. Inhibition of VEGF signaling has been investigated in a wide variety of solid tumors, with the most studied agent being bevacizumab, a monoclonal antibody that acts by via binding to and sequestering VEGF-A.

In UDT adenocarcinoma, limited retrospective data exist to suggest that VEGF overexpression may be associated with sensitivity to cisplatin [78]; however, VEGF signaling has primarily been examined in this disease as a potential target for intervention. Initial phase II studies indicated safety of VEGF targeting in combination with standard care, as well as some modest activity [79, 80]. Despite this early data, the AVAGAST trial found no benefit to the addition of bevacizumab to chemotherapy in the advanced first-line setting [81]. However, in a subset analysis of this trial, high circulating levels of VEGF-A, as well as low tumor neuropillin (a receptor known to bind to VEGF-A), were associated with a trend to improved outcome, further underscoring the importance of patient selection for this type of trial [82].

Other targets under development

Several additional targetable proteins have been investigated in the context of UDT adenocarcinoma. Mammalian target of rapamycin (mTOR) is a serine/threonine kinase activated by multiple inputs associated with cellular growth and survival. mTOR inhibition, as monotherapy, has been investigated in two phase II trials in heavily pretreated gastric cancer. In both trials, modest tumor responses were observed [83, 84]. High levels of phosphorylated S6 protein (a downstream target for inhibition by mTOR) were associated with improved response to this therapy [84]. A subsequent phase III randomized trial – GRANITE -1 – showed improved progression-free survival with mTOR inhibition alone, although no improvement in overall survival [85]. Moreover, it remains to be seen whether this treatment can safely be combined with standard therapy.

Another target investigated in UDT adenocarcinoma is c-Met, a gene which encodes the hepatocyte growth factor receptor. Although not commonly upregulated in UDT adenocarcinoma, case studies have shown some sustained responses to MET inhibition in those patients with c-MET amplification [86]. However, Shah and colleagues found no effect of c-MET inhibition as monotherapy in an unselected gastric cancer population [87]. Conversely, Cecchi and colleagues found significant benefit to c-MET inhibition in combination with chemotherapy [88]. This effect appeared to be most prominent in patients with c-MET amplification, underscoring the importance of correct patient selection for investigational treatments. No studies have examined the combination of c-MET inhibition and chemoradiotherapy thus far.

New horizons in predictive biomarkers for adenocarcinoma of the UDT

Recent advances in technology have allowed, for the first time, a broad overview of the genetic alterations associated with adenocarcinoma of the UDT. Historically, genetic sequencing of these tumors have been limited to small subsets of possibly mutated genes. However, with the availability of cost-effective whole-exome sequencing, the possibility of personalized medicine based upon the genetic composition of an individual tumor seems close to becoming a reality.

Recently, several groups have published the result of whole-exome sequencing in UDT adenocarcinoma [89–91]. The most common mutated gene in these studies is, not surprisingly, *TP53*. This gene is mutated in approximately 70% of all samples from either the stomach or esophagus. Additionally, mutations were commonly found in *PIK3CA* and *ARID1A* in tumors from both sub-sites. The latter gene encodes AT-rich interactive domain-containing protein 1A (ARIDA1A), a protein that modulates chromatin structure and, ultimately, transcription of repressed genes. Inhibition of ARID1A *in vitro* leads to increased cellular proliferation, while its forced expression reverses this effect [91]. Multiple additional genes are mutated or altered in UDT adenocarcinoma, albeit with significantly different frequency, depending upon the sub-site, such as *FAT4* in gastric adenocarcinoma and *CDKN2A* in esophageal adenocarcinoma. Although this work lays the foundation by profiling the mutational landscape, it remains to be seen whether the observed genetic alterations can predict response to current clinical therapy.

Conclusions

A wealth of possible biomarkers for sensitivity to current therapy for UDT adenocarcinoma have been examined although, as yet, none have proven their clinical usefulness in a prospective setting. In order to guide therapy in this disease, a prospective predictive biomarker must have a high degree of sensitivity and specificity. As such, any one single marker, aside from providing information regarding targetable pathways, is unlikely to suffice. Currently, work being performed using panels of biomarkers provides the best hope of generating a truly predictive framework to guide clinicians in the care of these patients. With the addition of targeted therapy and high-throughput sequencing, the dream of truly individualized care of patients with UDT adenocarcinoma is closer to being realized than ever before.

References

1. Jemal A, Bray F, Center MM, Ferlay J, Ward E, Forman D (2011). Global cancer statistics. *CA: A Cancer Journal for Clinicians* **61**(2), 69–90.
2. Souza RF, Spechler SJ (2005). Concepts in the Prevention of Adenocarcinoma of the Distal Esophagus and Proximal Stomach. *CA: A Cancer Journal for Clinicians* **55**(6), 334–51.
3. Yang P, Zhou Y, Chen B, Wan H-W, Jia G-Q, Bai H-L, *et al.* (2009). Overweight, obesity and gastric cancer risk: results from a meta-analysis of cohort studies. *European Journal of Cancer* **45**(16), 2867–73.
4. Van Hagen P, Hulsshof M, van Lansschot JJB, Styerberg EW, Henegouwen MIVB, Wijnhoven BP, *et al.* (2012). Preoperative chemoradiotherapy for esophageal or junctional Cancer. *New England Journal of Medicine* **366**, 2074–84.
5. Tepper JE, Krasna MJ, Niedzwieki D, Hollis D, Reed CE, Goldberg R, *et al.* (2008). Phase III trial of trimodality therapy with cisplatin, fluorouracil, radiotherapy, and surgery compared with surgery alone for esophageal cancer: CALGB 9781. *Journal of Clinical Oncology* **26**, 1086–92.
6. Cunningham D, Allum WH, Stenning SP, Thompson JN, Van de Velde CJH, Nicolson M, *et al.* (2006).

Perioperative chemotherapy versus surgery alone for resectable gastroesophageal cancer. *New England Journal of Medicine* **355**(1), 11–20.
7. Lee J, Lim DH, Park SH, Park JO, Park YS, Lim HY, *et al.* (2011). Phase III trial comparing capecitabine plus cisplatin versus capecitabine plus cisplatin with concurrent capecitabine radiotherapy in completely resected gastric cancer with D2 lymph node dissection: the ARTIST trial. *Journal of Clinical Oncology* **30**, 268–73.
8. Das P, Jiang Y, Lee JH, Bhutani MS, Ross WA, Mansfield PF, *et al.* (2010). Multimodality approaches to localized gastric cancer. *Journal of the National Comprehensive Cancer Network* **8**(4), 417–25.
9. Monjazeb AM, Blackstock AW (2013). The impact of multimodality therapy of distal esophageal and gastroesophageal junction adenocarcinomas on treatment-related toxicity and complications. *Seminars in Radiation Oncology* **23**(1), 60–73.
10. Ajani JA, Correa AM, Hofstetter WL, Rice DC, Blum MA, Suzuki A, *et al.* (2012). Clinical parameters model for predicting pathologic complete response following preoperative chemoradiation in patients with esophageal cancer. *Annals of Oncology* **23**(10), 2638–42.
11. Wong R, Walker-Dilks C, Raifu A (2012). Evidence-based guideline recommendations on the use of positron emission tomography imaging in oesophageal cancer. *Clinical Oncology* **24**(2), 86–104.
12. Vallböhmer D, Brabender J, Grimminger P, Schröder W, Hölscher AH (2011). Predicting response to neoadjuvant therapy in esophageal cancer. *Expert Review of Anticancer Therapy* **11**(9), 1449–55.
13. Metzger R, Leichman CG, Danenberg KD, Danenberg PV, Lenz HJ, Hayashi K, *et al.* (1998). ERCC1 mRNA levels complement thymidylate synthase mRNA levels in predicting response and survival for gastric cancer patients receiving combination cisplatin and fluorouracil chemotherapy. *Journal of Clinical Oncology* **16**(1), 309–16.
14. Fareed KR, Al-Attar A, Soomro IN, Kaye PV, Patel J, Lobo DN, *et al.* (2010). Tumour regression and ERCC1 nuclear protein expression predict clinical outcome in patients with gastro-oesophageal cancer treated with neoadjuvant chemotherapy. *British Journal of Cancer* **102**(11), 1600–7.
15. Chen L, Li G, Li J, Fan C, Xu J, Wu B, *et al.* (2013). Correlation between expressions of ERCC1/TS mRNA and effects of gastric cancer to chemotherapy in the short term. *Cancer Chemotherapy and Pharmacology* **71**(4), 921–8.
16. Huang J, Zhou Y, Zhang H, Qu T, Mao Y, Zhu H, *et al.* (2013). A phase II study of biweekly paclitaxel and cisplatin chemotherapy for recurrent or metastatic

esophageal squamous cell carcinoma: ERCC1 expression predicts response to chemotherapy. *Medical Oncology* **30**(1), 343.

17. Yamada Y, Boku N, Nishina T, Yamaguchi K, Denda T, Tsuji A, et al. (2013). Impact of excision repair cross-complementing gene 1 (ERCC1) on the outcomes of patients with advanced gastric cancer: correlative study in Japan Clinical Oncology Group Trial JCOG9912. *Annals of Oncology* **24**(10), 2560–5.

18. De Dosso S, Zanellato E, Nucifora M, Boldorini R, Sonzogni A, Biffi R, et al. (2013). ERCC1 predicts outcome in patients with gastric cancer treated with adjuvant cisplatin-based chemotherapy. *Cancer Chemotherapy and Pharmacology* **72**(1), 159–65.

19. Warnecke-Eberz U, Metzger R, Miyazono F, Baldus SE, Neiss S, Brabender J, et al. (2004). High specificity of quantitative excision repair cross-complementing 1 messenger RNA expression for prediction of minor histopathological response to neoadjuvant radiochemotherapy in esophageal cancer. *Clinical Cancer Research* **10**(11), 3794–9.

20. Joshi M-BM, Shirota Y, Danenberg KD, Conlon DH, Salonga DS, Herndon JE 2nd, et al. (2005). High gene expression of TS1, GSTP1, and ERCC1 are risk factors for survival in patients treated with trimodality therapy for esophageal cancer. *Clinical Cancer Research* **11**(6), 2215–21.

21. Kim MK, Cho K-J, Kwon GY, Park S-I, Kim YH, Kim JH, et al. (2008). ERCC1 predicting chemoradiation resistance and poor outcome in oesophageal cancer. *European Journal of Cancer* **44**(1), 54–60.

22. Langer R, Specht K, Becker K, Ewald P, Bekesch M, Sarbia M, et al. (2005). Association of Pretherapeutic Expression of Chemotherapy-Related Genes with Response to Neoadjuvant Chemotherapy in Barrett Carcinoma. *Clinical Cancer Research* **11**(20), 7462–9.

23. Langer R, Ott K, Feith M, Lordick F, Specht K, Becker K, et al. (2010). High pretherapeutic thymidylate synthetase and MRP-1 protein levels are associated with nonresponse to neoadjuvant chemotherapy in oesophageal adenocarcinoma patients. *Journal of Surgical Oncology* **102**(5), 503–8.

24. Yang L, Francois F, Pei Z (2012). Molecular Pathways: Pathogenesis and clinical implications of microbiome alteration in esophagitis and Barrett's esophagus. *Clinical Cancer Research* **18**(8), 2138–44.

25. Li F, Sethi G (2010). Targeting transcription factor NF-kappaB to overcome chemoresistance and radioresistance in cancer therapy. *Biochimica et Biophysica Acta* **1805**(2), 167–80.

26. Izzo JG, Malhotra U, Wu TT, Ensor J, Luthra R, Lee JH, et al. (2006). Association of activated transcription factor nuclear factor kB with chemoradiation resistance and

poor outcome in esophageal carcinoma. *Journal of Clinical Oncology* **24**, 748–54.

27. Abdel-Latif MMM, O'Riordan J, Windle HJ, Carton E, Ravi N, Kelleher D, et al. (2004). NF-kappaB activation in esophageal adenocarcinoma: relationship to Barrett's metaplasia, survival, and response to neoadjuvant chemoradiotherapy. *Annals of Surgery* **239**(4), 491–500.

28. Izzo JG, Wu X, Wu T-T, Huang P, Lee J-S, Liao Z, et al. (2009). Therapy-induced expression of NF-kappaB portends poor prognosis in patients with localized esophageal cancer undergoing preoperative chemoradiation. *Diseases of the Esophagus* **22**(2), 127–32.

29. Abdel-Latif MMM, O'Riordan JM, Ravi N, Kelleher D, Reynolds JV (2005). Activated nuclear factor-kappa B and cytokine profiles in the esophagus parallel tumor regression following neoadjuvant chemoradiotherapy. *Diseases of the Esophagus* **18**(4), 246–52.

30. Lee BL, Lee HS, Jung J, Cho SJ, Chung H-Y, Kim WH, et al. (2005). Nuclear Factor-κB Activation Correlates with Better Prognosis and Akt Activation in Human Gastric Cancer. *Clinical Cancer Research* **11**(7), 2518–25.

31. Freed-Pastor WA, Prives C (2012). Mutant p53: one name, many proteins. *Genes & Development* **26**(12), 1268–86.

32. Oren M, Rotter V (2010). Mutant p53 gain-of-function in cancer. *Cold Spring Harbor Perspectives in Biology* **2**(2), a001107.

33. Ribeiro U Jr, Finkelstein SD, Safatle-Ribeiro AV, Landreneau RJ, Clarke MR, Bakker A, et al. (1998). p53 sequence analysis predicts treatment response and outcome of patients with esophageal carcinoma. *Cancer* **83**(1), 7–18.

34. Gibson MK, Abraham SC, Wu T-T, Burtness B, Heitmiller RF, Heath E, et al. (2003). Epidermal Growth Factor Receptor, p53 Mutation, and Pathological Response Predict Survival in Patients with Locally Advanced Esophageal Cancer Treated with Preoperative Chemoradiotherapy. *Clinical Cancer Research* **9**(17), 6461–8.

35. Beardsmore DM, Verbeke CS, Davies CL, Guillou PJ, Clark GWB (2003). Apoptotic and proliferative indexes in esophageal cancer: predictors of response to neoadjuvant therapy [corrected]. *Journal of Gastrointestinal Surgery* **7**(1), 77–86 (discussion 86–87).

36. Duhaylongsod FG, Gottfried MR, Iglehart JD, Vaughn AL, Wolfe WG (1995). The significance of c-erb B-2 and p53 immunoreactivity in patients with adenocarcinoma of the esophagus. *Annals of Surgery* **221**(6), 677–683 (discussion 683–684).

37. Sirak I, Petera J, Hatlova J, Vosmik M, Melichar B, Dvorak J, et al. (2009). Expression of p53, p21 and p16 does not correlate with response to preoperative chemoradiation in gastric carcinoma. *Hepatogastroenterology* **56**(93), 1213–8.

38. Ott K, Vogelsang H, Mueller J, Becker K, Müller M, Fink U, et al. (2003). Chromosomal instability rather than p53 mutation is associated with response to neoadjuvant cisplatin-based chemotherapy in gastric carcinoma. *Clinical Cancer Research* **9**(6), 2307–15.

39. Robles AI, Harris CC (2010). Clinical Outcomes and Correlates of TP53 Mutations and Cancer. *Cold Spring Harbor Perspectives in Biology* (Internet) **2**(3). Available from: http://cshperspectives.cshlp.org/content/2/3/a001016.abstract

40. Muller PAJ, Vousden KH (2013). p53 mutations in cancer. *Nature Cell Biology* **15**(1), 2–8.

41. Harpole DH Jr, Moore MB, Herndon JE 2nd, Aloia T, D'Amico TA, Sporn T, et al. (2001). The prognostic value of molecular marker analysis in patients treated with trimodality therapy for esophageal cancer. *Clinical Cancer Research* **7**(3), 562–9.

42. Miyazaki I, Kawai T, Harada Y, Moriyasu F (2010). A predictive factor for the response to S-1 plus cisplatin in gastric cancer. *World Journal of Gastroenterology* **16**(36), 4575–82.

43. Hashiguchi K, Kitajima Y, Kai K, Hiraki M, Nakamura J, Tokunaga O, et al. (2010). A quantitative evaluation of the determinant proteins for S-1 responsiveness in a biopsy specimen assists in patient selection to neoadjuvant therapy in cases of advanced gastric cancer. *International Journal of Oncology* **37**(2), 257–64.

44. Langer R, Specht K, Becker K, Ewald P, Ott K, Lordick F, et al. (2007). Comparison of pretherapeutic and posttherapeutic expression levels of chemotherapy-associated genes in adenocarcinomas of the esophagus treated by 5-fluorouracil- and cisplatin-based neoadjuvant chemotherapy. *American Journal of Clinical Pathology* **128**(2), 191–7.

45. Takara K, Sakaeda T, Okumura K (2006). An update on overcoming MDR1-mediated multidrug resistance in cancer chemotherapy. *Current Pharmaceutical Design* **12**(3), 273–86.

46. Robey-Cafferty SS, Rutledge ML, Bruner JM (1990). Expression of a multidrug resistance gene in esophageal adenocarcinoma. Correlation with response to chemotherapy and comparison with gastric adenocarcinoma. *American Journal of Clinical Pathology* **93**(1), 1–7.

47. Gürel S, Yerci O, Filiz G, Dolar E, Yilmazlar T, Nak SG, et al. (1999). High expression of multidrug resistance-1 (MDR-1) and its relationship with multiple prognostic factors in gastric carcinomas in patients in Turkey. *Journal of International Medical Research* **27**(2), 79–84.

48. Sakai NS, Samia-Aly E, Barbera M, Fitzgerald RC (2013). A review of the current understanding and clinical utility of miRNAs in esophageal cancer. *Seminars in Cancer Biology* **23**(6 Pt B), 512–21.

49. Lynam-Lennon N, Reynolds JV, Marignol L, Sheils OM, Pidgeon GP, Maher SG (2012). MicroRNA-31 modulates tumour sensitivity to radiation in oesophageal adenocarcinoma. *Journal of Molecular Medicine* **90**(12), 1449–58.

50. Ko MA, Zehong G, Virtanen C, Guindi M, Waddell TK, Keshavjee S, et al. (2012). MicroRNA Expression Profiling of Esophageal Cancer Before and After Induction Chemoradiotherapy. *Nnals of Thoracic Surgery* **94**(4), 1094–103.

51. Skinner HD, Xu E, Lee JH, Bhutani MS, Weston B, Suzuki A, et al. (2013). A validated miRNA expression profile for response to neoadjuvant therapy in esophageal cancer. *Journal of Clinical Oncology* **31**(suppl; abstr 4078).

52. Gerlinger M, Rowan AJ, Horswell S, Larkin J, Endesfelder D, Gronroos E, et al. (2012). Intratumor heterogeneity and branched evolution revealed by multiregion sequencing. *New England Journal of Medicine* **66**(10), 883–92.

53. Hildebrandt MAT, Yang H, Hung MC, Izzo JG, Huang M, Lin J, et al. (2009). Genetic variations in the PI3K/PTEN/mTOR pathway are associated with clinical outcomes in esophageal cancer patients treated with chemoradiotherapy. *Journal of Clinical Oncology* **27**, 857–71.

54. Yoon HH, Catalano PJ, Murphy KM, Skaar TC, Philips S, Powell M, et al. (2011). Genetic variation in DNA-repair pathways and response to radiochemotherapy in esophageal adenocarcinoma: a retrospective cohort study of the Eastern Cooperative Oncology Group. *BMC Cancer* **11**, 176.

55. Stocker G, Ott K, Henningsen N, Becker K, Hapfelmeier A, Lordick F, et al. (2009). CyclinD1 and interleukin-1 receptor antagonist polymorphisms are associated with prognosis in neoadjuvant-treated gastric carcinoma. *European Journal of Cancer* **45**(18), 3326–35.

56. Kim JG, Sohn SK, Chae YS, Song HS, Kwon K-Y, Do YR, et al. (2009). TP53 codon 72 polymorphism associated with prognosis in patients with advanced gastric cancer treated with paclitaxel and cisplatin. *Cancer Chemotherapy and Pharmacology* **64**(2), 355–60.

57. Shirai O, Ohmiya N, Taguchi A, Nakamura M, Kawashima H, Miyahara R, et al. (2010). P53, p21, and p73 gene polymorphisms in gastric carcinoma. *Hepatogastroenterology* **57**(104), 1595–601.

58. Takahashi H, Kaniwa N, Saito Y, Sai K, Hamaguchi T, Shirao K, et al. (2013). Identification of a candidate single-nucleotide polymorphism related to chemotherapeutic response through a combination of knowledge-based algorithm and hypothesis-free genomic data. *Journal of Bioscience and Bioengineering* **116**(6), 768–73.

59. Azim HA Jr, Michiels S, Zagouri F, Delaloge S, Filipits M, Namer M, et al. (2013). Utility of prognostic genomic

tests in breast cancer practice: The IMPAKT 2012 Working Group Consensus Statement. *Annals of Oncology* **24**(3), 647–54.

60. Ajani JA, Wang X, Hayashi Y, Maru D, Welsh J, Hofstetter W, *et al.* (2011). Validated biomarker signatures that predict pathologic response to preoperative chemoradiation therapy (CTRT) with high specificity and desirable sensitivity levels in patients with esophageal cancer (EC). *Journal of Clinical Oncology* **29**(15 (suppl)).

61. Ong C-AJ, Shapiro J, Nason KS, Davison JM, Liu X, Ross-Innes C, *et al.* (2013). Three-gene immunohistochemical panel adds to clinical staging algorithms to predict prognosis for patients with esophageal adenocarcinoma. *Journal of Clinical Oncology* **1**(12), 1576–82.

62. Kim HK, Choi IJ, Kim CG, Kim HS, Oshima A, Yamada Y, *et al.* (2012). Three-gene predictor of clinical outcome for gastric cancer patients treated with chemotherapy. *Pharmacogenomics Journal* **12**(2), 119–27.

63. Kim HK, Choi IJ, Kim CG, Kim HS, Oshima A, Michalowski A, *et al.* (2011). A gene expression signature of acquired chemoresistance to cisplatin and fluorouracil combination chemotherapy in gastric cancer patients. *PloS One* **6**(2), e16694.

64. Slamon D, Eiermann W, Robert N, Pienkowski T, Martin M, Press M, *et al.* (2011). Adjuvant trastuzumab in HER2-positive breast cancer. *New England Journal of Medicine* **65**(14), 1273–83.

65. Yoon HH, Shi Q, Sukov WR, Wiktor AE, Khan M, Sattler CA, *et al.* (2012). Association of HER2/ErbB2 expression and gene amplification with pathologic features and prognosis in esophageal adenocarcinomas. *Clinical Cancer Research* **8**(2), 546–54.

66. Chan DSY, Twine CP, Lewis WG (2012). Systematic review and meta-analysis of the influence of HER2 expression and amplification in operable oesophageal cancer. *Journal of Gastrointestinal Surgery* **16**(10), 1821–9.

67. Yoon HH, Shi Q, Sukov WR, Lewis MA, Sattler CA, Wiktor AE, *et al.* (2012). Adverse prognostic impact of intratumor heterogeneous HER2 gene amplification in patients with esophageal adenocarcinoma. *Journal of Clinical Oncology* **32**, 3932–8.

68. Okines AFC, Thompson LC, Cunningham D, Wotherspoon A, Reis-Filho JS, Langley RE, *et al.* (2013). Effect of HER2 on prognosis and benefit from peri-operative chemotherapy in early oesophago-gastric adenocarcinoma in the MAGIC trial. *Annals of Oncology* **24**(5), 1253–61.

69. Phillips BE, Tubbs RR, Rice TW, Rybicki LA, Plesec T, Rodriguez CP, *et al.* (2013). Clinicopathologic features and treatment outcomes of patients with human epidermal growth factor receptor 2-positive adenocarcinoma of the esophagus and gastroesophageal junction. *Diseases of the Esophagus* **26**(3), 299–304.

70. Safran H, Dipetrillo T, Akerman P, Ng T, Evans D, Steinhoff M, *et al.* (2007). Phase I/II study of trastuzumab, paclitaxel, cisplatin and radiation for locally advanced, HER2 overexpressing, esophageal adenocarcinoma. '*International Journal of Radiation Oncology • Biology • Physics* **7**(2), 405–9.

71. Grávalos C, Gómez-Martín C, Rivera F, Alés I, Queralt B, Márquez A, *et al.* (2011). Phase II study of trastuzumab and cisplatin as first-line therapy in patients with HER2-positive advanced gastric or gastroesophageal junction cancer. *Clinical and Translational Oncology* **13**(3), 179–84.

72. Iqbal S, Goldman B, Fenoglio-Preiser CM, Lenz HJ, Zhang W, Danenberg KD, *et al.* (2011). Southwest Oncology Group study S0413: a phase II trial of lapatinib (GW572016) as first-line therapy in patients with advanced or metastatic gastric cancer. *Annals of Oncology* **22**(12), 2610–5.

73. Bang Y-J, Van Cutsem E, Feyereislova A, Chung HC, Shen L, Sawaki A, *et al.* (2010). Trastuzumab in combination with chemotherapy versus chemotherapy alone for treatment of HER2-positive advanced gastric or gastro-oesophageal junction cancer (ToGA): a phase 3, open-label, randomised controlled trial. *The Lancet* **76**(9742), 687–97.

74. Waddell T, Chau I, Cunningham D, Gonzalez D, Okines AFC, Frances A, *et al.* (2013). Epirubicin, oxaliplatin, and capecitabine with or without panitumumab for patients with previously untreated advanced oesophagogastric cancer (REAL3): a randomised, open-label phase 3 trial. *Lancet Oncology* **14**(6), 481–9.

75. Chan JA, Blaszkowsky LS, Enzinger PC, Ryan DP, Abrams TA, Zhu AX, *et al.* (2011). A multicenter phase II trial of single-agent cetuximab in advanced esophageal and gastric adenocarcinoma. *Annals of Oncology* **22**(6), 1367–73.

76. Ilson DH, Kelsen D, Shah M, Schwartz G, Levine DA, Boyd J, *et al.* (2011). A phase 2 trial of erlotinib in patients with previously treated squamous cell and adenocarcinoma of the esophagus. *Cancer* **17**(7), 1409–14.

77. Lordick F, Kang Y-K, Chung H-C, Salman P, Oh SC, Bodoky G, *et al.* (2013). Capecitabine and cisplatin with or without cetuximab for patients with previously untreated advanced gastric cancer (EXPAND): a randomised, open-label phase 3 trial. *Lancet Oncology* **14**(6), 490–9.

78. Boku N, Ohtsu A, Nagashima F, Shirao K, Koizumi W (2007). Relationship between expression of vascular endothelial growth factor in tumor tissue from gastric cancers and chemotherapy effects: comparison between S-1 alone and the combination of S-1 plus CDDP. *Japanese Journal of Clinical Oncology* **37**(7), 509–14.

79. Shah MA, Ramanathan RK, Ilson DH, Levnor A, D'Adamo D, O'Reilly E, *et al.* (2006). Multicenter phase

II study of irinotecan, cisplatin, and bevacizumab in patients with metastatic gastric or esophageal junction adenocarcinoma. *Journal of Clinical Oncology* **24**, 5201–6.

80. Moehler M, Mueller A, Hartmann JT, Ebert MP, Al-Batran SE, Reimer P, *et al.* (2011). An open-label, multicentre biomarker-oriented AIO phase II trial of sunitinib for patients with chemo-refractory advanced gastric cancer. *European Journal of Cancer* **47**(10), 1511–20.

81. Ohtsu A, Shah MA, Van Cutsem E, Rha SY, Sawaki A, Park SR, *et al.* (2011). Bevacizumab in combination with chemotherapy as first-line therapy in advanced gastric cancer: a randomized, double-blind, placebo-controlled phase III study. *Journal of Clinical Oncology* **9**(30), 3968–76.

82. Van Cutsem E, de Haas S, Kang Y-K, Ohtsu A, Tebbutt NC, Ming Xu J, *et al.* (2012). Bevacizumab in combination with chemotherapy as first-line therapy in advanced gastric cancer: a biomarker evaluation from the AVA-GAST randomized phase III trial. *Journal of Clinical Oncology* **30**(17), 2119–27.

83. Doi T, Muro K, Boku N, Yamada Y, Nishina T, Takiuchi H, *et al.* (2010). Multicenter phase II study of everolimus in patients with previously treated metastatic gastric cancer. *Journal of Clinical Oncology* **8**(11), 1904–10.

84. Yoon DH, Ryu M-H, Park YS, Lee HJ, Lee C, Ryoo B-Y, *et al.* (2012). Phase II study of everolimus with biomarker exploration in patients with advanced gastric cancer refractory to chemotherapy including fluoropyrimidine and platinum. *British Journal of Cancer* **06**(6), 1039–44.

85. Van Cutsem E, Yeh K, Bang Y, Shen L, Ajani J, Bai Y, *et al.* (2012). Phase III trial of everolimus (EVE) in previously treated patients with advanced gastric cancer (AGC): GRANITE-1. *Journal of Clinical Oncology* **30**(4 (Suppl)).

86. Lennerz JK, Kwak EL, Ackerman A, Michael M, Fox SB, Bergethon K, *et al.* (2011). MET amplification identifies a small and aggressive subgroup of esophagogastric adenocarcinoma with evidence of responsiveness to crizotinib. *Journal of Clinical Oncology* **9**(36), 4803–10.

87. Shah MA, Wainberg ZA, Catenacci DVT, Hochster HS, Ford J, Kunz P, *et al.* (2013). Phase II study evaluating 2 dosing schedules of oral foretinib (GSK1363089), cMET/VEGFR2 inhibitor, in patients with metastatic gastric cancer. *PloS One* **8**(3), e54014.

88. Cecchi F, Rabe DC, Bottaro DP (2012). Targeting the HGF/MET signalling pathway in cancer therapy. *Expert Opinion on Therapeutic Targets* **16**(6), 553–72.

89. Dulak AM, Stojanov P, Peng S, Lawrence MS, Fox C, Stewart C, *et al.* (2013). Exome and whole-genome sequencing of esophageal adenocarcinoma identifies recurrent driver events and mutational complexity. *Nature Genetics* **45**(5), 478–86.

90. Agrawal N, Frederick MJ, Pickering CR, Bettegowda C, Chang K, Li RJ, *et al.* (2011). Exome sequencing of head and neck squamous cell carcinoma reveals inactivating mutations in NOTCH1. *Science* **33**(6046), 1154–7.

91. Zang ZJ, Cutcutache I, Poon SL, Zhang SL, McPherson JR, Tao J, *et al.* (2012). Exome sequencing of gastric adenocarcinoma identifies recurrent somatic mutations in cell adhesion and chromatin remodeling genes. *Nature Genetics* **44**(5), 570–4.

CHAPTER 11

Pancreatic Cancer

Sam C Wang and Peter J Allen

Department of Surgery, Memorial Sloan-Kettering Cancer Center, New York, NY, USA

Introduction

Pancreatic ductal adenocarcinoma (PDA) is the fourth leading cause of cancer death in the United States. During 2013, there will be an estimated 45 220 new cases and 38 460 deaths, clearly demonstrating the lethality of the disease [1–3].

Surgical resection of the primary tumor is the only chance for long-term survival. However, up to 80% of patients present with locally advanced or metastatic disease that precludes operation [4–6]. Overall median survival for the highly selected patients who can undergo resection is still only approximately 24 months, with actual five-year survival rates typically reported to be less than 10%. (Figure 11.1) [7–9]. The dismal prognosis of patients who undergo resection suggests that the majority of the patients present with undetectable systemic disease at the time of operation. Unfortunately, current chemotherapeutic regimens are not successful in preventing recurrent disease in the majority of patients.

Many of the patients who do experience long-term survival have a subset of invasive carcinoma that arose from mucinous cystic neoplasms (MCN) or intraductal papillary mucinous neoplasms (IPMN). Five-year survival for these patients ranges from approximately 50% to 70%, depending on the histologic subtype [10–13]. Unfortunately, the great majority of pancreatic cancer patients suffer from pancreatic ductal adenocarcinoma, which is the most deadly form of

pancreatic cancer, while only a small subset develop carcinoma in the setting of MCN and IPMN.

The overall survival in patients undergoing resection with curative intent has remained unchanged over the past 30 years, despite remarkable improvement in surgical technique and pre-operative care. At our institution, 30-day postoperative mortality has decreased from 4.9% in the 1980s to 1.3% in the 2000s, with median lengths of stay improving from 22 days to 8 days during the same timeframe [14–16]. Despite such improvements, complication rates following pancreatectomy remain significant, so any consideration for operation must be made carefully [10, 17–19].

The use of biomarkers in cancer care is rapidly accelerating, as the field strives for "personalized" treatments. Biomarkers can be broadly classified as diagnostic, prognostic, or predictive. Diagnostic markers detect newly onset, recurrent, or progressing disease. Prognostic markers project the natural history of the disease, and may predict staging, recurrence patterns, or survival. Finally, predictive markers forecast response to a given systemic therapy.

Biomarkers may potentially improve outcomes for pancreatic cancer patients in the following manner:

1 Early detection of cancer before it has metastasized
2 Identify precancerous lesions to facilitate prophylactic resections

Biomarkers in Cancer Screening and Early Detection, First Edition. Edited by Sudhir Srivastava.
© 2017 John Wiley & Sons, Inc. Published 2017 by John Wiley & Sons, Inc.

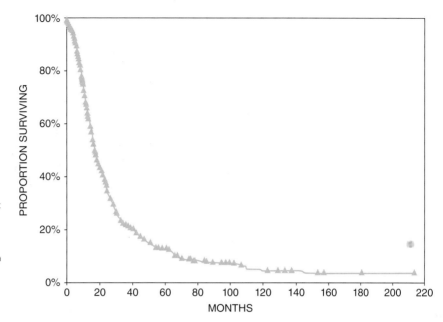

Figure 11.1
Overall survival for 812 pancreatic cancer patients who underwent pancreatectomy (1983–2004). For a color version of this figure please see color plate section.

3 Provide prognostic information to facilitate informed clinical decision making
4 Identify patients who may preferentially respond to one systemic therapy over another
5 Place patients into more uniform prognostic categories to allow for better stratification in clinical trials

Recently, Harsha *et al.* catalogued all molecules that have been published as potential PDA biomarkers. They found 2325 papers, implicating more than 2500 genes [20–22]. Despite such an astounding number of potential markers, the cancer antigen 19-9 (CA 19-9), a sialylated Lewis blood antigen, remains the only FDA approved marker for pancreatic cancer. An estimated 5–15% of the population lacks the necessary enzymes to produce CA 19-9 [23–27]. However, the recent Radiation Therapy Oncology Group (RTOG) trial 9704, which was a randomized phase III trial comparing the use of either continuous infusion 5-fluorouracil or gemcitabine before and after adjuvant chemoradiotherapy, with 5-fluorouracil in patients with resected pancreatic adenocarcinoma, found that 34% of the enrollees lacked Lewis antigen. This finding suggests that a much higher than expected portion of the population may lack the ability to produce CA 19-9 [28–30].

Table 11.1 Notable reference papers.

Fong *et al.* [34, 35]	Review of pancreatic cancer biomarkers
Costello *et al.* [35, 37]	Review of pancreatic cancer biomarkers
Ballehaninna *et al.* [32, 39]	Review of serum CA 19-9 as biomarker for pancreatic cancer
Harsha *et al.* [22, 41]	Compendium of potential pancreatic cancer biomarkers

This chapter will provide a summary of the current state of biomarkers in pancreatic cancer, focusing on CA 19-9 as it is the most extensively studied PDA biomarker [31, 32]. We will focus on clinical utility of these assays, since the ultimate determination of the usefulness of a given assay is whether the result guide management or improve outcome for PDA patients. For even more detailed discussion on the topic, we provide a list of recent review articles in the literature detailing novel biomarkers for pancreatic cancer (Table 11.1) [33–35].

Diagnostic markers

CA 19-9 for PDA

Serum CA 19-9 has been evaluated as a population screening tool in an attempt to detect early stage pancreatic cancer. The ideal screening test has both an exceedingly high sensitivity and specificity, so that there will be few false negatives (missed diagnosis) and few false positives (resulting in unnecessary interventions). However, in reality, increased sensitivity is obtained by sacrificing specificity, or vice versa, so the acceptable tradeoff between false negatives and false positives must be determined *a priori*.

Goonetilleke and Siriwardena analyzed 26 manuscripts with a total of 2283 pancreatic cancer patients, and found that elevated CA 19-9 correctly diagnosed PDA with a median sensitivity of 79% (70–90%) and median specificity of 82% (68–91%) [36, 37]. However, the retrospective nature of that study, and the inherent selection bias, likely overestimates the utility of the test.

Because the incidence of pancreatic cancer is so low, the relatively low sensitivity and specificity of CA 19-9 renders it an ineffective screening tool. Two large population-based studies from Asia showed that the positive predictive value (PPV) of CA 19-9 is in the range of 0.5% ($N = 5343$) [38, 39] to 0.9% ($N = 70\ 940$) [40, 41]. Even when applied to a more selected group of 8756 patients who were older than 40 years of age and presented with gastrointestinal complaints, jaundice, or diabetes, only 1.8% of patients with an abnormal CA 19-9 were found to have cancer [2, 42, 43]. However, jaundiced patients made up a very small minority of the cohort.

These studies demonstrate the lack of practical utility of CA 19-9 as a screening biomarker. An effective diagnostic biomarker needs to be able to identify patients at a time when therapeutic intervention can result in cure or significantly prolonged survival. The exceedingly low PPV of CA 19-9 renders it unusable as a screening modality as previously described.

In addition, even though elevated CA 19-9 does confirm the diagnosis at a reasonable sensitivity and specificity in large group of patients with known PDA, this offers very little practical value. The initial management of a patient who presents with clinical signs and symptoms of pancreatic cancer, such as painless jaundice, back pain, and/or weight loss, should not be altered by the CA 19-9 value. Diagnostic testing for PDA is not discontinued in the jaundiced patient with a

normal CA 19-9 and, alternatively, a diagnosis is not confirmed with an elevated value in that same patient.

Although tissue diagnosis can be challenging, treatment recommendations regarding surgical resection in this group is generally based on radiographic features at the time of presentation. Legmann *et al.* showed that dual-phased CT imaging diagnosed PDA with a 93% sensitivity [5, 44], while DeWitt *et al.* demonstrated 86% sensitivity with a multi-detector CT with a quad-channel scanner [8, 45, 46]. Furthermore, both of these studies found the sensitivity and specificity of endoscopic ultrasound to be 86% and 98%, respectively, providing a high quality alternative diagnostic modality if the CT scan is equivocal. If a solid pancreatic mass with proximal pancreatic ductal dilation is identified incidentally in an asymptomatic patient, the likely management recommendation is resection. In patients who are fit for pancreatectomy, there are not any solid pancreatic lesions that should be observed. Thus, CA 19-9 value is also irrelevant in guiding management in this situation.

One instance where CA 19-9 may be useful in the diagnostic setting is identifying recurrence or progression of disease after treatment (this use may also be cross-classified as prognostic test – see below). Zerbi *et al.* performed short-interval CA 19-9 monitoring in a small series of post-pancreatectomy patients. In all seven patients whose CA 19-9 normalized, elevation of the markers preceded radiographic identification of recurrence [11, 47], Glenn *et al.* also found that elevated CA 19-9 preceded radiographic recurrence in all 11 patients who underwent serial marker measurements [15, 40].

The marker has also been used a surrogate for disease burden or response in clinical trials for therapy. For example, Ahmed *et al.* studied the use of cisplatin, cytarabine, caffeine, and continuous intravenous infusion 5-fluorouracil in a phase II study in advanced pancreatic cancer patients. They found that stable or decreasing CA 19-9 is associated with improved survival [17, 48]. Similarly, Rocha Lima *et al.* found that patients given irinotecan plus gemcitabine have improved CA 19-9 and radiographic response, compared with untreated patients [21, 49].

This concept of elevated CA 19-9 as a marker for extensive disease burden has been applied in large clinical trials. In the CONKO-001 trial, which was an open, multicenter, randomized controlled trial comparing adjuvant gemcitabine and observation after R0 or R1 resection for pancreas cancer, patients with CA 19-9 levels greater than 2.5 times normal were excluded from the study, with the assumption that the patient had a high burden of disease [24, 50].

Other markers for PDA

Serum carcinoembryonic antigen (CEA) and CA-125 have also been studied as potential diagnostic markers for PDA. However, compared with CA 19-9, both markers have lower sensitivity and specificity. Haglund *et al.* compared the utility of serum CA 19-9 against CEA and CA-125 in a cohort of patients with pancreatic cancer, pancreatitis, benign biliary disease, and jaundice due to hepatitis or cirrhosis. He found sensitivity and specificity of CA 19-9 for diagnosing PDA was 78% and 78%, while they were 54% and 76% for CEA, and 45% and 76% for CA-125, respectively. PPV and NPV for CA 19-9 were 75% and 81%, for CEA 68% and 81%, and for CA-125 were 63% and 61%. He did find that, as multiple tests were positive, specificity and PPV increased accordingly [29, 51]. Benini *et al.* also compared these three markers and found that, while all three markers had approximately 90% specificity for diagnosing PDA from non-malignant gastrointestinal disease and other types of malignancies, the sensitivity for CA 19-9 was the highest, at 55.9%. The sensitivity of CA 125 and CEA were only 33.8% and 39.7%, respectively [2, 31].

Other modalities under study to differentiate PDA patients from non-cancer cohorts include urine metabolome [5, 33], salivary transcriptome [8, 36], and microRNA expression [11, 12, 38].

Markers for cystic lesions

With the ever-increasing use of cross-sectional imaging, more and more pancreatic cystic neoplasms are being detected incidentally [15, 40]. The differential diagnosis for a cystic lesion of the pancreas is broad, and includes non-neoplastic pseudocysts, benign neoplastic cysts, premalignant cysts, and cystic lesions with invasive carcinoma. Ideally,

surgical treatment of these lesions is reserved for those lesions that are either pre-malignant or invasive. Even though our ability to differentiate histology using radiographic and endoscopic techniques is improving, too often the diagnosis is made only after pancreatectomy. This dilemma is especially acute in smaller lesions (<3 cm).

Detailed discussions of various types of pancreatic cysts are beyond the scope of this chapter, and are well reviewed in the literature [17, 18, 42, 43]. However, we will briefly describe the most commonly encountered types of cysts. Non-neoplastic cysts are most often pseudocysts that form as a complication from pancreatitis. Serous cystadenomas (SCA) are the most common benign neoplastic cysts, which do not need resection unless symptomatic. Premalignant cystic lesions include intraductal papillary mucinous neoplasms (IPMN) and mucinous cystic neoplasms (MCN). Both IPMN and MCN produce mucin (and are thus both also known as mucinous lesions) and may progress to invasive ductal adenocarcinoma or cystadenocarcinomas. IPMNs can be further categorized into branch duct (BD-IPMN) and main duct (MD-IPMN), depending on their radiographic appearance.

Cyst fluid biomarkers have been highly successful in guiding management of cystic neoplasms of the pancreas by differentiating non-mucinous from mucinous lesions. This distinction is essential, as non-mucinous cysts (pseudocysts and SCA) do not have malignant potential, while some mucinous lesions (MCN and IPMN) may progress to cancer. In a prospective, multicenter trial, Brugge *et al.* found that cyst fluid CEA most accurately diagnosed mucinous lesions over CA 72-4, CA 125, CA 19-9, and CA 15-3. They found that, at the optimal cutoff of 192 ng/mL, the receiver operating characteristics area under the curve was 0.79, while sensitivity and specificity were 73% and 84%, respectively [21, 44].

Previously, many authors have argued for resection of all cystic neoplasms [24–26, 45, 46]. However, improved ability to distinguish mucinous from non-mucinous lesions has allowed for a more selective approach. While the general consensus is that all MCNs should be resected [29, 47], controversy remains regarding IPMNs. Most groups, including ours, have moved to a more selective approach with IPMNs, as it has become clear over time that lesions lacking suspicious features rarely harbor malignancy [31, 40]. The modified Sendai Criteria, which is an international consensus guideline, supports observation of BD-IPMNs if they lack worrisome features such as main duct diameter greater than 5 mm, mural nodularity, or suspicious/malignancy cytology on endoscopic ultrasound (EUS). However, some groups continue to advocate a more aggressive approach to even small BD-IPMN, as their experience has shown that these lesions have a significant risk of malignant progression [33, 34, 48].

It is precisely in these equivocal clinical situations where biomarkers can be helpful. Our group recently reported that IPMN patients with high-grade dysplasia or carcinoma (high risk lesions) had significantly higher cyst mucin 2 (MUC2) and mucin 4 (MUC4) and serum mucin 5AC levels than IPMN patients with low-grade or moderate dysplasia (low risk) [36, 49]. Furthermore, we also found that cyst fluid interleukin 1β (IL1β) can distinguish low risk from high risk IPMNs. Using 1.26 pg/mL at the cutoff, the sensitivity and specificity were 79% and 95%, respectively, to distinguish low- from high-risk cysts and PPV of 71% for correctly diagnosing high-risk cysts, and a NPV of 75% for correctly identifying low-risk cysts [38, 50].

Other groups have analyzed cyst fluid DNA content as a potential diagnostic biomarker for cystic lesions of the pancreas. In a pilot study, Khalid *et al.* found that *KRAS* mutations detected in cyst fluids is significantly associated with high-risk cysts [40, 51]. However, a follow-up study with a larger patient population found that, even though cyst fluid with detectable *KRAS* mutation differentiated mucinous from non-mucinous lesions, it no longer distinguished high-risk and low-risk cysts [42, 52]. Another group used the commercially available PathFinderTG test to evaluate the diagnostic capability of cyst *KRAS* mutations. Shen *et al.* found that the PathFinderTG assay correlated well with the clinical assessment by experts, regarding the malignancy status of 35 cysts. However, not all of these samples were resected, so there was often no pathologic gold standard available to confirm the diagnosis [53].

More recently, Wu *et al.* analyzed cyst fluid DNA from 19 IPMN samples, and found that only two genes were mutated in more than one sample. As expected, *KRAS* mutations were present in a majority of patients (73.7%). However, *GNAS*, a gene previously not known to be associated with pancreas tumors, was mutated in 31.6% of IPMN. A study of 84 IPMN cysts fluid found that *GNAS* was mutated in 61% of tumors, while no mutation was found in 44 SCA, 21 MCN, and 95 PDA patient samples. However, *GNAS* mutation status did not appear to differentiate high-risk from low-risk lesions [54].

Prognostic markers

CA 19-9 for PDA

Serum CA 19-9 has also been extensively evaluated as a prognostic marker for PDA patients. Stratifying a patient into a favorable or unfavorable cohort may potentially alter management decisions. For example, several reports have noted that an elevated pre-operative CA 19-9 is associated with an increased likelihood of finding radiographically occult metastatic disease at staging laparoscopy in PDA patients being taken to the operating room for resection [11, 55]. In a study from our institution, 40 of 262 patients who had preoperative CA 19-9 measured, and underwent staging laparoscopy, were found to have metastatic disease. Patients with CA 19-9 greater than 130 U/mL had a significantly higher chance of having metastatic disease (HR = 2.7, 95% CI = 1.3–5.4). Patients with lesions in the tail of the pancreas and an elevated CA19-9 were at the highest risk for radiographic occult metastatic disease, with 35% of patients in this group found to be unresectable at time of laparoscopy. In this group of patients, it may be reasonable to perform the laparoscopy as a separate procedure.

Recently, Hartwig *et al.* published the Heidelburg experience with 1626 consecutive patients who underwent attempted resection for pancreatic adenocarcinoma. They found that preoperative CA 19-9 level was the strongest predictor for resectability on multivariate analysis. For patients with CA 19-9 <250 U/mL, approximately 80% of the patients underwent resection. However, when CA 19-9 was >1000 U/mL, the resectability rate was 60% or lower [15, 40, 56]. These studies suggest that patients with elevated CA 19-9 levels should undergo high-quality preoperative imaging and diagnostic laparoscopy to minimize the risk of undergoing unnecessary laparotomy.

Many studies have also shown that an increased CA 19-9 level is associated with higher pathologic staging and decreased survival. For example, Ferrone *et al.* reviewed the Massachusetts General Hospital (MGH) experience, and noted that the median preoperative CA 19-9 level was progressively higher in more advanced staged patients [17, 48, 57]. Similarly, a cooperative group in Australia also found a significant correlation between higher CA 19-9 and increased pathologic stage in 202 consecutive patients who underwent resection [21, 23, 49]. In addition, both groups noted that CA 19-9 levels above a given elevated value were associated with worse disease specific survival.

Interestingly, both groups also found that postoperative reduction in CA 19-9 is a useful prognostic indicator. Ferrone *et al.* found on multivariate analysis that an increase in CA 19-9 post-operatively (RR = 2.9), or a post-resection level >200 U/mL (RR = 2.7) are associated with a lower chance for survival than even if the patient had lymph node involvement (RR = 2.5) [24,50,57] Humphris *et al.* found that patients with CA 19-9 >120 U/mL within three months of resection had significantly worse survival than patients with lower values (HR = 1.9, 95% CI 1.3–2.9) [23,29,51].

The challenge with any prognostic marker is properly incorporating the information it provides into clinical decision-making. The MGH group suggests that CA 19-9 should be used to stratify patients in adjuvant trials. Hartwig *et al.* recommended that patients with highly elevated CA 19-9 should undergo extensive workup to exclude distant disease, and should be considered for neoadjuvant therapy.

Investigational markers for PDA

The expression profiles of a variety of genes have been shown to be potential prognostic markers for PDA patients [22, 52]. For example, Oshima *et al.* studied 106 resected samples, and reported that *DPC4/SMAD4* loss was associated with worse survival on multivariate analysis. Patients with increasing number of loss amongst tumor suppressor *p16 (CDKN2A/Ink4A), TP53,* and *DPC4/SMAD4* had poorer survival [1, 53]. Reid-Lombardo *et al.* found that various single

nucleotide polymorphisms (SNPs) in inflammatory pathway genes were associated with survival differences in patients, based on resectable, locally unresectable, and metastatic disease. For example, certain SNPs in *MAPK8IP1* and *SOCS3* were associated with a ten- and six-month overall survival advantage in patients undergoing curative resections, respectively. SNPs in other inflammatory genes were also noted to be associated with improved survival in patients with locally advanced or metastatic disease [4, 54].

While the results of these studies are informative, they are unlikely to alter management. One example where a prognostic marker may guide treatment is based on a study by Iacobuzio-Donahue *et al.*, who found that *DPC4* status in the primary tumor is associated with recurrence pattern. This group reported on autopsy results of 76 PDA patients, and found that 72% of tumors in patients who recurred in widely metastatic patterns lacked *DPC4*, compared with only 35% of patients who died of locally destructive disease [7, 55].

These results are intriguing, as they argue that patients with intact *DPC4* may benefit from additional local therapy, such as radiation. However, when our group tried to validate this finding with a PDA cohort treated at Memorial Sloan-Kettering Cancer Center, we did not find the same association. In this study, we constructed a tissue microarray (TMA) composed of 58 short-term survivors, and compared them to 79 long-term survivors, as defined by death within one year of resection and survival of at least 30 months, respectively [10, 56]. We found that 40 patients had loss of *DPC4*, but did not find an association between *DPC4* status of the primary tumor and recurrence pattern [14, 57].

Our group has taken several targeted approaches in identifying prognostic biomarkers. Using the differential survival TMA, we compared patients from the two ends of the survival curve, and hypothesized that we can identify differentially expressed proteins associated with these survival extremes. We identified mucin 1 (MUC1) and mesothelin (MSLN) as excellent prognostic markers for survival, outstripping traditional pathologic factors such as tumor size, lymph node involvement, and grade [10, 23].

We also tested molecules based on results garnered from murine model of PDA. In Fukuda *et al.*, matrix metalloproteinase 7 (MMP7) was found to play an important role in the progression of PDA [20, 57]. The group studied genetically engineered mice harboring pancreas-specific activating Kras mutation and heterozygous loss of p53 resulting in PDA formation at 100% penetrance. When MMP7 was knocked out in these mice, these animals had smaller primary tumors, less gross lymph node involvement, and a lower rate of liver metastasis. Based on this finding, the group measured serum MMP7 in human PDA patients, and found that elevated MMP7 level was associated with stage IV disease.

While interesting, the finding does not have much practical value, as the stage IV patients in the study had known metastatic disease. It would be more useful if the marker could help in prognosis or management. Thus, we are measuring MMP7 in patients who are deemed to be resectable on pre-operative workup. In this population, we know that approximately 10–20% of these patients will be unresectable at the time of operation, due to locally advanced disease or occult distant metastasis. It is our hope that MMP7 will be able to identify these patients, so as to avoid an unnecessary operation, with the resultant delay in systemic therapy.

Predictive markers

Many groups have suggested that post-resection CA 19-9 levels may predict response to adjuvant chemotherapy. For example, Humphris *et al.* found there was a significant improvement in median survival for the 48 patients whose post-resection CA 19-9 was <90 U/mL if they underwent adjuvant chemotherapy, compared with the 23 patients who did not receive treatment. However, if the patients' CA 19-9 was >90 U/mL, there was no survival difference between treated and non-treated groups ($N = 19$ and 16, respectively) [23].

The Hu antigen R (HuR) has recently been described as another predictive marker for gemcitabine response. HuR is a mRNA binding protein that regulates expression of deoxycytidine kinase, which the enzyme that metabolizes gemcitabine into its active forms. Richards *et al.* stratified 24 patients treated with gemcitabine based on HuR expression levels, and found that the higher

expression is associated with longer overall survival [22, 28].

Predictive biomarkers based on tumor genotyping have been extremely successful in guiding management in various types of cancer. These include hormone receptors in breast cancer, BRAF in melanoma, or epidermal growth factor receptor in non-small cell lung cancer. Unfortunately, such molecular targets remain elusive for pancreatic cancer. However, a breakthrough may be on the horizon for the 5–10% of pancreatic cancer patients whose tumors develop in the setting of *BRCA1* or *BRCA2* mutations [3, 58, 59], which may predict improved responses to poly ADP-ribose polymerase (PARP) inhibition.

The protein products of the two *BRCA* genes are essential components in the repair of double-stranded DNA breaks through homologous joining, while the PARP protein plays an important role in single-stranded repair mechanisms. Inhibition of PARP leads to the accumulation of single-stranded breaks, which further results in double-stranded breaks. Thus, it is thought that PARP inhibition will result in synthetic lethality in tumors that develop in the setting of BRCA deficiency. Indeed, recent studies in breast and ovarian cancer patients have shown that patients with *BRCA* mutations may have a more favorable response to PARP inhibition [6, 60]. As we gain more comprehensive understanding of the genetic changes that drive pancreatic carcinogenesis, rational uses of targeted therapy, such as PARP inhibition in the setting of *BRCA* mutation, will hopefully improve outcomes for PDA patients.

Investigational markers for PDA

Several lines of investigational predictive markers have focused on the molecular machinery involved in the intracellular transport and processing of gemcitabine [9, 61, 62]. Marechal *et al.* compared 243 patients who received gemcitabine with 191 patients who did not. Patients who highly expressed human equilibrative nucleoside transporter 1 (hENT1), which is a membrane transporter that allows gemcitabine to enter cells, or deoxycytidine kinase (dCK), which the rate-limiting enzyme in the processing of gemcitabine into the active metabolite, have longer survival after gemcitabine treatment than non-treated patients.

Of the low-expressing group, adjuvant gemcitabine did not affect survival length [12, 13, 61]. Farrell *et al.* also reported the predictive power of hENT1 status. Using samples from the RTOG 9704 trial, they found that hENT1 expression was associated with improved overall survival and disease-free survival in patients who received gemcitabine, but not in those who were treated with 5-FU [16,62].

MicroRNAs (miRNAs) have also emerged as a potential source for predictive markers. Hwang *et al.* found that miR-21 expression is associated with improved survival in 52 patients who received post-resection adjuvant therapy. No such association was seen in the 27 patients who did not undergo adjuvant treatment [18,19,63]. Pries *et al.* found that miR-10b expression in EUS-aspirated cancer cells was associated with improved response to neoadjuvant therapy [22,64].

Future directions

Despite the identification of more than 2500 genes as potential biomarker for PDA [22, 25–27], CA 19-9 remains the only FDA-approved assay that is in clinical use. However, the most recent consensus statement by the American Society of Clinical Oncology (ASCO) from 2006 recommends against the use of CA 19-9 *alone* to determine operability, provide evidence of recurrent, or monitor for response to therapy. In contrast, the most recent National Comprehensive Network (NCCN) guidelines for pancreatic adenocarcinoma published in January, 2013 recommends measuring CA 19-9 pre-operatively, post-operatively before initiation of chemotherapy, and for surveillance. The recommendation was only Class 2B, which is a category where the recommendation is based upon lower-level evidence, but there is consensus on the NCCN panel that the intervention is appropriate. The relative lack of enthusiasm for CA 19-9 as a biomarker demonstrates that more robust biomarker targets must be identified.

The "holy grail" of cancer therapy is prevention. However, due to the low prevalence of pancreatic cancer and the significant morbidity of pancreatic resection, any proposed screening assay must have exceedingly low false positive rates. The majority of PDA are thought to arise from precursor lesions known as pancreatic intraepithelial

neoplasia (PanIN) that progress in a step-wise fashion to frank carcinoma with the accumulation of genetic mutations in key oncogenes or tumor suppressors [30,65]. Thus, highly dysplastic PanINs are a prime target for diagnostic biomarker development. Patients discovered to have high risk PanINs can be counseled regarding prophylactic pancreatic resection. Similarly, if biomarkers can be identified to differentiate IPMN harboring high-grade dysplasia or carcinoma from low risk IPMNs, outcomes will be improved by preventing a pancreatic cancer from forming at all.

Finally, the dismal prognosis for pancreatic cancer patients is directly related to the lack of effective systemic therapy. The relatively short survival in patients who underwent putative curative resections, and the exceedingly low number of long-term disease-free survivors, suggests that systemic micrometastases are present at the time of operation in a large majority of patients, and that these sites of distant disease were not eradicated by adjuvant therapy. Predictive biomarkers that can predict responsiveness to current available therapies will be valuable to extend survival.

Despite the remarkable improvement in patient selection resulting from improved cross-sectional imaging technology and operative mortality in the past 30 years, the survival curve for pancreatic cancer patients has not improved [32, 66]. A new paradigm must be developed. There does exist a small cohort of long-term survivors (see Figure 11.1) that should serve as a focus of future studies to determine if there are *actionable* alterations for their biologic exceptionalism – be it in tumor genetics, epithelial-stromal interaction, inherent immunity, etc. We hypothesize that understanding the biology underlying the tumors in these unique long-term survivors will lead to new breakthroughs in systemic treatments that will truly bend the survival curve in the patients' favor.

References

1. Oshima M, Okano K, Muraki S, Haba R, Maeba T, Suzuki Y, *et al.* (2013). Immunohistochemically Detected Expression of 3 Major Genes (CDKN2A/p16, TP53, and SMAD4/DPC4) Strongly Predicts Survival in Patients With Resectable Pancreatic Cancer. *Annals of Surgery* **258**(2), 336–46.

2. Satake K, Takeuchi T, Homma T, Ozaki H (1994). CA19-9 as a screening and diagnostic tool in symptomatic patients: the Japanese experience. *Pancreas* **9**(6), 703–6.

3. Siegel R, Naishadham D, Jemal A (2013). Cancer statistics, 2013. *CA: A Cancer Journal for Clinicians* **63**(1), 11–30.

4. Reid-Lombardo KM, Fridley BL, Bamlet WR, Cunningham JM, Sarr MG, Petersen GM (2013). Survival Is Associated With Genetic Variation in Inflammatory Pathway Genes Among Patients With Resected and Unresected Pancreatic Cancer. *Annals of Surgery* **257**(6), 1096–102.

5. Legmann P, Vignaux O, Dousset B, Baraza AJ, Palazzo L, Dumontier I, et al. (1998). Pancreatic tumors: comparison of dual-phase helical CT and endoscopic sonography. American Journal of Roentgenology. *American Roentgen Ray Society* **170**(5), 1315–22.

6. Sener SF, Fremgen A, Menck HR (1999). Pancreatic cancer: a report of treatment and survival trends for 100,313 patients diagnosed from 1985–1995, using the National Cancer Database. *Journal of the American College of Surgeons* **189**(1), 1–7.

7. Iacobuzio-Donahue CA, Fu B, Yachida S, Luo M, Abe H, Henderson CM, et al. (2009). DPC4 Gene Status of the Primary Carcinoma Correlates With Patterns of Failure in Patients With Pancreatic Cancer. *Journal of Clinical Oncology* **27**(11), 1806–13.

8. DeWitt J, Devereaux B, Chriswell M, McGreevy K, Howard T, Imperiale TF, et al. (2004). Comparison of endoscopic ultrasonography and multidetector computed tomography for detecting and staging pancreatic cancer. *Annals of Internal Medicine* **141**(10), 753–63.

9. Winter JM, Brennan MF, Tang LH, D'Angelica MI, DeMatteo RP, Fong Y, et al. (2011). Survival after Resection of Pancreatic Adenocarcinoma: Results from a Single Institution over Three Decades. *Annals of Surgical Oncology* **19**(1), 169–75.

10. Winter JM, Tang LH, Klimstra DS, Brennan MF, Brody JR, Rocha FG, et al. (2012). A Novel Survival-Based Tissue Microarray of Pancreatic Cancer Validates MUC1 and Mesothelin as Biomarkers. *PLoS One* **7**(7), e40157.

11. Beretta E, Malesci A, Zerbi A, Mariani A, Carlucci M, Bonato C, et al. (1987). Serum CA 19-9 in the postsurgical follow-up of patients with pancreatic cancer. *Cancer* **60**(10), 2428–31.

12. Crippa S, Salvia R, Warshaw AL, Domínguez I, Bassi C, Falconi M, et al. (2008). Mucinous Cystic Neoplasm of the Pancreas is Not an Aggressive Entity. *Annals of Surgery* **247**(4), 571–9.

13. Yopp AC, Katabi N, Janakos M, Klimstra DS, D'Angelica MI, DeMatteo RP, et al. (2011). Invasive Carcinoma Arising in Intraductal Papillary Mucinous Neoplasms of the Pancreas. *Annals of Surgery* **253**(5), 968–74.

14. Winter JM, Tang LH, Klimstra DS, Liu W, Linkov I, Brennan MF, et al. (2013). Failure Patterns in Resected Pancreas Adenocarcinoma. *Annals of Surgery* **258**(2), 331–5.

15. Glenn J, Steinberg WM, Kurtzman SH, Steinberg SM, Sindelar WF (1988). Evaluation of the utility of a radioimmunoassay for serum CA 19-9 levels in patients before and after treatment of carcinoma of the pancreas. *Journal of Clinical Oncology* **6**(3), 462–8.

16. Winter JM, Brennan MF, Tang LH, D'Angelica MI, DeMatteo RP, Fong Y, et al. (2011). Survival after Resection of Pancreatic Adenocarcinoma: Results from a Single Institution over Three Decades. *Annals of Surgical Oncology* **19**(1), 169–75.

17. Ahmed S, Vaitkevicius VK, Zalupski MM, Du W, Arlauskas P, Gordon C, et al. (2000). Cisplatin, Cytarabine, Caffeine, and Continuously Infused 5-Fluorouracil (PACE) in the Treatment of Advanced Pancreatic Carcinoma: A Phase II Study. *American Journal of Clinical Oncology* **23**(4), 420.

18. Winter JM, Cameron JL, Campbell KA, Arnold MA, Chang DC, Coleman J, et al. (2006). 1423 pancreaticoduodenectomies for pancreatic cancer: A single-institution experience. *Journal of Gastrointestinal Surgery* **10**(9), 1199–210–discussion1210–1.

19. Kooby DA, Gillespie T, Bentrem D, Nakeeb A, Schmidt MC, Merchant NB, et al. (2008). Left-sided pancreatectomy: a multicenter comparison of laparoscopic and open approaches. *Annals of Surgery* **248**(3), 438–46.

20. Fukuda A, Wang SC, Morris JP, Folias AE, Liou A, Kim GE, et al. (2011). Stat3 and MMP7 contribute to pancreatic ductal adenocarcinoma initiation and progression. *Cancer Cell* **19**(4), 441–55.

21. Rocha Lima CMS, Savarese D, Bruckner H, Dudek A, Eckardt J, Hainsworth J, et al. (2002). Irinotecan plus gemcitabine induces both radiographic and CA 19-9 tumor marker responses in patients with previously untreated advanced pancreatic cancer. *Journal of Clinical Oncology* **20**(5), 1182–91.

22. Harsha HC, Kandasamy K, Ranganathan P, Rani S, Ramabadran S, Gollapudi S, et al. (2009). A Compendium of Potential Biomarkers of Pancreatic Cancer. *PLOS Medicine* **6**(4), e1000046.

23. Humphris JL, Chang DK, Johns AL, Scarlett CJ, Pajic M, Jones MD, et al. (2012). The prognostic and predictive value of serum CA19.9 in pancreatic cancer. *Annals of Oncology* **23**(7), 1713–22.

24. Oettle H, Post S, Neuhaus P, Gellert K, Langrehr J, Ridwelski K, et al. (2007). Adjuvant chemotherapy with gemcitabine vs observation in patients undergoing curative-intent resection of pancreatic cancer. *JAMA* **297**(3), 267–77. Available from: http://jama.jamanetwork.com/article.aspx?articleid=205145

25. Tempero MA, Uchida E, Takasaki H, Burnett DA, Steplewski Z, Pour PM (1987). Relationship of carbohydrate antigen 19-9 and Lewis antigens in pancreatic cancer. *Cancer Research* **47**(20), 5501–3.

26. Lamerz R (1999). Role of tumour markers, cytogenetics. *Annals of Oncology* **10**(suppl 4), S145–9.

27. Narimatsu H, Iwasaki H, Nakayama F, Ikehara Y, Kudo T, Nishihara S, *et al.* (1998). Lewis and secretor gene dosages affect CA19-9 and DU-PAN-2 serum levels in normal individuals and colorectal cancer patients. *Cancer Research* **58**(3), 512–8.

28. Richards NG, Rittenhouse DW, Freydin B, Cozzitorto JA, Grenda D, Rui H, *et al.* (2010). HuR Status is a Powerful Marker for Prognosis and Response to Gemcitabine-Based Chemotherapy for Resected Pancreatic Ductal Adenocarcinoma Patients. *Annals of Surgery* **128**, 96–104.

29. Haglund C (1986). Tumour marker antigen CA125 in pancreatic cancer: a comparison with CA19-9 and CEA. *British Journal of Cancer* **54**(6), 897–901.

30. Berger AC, Garcia M, Hoffman JP, Regine WF, Abrams RA, Safran H, *et al.* (2008). Postresection CA 19-9 Predicts Overall Survival in Patients With Pancreatic Cancer Treated With Adjuvant Chemoradiation: A Prospective Validation by RTOG 9704. *Journal of Clinical Oncology* **26**(36), 5918–22.

31. Benini L, Cavallini G, Zordan D, Rizzotti P, Rigo L, Brocco G, *et al.* (1988). A Clinical Evaluation of Monoclonal (CA19-9, CA50, CA 12-5) and Polyclonal (CEA, TPA) Antibody-Defined Antigens for the Diagnosis of Pancreatic Cancer. *Pancreas* **3**(1), 61.

32. Ballehaninna U, Chamberlain RS (2012). The clinical utility of serum CA 19-9 in the diagnosis, prognosis and management of pancreatic adenocarcinoma: An evidence based appraisal. *Journal of Gastrointestinal Oncology* **3**(2), 105–19.

33. Napoli C, Sperandio N, Lawlor RT, Scarpa A, Molinari H, Assfalg M (2012). Urine Metabolic Signature of Pancreatic Ductal Adenocarcinoma by 1H Nuclear Magnetic Resonance: Identification, Mapping, and Evolution. *Journal of Proteome Research* **11**(2), 1274–83.

34. Fong ZV, Winter JM (2012). Biomarkers in Pancreatic Cancer. *The Cancer Journal* **18**(6), 530–8.

35. Costello E, Greenhalf W, Neoptolemos JP (2012). New biomarkers and targets in pancreatic cancer and their application to treatment. *Nature Reviews Gastroenterology and Hepatology* **9**(8), 435–44.

36. Zhang L, Farrell JJ, Zhou H, Elashoff D, Akin D, Park N-H, *et al.* (2010). Salivary transcriptomic biomarkers for detection of resectable pancreatic cancer. *Gastroenterology* **138**(3), 949–57.e1–7.

37. Goonetilleke KS, Siriwardena AK (2007). Systematic review of carbohydrate antigen (CA 19-9) as a biochemical marker in the diagnosis of pancreatic cancer. *European Journal of Surgical Oncology* **33**(3), 266–70.

38. Bauer AS, Keller A, Costello E, Greenhalf W, Bier M (2012). Diagnosis of pancreatic ductal adenocarcinoma and chronic pancreatitis by measurement of microRNA abundance in blood and tissue. *PLoS One* **7**(4), e34151.

39. Chang C-Y, Huang S-P, Chiu H-M, Lee Y-C, Chen M-F, Lin J-T (2006). Low efficacy of serum levels of CA 19-9 in prediction of malignant diseases in asymptomatic population in Taiwan. *Hepatogastroenterology* **53**(67), 1–4.

40. Gaujoux S, Brennan MF, Gonen M, D'Angelica MI, DeMatteo R, Fong Y, *et al.* (2011). Cystic Lesions of the Pancreas: Changes in the Presentation and Management of 1,424 Patients at a Single Institution over a 15-Year Time Period. *Journal of the American College of Surgeons* **212**(4), 590–600.

41. Kim JE, Lee KT, Lee JK, Paik SW (2004). Clinical usefulness of carbohydrate antigen 19-9 as a screening test for pancreatic cancer in an asymptomatic population. *Journal of Gastroenterology and Hepatology* **19**(2), 182–6.

42. Allen PJ, Brennan MF (2007). The Management of Cystic Lesions of the Pancreas. *Advances in Surgery* **41**, 211–28.

43. Klöppel G, Kosmahl M (2001). Cystic lesions and neoplasms of the pancreas: the features are becoming clearer. *Pancreatology* **1**, 648–655

44. Brugge WR, Lewandrowski K, Lee-Lewandrowski E, Centeno BA, Szydlo T, Regan S, *et al.* (2004). Diagnosis of pancreatic cystic neoplasms: a report of the cooperative pancreatic cyst study. *Gastroenterology* **126**(5), 1330–6.

45. Horvath KD, Chabot JA (1999). An aggressive resectional approach to cystic neoplasms of the pancreas. *The American Journal of Surgery* **178**, 269–274.

46. Ooi LL, Ho GH, Chew SP, Low CH, Soo KC (1998). Cystic tumours of the pancreas: a diagnostic dilemma. *Australian and New Zealand Journal of Surgery* **68**(12), 844–6.

47. Tanaka M, Fernández-del Castillo C, Adsay V, Chari S, Falconi M, Jang J-Y, *et al.* (2012). International consensus guidelines 2012 for the management of IPMN and MCN of the pancreas. *Pancreatology* **12**(3), 183–97.

48. Fritz S, Klauss M, Bergmann F, Hackert T, Hartwig W, Strobel O, *et al.* (2012). Small (Sendai Negative) Branch-Duct IPMNs. *Annals of Surgery* **256**(2), 313–20.

49. Maker AV, Katabi N, Gönen M, DeMatteo RP, D'Angelica MI, Fong Y, *et al.* (2010). Pancreatic Cyst Fluid and Serum Mucin Levels Predict Dysplasia in Intraductal Papillary Mucinous Neoplasms of the Pancreas. *Annals of Surgical Oncology* **18**(1), 199–206.

50. Maker AV, Katabi N, Qin LX, Klimstra DS, SCHATTNER M, Brennan MF, *et al.* (2011). Cyst Fluid

Interleukin-1 (IL1) Levels Predict the Risk of Carcinoma in Intraductal Papillary Mucinous Neoplasms of the Pancreas. *Clinical Cancer Research* **17**(6), 1502–8.

51. Khalid A, McGrath KM, Zahid M, Wilson M, Brody D, Swalsky P, *et al.* (2005). The role of pancreatic cyst fluid molecular analysis in predicting cyst pathology. *Clinical Gastroenterology and Hepatology* **3**(10), 967–73.

52. Khalid A, Zahid M, Finkelstein SD, LeBlanc JK, Kaushik N, Ahmad N, *et al.* (2009). Pancreatic cyst fluid DNA analysis in evaluating pancreatic cysts: a report of the PANDA study. *Gastrointestinal Endoscopy* **69**(6), 1095–102.

53. Shen J, Brugge WR, DiMaio CJ, Pitman MB (2009). Molecular analysis of pancreatic cyst fluid. *Cancer Cytopathology* **117**(3), 217–27.

54. Wu J, Matthaei H, MAITRA A, Dal Molin M, Wood LD, Eshleman JR, *et al.* (2011). Recurrent GNAS Mutations Define an Unexpected Pathway for Pancreatic Cyst Development. *Science Translational Medicine* **3**(92), 92ra66–6.

55. Maithel SK, Maloney S, Winston C, Gönen M, D'Angelica MI, DeMatteo RP, *et al.* (2008). Preoperative CA 19-9 and the Yield of Staging Laparoscopy in Patients with Radiographically Resectable Pancreatic Adenocarcinoma. *Annals of Surgical Oncology* **15**(12), 3512–20.

56. Hartwig W, Strobel O, Hinz U, Fritz S, Hackert T, Roth C, *et al.* (2013). CA19-9 in Potentially Resectable Pancreatic Cancer: Perspective to Adjust Surgical and Perioperative Therapy. *Annals of Surgical Oncology* **20**(7), 2188–96.

57. Ferrone CR, Finkelstein DM, Thayer SP, Muzikansky A, Fernandez-del Castillo C, Warshaw AL (2006). Perioperative CA19-9 levels can predict stage and survival in patients with resectable pancreatic adenocarcinoma. *Journal of Clinical Oncology* **24**(18), 2897–902.

58. Hahn SA, Greenhalf B, Ellis I, Sina-Frey M, Rieder H, Korte B, *et al.* (2003). BRCA2 germline mutations in familial pancreatic carcinoma. *Journal of the National Cancer Institute* **5**(3), 214–21.

59. Lowery MA, Kelsen DP, Stadler ZK, Yu KH, Janjigian YY, Ludwig E, *et al.* (2011). An Emerging Entity: Pancreatic Adenocarcinoma Associated with a Known BRCA Mutation: Clinical Descriptors, Treatment Implications, and Future Directions. *The Oncologist* **16**(10), 1397–402.

60. Gelmon KA, Tischkowitz M, Mackay H, Swenerton K, Robidoux A, Tonkin K, *et al.* (2011). Olaparib in patients with recurrent high-grade serous or poorly differentiated ovarian carcinoma or triple-negative breast cancer: a phase 2, multicentre, open-label, non-randomised study. *Lancet Oncology* **12**(9), 852–61.

61. Marechal R, Bachet JB, Mackey JR, Dalban C, Demeter P, Graham K, *et al.* (2012). Levels of Gemcitabine Transport and Metabolism Proteins Predict Survival Times of Patients Treated With Gemcitabine for Pancreatic Adenocarcinoma. *Gastroenterology* **143**(3), 664–6.

62. Farrell JJ, Elsaleh H, Garcia M, Lai R, Ammar A, Regine WF, *et al.* (2009). Human Equilibrative Nucleoside Transporter 1 Levels Predict Response to Gemcitabine in Patients With Pancreatic Cancer. *Gastroenterology* **b**(1), 187–95.

63. Hwang J-H, Voortman J, Giovannetti E, Steinberg SM, Leon LG, Kim Y-T, *et al.* (2010). Identification of microRNA-21 as a biomarker for chemoresistance and clinical outcome following adjuvant therapy in resectable pancreatic cancer. *PLoS One* **5**(5), e10630.

64. Preis M, Gardner TB, Gordon SR, Pipas JM (2011). MicroRNA-10b expression correlates with response to neoadjuvant therapy and survival in pancreatic ductal adenocarcinoma. *Clinical Cancer Research* **17**(17), 5812–21.

65. Morris JP, Wang SC, Hebrok M (2010). KRAS, Hedgehog, Wnt and the twisted developmental biology of pancreatic ductal adenocarcinoma. *Nature Reviews Cancer* **10**(10), 683–95.

66. Allen PJ (2007). Pancreatic Adenocarcinoma: Putting a Hump in Survival. *Journal of the American College of Surgeons* **205**(4), S76–S80.

CHAPTER 12

Colon Cancer

Paul D Wagner

Cancer Biomarkers Research Group, Division of Cancer Prevention, National Cancer Institute,
National Institutes of Health, Rockville, MD, USA

Importance of colorectal cancer screening

In the United States, colorectal cancer is the third most common cancer among both men and women, and the second most common cause of cancer death in men and women combined, second only to lung cancer mortality. The American Cancer Society estimated that, in 2013, there were 140 000 new cases of colorectal cancer (100 000 colon cancer and 40 000 rectal cancers) and 50 000 deaths from colorectal cancer (26 000 men and 24 000 women) [1]. The lifetime risk of developing colorectal cancer in the USA is about 1 in 20. Increased age, male sex and black race are associated with increasing incidence of colorectal cancer. Over the past several decades, the incidence rate of colorectal cancer and deaths due to this cancer have been declining in the US. From 2001 to 2010, the incidence rate of colorectal cancer decreased 3.8% per year in men, and 3.2% per year in women. During the same time period, deaths due to colorectal cancer declined by about 3% in both men and women [2].

Colorectal cancers develop from noncancerous polyps, and usually take 10–15 years to develop [3]. This long preclinical phase makes colorectal cancer amenable to screening, and a significant fraction of the decline in both the colorectal cancer incidence and mortality can be attributed to screening and early detection. The five-year survival is 93% for stage I, 78% for stage II (confined within the wall of the colon), 64% for stage III (spread to regional lymph nodes), and 8% for stage IV (metastasized to distant sites). Currently, only about 40% of colorectal cancers in the US are detected early (US National Cancer Institute's Surveillance, Epidemiology, and End Results (SEER) Program (http://seer.cancer.gov/statfacts/html/colorect.html). The burden of this disease could be reduced by increasing the fraction of these cancer detected at an early stage.

As early stage colorectal cancer and its precursors, adenomatous polyps and adenomas, are asymptomatic, this can only be achieved by screening. Currently, about 40% of the US population is not screened within the recommended time intervals [4]. Improved screening methods, with improved accuracy and/or patient acceptability, are needed to increase the fraction of colorectal cancers detected early, and to increase the detection of advanced adenomas. One-third to one-half of all individuals will develop adenomas, and 10% of adenomas progress to cancer [1]. Removal of adenomas will prevent their progression.

Current screening modalities

The US Prevention Services Task Force (USPSTF) recommends screening for colorectal cancer in patients between 50 and 75 years using fecal occult blood tests (annually), flexible sigmoidoscopy (every five years) or colonoscopy (every ten years) [5]. As of 2014, USPSTF concluded that the evidence is insufficient to assess the benefits and harms of computed tomographic colonography

Biomarkers in Cancer Screening and Early Detection, First Edition. Edited by Sudhir Srivastava.
© 2017 John Wiley & Sons, Inc. Published 2017 by John Wiley & Sons, Inc.

(virtual colonoscopy) and fecal DNA testing as screening modalities for colorectal cancer.

Colonoscopy allows for direct vision of the rectum and colon, and is considered the gold standard for colorectal cancer screening, as it examines the entire colon, detects both cancer and polyps, and allows for the polyps to be removed and biopsied. However, there are limitations, including expense, and requirement for full bowel preparation. It also usually requires sedation, and misses about 5% of cancers, and in the US, there are about four perforations of the colon per 10 000 procedures and 25 adverse events per 10 000 procedures, most of which are in those patients who had a polypectomy [6].

Flexible sigmoidoscopy allows for direct visual examination of the rectum and the lowest third of the colon. Advantages over colonoscopy are that flexible sigmoidoscopy does not require sedation and has fewer serious complications – 3.4 per 10 000 procedures. Limitations include that it only examines one-third of the colon and, if a polyp or tumor is found, it must be followed by colonoscopy to examine the entire colon. In the Prostate, Lung, Colorectal and Ovarian Cancer Screening Trial (PLCO), sigmoidoscopy was shown to reduce incidence of colorectal cancer by 21%, and mortality from colorectal cancer by 26% [7]. Mortality from distal colorectal cancer was reduced by 50%, but mortality from proximal colorectal cancer was unaffected.

Fecal occult blood tests (FOBT) test for the presence of blood in stools, resulting from bleeding by colorectal cancers or large polyps in the colon. There are two types of fecal occult blood tests; the older guaic-base test (gFOBT), which detects heme, and the fecal immunological test (FIT), which detects human globin. The detection of heme is dependent on its peroxidase activity, and peroxidases from dietary source such as red meat and certain fruits and vegetables can cause a false positive gFOBT. The detection of human globin by FIT is more specific, as it is not subject to interference by diet. A positive gFOBT or FIT results in the patient being referred for colonoscopy.

The sensitivity gFOBT for colorectal cancer is 12–40%, depending on the stage of the cancer (the earlier the stage the lower the sensitivity), and the specificity of gFOBT is approximately 95%. The sensitivity FIT in a recent large trial was 74% for cancer and 42% for advanced adenomas [8]. The primary advantages of these tests are that they are non-invasive and relatively inexpensive. The main limitations are poor patient compliance and relatively low sensitivities for early stage cancers and advanced adenomas. gFOBT misses more than 60% of the cancers, and even a higher fraction of the advanced adenomas. FIT misses 25% of the cancers and 60% of the advanced adenomas. However, as gFOBT and FIT assays are recommended to be performed annually, a cancer missed one year may be detected in subsequent screens. Conversely, annual screening results in an increase in false positives, resulting in patients having unnecessary colonoscopies.

Despite its low sensitivity, regular screening with gFOBT has been shown to result in a 15–33% reduction in mortality due to colorectal cancer [9]. Similar trials have not been performed with FIT but, given its superior accuracy, it seems likely that screening with FIT would result in a comparable, if not larger, decrease in mortality.

Desirable properties of biomarkers for screening/early detection of colorectal cancer

Most current research on biomarkers for colorectal cancer screening/early detection is to develop a biomarker to determine which patients need to have a colonoscopy. Indeed, this is how the fecal occult blood tests are currently used. The goal is to develop a biomarker, or a panel of biomarkers, with sensitivities better than, or additive with, gFOBT or FIT (fewer missed cancers and advanced adenomas) – that is, sensitivity greater than 75% for early stage cancers, and 45% for advanced adenomas and specificities comparable to that of FIT – that is, greater than 90%. Other desirable properties include being of low cost, and measurable in specimens obtained noninvasively, such as stool, blood or urine. A blood- or urine-based biomarker might be more acceptable to patients than a stool-based biomarker, resulting an increase in compliance to screening schedules.

There are active research programs to discover and develop protein, DNA, RNA and metabolomic biomarkers for colorectal cancer detectable in stool and blood and, to a lesser extent, in urine. A PubMed search for colorectal cancer and screening biomarkers gives 900–1000 publications per year yet, to date, only gFOBT and FIT are recommended by USPTF for screening. Most biomarker publications describe discovery and/or pilot studies, and many report sensitivities and specificities that exceed those of gFOBT or FIT. However, despite these promising preliminary results, their reported sensitivities and specificities are usually considerably less when assayed on new specimens, and they are not pursued further.

Rather than discuss the numerous reported biomarkers for colorectal cancer screening/early detection, an overview of the classes of biomarkers, types of specimens in which they are measured, and a few selected examples will be presented. In 2014, the US Food and Drug Administration (FDA) approved a DNA based biomarker assay in stool for colorectal cancer screening and in 2016 a DNA based biomarker assay in blood for colorectal cancer screening (both are described below in detail).

Biomarker discovery, verification and validation

The first step to enhance the translation of biomarkers into useful diagnostic assays is to improve the discovery process. Recurrent problems in biomarker discovery research occur in both biospecimens used and study design [10].

Biospecimens:

- Differences in age, sex, ethnicity, and confounding conditions of cases and controls can result in biomarkers that reflect these differences, rather than the presence of cancer.
- Differences in sample collections, processing times, and storage can result in biomarkers that reflect these differences, rather than the presence of cancer (e.g., cancers collected and stored for years and cases recently collected).
- Cases and controls collected under different conditions (e.g. controls collected during a routine office visit and cases collected immediately prior to surgery).

Study design:

- Biomarker discovery is undertaken without consideration of the biomarkers potential clinical use.

- Classifier results from overfitting. This frequently occurs when the discovery involves a small number of samples and large number of variables (e.g., microarrays and mass spectrometry profiles), which can result in a statistical model that describes random error or noise, and not a panel of biomarkers that discriminates cases from controls. An independent test set of specimens can be used to help rule out the possibility that the classifier results from overfitting.
- Discovery of biomarkers for screening or early detection should preferably be done using early stage cancers or preneoplastic lesions (e.g., advanced adenomas) or body fluids from patients with early stage disease or preneoplastic lesions.
- Failure to account for lack of tissue specificity. Other tissues produce the biomarker, resulting in high biomarker levels in healthy patients.

A number of reviews discuss in detail problems associated with study design and biospecimen collection [11–14].

After sufficient preliminary data has been obtained to demonstrate the potential clinical use of a biomarker or panel of biomarkers, which usually involves several independent sets of experiments, the validation process begins. This process consists of two steps: a pre-validation or verification study; followed by a validation trial. Verification involves both analytical validation of the assay, and an independent evaluation of the biomarker's clinical performance. Analytical or assay validation includes optimization and determination of the accuracy, reproducibility and reliability of the assay.

Verification of the clinical performance of the biomarker can be achieved by performing the assay on a new set of specimens, for which the investigators are blinded [15]. Results from a verification study should answer the questions, "does the biomarker accurately and reliably distinguish those with cancer from those without it", and "how does its performance compare to the currently used biomarker, if any". Most biomarkers evaluated in a verification study do not progress to a validation trial, primarily due to lack of performance when assayed using independently collected specimens. Only after the performance of the biomarker has been verified, using an independent set of blinded specimens, should a biomarker validation trial be undertaken. Whether the validation trial is retrospective or prospective, the study must be well designed, conducted following a standard operating procedure, and sufficiently powered. The National Cancer Institute's Early Detection Research Network (EDRN) has published guidelines to help improve the process of biomarker discovery, verification and validation [16, 17].

Stool-based biomarkers

Colorectal cancer biomarkers detectable in the stool come primarily from colonocytes that are shed into the fecal stream. DNA mutations and methylated DNA detected in stool provide information on the presence of cancer and adenomas in the colon and rectum. These DNA biomarkers are based on knowledge of the mutations and epigenetic changes that occur within these cells that contribute to carcinogenesis. Most of the biomarker research using stool has been on DNA mutations (e.g. *Kras, APC, p53*) and methylation of tumor suppressor genes. As no single gene is mutated in all colorectal cancers, efforts have focused on forming panels. *APC* mutations are found in 85%, *Kras* mutations in 35–45% and *p53* in 35–45% of colorectal cancers [18]. *APC* and *Kras* mutations are also found in a significant fraction of adenomas.

Attempts to develop stool-based DNA biomarkers began in the 1990s, and very promising results have recently been published [8] and submitted to the US FDA for approval. The current panel consists of *Kras* mutations, aberrant *NDG4* and *BMP3* methylation, and a hemoglobin immunoassay. *Kras* is an oncogene and *NDG4* (N-Myc downstream-regulated gene 4) and *BMP3* (bone morphogenetic protein 3) are tumor-suppressor genes. Biomarkers in this panel differ from those in a panel previously developed by these investigators, which had 52% sensitivity for colorectal cancer and 41% for cancer plus advanced adenomas with a specificity of 94% [19]. The new panel has a sensitivity of 92.3% for the detection of colorectal cancer, and 42.4% for the detection of advanced adenomas [8]. This is significantly better than performance of FIT assayed on the same specimens – sensitivity of 73.8% for colorectal cancer and 23.8% for advanced

adenomas. FIT did give better specificity (94.9%) than the DNA test (89.8%).

In 2014, the FDA approved this panel (Cologuard by Exact Sciences Corp) for non-invasive colorectal cancer screening. While recommendations of the Advisory Committee are not binding, they are considered in FDA's review process. Despite the very high sensitivity of Cologuard for colorectal cancer, the sensitivity for advanced adenomas is significantly less; nearly 60% of these lesions were not detected. This a concern, as the projected ten-year cumulative risk for progression from advanced adenoma to cancer is about 25% at age 55 years [20]. Another concern is Cologuard's false positive rate of 10% – double that of FIT. Additional research is needed to determine the frequency at which this test should be performed [21]. As with any new screening test, other issues that need to be addressed include cost, patient acceptance and compliance.

Several other DNA based-stool tests are under development. For example, data from pilot studies indicate that methylated *VIM* (vimentin) in stool has a sensitivity of 46% and specificity of 90% [22]. The biomarker appears to be as sensitive for early stage cancers (I and II) as it is for late stage cancers (III and IV). An improved assay gives 75% sensitivity for colorectal cancer and a specificity of about 90%. The detection rate for general population screening is being determined as part of a prospective biomarker validation trial sponsored by NCI EDRN.

Microbiome

The human microbiome is the collection of microbes (bacteria, viruses, and single-cell eukaryotes) living in and on the human body. In a healthy human adult, microbes are estimated to outnumber human cells by ten to one. The human colon contains trillions of bacteria that play major roles in food digestion, protection against pathogens and disease, and development of innate and cell mediated immunity. Several studies indicate that a change in or imbalance (dysbiosis) in gut microbiome can contribute to the development of adenomas and colorectal cancer [23].

There are several mechanisms by which bacteria in the colon may alter susceptibility to cancer, including activation of the innate immune system, modulation of inflammation, and influencing gene expression. There are several reports that there are differences in the microbiome in stools from patients with colorectal cancer and from those without cancer. For example, a taxonomy-based analysis found that the risk of colorectal cancer was associated with decreased bacterial diversity in feces; depletion of Gram-positive, fiber-fermenting Clostridia; and increased presence of Gram-negative, proinflammatory *Fusobacterium* and *Porphyromonas* [24]. These changes are thought to contribute cancer development, and may be useful in determining the risk of developing colorectal cancer and in cancer prevention.

Blood-based biomarkers

A significant amount of research has been devoted to the discovery and development of blood-based biomarkers for early detection/screening of colorectal cancer. Serum and plasma from patients are more readily available than stool, and a blood-based test is likely to be more acceptable to patients than a stool-based test. To date only one has been approved by the US FDA for early detection of colorectal cancer, and few have met the requirements established by the Clinical Laboratory Improvement Amendments of 1988 (CLIA) law.

The difficulties of using blood as a source of cancer biomarkers include the presence of cell products from many different organs, immune response proteins and hormones, and the low amounts of biomarkers shed by the tumors into the blood, especially from early stage cancers [25]. Nevertheless, there are many examples of blood-based cancer biomarkers, including PSA for prostate cancer, CA-125 for ovarian cancer, CA19-9 for pancreatic cancer, alpha-fetoprotein (AFP) for liver cancer, and carcinoembryonic antigen (CEA) and CA19-9 to monitor colorectal cancer prognosis and response to surgery. CEA and CA19-9 are not useful for colorectal cancer screening, as their sensitivities for early stage cancer are too low. Blood-based biomarkers include proteins, DNA, and RNA. Recent advances in detection methods have expanded the potential number of candidate biomarkers.

Proteins

A large number of potential protein biomarkers for early detection of colorectal have been reported in the literature [26]. Many of these have low sensitivity for the detection of early stage colorectal cancer and have not been pursued. Others were initially reported to have very high sensitivity and specificity, but these results were only reported in a single study, or the sensitivity and specificity were significantly less when analyzed in a different set of specimens. For example, initial results for TIMP1 (tissue inhibitor of metalloproteinase) gave 56% sensitivity for early stage cancer with a specificity of 90%. A subsequent study by the same group of investigators reported no distinction between adenomas and normal [27]. A review in 2007 provided an overview of the status of 52 blood-based protein biomarkers, and concluded that larger prospective studies were needed to verify those that have given promising results [28].

Mass spectrometry protein profiling

There have been a number of reports that mass spectrometric profiles of plasma or sera could be used to distinguish with high accuracy patients with cancer from those without. The methods used for this profiling, surface-enhanced laser desorption/ionization time-of-flight mass spectrometry (SELDI-TOF-MS), and matrix-assisted laser desorption/ionization time-of-flight mass spectrometry (MALDI-TOF-MS), are high throughput techniques. However, most of these proteomic classifiers likely resulted from overfitting or other mythological problems.

Today, mass spectrometric techniques for protein expression profiling are used primarily for biomarker discovery [29]. Once proteins or peptides are identified by these technologies, targeted quantitative assays need to be developed that are suitable for the examination of a large number of biospecimens. These could be either immunochemical methods (e.g. ELISA), or mass spectrometry-based methods such as multiple-reaction monitoring (MRM) [30]. These assays are used to examine whether the discovered candidate biomarkers are present at concentrations that discriminate patients with cancer from healthy individuals, either independently or as part of a panel.

Other methods being used to discover protein biomarkers for colorectal cancer include peptide and antibody arrays. As with mass spectrometry based discovery, biomarkers identified by these high throughput methods need to be verified, using more targeted assays and larger numbers of specimens [31].

Glycosylated proteins are another source of potential biomarkers, as aberrant glycosylation is common to many cancer cells, and these proteins are frequently released into the blood [32]. One example is a specific glycosylated form of haptoglobin that is made in colon cancer cells but not in normal colon epithelium. This potential biomarker was found at 10–30 times higher levels in the serum of colon cancer patients, compared with healthy controls, and patients with adenomas have slightly higher levels of this protein than controls. There is only a small increase in total haptoglobin in the blood of colon cancer patients. The investigators' hypothesis is that this glycoslyated form of haptoglobin results from a tumor-specific ectopic expression of the haptoglobin protein, combined with colon-specific glycosylation. Pilot data using blinded specimens gave a sensitivity of 75% at specificity 80% [33]. The detection rate for general population screening is being determined as part of a prospective biomarker validation trial sponsored by NCI EDRN.

Circulating tumor DNA

Cell-free circulating tumor DNA (ctDNA) results from the release of DNA directly from the cancer cells into the blood, or from circulating tumor cells. ctDNAs contain the same point mutations and rearrangements as the tumor and are, therefore, specific for cancer. In contrast, many protein biomarkers are not cancer-specific. It has been reported that ctDNA can be detected in plasma of 73% of patients with localized colorectal cancer [34]. While this is an intriguing result, for this approach to useful for screening, a panel of genes that would encompass the diversity mutations present in colorectal cancer and advanced adenomas would have to be developed and tested.

Methylated DNA

An example of a methylated DNA biomarker for colorectal cancer that can be measured in blood is methylated *SEPT9*. Greater than 90% of colorectal cancers contain methylated *SEPT9*, and decreased *SEPT9* expression enhances call proliferation, cell movement, and angiogenesis. In a prospective screening trial of almost 7000 asymptomatic patients, the sensitivity of methylated *SEPT9* in plasma was 48.2%, with a specificity of 91.5%. Sensitivities for stage I and stage II cancers were respectively 35% and 63%. The sensitivity for advanced adenomas was 11.2% [35].

Although the sensitivity of methylated *SEPT9* is less than that of the DNA stool-based panel discussed above, the ability to measure this biomarker in plasma may make it more acceptable to patients and increase compliance. In 2014, an Advisory Committee to the US FDA supported the view that the product's (Epi proColon by Epigenomics AG) benefits outweigh its risks and in 2016, approved this test. Other possible blood-based methylated DNA biomarkers include *IRF4*, *BCAT1* and *IKZF1* [36].

mRNAs

Circulating mRNAs have also been investigated as biomarkers for colorectal cancer, as there are large and significant changes in gene expression in colon cancer tissues. Perhaps the most advanced is a panel of seven mRNAs; ANXA3, CLEC4D, LMNB1, PRRG4, TNFAIP6, AND VN1, which are overexpressed from 1.31- to 1.67-fold in colorectal cancer patients, and IL2RB, which is underexpressed. The assay produces a risk score that predicts the presence of colon cancer with a sensitivity of 72% and a specificity of 70% [37]. The sensitivity by stage was not reported (equal amounts of stage I, II and III were used to validate the assay), nor has its sensitivity for advanced adenomas been reported. This test was developed by GeneNews Ltd and is available in New York, New Jersey and Pennsylvania from Enzo Clinical Labs as ColonSentry. Its performance characteristics are in adherence with CLIA requirements. The FDA has determined that FDA approval is not necessary.

MicroRNAs (miRNAs)

MiRNAs are small noncoding RNAs (about 22 nucleotides long), and they have a role in post-transcriptional regulation of gene expression. MiRNAs bind to complementary sequences in the target

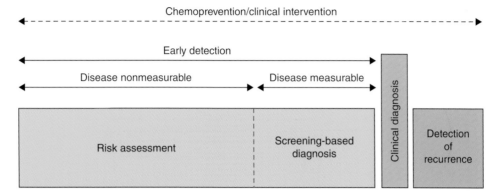

Figure 1.1 Biomarker application in the clinic. A long window of opportunity for chemoprevention or any clinical intervention is divided into sub-windows, based on whether a risk assessment is made when the disease is non-measureable, or an early diagnosis is made based on screening for measurable characteristics of the tumor, or a clinical diagnosis is made when the disease is symptomatic or has recurred. Adapted from [13].

Biomarkers in Cancer Screening and Early Detection, First Edition. Edited by Sudhir Srivastava.
© 2017 John Wiley & Sons, Inc. Published 2017 by John Wiley & Sons, Inc.

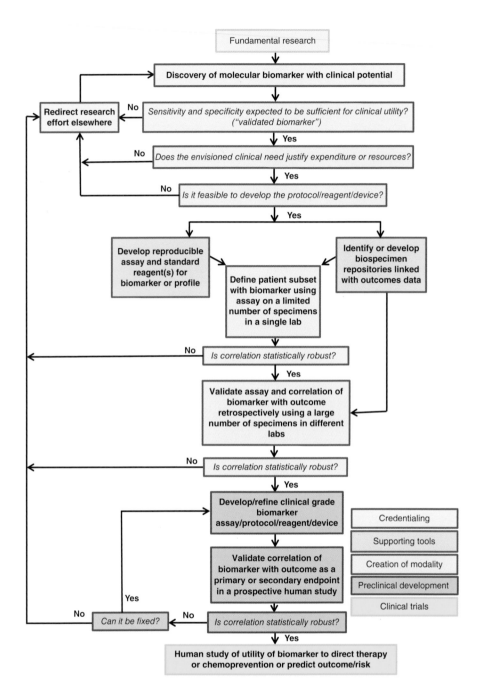

Figure 1.2 Biospecimen-Based Assessment Modality (BM) Pathway. The BM pathway is depicted as a flowchart, a schematic process representation widely used in engineering. The origin of the process is at the top. Fonts in bold indicate activity steps. Fonts in italics indicate conditional tests or decision steps. Unidirectional arrows represent the direction of the activity sequence and the direction of transfer of supporting tools from their parallel development paths to the main path of modality development. For each activity or decision point, it is understood that there are many more variations that can occur, and that not all steps may occur in each instance.

The pathway does not address the ways in which insights gained from late-stage clinical trials can influence the development process. Biospecimen-based assessment devices can be used for screening, early detection, diagnosis, prediction, prognosis, or response assessment. The pathways are conceived, not as comprehensive descriptions of the corresponding real-world processes, but as tools designed to serve specific purposes, including research program and project management, coordination of research efforts, and professional and lay education and communication [39].

Normal Cell

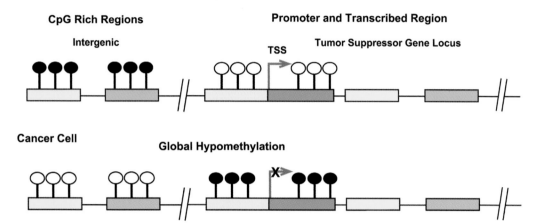

CpG Rich Regions

Promoter and Transcribed Region

Intergenic

Tumor Suppressor Gene Locus

TSS

Cancer Cell

Global Hypomethylation

Figure 2.1 Global hypomethylation: The diagram represents the hypo- and hyper-methylation of tumorsuppressor gene loci and intergenic regions, respectively, within the genome. In cancer cells, hypomethylation of intergenic CpG sequences and aberrant hypermethylation of tumor suppressor gene loci are hallmarks of the cancer epigenome.

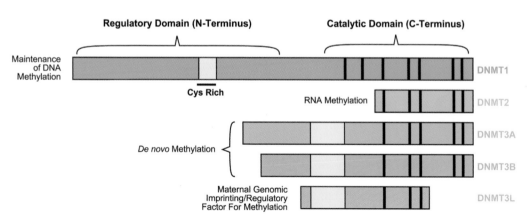

Regulatory Domain (N-Terminus)

Catalytic Domain (C-Terminus)

Maintenance of DNA Methylation

Cys Rich

DNMT1

RNA Methylation

DNMT2

De novo Methylation

DNMT3A

DNMT3B

Maternal Genomic Imprinting/Regulatory Factor For Methylation

DNMT3L

Figure 2.2 DNA Methyltransferases. Schematic diagram of the three main DNA methyltransferase families mammalian; DNMT1; DNMT2 and DNMT3. The DNMT1 is the largest enzyme ($\approx$ 200 kDa), composed of a C-terminal catalytic domain and a large N-terminal regulatory domain with several functions. The DNMT2 (391 aa) lacks the N-terminal domain. The DNMT3 family belongs to three enzymes, DNMT3A (912 aa), DNMT3B (865 aa) and DNMT3L (387 aa). The N-terminus of DNMT3A and 3B are divergent, as opposed to the C-terminus, which is highly similar. The DNMT3L is closely related to C-terminus of DNMT3A and 3B, but lacks the DNA cytocine-methyltransferase motifs (modified figure from [16]).

Normal Cell

Promoter

Normal Transcript

Cancer Cell

Promoter

Alternatively Spliced Transcript

Figure 2.3 Alternatively spliced transcript. The schematic diagram represents the intronic hypo- and hyper-methylation in normal or cancer cells by creating alternatively spliced transcripts. Alternatively, alterations of methylation patterns may also result in gene silencing and altered chromatin structure.

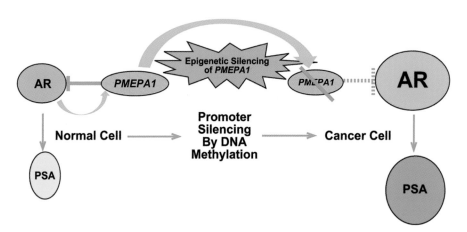

Figure 2.4 Silencing of the PMEPA1 gene disrupts a negative control over AR, leading to enhanced AR activity and resulting in elevated levels of PSA. Silencing of the PMEPA1 gene leads to enhanced AR activity in prostate cancer, by eliminating a negative regulatory control of AR protein levels. PMEPA1 facilitates AR protein degradation, which can be monitored by the detection of PSA, a tightly AR-regulated gene.

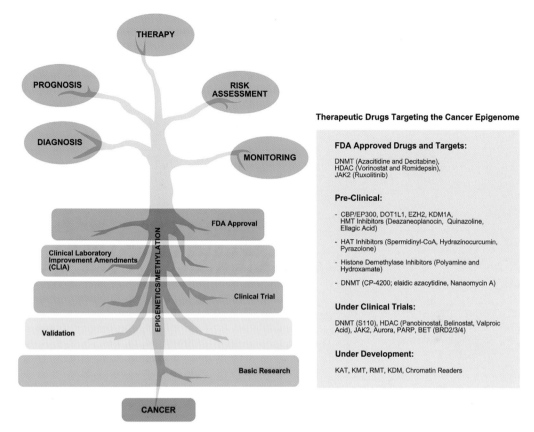

Figure 2.5 Cancer epigenome: biomarkers and therapeutic targets. The model represents the process of developing epigenetic biomarkers for diagnosis, prognosis, risk assessment, treatment response monitoring and therapeutic targets in cancer. FDA approved, pre-clinical and currently evaluated therapeutic drugs and targets are shown in the right panel.

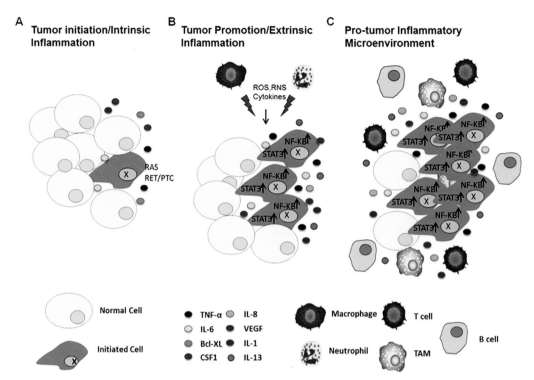

A Tumor initiation/Intrinsic Inflammation

B Tumor Promotion/Extrinsic Inflammation

C Pro-tumor Inflammatory Microenvironment

Figure 4.1 Co-evolution of cancer and its inflammatory microenvironment. **A.** Oncogenic mutations (e.g. Ras, RET/PTC) or other initiators of malignant transformation change the transcriptional program of initiated cells, including *de novo* transcription of inflammatory cytokines (intrinsic inflammation). **B.** These cytokines attract the cells of the innate immune system (e.g. macrophages and neutrophils), which produce their own cytokines and other inflammatory molecules (ROS, RNS) (extrinsic inflammation) that promote tumor development and tumor cell survival. **C.** The growing tumor attracts many cells of the immune system, creating a pro-tumor inflammatory microenvironment. Tumor-specific T cells and B cells are also present, but their function is compromised by the immunosuppressive effect of the tumor microenvironment.

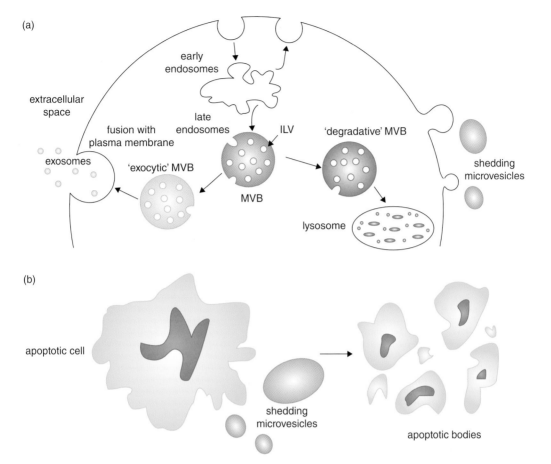

(a)

early
endosomes

extracellular
space

fusion with   late
plasma membrane   endosomes   ILV   'degradative' MVB

exosomes   shedding
                'exocytic' MVB   microvesicles

MVB

lysosome

(b)

apoptotic cell

shedding
microvesicles

apoptotic bodies

Figure 5.1 Schematic representation of biogenesis of extracellular vesicles. **A**. Release of exosomes and shedding microvesicles. Cytosolic components are trapped within intraluminal vesicles (ILVs) formed by invagination of endosomal membranes and contained within larger multivesicular bodies (MVBs). MVBs can release the ILVs into the extracellular space upon exocytic fusion with the plasma membrane (the released vesicles are defined as exosomes), or may be targeted for ubiquitination-dependent lysomal degradation. The role of the endosomal sorting complex responsible for transport (ESCRT) machinery in exosome biogenesis is unclear. There is support for both an ESCRT-dependent and an ESCRT-independent mechanism [19–22]. New studies may provide insights into the mechanisms governing MVB trafficking to the plasma membrane [23, 24]. Currently, it is not known whether there are MVB-independent mechanisms of exosome formation. The shedding microvesicles are formed directly by blebbing of the plasma membrane. **B**. Apoptotic bodies are vesicles with nuclear and cytoplasmic contents of apoptotic or dying cells. *Source:* Mathivanan 2010 [8]. Reproduced with permission of Elsevier.

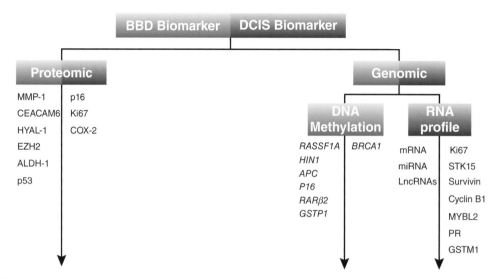

Figure 7.2 Candidate risk biomarkers for progression from benign breast disease/ductal carcinoma *in situ* to invasive breast carcinoma. Red indicates proteomic and genomic markers of benign breast disease; blue indicates proteomic and genomic markers of ductal carcinoma in situ. This figure is courtesy of Andrew K. Godwin.

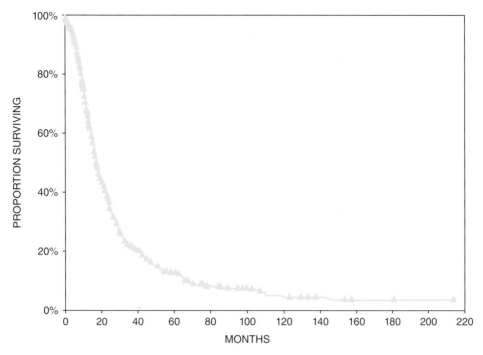

Figure 11.1 Overall survival for 812 pancreatic cancer patients who underwent pancreatectomy (1983–2004).

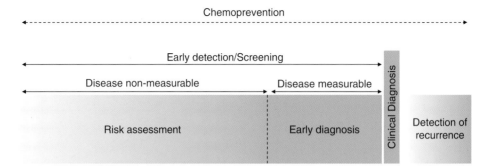

Figure 14.1 Clinical contexts for biomarker development in early detection of lung cancer. This diagram illustrates four clinical contexts within four windows of time. The period during which lung cancer is non-measurable and precedes the diagnosis characterizes the context of *risk assessment*. It represents a long window of time, during which the disease develops and corresponds to an opportunity for chemoprevention. When the disease becomes measurable but remains asymptomatic, we enter the context of *early diagnosis*. Two other clinical contexts relate to *clinical diagnosis* – that is, when the disease is measurable and patients symptomatic – and to *detection of recurrence*. These windows of time correspond to the different contexts for which different biomarker targets can be developed. Adapted from Hassanein *et al.*, 2011 [135]. Reprinted with permission of the American Thoracic Society. Copyright © 2012, American Thoracic Society.

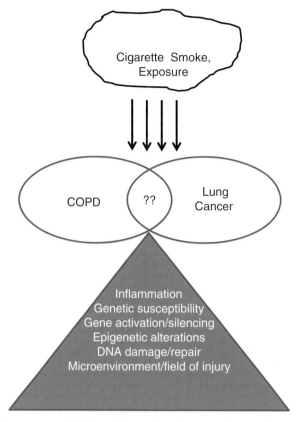

Figure 15.1 Link between lung cancer and COPD. Pathogenetic mechanisms responsible for the lung cancer-COPD association are poorly understood. Biomarkers common to both disease processes fall into many categories, but all require further validation.

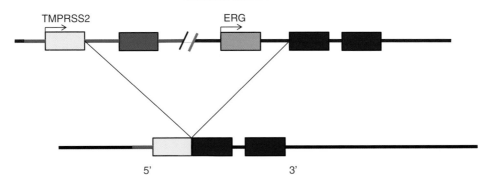

Figure 16.1 Example of a genomic rearrangement on chromosome 21 that juxtaposed an androgen responsive promoter and a noncoding exon of the TMPRSS2 gene to an ETS gene family member, ERG. The rearrangement caused the aberrant expression of the ERG proto-oncogene.

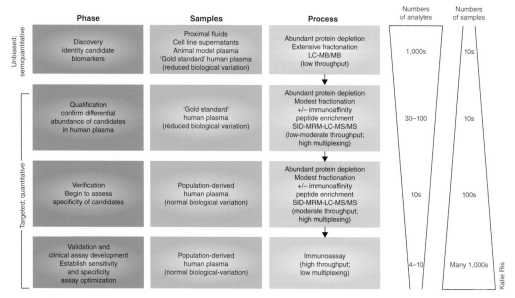

Figure 17.1 In this figure, illustrating process flow for development of biomarker candidates, the word "validation" appears in the bottom row in the fourth "phase." In phases 2 and 3, the concept of validity (i.e., "how valid is the study result") is relevant, even if the word "validation" is not used.

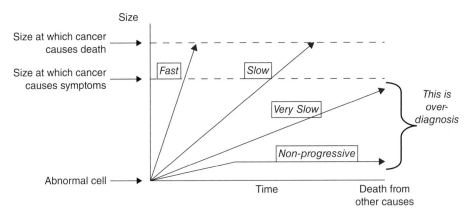

Figure 18.1 The heterogeneity of cancer progression is reflected in the variation in growth rate of similarly appearing cancers. Growth rate contributes to whether, and when, an occult cancer within the preclinical reservoir becomes clinically symptomatic within the individual's lifetime.

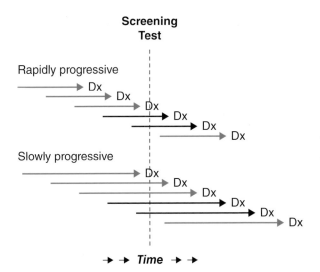

Figure 18.2 Periodic screening selectively detects slowly progressing cancers. Many of these might never have become clinically symptomatic and are, therefore, overdiagnoses.

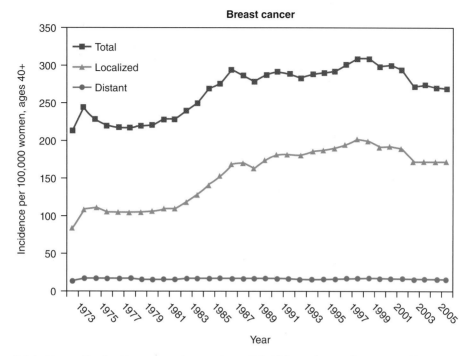

Figure 18.3 Incidence of localized breast cancer increases in parallel with increasing use of mammographic screening during the 1980s and 1990s. Distant disease remains constant, suggesting overdiagnosis. Adapted from [3].

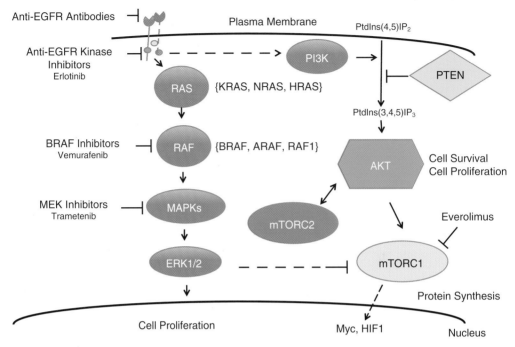

Figure 19.1 Predictive markers in human cancers. The common markers are depicted that are the targets of specific therapies, as indicated by the (⊣). The dashed brown receptor kinase indicates a mutation in the receptor that may cause constitutive activation of that receptor with consequent activation of the downstream molecules.

While EGFR is depicted, other receptors, such as the Insulin Growth Factor Receptor (IGFR), the Platelet Derived Growth Factor Receptor (PDGFR), and so on, may also be activated by mutation or even fusion with other genes. Arrows denote stimulation of the molecular marker.

mRNAs, resulting in the destruction of the mRNA. Altered expressions of miRNAs are associated with cancer and, over the last decade, there have been numerous reports demonstrating that cancer cells have different miRNAs profiles than normal cells. MiRNAs can be readily measured in blood and are more stable than either DNA or mRNA. This stability is thought to result from miRNAs being protected from degradation by being packaged into lipid vesicles, or by being bound to protein or lipoprotein complexes.

The stability and relatively high abundance in blood make miRNAs an attractive source of cancer biomarkers, and there are a large number of publications on the potential use of panels of miRNAs measured in blood as biomarkers for colorectal cancer. Many of these panels have been reported to have high sensitivities (83–91%) and specificities (70–95%) [38]. For example, a panel of six miRNAs (miR-21, let-7g, miR-31, mir-92a, miR-181b and miR-203) was reported to have a sensitivity of 96.4% and specificity of 88.1% for colorectal cancer; about half of the cancers examined were stage I and II [39]. As with most biomarkers, a well-designed and powered validation trial, using a predefined panel of miRNAs, is required before these panels can be used for screening.

Metabolomics

The metabolome is the complete set of small-molecule metabolites (metabolic intermediates, secondary metabolites, hormones and other signaling molecules) in a biological sample. Metabolomics is the measurement and analysis of these metabolites in cells, tissues, organs or bodily fluids. There have been several studies to determine whether metabolomics, or metabolic profiling of stool or blood, can be used to detect colorectal cancer. Thus far, results in blood have been mixed, with some reporting no overall association between serum metabolites and colorectal cancer [40], while others report promising sensitivities and specificities (82.8% sensitivity for stage 0–2 colorectal cancer at 81% specificity) [41]. It has been reported that stool samples from patients with colorectal cancer contain higher concentrations of amino acids, and stool samples from healthy patients contain higher concentrations of poly- and monounsaturated fatty acids

and ursodeoxycholic acid [42]. These differences in the stool metabolome are thought to reflect differences in the intestinal microbiome of patients with colorectal cancer.

Urine-based biomarkers

In addition to stool and blood, urine has been used a potential source of biomarkers for a variety of cancers, including colorectal cancer. Research on urinary biomarkers for colorectal cancer is not as extensive or as well developed as that on blood and stool based biomarkers.

DNA

Several studies have demonstrated that urine contains short-length DNAs derived from the circulation, and that these DNAs can originate from organs and tumors distal to the urinary tract. The concentration of DNA in the urine is similar to that in the serum, and mutated *Kras* was detected in the urine of 95% of patients with *Kras* containing tumors, but only in the serum of 35% of these same patients [43]. Methylated DNA can also be detected in urine. In a pilot study, methylated *VIM* was detected in the urine of 75% of patients with colorectal cancer, and in 10% of healthy patients [44] – comparable to the results for methylated *VIM* measured in stool.

Metabolomics

There have been several studies to determine whether metabolomics or metabolic profiling of urine can be used to detect colorectal cancer. For example, one-dimensional nuclear magnetic resonance spectra of urine were used to generate a diagnostic metabolomic profile for colonic adenomas, which gave a sensitivity of 82.7% and specificity of 51.2% [45]. Two different FIT tests performed on stool from the same patients gave sensitivities of 7.6% and 11.8% for colonic adenomas.

The enzyme cyclooxygenase-2 is expressed in a majority of colorectal cancers, and plays an important role in prostaglandin production [46]. PGE-M, the urinary metabolite of prostaglandin E(2), is increased in patients with colorectal cancers or large adenomas, suggesting that urinary PGE-M is potentially a useful biomarker for the detection of colorectal cancer and advanced adenomas. In a nested case-control study, urinary PGE-M was measured in 150 cohort members who developed colorectal cancer, and 150 matched controls. The relative risk increased from 1.0 to 2.5, 4.5, and 5.6 with increasing urinary PGE-M quartiles [47]. Urinary PGE-M was also analyzed in a case control study that included 224 cases with at least one advanced adenoma, 152 cases with multiple small tubular adenomas, 300 cases with only a single small tubular adenoma, and 364 polyp-free controls. Patients with the highest quartile level of PGE-M were 2.5-fold more likely to have advanced or multiple small tubular adenomas than those with the lowest level of PGE-M [48].

Proteins

Urine contains highly soluble low molecular weight proteins and peptides (< 30 kDa), and the composition of proteins in urine is qualitatively similar to that of blood, but more dilute. Polypeptides in urine are relatively stable compared to those in sera or plasma, and do not undergo significant proteolysis within several hours of collection. A review of the literature reported a consensus list of 443 proteins found in urine [49]. SELDI and MALDI TOF profiling have been used to identify protein biomarkers in urine for colorectal cancer. In one study, MALDI and SELDI spectra were generated using urine from 67 patients with colorectal cancer (45 early and 22 late stage cancers), as well as 72 control subjects. A classifier was developed that identified colorectal cancer with 78% sensitivity at 87% specificity. Three of the discriminatory peptides were an 1885 Da fragment of fibrinogen, hepcidin-20 and beta2-microglobulin [50].

Conclusion

As discussed in this chapter, there are a number of promising biomarkers in the pipeline, ranging from very preliminary results obtained using a few specimens, to two recently approved by the US FDA examined thousands of patients. A recurrent theme for most biomarker discovery, no matter the technology or source of specimens, is that the initial sensitivity and specificity rarely hold up on repetition in different set of specimens, or when examined by a differ set of investigators. The performance of the biomarker must be validated

using an independent set of blinded specimens, and preferably compared directly to the currently used biomarker – that is, FIT for colorectal cancer.

References

1. American Cancer Society (2016). *Colorectal Cancer Facts & Figures 2014–2016.* http://www.cancer.org/research/cancerfactsstatistics/colorectal-cancer-facts-figures.
2. Siegel R, Ma J, Zou Z, Jemel A (2014). Cancer statistics, 2014. *CA: A Cancer Journal for Clinicians* **64**(1), 9–29.
3. Kinzler KW, Vogelstein B (2002). Colorectal tumors. In: Vogelstein B, Kinzler KW (eds). *The genetic basis of human cancer,* 2nd edition, pp. 583–612. New York: McGraw-Hill.
4. Centers for Disease Control and Prevention (CDC) (2013). Vital Signs: Colorectal Cancer Screening Test Use-United States, 2012. *Morbidity and Mortality Weekly Report (MMWR)* **62**(44), 881–8.
5. U.S. Preventive Services Task Force (2016). http://www.uspreventiveservicestaskforce.org/recommendations.htm
6. Fisher DA, Maple JT, Ben-Menachem T, *et al.* (2011). Complications of colonoscopy. *Gastrointestinal Endoscopy* **74**(40), 45–52.
7. Schoen RE, Pinsky PF, Weissfeld JL, *et al.* (2012). Colorectal-cancer incidence and mortality with screening flexible sigmoidoscopy. *New England Journal of Medicine* **366**(25), 2345–57.
8. Imperiale TF, Ransohoff DF, Itzkowitz SH, *et al.* (2014). Multitarget stool DNA testing for colorectal-cancer screening. *New England Journal of Medicine* **370**(14), 1287–97.
9. Levin B, Lieberman DA, McFarland B, *et al.* (2008). Screening and surveillance for the early detection of colorectal cancer and adenomatous polyps, 2008: a joint guideline from the American Cancer Society, the US Multi-Society Task Force on Colorectal Cancer, and the American College of Radiology. *Gastroenterology* **134**(5), 1570–95
10. Wagner PD, Srivastava S (2012). New paradigms in translational science research in cancer biomarkers. *Translational Research* **159**(4), 343–53.
11. Baker SG, Kramer BS, McIntosh M, *et al.* (2006). Evaluating markers for the early detection of cancer: overview of study designs and methods. *Clinical Trials* **3**, 43–56.
12. Brenner DE, Normolle DP (2007). Biomarkers for cancer risk, early **detection**, and prognosis: the validation conundrum. *Cancer Epidemiology, Biomarkers & Prevention* **16**, 1918–20.
13. Dunn BK, Wagner PD, Anderson D, Greenwald P (2010). Molecular markers for early detection. *Seminars in Oncology* **37**, 224–42.

14. Ransohoff DF, Gourlay ML (2010). Sources of bias in specimens for research about molecular markers for cancer. *Journal of Clinical Oncology* **28**, 698–704.

15. Feng Z, Kagan J, Pepe M, *et al.* (2013). The Early Detection Research Network's specimen reference sets: paving the way for rapid evaluation of potential biomarkers. *Clinical Chemistry* **59**(1), 68–74.

16. Pepe MS, Etzioni R, Feng Z, *et al.* (2001). Phases of biomarker development for early detection of cancer. *Journal of the National Cancer Institute* **93**(14), 1054–61.

17. Pepe MS, Feng Z, Janes H, *et al.* (2008). Pivotal evaluation of the accuracy of a biomarker used for classification or prediction: standards for study design. *Journal of the National Cancer Institute* **100**(20), 1432–8.

18. Markowitz DS, Bertagnolli MM (2009). Molecular basis of colon cancer. *New England Journal of Medicine* **361**, 2449–60.

19. Imperiale TF, Ransohoff DF, Itzkowitz SH, *et al.* (2004). Fecal DNA versus fecal occult blood for colorectal-cancer screening in an average-risk population. *New England Journal of Medicine* **351**(26), 2704–14.

20. Brenner H, Hoffmeister M, Stegmaier C, *et al.* (2007). Risk of progression of advanced adenomas to colorectal cancer by age and sex: estimates based on 840,149 screening colonoscopies. *Gut* **56**(11), 1585–89.

21. Robertson DJ, Dominitz JA (2014). Stool DNA and colorectal-cancer screening. *New England Journal of Medicine* **370**(14), 1350–1.

22. Chen WD, Han ZJ, Skoletsky J, *et al.* (2005). Detection in fecal DNA of colon cancer-specific methylation of the nonexpressed vimentin gene. *Journal of the National Cancer Institute* **97**(15), 1124–32.

23. Dulal S, Keku TO (2014). Gut microbiome and colorectal adenomas. *The Cancer Journal* **20**(3), 225–31.

24. Ahn J, Sinha R, Pei Z, *et al.* (2013). Human gut microbiome and risk for colorectal cancer. *Journal of the National Cancer Institute* **105**(24), 1907–11.

25. Hori SS, Gambhir SS (2011). Mathematical model identifies blood biomarker-based early cancer detection strategies and limitations. *Science Translational Medicine* **3**, 109ra116.

26. Wang K, Huang C, Nice EC (2014). Proteomics, genomics and transcriptomics: their emerging roles in the discovery and validation of colorectal cancer biomarkers. *Expert Review of Proteomics* **11**(2), 179–205.

27. Holten-Andersen MN, Fenger C, Nielsen HJ, *et al.* (2004). Plasma TIMP-1 in patients with colorectal adenomas: a prospective study. *European Journal of Cancer* **40**, 2159–64

28. Hundt S, Haug U, Brenner H (2007). Blood markers for early detection of colorectal cancer: a systematic review. *Cancer Epidemiology, Biomarkers & Prevention* **16**(10), 1935–53.

29. Gemoll T, Roblick UJ, Auer G, *et al.* (2010). SELDI-TOF serum proteomics and colorectal cancer: a current overview. *Archives of Physiology and Biochemistry* **116**(4–5), 188–96.

30. Boja ES, Rodriguez H (2012). Mass spectrometry-based targeted quantitative proteomics: achieving sensitive and reproducible detection of proteins. *Proteomics* **12**(8), 1093–110.

31. Lee JR, Magee DM, Gaster RS, *et al.* (2013). Emerging protein array technologies for proteomics. *Expert Review of Proteomics* **10**(1), 65–75.

32. Kuzmanov U, Kosanam H, Diamandis EP (2013). The sweet and sour of serological glycoprotein tumor biomarker quantification. *BMC Medicine* **11**, 31 doi: 10.1186/1741-7015-11-31.

33. Bresalier RS, Byrd JC, Tessler D, *et al.* (2004). A circulating ligand for galectin-3 is a haptoglobin-related glycoprotein elevated in individuals with colon cancer. *Gastroenterology* **127**(3), 741–8.

34. Bettegowda C, Sausen M, Leary RJ, *et al.* (2014). Detection of circulating tumor DNA in early- and late-stage human malignancies. *Science Translational Medicine* **6**, 224ra24.

35. Church TR, Wandell M, Lofton-Day C, *et al.* (2014). Prospective evaluation of methylated SEPT9 in plasma for detection of asymptomatic colorectal cancer. *Gut* **63**(2), 317–25.

36. Mitchell SM, Ross JP, Drew HR, *et al.* (2014). A panel of genes methylated with high frequency in colorectal cancer. *BMC Cancer* **14**, 54.

37. Marshall KW, Mohr S, Khettabi FE, *et al.* (2010). A blood-based biomarker panel for stratifying current risk for colorectal cancer. *International Journal of Cancer* **126**(5);1177–86.

38. Ganepola AP, Nizin J, Rutledge JR, Chang DH (2014). Use of blood-based biomarkers for early diagnosis and surveillance of colorectal cancer. *World Journal of Gastrointestinal Oncology* **6**(4), 83–97.

39. Wang J, Huang S-k, Zhao M, *et al.* (2014). Identification of a circulating microRNA signature for colorectal cancer detection. *PLoS One* **9**(4), e87451. doi:10.1371/journal.pone.0087451

40. Cross AJ, Moore SC, Boca S, *et al.* (2014). A prospective study of serum metabolites and colorectal cancer risk. *Cancer*. doi: 10.1002/cncr.28799. Epub ahead of print

41. Nishiumi S, Kobayashi T, Ikeda A, *et al.* (2012). A Novel Serum Metabolomics-Based Diagnostic Approach for Colorectal Cancer. *PLoS One* **7**(7), e40459. doi:10.1371/journal.pone.0040459

42. Weir TL, Manter DK, Sheflin AM, *et al.* (2013). Stool microbiome and metabolome differences between colorectal cancer patients and healthy adults. *PLoS One* **8**(8), e70803. doi: 10.1371/journal.pone.0070803.

43. Su YH, Wang M, Brenner DE, *et al.* (2008). Detection of mutated K-ras DNA in urine, plasma, and serum of patients with colorectal carcinoma or adenomatous polyps. *Annals of the New York Academy of Sciences* **1137**, 197–206.

44. Song BP, Jain S, Lin SY, *et al.* (2012). Detection of hyper-methylated vimentin in urine of patients with colorectal cancer. *Journal of Molecular Diagnostics* **14**(2), 112–9.

45. Wang H, Tso V, Wong C, Sadowski D, Fedorak RN (2014). Development and validation of a highly sensitive urine-based test to identify patients with colonic adeno-matous polyps. *Clin Transl Gastroenterology* **5**(3), e54.

46. Anderson WF, Umar A, Hawk ET (2003). Cyclooxy-genase inhibition in cancer prevention and treatment. *Expert Opinion on Pharmacotherapy* **4**(12), 2193–204.

47. Cai Q, Gao YT, Chow WH, *et al.* (2006). Prospective study of urinary prostaglandin E2 metabolite and col-orectal cancer risk. *Journal of Clinical Oncology* **24**(31), 5010–6

48. Shrubsole MJ, Cai Q, Wen W, *et al.* (2012). Uri-nary prostaglandin E2 metabolite and risk for col-orectal adenoma. *Cancer Prevention Research* **5**, 336–42.

49. Casado-Vela J, Gómez del Pulgar T, Cebrián A, *et al.* (2011). Human urine proteomics: building a list of human urine cancer biomarkers. *Expert Review of Pro-teomics* **8**(3), 347–60.

50. Ward DG, Nyangoma S, Joy H, *et al.* (2008). Proteomic profiling of urine for the detection of colon cancer. *Proteome Science* **6**, 19.

CHAPTER 13

Prognostic and Predictive Biomarkers for Colorectal Cancer

Upender Manne,[1] Balananda-Dhurjati Kumar Putcha,[2] Temesgen Samuel,[3] and Sudhir Srivastava[4]

[1] Department of Pathology and Comprehensive Cancer Center, University of Alabama Birmingham, AL, USA

[2] Department of Pathology, University of Alabama, Birmingham, AL, USA

[3] Centre for Cancer Research and Department of Pathobiology, Tuskegee University, Tuskegee, AL, USA

[4] Cancer Biomarkers Research Group, Division of Cancer Prevention, National Cancer Institute, National Institutes of Health, Bethesda, MD, USA

Introduction

Recent advances in our understanding of cancer pathobiology and the key molecular pathways in oncogenesis, and improved strategies of cancer biomarker development, have resulted in the identification of several candidate molecular biomarkers. However, most of these candidates fail to reach the clinic because the causes of tumor development, rates of progression, and responses to therapeutic interventions are unique to individual patients. Furthermore, various factors, including cellular and molecular heterogeneity within tumors, varying host immune responses, diet, environmental exposure, lifestyle, and patient demographics influence the effectiveness of cancer biomarkers. Thus, the *"one size fits all"* approach is obsolete, and there is a need to design strategies to develop effective biomarkers by applying principles of individualized cancer care.

Definitions and types of biomarkers

A tumor marker is also referred to as a "cancer biomarker." It is a characteristic that is objectively measured and evaluated as an indicator of normal biologic processes, pathogenic processes, or pharmacologic responses to a therapeutic intervention. A biomarker is either produced by the tumor, or by the body, in response to cancer, and it can be measured by genetic, proteomic, or cellular or molecular substances found in higher than normal amounts in the blood, urine, or body tissues of a cancer patient. Biomarkers are measurable and reliable indicators, utilized to assess the disease process or outcome, or to estimate whether a drug used in the treatment was effective or not [1].

Based on their utility, biomarkers can be divided into the following categories:

1 *Early detection*, if used for screening patients to find cancer early.
2 *Diagnostic*, if used to assess the presence or absence of cancer.
3 *Prognostic*, if used to assess the survival probabilities of patients or to detect an aggressive phenotype and determine how the cancer will behave (natural history of cancer).
4 *Predictive*, if used to predict whether the drug and other therapies will be effective or to monitor the effectiveness of treatment (likelihood of cancer response to a particular therapy).

Biomarkers in Cancer Screening and Early Detection, First Edition. Edited by Sudhir Srivastava.

© 2017 John Wiley & Sons, Inc. Published 2017 by John Wiley & Sons, Inc.

5 *Target*, if used to identify the molecular targets of novel therapies and to determine which molecular markers are affected by therapy.

Surrogate endpoints are biomarkers used to substitute for clinical endpoints, which can be used to measure clinical benefit, harm, or lack of benefit or harm. Surrogates can replace traditional endpoints, such as incidence of disease, mortality due to disease, or the recurrence or relapse of disease. *Companion diagnostic* is a biomarker-based diagnostic test that aids in stratifying patients into subsets with distinct clinical outcomes (susceptibility/risk/therapy response). This test can be an *in vitro* diagnostic device or imaging tool.

The advantages of biomarkers are well recognized by the research, medical, and pharmaceutical communities. By replacing clinical endpoints, biomarkers can reduce time and costs for Phase I and Phase II clinical trials. They can also be helpful in redefining diseases and their therapies by shifting the emphasis from traditional practices of depending on symptoms and morphology to a more rational, objective, and molecular basis.

Biomarkers of colorectal cancers (CRCS)

Race/ethnicity-based biomarkers

To develop effective cancer biomarkers, there is a need to understand the pathobiology of cancers. In regard to CRCs, the findings of earlier efforts, focused on identifying molecular bases for racial/ethnic disparities, are inconclusive and are not useful clinically, because of the confounding effect of population admixture and the molecular/genetic heterogeneity of these cancers. Furthermore, investigations performed by us and others show different biologic consequences based on pathologic stage, tumor location, and the race/ethnicity of CRC patients. Thus, there is a need to identify and validate 'early detection' markers (assessing risk of premalignant lesions to progress to invasive carcinomas), 'predictive' factors (allowing patients to receive treatments to which they are most likely to respond), and 'prognostic' factors (providing better information on the likely course of the disease and patient survival).

To evaluate effects of race/ethnicity, these steps should be accomplished with large tissue cohorts of CRCs collected from African Americans, Hispanics, Caucasians and other groups of rural-urban and Northern-Southern populations of the USA. The tissues should be well characterized for histologic, pathologic, clinical, and epidemiologic features. Such biomarker studies yield results suggesting that biologically based differences in patient demographic (age/race/ethnicity/age) groups relate to cancer outcomes. Further, the data may provide a rationale for evaluation of population-based biomarkers in the *personalization of cancer therapies*.

Exosomes as biomarkers

Exosomes are membrane-bound extracellular vesicles, about 30–150 nm in size, that originate from the extrusions of cell membranes, and are distinct in their contents in relation to normal and pathological circumstances [2, 3]. The relevance of exosomes in cell-cell communication, especially for their role in modulating immunity, has been evaluated. Exosomes are also produced by cancer cells, and the roles of their cargoes in mediating various cancer-associated processes such as transformation, angiogenesis, immune cell modulation, and metastasis have been identified [4–7]. Therefore, as structures released into body fluids and circulation, exosomes have become attractive to cancer researchers for their potential as carriers of diagnostic, predictive, or prognostic biomarkers [8].

Exosomes, which can be separated by physical methods, carry cargoes that are specific to the cells from which they originated. These facts endow exosomes and other extracellular vesicles with high clinical significance as potential biomarkers for prediction, prognosis, and establishment of personalized therapies. Identification of exosomes in body fluids is of minimal clinical importance, as these are also released under non-pathological states. Rather, the contents of exosomes – including miRNA, RNA, DNA, proteins, and lipids – may prove to be useful, as they bear specific markers of their tissues of origin and are readily distributed through the body fluids.

Although there is considerable interest in exosomes and unfinished studies of microvesicles, there is no regulatory agency-approved, exosome-based diagnostic, prognostic, or predictive clinical test for colon cancer [9]. Nevertheless, a few molecular biomarkers that have potential value in these areas are under investigation (Table 13.1) [10–13].

Table 13.1 Candidate biomarkers of colorectal cancer.

	Candidate individual molecules or sets of molecules	Potential clinical utility in CRC	Remark	References
Exosome Associated	Mir-18	Screening/diagnostic		[10]
	Let-7a, mir-1229, mir-1246, mir-150, mir-21, mir-223, mir-23a	Screening/diagnostic		[11]
	MET, S100A8, S100A9, TNC	Not defined yet	Involved in metastasis	[12]
	EFNB2, JAG1, SRC, TNIK	Not defined yet	Involved in signal transduction	[12]
	CAV1, FLOT1, FLOT2, PROM1	Not defined yet	Involved in lipid biology	[12]
Metabolome	2-hydroxybutyrate, aspartic acid, kynurenine, and cystamine	Diagnostic	Better sensitivity and accuracy than CEA	[18]
	3-hydroxybutyric acid, L-valine, L-threonine, 1-deoxyglucose, and glycine	Diagnostic		[21]
	A panel consisting of citrate, hippurate, p-cresol, 2-aminobutyrate, myristate, putrescine, and kynurenate;	Diagnostic		[22]
	Alanine, citrate, creatine, glutamine, peptide NHs, lactate, leucine, pyruvate, tyrosine, 3-hydroxybutyrate, acetate, formate, glycerol, lipid (–CH2–OCOR), N-acetyl signal of glycoproteins, phenylalanine, and proline;	Diagnostic		[23]
	Hydroxylated polyunsaturated ultra-long chain fatty acid metabolites	Diagnostic		[24]
	Glucose, inositol, hypoxanthine, xanthine, uric acid and deoxycholic acid	Diagnostic		[25]
	L-valine, 5-oxo-l-proline, 1-deoxyglucose, D-turanose, D-maltose, arachidonic acid, hexadecanoic acid, and l-tyrosine	Diagnostic		[26]
	Proline, cysteine, acetate and butyrate	Diagnostic		[27]
	L-alanine, glucuronoic lactone, and L-glutamine	Diagnostic		[28]
miRNA	miR-21, miR-92, and miR-135	Diagnosis/Prognosis	83% sensitivity, 85% specificity (miR-92)	[37–40]
	miR-200b, let-7, miR-140, miR-143, and miR-192	Predictive		[56–59]
Genetic alterations	Loss of chromosome 18q	Prognostic		[64,65]
	MSI	Diagnostic/Predictive		[66,67]
	Multi-gene assays (ColoGuidePro, Onco type DX test™, ColoPrint®,	Prognostic/Predictive		[68–72]
	Mutations in KRAS, BRAF, PIC3CA, TP53, UGT1A1, and DYPD	Predictive		[73–81]
	CEA	Diagnostic/Predictive		[82,83]
Methylation markers	Hypermethylation of Vimentin (hV)	Detection	83% sensitivity, 82% specificity	[86]
	Hypermethylation of the MLH1 promoter	Risk		[87,88]
	Hypermethylation of plasma septin-9	Detection	Poor sensitivity in prospective trials	[89]
	CpG island methylator phenotype	Prognostic		[91]

Similarly, exosomes isolated from the ascites fluid of CRC patients contain hundreds of proteins [14], some of which may be developed as biomarkers for CRC in general, or for a subset of CRC patients. Overall, the clinical potentials for these and other exosome-associated molecules as biomarkers for CRCs remain to be established. Since exosomes can be obtained from patients non-invasively, by collecting blood, urine, saliva, or other body fluids, and these microvesicles hold promising potential as sources of diagnostic, prognostic, and/or predictive biomarkers.

The metabolome as a source of biomarkers for CRCs

The metabolome, defined as the set of metabolites of less than 2000 Da molecular mass existing within a biological unit ranging from a cell to a whole animal [15,16], presents a unique source of biomarkers that reflect the physiological or pathological state at a given time. These molecules are generally released into the microenvironment in which the biological unit finds itself and, thus, into the circulation at large. Their presence in the circulation, and the ease of collecting samples, makes them attractive targets for biomarker development.

With technological advances in methods to detect small molecules, as well as increased high-throughput and bioinformatics capabilities to analyze thousands of metabolites simultaneously, metabolomics holds great promise to enhance the discovery of metabolites for the diagnosis, prediction, and prognosis of a variety of cancers [17]. As a recent entrant into the field of cancer biology, metabolomics has not yet reached a stage for clinical trials or routine clinical use. Nevertheless, there is a potential for application of this powerful tool and resource in the clinical oncology of CRCs.

To date, the metabolomic features of CRCs include dysregulated mechanisms and pathways that can be exploited to establish a systematic methodology, and to allow development of biomarkers. A prediction model, based on mass spectrometric analysis of the serum metabolome, identified a set of metabolites, including 2-hydroxybutyrate, aspartic acid, kynurenine, and cystamine; its sensitivity, specificity, and accuracy were 85.0%, 85.0%, and 85.0%, respectively. In contrast, the sensitivity, specificity, and accuracy of the CRC marker carcinogenic embryonic antigen (CEA) were 35.0%, 96.7%, and 65.8%, respectively, and those of the marker CA19-9 were 16.7%, 100%, and 58.3%, respectively [18].

These results show that, although there is less sensitivity relative to CEA-based testing, the metabolomics set of biomarkers have superior values for sensitivity and accuracy. Moreover, the metabolite sets showed higher sensitivity for the detection of early stage CRCs. Of note, serum metabolite composition may differ between localized and metastatic CRCs, or even between liver-only metastasis and extrahepatic metastasis, opening the possibility of identifying patients at different stages of CRC [19].

In addition to liquid biopsies, solid-tissue biopsies could also be used for metabolic profiling of CRCs. Mass spectrometric analysis of tumor tissue identified a distinct type of metabolite profile associated with CRCs relative to that of normal tissue, and led to the identification of chemically diverse marker metabolites which were associated with dysregulated biochemical processes [20]. These include: glycolysis; the Krebs cycle; osmoregulation; steroid biosynthesis; eicosanoid biosynthesis; bile acid biosynthesis; and lipid, amino acid, and nucleotide metabolism. Some metabolites were found to be distinct between normal and CRC patients so, therefore, several studies have suggested metabolites as candidate diagnostic biomarkers (Table 13.1) [21–28]. Other metabolites yet to be identified, but expected to be validated in the future, will add to the arsenal of metabolomics tools for the detection, prediction, and prognosis of CRCs.

Although metabolomics appears to be a powerful tool for ultimate clinical use in CRC oncology, substantial challenges need to be overcome. The most fundamental challenge is the dynamic nature of metabolic processes and their susceptibility to a range of factors that are independent of CRC pathology, but which result from endogenous or exogenous factors. For example, although stools provide a direct, non-invasive source of the gastrointestinal metabolome [29], the inter-personal variation in gut microbiota, which has a significant effect on the outcomes of the digestive process, could make it difficult to separate pathological changes from gut microenvironment effects.

Additionally, the effects of genetic background, time of day, health, nutritional status, and other spatial or temporal variations, may pose challenges. Therefore, standardized protocols and combinations of biomarkers of high individual scores, in conjunction with appropriate algorithms, are needed to establish biomarker platforms for universal CRCs or for subgroup-oriented clinical use [30].

The kinome

The kinome, defined as the protein kinase complement of the human genome, contains nine broad groups of genes [31]. Protein tyrosine kinases (PTKs), subsets of the kinome, are regulators of intracellular signal-transduction pathways, mediating development and multicellular communication in metazoans. Normally, their activity is tightly controlled and regulated [32]. Since mutations in PTKs are rare in CRCs, most research and clinical efforts that involve these kinases are geared towards targeting them for therapy, rather than for biomarker applications. Currently, the only candidate kinase considered for clinical CRC biomarker application is the serine-threonine-kinase, BRAF [33]. BRAF mutations, the most common being V600E, occur in a small percentage of CRC tumors, but the existence of this mutation is associated with poor survival [34], suggesting the prognostic potential for the status of BRAF mutation.

miRNAs as biomarkers

MicroRNAs (miRNAs), small non-coding RNAs of ~17–27 nucleotides, negatively regulate gene expression at the post-transcriptional level, through direct interaction with the 3'UTR of the target mRNA. There is abnormal expression of miRNAs in several human cancers, including CRCs. Aberrantly expressed miRNAs contribute to the development and progression of cancers by targeting tumor suppressors or oncogenes [35].

miRNAs are stable in feces, serum, plasma, and urine, making them possibly minimally invasive and sensitive biomarkers [36]. The stability of miRNAs in these sources might be due to their encapsulation in extracellular membrane-enclosed vesicles or exosomes. Upregulation of miR-135, which targets and reduces levels of the adenomatous polyposis coli protein, is an early event in CRC and is a potential biomarker for early detection [37]. Serum

miR-21 was also shown to be a potential biomarker for diagnosis and prognosis of CRC [38]. Expression levels of miR-92a can be used to distinguish CRC from healthy controls with 83.0% sensitivity and 84.7% specificity [39, 40].

The prognostic value of single and large-scale miRNA panels has been assessed [41]. There is high expression of miR-21, which has been extensively studied, in breast cancer, CRC, lung cancer, glioblastoma, and chronic lymphocytic leukemia [42–46]. In patients with CRCs, serum levels of miR-21 increase with the stage of the disease [47]. The prognostic significance of miR-21 overexpression has been established for various types of cancer [48–51]. Our studies on CRCs have found that high expression of miR-21 is associated with poor prognosis for patients, especially for non-Hispanic Caucasians [52]. High serum levels of miR-21 are present in breast, colorectal, and pancreatic cancers.

Serum/plasma miRNAs are potential prognostic biomarkers for CRCs and other gastric carcinomas [53]. Particularly in CRCs, serum miR-21 expression is a strong diagnostic and prognostic biomarker. Additionally, reductions in serum miR-21 levels are observed after surgical removal of CRC tumors [47, 54]. miRNA expression profiles are distinctly different in CRC patients with microsatellite instability (MSI), relative to those with microsatellite stability (MSS) [55]. This may have implications in CRC prognosis and patient treatment decisions, as patients with MSI have a favorable prognosis relative to those with MSS.

Expression of miRNAs is altered upon treatment of CRC cell lines with 5-fluorouracil (5-FU). 5-FU reduces miR-200b, which reduces the levels of protein tyrosine phosphatase PTPN12 which, in turn, downregulates oncogenes, including c-ABL and RAS, resulting in decreased cell proliferation [56]. Further, altered miRNA levels can modulate efficacy of biological and cytotoxic reagents. KRAS mutations reduce the efficacy of anti-EGFR treatment. However, patients exhibiting KRAS mutations and high let-7 have increased survival benefit from anti-EGFR therapy, as let-7 targets KRAS and reduces its expression.

Since they modulate drug targets directly or indirectly, other miRNAs have emerged as potential predictive biomarkers for CRCs. miR-140 and miR-143 sensitize CRC cells to 5-FU [57, 58], and miR-192 downregulates the anticancer target, dihydrofolate reductase [59]. Additional mechanisms that alter response to therapy include single nucleotide polymorphisms (SNPs) in miRNA binding sites within the target mRNA. In metastatic CRC cancer patients, the LCS6 polymorphism in the let-7 binding site within the 3'UTR of KRAS has predicted response to anti-EGFR-based therapy [60]. Similarly, SNPs in the 3'UTRs of base-excision repair (BER) genes have altered CRC prognosis and response to 5-FU [61].

Plasma miR-205 and let-7f are potential diagnostic biomarkers, especially for early-stage epithelial ovarian cancer (EOC). Let-7f is also a potential prognostic biomarker for late-stage EOC [62]. The tissue origin of metastatic cancer can be established based on expression of a library of 48 miRNAs [63].

Genetic alterations as biomarkers

Genetic abnormalities, including chromosomal and gene alterations and dysregulation of gene and protein expression, provide useful information for optimal care and outcomes of CRC patients. Chromosomal instability is frequently observed in CRCs. Loss of chromosome 18q is associated with a poor prognosis for CRC patients [64, 65]. MSI occurs in about 15–20% of sporadic CRC cases and in > 95% of patients with the Lynch syndrome [66,67]. In CRCs, detection of MSI helps to identify patients who might benefit from surgery alone [67].

Multi-gene assays are likely to provide more robust information and serve as strong prognostic and predictive biomarkers. Several gene expression signatures have been developed to assess prognosis of CRC patients [68–70]. A seven-gene expression prognostic test, ColoGuidePro, was developed for stage II and III CRC patients [71]. Recurrence score assays, such as the Onco type DX test™, which is based on gene expression profiling, were designed for determination of risk of recurrence for stage II and III CRCs, and for breast and prostate cancer patients after surgery. Similarly, ColoPrint® was effective in determining recurrence risk in stage II CRC patients, and in identifying patients who can be safely managed without chemotherapy [72]. These assays were validated in large patient series.

Predictive biomarkers aid in distinguishing patients who respond to cytotoxic and biological agents from those who are non-responders. For example, in metastatic CRC patients, mutations in KRAS and BRAF serve as biomarkers for determining efficacy of anti-EGFR therapies involving panitumumab or cetuximab [73–75]. Similarly, the PIC3CA mutation is a potential predictive biomarker for determining longer survival of CRC patients with regular use of aspirin after diagnosis [76]. Another potential predictive biomarker for CRC is high levels of microsatellite instability (MSI-H), which may be due to a less aggressive nature of tumors or to a higher sensitivity of MSI-H patients to 5-FU, a standard chemotherapeutic agent for CRCs. Mutations in TP53 and DYPD decrease the therapeutic response to 5-FU [77–79]. Variations of the uridine diphosphate-glucuronosyltransferase 1A (UGT1A1) gene have predictive value for side-effects and for the efficacy of irinotecan [80, 81]. However, prospective trials are required to determine the clinical utility of these mutations in identifying patients who are likely to suffer serious side-effects of 5-FU toxicity.

CEA, one of the first known tumor biomarkers, is widely used for CRC patients [82,83]. Elevated CEA is detected in CRC tissues and in serum or plasma of the patients. CEA levels increase with stage of the disease [83]. Although CEA is used to detect recurrence of CRCs, its specificity as a biomarker is limited, as CEA levels are also elevated in patients with epithelial tumors of non-intestinal origin, in patients with liver disease, and in smokers [84, 85].

Fecal biomarkers for CRC include fecal blood, detected by the fecal occult blood test, and detection of mutations and hypermethylation of genes for fecal DNA shed from CRC cells. Several fecal DNA markers have been evaluated for CRC screening. For example, a simplified stool DNA test for hypermethylation of vimentin gene (hV) and a two-site DNA integrity assay (DY) showed high sensitivity (83%) and specificity (82%) for CRCs [86].

Epigenetic alterations of cancers include DNA methylation profiles, post-translational modification of histones, and miRNA expression patterns. Hypermethylation of the MLH1 promoter was observed in the serum of MSI-positive, sporadic CRC patients, while subsequent studies showed that it is associated with higher risk of death

[87, 88]. A multi-center clinical trial of a screening test for CRC relating to hypermethylation of plasma septin-9 (mSEPT9) showed that the test could detect CRC in asymptomatic, average-risk individuals. However, this method may not be widely applicable, due to its poor sensitivity [89,90]. Hypermethylation of the *DYPD* (dihydropyrimidine dehydrogenase) gene has been proposed to be a mechanism for severe 5-FU toxicity [91]. However, DYPD promoter methylation is not an important prognostic factor for severe toxicity to 5-FU [92].

CpG island methylator phenotype (CIMP) has been implicated in a poor prognosis for CRC patients [93]. However, different subgroups of CIMP also exhibit MSI and mutations in *BRAF*, *KRAS*, and *TP53* [94, 95]. Therefore, the association between the CIMP phenotype and CRC prognosis remains controversial. A highly sensitive Methyl-BEAMing technology was developed for absolute quantification of methylation in DNA samples [96]. For early-stage CRCs, the sensitivity of this approach was four-fold higher than that for measurement of CEA levels.

Companion diagnostics

Companion diagnostics are *in vitro* tests or imaging tools (medical devices) that help oncologists to: stratify cancer patients into sub-groups, based on their responses to a specific therapy; decide appropriate doses; design optimal treatment plans; and develop post-surgery intervention strategies, including diet, therapy, and/or exercise, tailored specifically to the patient. A companion diagnostic may identify patients who are more likely to benefit or have risk of serious adverse side-effects from a particular therapeutic agent. The *Personalized Medicine* branch of the Food and Drug Administration (FDA), which clears or approves these biomarker-based tests, suggests that companion diagnostic devices are essential to the safe and effective use of drugs (http://www.fda.gov/MedicalDevices.htm).

Only biomarker based-companion diagnostic devices that demonstrate robustness and both analytic and clinical utility pass through the regulatory approval processes of the FDA. Thus far, FDA has cleared/approved 19 companion diagnostic tests for selection of drugs to treat various cancers (fda.gov);

most are nucleic acid-based. The development of companion diagnostic devices is a continuous process as new approaches, including next-generation sequencing of multiple genes, are evolving. These deep-sequencing techniques are helping to identify the presence of low-incidence and high-penetrance biomarker mutations [97].

For example, FDA has approved the *therascreen KRAS RGQ PCR Kit* (QIAGEN, Manchester, UK), a companion diagnostic test to identify metastatic CRC patients (with Stage III or IV) suitable for treatment with Erbitux (cetuximab) and Vectibix (panitumumab). This test is a real-time qualitative PCR assay, conducted on DNA extracted from formalin-fixed paraffin-embedded CRC tissues, for the detection of seven somatic mutations in the *Kras* gene. Patients who exhibit mutation(s) in *Kras* are potentially non-responsive to Erbitux and Vectibix therapy [98,99].

In some instances, multiple companion diagnostic tests approved by the FDA are available to assess the status of a biomarker. For example, multiple companion diagnostic tests are used to assess overexpression of human epidermal growth factor receptor-2 (HER2/ErbB2/c-neu) (increased expression of protein or gene amplification) in breast cancer tissues, to identify patients with aggressive disease and to be candidates for Herceptin therapy. These tests have been improved as scientists resolved the technical difficulties in utilizing these devices.

Challenges and future directions

Despite the huge potential, several prognostic and predictive biomarkers are not in clinical practice, due to various challenges. Failure in developing effective molecular cancer biomarkers is due, in part, to: a lack of uniformity in implementation and interpretation of assay results; diversity of assay methods (platforms); heterogeneity in genetic alterations; admixture in study populations (patient race/ethnicities and demographics); and diversity in pathobiology of disease (geography-specific disease forms). Other reasons include the lack of: standardization of sample collection, processing, and stabilization techniques; standard specimen reference sets in specimen selection, collection, procession, and storage; statistical competence; and adequate clinical validation tools. Moreover, the field of cancer biomarker development is challenging, because of our lack of understanding of the molecular pathogenesis of cancers, and because advancements in developing new assay platforms are continuing to emerge.

Because biologically based differences in racial/ethnic and demographic (age/gender) groups have implications on clinical presentation and cancer outcomes [52, 100–103], approaches to develop biomarkers should progress through population-based studies. Such biomarker studies provide a strong rationale and foundation for *personalization of cancer therapies*. To validate the clinical utility of molecular biomarkers, biomarker development studies should be conducted in both academic and community settings, so there should be an emphasis in establishing collaborations with community oncologists to form tissue/patient data consortia. To aid in performing cancer biomarker development studies, such academic-community based efforts will:

a enhance translational cancer research for rapid incorporation of molecular advancements and pivotal trial data into community practice; and

b facilitate the integration of biomarker profiles and epidemiological, nutritional, and behavioral research, in order to have maximum impact of molecular biomarker testing and to help in providing personalized medicine.

Overall, integration of biomarkers into routine clinical practice requires combined efforts from experts from both academic cancer research centers and community cancer care givers. These experts include translational cancer biologists, pathologists, medical oncologists, surgical oncologists, gastroenterologists, community physicians, bioinformaticists, computational biologists, biostatisticians, epidemiologists, nutritionists, and behavioral scientists. Further, to address the moral, ethical, and social issues related to cancer biomarker development, there is a need to involve bioethicists and social scientists for their effective implementation.

Acknowledgements

We thank Dr. Donald L. Hill, Division of Preventive Medicine, University of Alabama at Birmingham, AL, for his critical review of this manuscript. This study is supported in part by grants from the NIH (U54-CA118948) to Dr. Manne and GM109314 to Dr. Samuel.

References

1. Atkinson AJ, Magnason WG, Colburn WA, DeGruttola VG, DeMets DL, Downing GJ, et al. (2001). NCI-FDA Biomarkers Definitions Working Group; Biomarkers and surrogate endpoints: preferred definitions and conceptual framework. *Clinical Pharmacology & Therapeutics* **69**(3), 89–95.

2. Harding CV, Heuser JE, Stahl PD (2013). Exosomes: looking back three decades and into the future. *Journal of Cell Biology* **200**(4), 367–71.

3. Pan BT, Johnstone RM (1983). Fate of the transferrin receptor during maturation of sheep reticulocytes *in vitro*: selective externalization of the receptor. *Cell* **33**(3), 967–78.

4. Kucharzewska P, Christianson HC, Welch JE, Svensson KJ, Fredlund E, Ringner M, et al. (2013). Exosomes reflect the hypoxic status of glioma cells and mediate hypoxia-dependent activation of vascular cells during tumor development. *Proceedings of the National Academy of Sciences of the United States of America* **110**(18), 7312–7.

5. Taylor DD, Gercel-Taylor C (2005). Tumour-derived exosomes and their role in cancer-associated T-cell signalling defects. *British Journal of Cancer* **92**(2), 305–11.

6. Yang M, Chen J, Su F, Yu B, Su F, Lin L, et al. (2011). Microvesicles secreted by macrophages shuttle invasion-potentiating microRNAs into breast cancer cells. *Molecular Cancer* **10**, 117.

7. Park JE, Tan HS, Datta A, Lai RC, Zhang H, Meng W, et al. (2010). Hypoxic tumor cell modulates its microenvironment to enhance angiogenic and metastatic potential by secretion of proteins and exosomes. *Molecular & Cellular Proteomics* **9**(6), 1085–99.

8. Raposo G, Stoorvogel W (2013). Extracellular vesicles: exosomes, microvesicles, and friends. *Journal of Cell Biology* **200**(4), 373–83.

9. Locker GY, Hamilton S, Harris J, Jessup JM, Kemeny N, Macdonald JS, et al. (2006). ASCO 2006 update of recommendations for the use of tumor markers in gastrointestinal cancer. *Journal of Clinical Oncology* **24**(33), 5313–27.

10. Komatsu S, Ichikawa D, Takeshita H, Morimura R, Hirajima S, Tsujiura M, et al. (2014). Circulating miR-18a: a sensitive cancer screening biomarker in human cancer. *In vivo (Athens, Greece)* **28**(3), 293–7.

11. Ogata-Kawata H, Izumiya M, Kurioka D, Honma Y, Yamada Y, Furuta K, et al. (2014). Circulating exosomal microRNAs as biomarkers of colon cancer. *PLoS One* **9**(4), e92921.

12. Ji H, Greening DW, Barnes TW, Lim JW, Tauro BJ, Rai A, *et al.* (2013). Proteome profiling of exosomes derived from human primary and metastatic colorectal cancer cells reveal differential expression of key metastatic factors and signal transduction components. *Proteomics* **13**(10–11), 1672–86.

13. Klein-Scory S, Kubler S, Diehl H, Eilert-Micus C, Reinacher-Schick A, Stuhler K, *et al.* (2010). Immunoscreening of the extracellular proteome of colorectal cancer cells. *BMC Cancer* **10**, 70.

14. Choi DS, Park JO, Jang SC, Yoon YJ, Jung JW, Choi DY, *et al.* (2011). Proteomic analysis of microvesicles derived from human colorectal cancer ascites. *Proteomics* **11**(13), 2745–51.

15. Pearson H. Meet the human metabolome (2007). *Nature* **446**(7131), 8.

16. Wishart DS, Jewison T, Guo AC, Wilson M, Knox C, Liu Y, *et al.* (2013). HMDB 3.0 –The Human Metabolome Database in 2013. *Nucleic Acids Research* **41**(Database issue), D801–7.

17. Malet-Martino M, Holzgrabe U (2011). NMR techniques in biomedical and pharmaceutical analysis. *Journal of Pharmaceutical and Biomedical Analysis* **55**(1), 1–15.

18. Nishiumi S, Kobayashi T, Ikeda A, Yoshie T, Kibi M, Izumi Y, *et al.* (2012). A novel serum metabolomics-based diagnostic approach for colorectal cancer. *PLoS One* **7**(7), e40459.

19. Farshidfar F, Weljie AM, Kopciuk K, Buie WD, Maclean A, Dixon E, *et al.* (2012). Serum metabolomic profile as a means to distinguish stage of colorectal cancer. *Genome Medicine* **4**(5), 42.

20. Mal M, Koh PK, Cheah PY, Chan EC (2012). Metabotyping of human colorectal cancer using two-dimensional gas chromatography mass spectrometry. *Analytical and Bioanalytical Chemistry* **403**(2), 483–93.

21. Ma Y, Zhang P, Wang F, Liu W, Yang J, Qin H (2012). An integrated proteomics and metabolomics approach for defining oncofetal biomarkers in the colorectal cancer. *Annals of Surgery* **255**(4), 720–30.

22. Cheng Y, Xie G, Chen T, Qiu Y, Zou X, Zheng M, *et al.* (2012). Distinct urinary metabolic profile of human colorectal cancer. *Journal of Proteome Research* **11**(2), 1354–63.

23. Bertini I, Cacciatore S, Jensen BV, Schou JV, Johansen JS, Kruhoffer M, *et al.* (2012). Metabolomic NMR fingerprinting to identify and predict survival of patients with metastatic colorectal cancer. *Cancer Research* **72**(1), 356–64.

24. Ritchie SA, Ahiahonu PW, Jayasinghe D, Heath D, Liu J, Lu Y, *et al.* (2010). Reduced levels of hydroxylated, polyunsaturated ultra long-chain fatty acids in the serum of colorectal cancer patients: implications for early screening and detection. *BMC Medicine* **8**, 13.

25. Ong ES, Zou L, Li S, Cheah PY, Eu KW, Ong CN (2010). Metabolic profiling in colorectal cancer reveals signature metabolic shifts during tumorigenesis. *Molecular & Cellular Proteomics* [Epub ahead of print].

26. Ma Y, Liu W, Peng J, Huang L, Zhang P, Zhao X, *et al.* (2010). A pilot study of gas chromatograph/mass spectrometry-based serum metabolic profiling of colorectal cancer after operation. *Molecular Biology Reports* **37**(3), 1403–11.

27. Monleon D, Morales JM, Barrasa A, Lopez JA, Vazquez C, Celda B (2009). Metabolite profiling of fecal water extracts from human colorectal cancer. *NMR in Biomedicine* **22**(3), 342–8.

28. Ikeda A, Nishiumi S, Shinohara M, Yoshie T, Hatano N, Okuno T, *et al.* (2012). Serum metabolomics as a novel diagnostic approach for gastrointestinal cancer. *Biomedical Chromatography* **26**(5), 548–58.

29. Weir TL, Manter DK, Sheflin AM, Barnett BA, Heuberger AL, Ryan EP (2013). Stool microbiome and metabolome differences between colorectal cancer patients and healthy adults. *PLoS One* **8**(8), e70803.

30. Reimers MS, Zeestraten EC, Kuppen PJ, Liefers GJ, van de Velde CJ (2013). Biomarkers in precision therapy in colorectal cancer. *Gastroenterology Report* **1**(3), 166–83.

31. Manning G, Whyte DB, Martinez R, Hunter T, Sudarsanam S (2002). The protein kinase complement of the human genome. *Science* **298**(5600), 1912–34.

32. Blume-Jensen P, Hunter T (2001). Oncogenic kinase signalling. *Nature* **411**(6835), 355–65.

33. Tejpar S, Bertagnolli M, Bosman F, Lenz HJ, Garraway L, Waldman F, *et al.* (2010). Prognostic and predictive biomarkers in resected colon cancer: current status and future perspectives for integrating genomics into biomarker discovery. *Oncologist* **15**(4), 390–404.

34. Samowitz WS, Sweeney C, Herrick J, Albertsen H, Levin TR, Murtaugh MA, *et al.* (2005). Poor survival associated with the BRAF V600E mutation in microsatellite-stable colon cancers. *Cancer Research* **65**(14), 6063–9.

35. Volinia S, Calin GA, Liu CG, Ambs S, Cimmino A, Petrocca F, *et al.* (2006). A microRNA expression signature of human solid tumors defines cancer gene targets. *Proceedings of the National Academy of Sciences of the United States of America* **103**(7), 2257–61.

36. Schwarzenbach H, Nishida N, Calin GA, Pantel K (2014). Clinical relevance of circulating cell-free microRNAs in cancer. *Nature Reviews Clinical Oncology* **11**(3), 145–56.

37. Nagel R, le Sage C, Diosdado B, van der Waal M, Oude Vrielink JA, Bolijn A, *et al.* (2008). Regulation of the

adenomatous polyposis coli gene by the miR-135 family in colorectal cancer. *Cancer Research* **68**(14), 5795–802.

38. Liu GH, Zhou ZG, Chen R, Wang MJ, Zhou B, Li Y, *et al.* (2013). Serum miR-21 and miR-92a as biomarkers in the diagnosis and prognosis of colorectal cancer. *Tumor Biology* **34**(4), 2175–81.

39. Ng EK, Chong WW, Jin H, Lam EK, Shin VY, Yu J, *et al.* (2009). Differential expression of microRNAs in plasma of patients with colorectal cancer: a potential marker for colorectal cancer screening. *Gut* **58**(10), 1375–81.

40. Huang Z, Huang D, Ni S, Peng Z, Sheng W, Du X (2010). Plasma microRNAs are promising novel biomarkers for early detection of colorectal cancer. *International Journal of Cancer* **127**(1), 118–26.

41. Bovell L, Putcha B, Samuel T, Manne U (2013). Clinical implications of microRNAs in cancer. *Biotechnic & Histochemistry* **88**(7), 388–96.

42. Schetter AJ, Leung SY, Sohn JJ, Zanetti KA, Bowman ED, Yanaihara N, *et al.* (2008). MicroRNA expression profiles associated with prognosis and therapeutic outcome in colon adenocarcinoma. *JAMA* **299**(4), 425–36.

43. Iorio MV, Ferracin M, Liu CG, Veronese A, Spizzo R, Sabbioni S, *et al.* (2005). MicroRNA gene expression deregulation in human breast cancer. *Cancer Research* **65**(16), 7065–70.

44. Chan JA, Krichevsky AM, Kosik KS (2005). MicroRNA-21 is an antiapoptotic factor in human glioblastoma cells. *Cancer Research* **65**(14), 6029–33.

45. Yanaihara N, Caplen N, Bowman E, Seike M, Kumamoto K, Yi M, *et al.* (2006). Unique microRNA molecular profiles in lung cancer diagnosis and prognosis. *Cancer Cell* **9**(3), 189–98.

46. Fulci V, Chiaretti S, Goldoni M, Azzalin G, Carucci N, Tavolaro S, *et al.* (2007). Quantitative technologies establish a novel microRNA profile of chronic lymphocytic leukemia. *Blood* **109**(11), 4944–51.

47. Toiyama Y, Takahashi M, Hur K, Nagasaka T, Tanaka K, Inoue Y, *et al.* (2013). Serum miR-21 as a diagnostic and prognostic biomarker in colorectal cancer. *Journal of the National Cancer Institute* **105**(12), 849–59.

48. Yan LX, Huang XF, Shao Q, Huang MY, Deng L, Wu QL, *et al.* (2008). MicroRNA miR-21 overexpression in human breast cancer is associated with advanced clinical stage, lymph node metastasis and patient poor prognosis. *RNA* **14**(11), 2348–60.

49. Markou A, Tsaroucha EG, Kaklamanis L, Fotinou M, Georgoulias V, Lianidou ES (2008). Prognostic value of mature microRNA-21 and microRNA-205 overexpression in non-small cell lung cancer by quantitative real-time RT-PCR. *Clinical Chemistry* **54**(10), 1696–704.

50. Ma XL, Liu L, Liu XX, Li Y, Deng L, Xiao ZL, *et al.* (2012). Prognostic role of microRNA-21 in non-small

cell lung cancer: a meta-analysis. *Asian Pacific Journal of Cancer Prevention* **13**(5), 2329–34.

51. Wu L, Li G, Feng D, Qin H, Gong L, Zhang J, *et al.* (2013). MicroRNA-21 expression is associated with overall survival in patients with glioma. *Diagnostic Pathology* **8**, 200.

52. Bovell LC, Shanmugam C, Putcha BD, Katkoori VR, Zhang B, Bae S, *et al.* (2013). The prognostic value of microRNAs varies with patient race/ethnicity and stage of colorectal cancer. *Clinical Cancer Research* **19**(14), 3955–65.

53. Komatsu S, Ichikawa D, Tsujiura M, Konishi H, Takeshita H, Nagata H, *et al.* (2013). Prognostic impact of circulating miR-21 in the plasma of patients with gastric carcinoma. *Anticancer Research* **33**(1), 271–6.

54. Kanaan Z, Rai SN, Eichenberger MR, Roberts H, Keskey B, Pan J, *et al.* (2012). Plasma miR-21: a potential diagnostic marker of colorectal cancer. *Annals of Surgery* **256**(3), 544–51.

55. Balaguer F, Moreira L, Lozano JJ, Link A, Ramirez G, Shen Y, *et al.* (2011). Colorectal cancers with microsatellite instability display unique miRNA profiles. *Clinical Cancer Research* **17**(19), 6239–49.

56. Rossi L, Bonmassar E, Faraoni I (2007). Modification of miR gene expression pattern in human colon cancer cells following exposure to 5-fluorouracil *in vitro*. *Pharmacological Research* **56**(3), 248–53.

57. Borralho PM, Kren BT, Castro RE, da Silva IB, Steer CJ, Rodrigues CM (2009). MicroRNA-143 reduces viability and increases sensitivity to 5-fluorouracil in HCT116 human colorectal cancer cells. *FEBS Journal* **276**(22), 6689–700.

58. Song B, Wang Y, Xi Y, Kudo K, Bruheim S, Botchkina GI, *et al.* (2009). Mechanism of chemoresistance mediated by miR-140 in human osteosarcoma and colon cancer cells. *Oncogene* **28**(46), 4065–74.

59. Song B, Wang Y, Kudo K, Gavin EJ, Xi Y, Ju J (2008). miR-192 Regulates dihydrofolate reductase and cellular proliferation through the p53-microRNA circuit. *Clinical Cancer Research* **14**(24), 8080–6.

60. Sebio A, Pare L, Paez D, Salazar J, Gonzalez A, Sala N, *et al.* (2013). The LCS6 polymorphism in the binding site of let-7 microRNA to the KRAS 3'-untranslated region: its role in the efficacy of anti-EGFR-based therapy in metastatic colorectal cancer patients. *Pharmacogenetics and Genomics* **23**(3), 142–7.

61. Pardini B, Rosa F, Barone E, Di Gaetano C, Slyskova J, Novotny J, *et al.* (2013). Variation within 3'-UTRs of base excision repair genes and response to therapy in colorectal cancer patients: A potential modulation of microRNAs binding. *Clinical Cancer Research* **19**(21), 6044–56.

62. Zheng H, Zhang L, Zhao Y, Yang D, Song F, Wen Y, et al. (2013). Plasma miRNAs as diagnostic and prognostic biomarkers for ovarian cancer. *PLoS One* **8**(11), e77853.

63. Rosenfeld N, Aharonov R, Meiri E, Rosenwald S, Spector Y, Zepeniuk M, et al. (2008). MicroRNAs accurately identify cancer tissue origin. *Nature Biotechnology* **26**(4), 462–9.

64. Fearon ER, Cho KR, Nigro JM, Kern SE, Simons JW, Ruppert JM, et al. (1990). Identification of a chromosome 18q gene that is altered in colorectal cancers. *Science* **247**(4938), 49–56.

65. Jen J, Kim H, Piantadosi S, Liu ZF, Levitt RC, Sistonen P, et al. (1994). Allelic loss of chromosome 18q and prognosis in colorectal cancer. *New England Journal of Medicine* **331**(4), 213–21.

66. Benatti P, Gafa R, Barana D, Marino M, Scarselli A, Pedroni M, et al. (2005). Microsatellite instability and colorectal cancer prognosis. *Clinical Cancer Research* **11**(23), 8332–40.

67. Merok MA, Ahlquist T, Royrvik EC, Tufteland KF, Hektoen M, Sjo OH, et al. (2013). Microsatellite instability has a positive prognostic impact on stage II colorectal cancer after complete resection: results from a large, consecutive Norwegian series. *Annals of Oncology* **24**(5), 1274–82.

68. Wang Y, Jatkoe T, Zhang Y, Mutch MG, Talantov D, Jiang J, et al. (2004). Gene expression profiles and molecular markers to predict recurrence of Dukes' B colon cancer. *Journal of Clinical Oncology* **22**(9), 1564–71.

69. Eschrich S, Yang I, Bloom G, Kwong KY, Boulware D, Cantor A, et al. (2005). Molecular staging for survival prediction of colorectal cancer patients. *Journal of Clinical Oncology* **23**(15), 3526–35.

70. Kennedy RD, Bylesjo M, Kerr P, Davison T, Black JM, Kay EW, et al. (2011). Development and Independent Validation of a Prognostic Assay for Stage II Colon Cancer Using Formalin-Fixed Paraffin-Embedded Tissue. *Journal of Clinical Oncology* **29**(35), 4620–6.

71. Sveen A, Agesen TH, Nesbakken A, Meling GI, Rognum TO, Liestol K, et al. (2012). ColoGuidePro: a prognostic 7-gene expression signature for stage III colorectal cancer patients. *Clinical Cancer Research* **18**(21), 6001–10.

72. Maak M, Simon I, Nitsche U, Roepman P, Snel M, Glas AM, et al. (2013). Independent validation of a prognostic genomic signature (ColoPrint) for patients with stage II colon cancer. *Annals of Surgery* **257**(6), 1053–8.

73. Amado RG, Wolf M, Peeters M, Van Cutsem E, Siena S, Freeman DJ, et al. (2008). Wild-type KRAS is required for panitumumab efficacy in patients with metastatic colorectal cancer. *Journal of Clinical Oncology* **26**(10), 1626–34.

74. Roth AD, Tejpar S, Delorenzi M, Yan P, Fiocca R, Klingbiel D, et al. (2010). Prognostic role of KRAS and BRAF in stage II and III resected colon cancer: results of the translational study on the PETACC-3, EORTC 40993, SAKK 60-00 trial. *Journal of Clinical Oncology* **28**(3), 466–74.

75. Prahallad A, Sun C, Huang S, Di Nicolantonio F, Salazar R, Zecchin D, et al. (2012). Unresponsiveness of colon cancer to BRAF(V600E) inhibition through feedback activation of EGFR. *Nature* **483**(7387), 100–3.

76. Liao X, Lochhead P, Nishihara R, Morikawa T, Kuchiba A, Yamauchi M, et al. (2012). Aspirin use, tumor PIK3CA mutation, and colorectal-cancer survival. *New England Journal of Medicine* **367**(17), 1596–606.

77. Raida M, Schwabe W, Hausler P, Van Kuilenburg AB, Van Gennip AH, Behnke D, et al. (2001). Prevalence of a common point mutation in the dihydropyrimidine dehydrogenase (DPD) gene within the 5'-splice donor site of intron 14 in patients with severe 5-fluorouracil (5-FU)- related toxicity compared with controls. *Clinical Cancer Research* **7**(9), 2832–9.

78. Bunz F, Hwang PM, Torrance C, Waldman T, Zhang Y, Dillehay L, et al. (1999). Disruption of p53 in human cancer cells alters the responses to therapeutic agents. *Journal of Clinical Investigation* **104**(3), 263–9.

79. Russo A, Bazan V, Iacopetta B, Kerr D, Soussi T, Gebbia N, et al. (2005). The TP53 colorectal cancer international collaborative study on the prognostic and predictive significance of p53 mutation: influence of tumor site, type of mutation, and adjuvant treatment. *Journal of Clinical Oncology* **23**(30), 7518–28.

80. Rouits E, Boisdron-Celle M, Dumont A, Guerin O, Morel A, Gamelin E (2004). Relevance of different UGT1A1 polymorphisms in irinotecan-induced toxicity: a molecular and clinical study of 75 patients. *Clinical Cancer Research* **10**(15), 5151–9.

81. Palomaki GE, Bradley LA, Douglas MP, Kolor K, Dotson WD (2009). Can UGT1A1 genotyping reduce morbidity and mortality in patients with metastatic colorectal cancer treated with irinotecan? An evidence-based review. *Genetics in Medicine* **11**(1), 21–34.

82. Gold P, Freedman SO (1965). Specific carcinoembryonic antigens of the human digestive system. *Journal of Experimental Medicine* **122**(3), 467–81.

83. Ballesta AM, Molina R, Filella X, Jo J, Gimenez N (1995). Carcinoembryonic antigen in staging and follow-up of patients with solid tumors. *Tumour Biology* **16**(1), 32–41.

84. Duffy MJ (2001). Carcinoembryonic antigen as a marker for colorectal cancer: is it clinically useful? *Clinical Chemistry* **47**(4), 624–30.

85. Loewenstein MS, Zamcheck N (1978). Carcinoembryonic antigen (CEA) levels in benign gastrointestinal disease states. *Cancer* **42**(3 Suppl), 1412–8.

86. Itzkowitz S, Brand R, Jandorf L, Durkee K, Millholland J, Rabeneck L, *et al.* (2008). A simplified, noninvasive stool DNA test for colorectal cancer detection. *American Journal of Gastroenterology* **103**(11), 2862–70.

87. Grady WM, Rajput A, Lutterbaugh JD, Markowitz SD (2001). Detection of aberrantly methylated hMLH1 promoter DNA in the serum of patients with microsatellite unstable colon cancer. *Cancer Research* **61**(3), 900–2.

88. Leung WK, To KF, Man EP, Chan MW, Bai AH, Hui AJ, *et al.* (2005). Quantitative detection of promoter hypermethylation in multiple genes in the serum of patients with colorectal cancer. *American Journal of Gastroenterology* **100**(10), 2274–9.

89. Church TR, Wandell M, Lofton-Day C, Mongin SJ, Burger M, Payne SR, *et al.* (2014). Prospective evaluation of methylated SEPT9 in plasma for detection of asymptomatic colorectal cancer. *Gut* **63**(2), 317–25.

90. Lofton-Day C, Model F, Devos T, Tetzner R, Distler J, Schuster M, *et al.* (2008). DNA methylation biomarkers for blood-based colorectal cancer screening. *Clinical Chemistry* **54**(2), 414–23.

91. Ezzeldin HH, Lee AM, Mattison LK, Diasio RB (2005). Methylation of the DPYD promoter: an alternative mechanism for dihydropyrimidine dehydrogenase deficiency in cancer patients. *Clinical Cancer Research* **11**(24 Pt 1), 8699–705.

92. Amstutz U, Farese S, Aebi S, Largiader CR (2008). Hypermethylation of the DPYD promoter region is not a major predictor of severe toxicity in 5-fluorouracil based chemotherapy. *Journal of Experimental & Clinical Cancer Research* **27**, 54.

93. Shen L, Toyota M, Kondo Y, Lin E, Zhang L, Guo Y, *et al.* (2007). Integrated genetic and epigenetic analysis identifies three different subclasses of colon cancer. *Proceedings of the National Academy of Sciences of the United States of America* **104**(47), 18654–9.

94. Samowitz WS, Albertsen H, Herrick J, Levin TR, Sweeney C, Murtaugh MA, *et al.* (2005). Evaluation of a large, population-based sample supports a CpG island methylator phenotype in colon cancer. *Gastroenterology* **129**(3), 837–45.

95. Ward RL, Cheong K, Ku SL, Meagher A, O'Connor T, Hawkins NJ (2003). Adverse prognostic effect of methylation in colorectal cancer is reversed by microsatellite instability. *Journal of Clinical Oncology* **21**(20), 3729–36.

96. Li M, Chen WD, Papadopoulos N, Goodman SN, Bjerregaard NC, Laurberg S, *et al.* (2009). Sensitive digital quantification of DNA methylation in clinical samples. *Nature Biotechnology* **27**(9), 858–63.

97. Nohaile M (2011). The biomarker is not the end. *Drug Discovery Today* **16**(19–20), 878–83.

98. Neuzillet C, Tijeras-Raballand A, de Mestier L, Cros J, Faivre S, Raymond E (2014). MEK in cancer and cancer therapy. *Pharmacology & Therapeutics* **141**(2), 160–71.

99. Ogino S, Meyerhardt JA, Cantor M, Brahmandam M, Clark JW, Namgyal C, *et al.* (2005). Molecular alterations in tumors and response to combination chemotherapy with gefitinib for advanced colorectal cancer. *Clinical Cancer Research* **11**(18), 6650–6.

100. Alexander D, Chatla C, Funkhouser E, Meleth S, Grizzle WE, Manne U (2004). Postsurgical disparity in survival between African Americans and Caucasians with colonic adenocarcinoma. *Cancer* **101**(1), 66–76.

101. Alexander D, Jhala N, Chatla C, Steinhauer J, Funkhouser E, Coffey CS, *et al.* (2005). High-grade tumor differentiation is an indicator of poor prognosis in African Americans with colonic adenocarcinomas. *Cancer* **103**(10), 2163–70.

102. Alexander DD, Waterbor J, Hughes T, Funkhouser E, Grizzle W, Manne U (2007). African-American and Caucasian disparities in colorectal cancer mortality and survival by data source: an epidemiologic review. *Cancer Biomarkers* **3**(6), 301–13.

103. Manne U, Weiss HL, Myers RB, Danner OK, Moron C, Srivastava S, *et al.* (1998). Nuclear accumulation of p53 in colorectal adenocarcinoma: prognostic importance differs with race and location of the tumor. *Cancer* **83**(12), 2456–67.

CHAPTER 14

Early Detection of Lung Cancer

Mohamed Hassanein,[1] Melinda C Aldrich,[2] Stephen A Deppen,[3] Karl E Krueger,[4] Eric L Grogan,[5] and Pierre P Massion[6]

[1] Division of Allergy, Pulmonary and Critical Care Medicine, Vanderbilt-Ingram Cancer Center, TN, USA

[2] Department of Thoracic Surgery and Division of Epidemiology, Vanderbilt University Medical Center, Nashville, TN, USA

[3] Department of Thoracic Surgery, Vanderbilt University Medical Centre, Nashville, TN, USA

[4] Division of Cancer Prevention, National Cancer Institute, National Institutes of Health, Rockville, MD, USA

[5] Veterans Affairs, Tennessee Valley Healthcare System, Nashville Campus, Department of Thoracic Surgery Medical Centre, Nashville, TN, USA

[6] Division of Allergy, Pulmonary and Critical Care Medicine, Vanderbilt-Ingram Cancer Centre, Veterans Affairs, Tennessee Valley Healthcare System, Nashville Campus, TN, USA

Introduction

Lung cancer is the leading cause of cancer-related deaths in the United States [1]. The annual mortality from lung cancer exceeds the annual rates for breast, prostate, and colon cancer combined, all of which have successful clinical screening tools for the detection of early stage disease [2]. Over 60% of lung cancer patients are diagnosed at advanced stages when metastasis has already occurred, by which stage a cure is unlikely [3]. For these patients with advanced disease, the five-year survival rate is less than 10%, in contrast to patients diagnosed with stage 1 lung cancer, where the five-year survival is greater than 70% [4]. Because of the improved prognosis with detecting this disease early, the search for diagnostic strategies for early lung cancer detection has intensified.

It has been difficult to demonstrate that the earlier lung cancer is diagnosed, the more the opportunity for improved survival increases. Screening trials for lung cancer performed in the 1970s–80s utilized chest x-ray and sputum cytology. Although these tests increased the number of lung cancers diagnosed, there was no concomitant improvement in lung cancer mortality [5,6]. The Early Lung Cancer Action Program (ELCAP) was a large lung cancer screening trial initiated in the 1990s, employing chest computed tomography (CT) imaging [7]. Use of this new imaging technology showed improved detection rate and survival, because more early stage lung cancers were being detected.

The promising results of this study prompted the design of the large randomized National Lung Screening Trial (NLST). This recently completed study generated much excitement in the clinical community, as low-dose CT screening showed a 20% relative reduction in lung cancer mortality, compared with chest x-ray screening, in patients at high risk for lung cancer followed up for a median of 6.5 years [8]. This represents the first large randomized screening study of lung cancer to show an improvement in overall survival, providing a glimmer of hope to improve survival in the management of this cancer. Based on the NLST results, a

Biomarkers in Cancer Screening and Early Detection, First Edition. Edited by Sudhir Srivastava.
© 2017 John Wiley & Sons, Inc. Published 2017 by John Wiley & Sons, Inc.

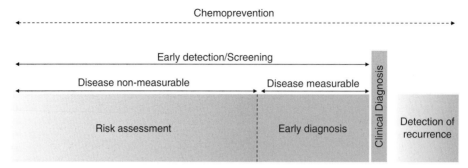

Figure 14.1 Clinical contexts for biomarker development in early detection of lung cancer. This diagram illustrates four clinical contexts within four windows of time. The period during which lung cancer is non-measurable and precedes the diagnosis characterizes the context of *risk assessment*. It represents a long window of time, during which the disease develops and corresponds to an opportunity for chemoprevention. When the disease becomes measurable but remains asymptomatic, we enter the context of *early diagnosis*. Two other clinical contexts relate to *clinical diagnosis* – that is, when the disease is measurable and patients symptomatic – and to *detection of recurrence*. These windows of time correspond to the different contexts for which different biomarker targets can be developed. Adapted from Hassanein *et al.*, 2011 [135]. Reprinted with permission of the American Thoracic Society. Copyright © 2012, American Thoracic Society. For a color version of this figure please see color plate section.

screening method that reduces lung cancer specific mortality by 20% could save over 11 000 lives annually in the USA. This benefit is much greater than the estimated 2300 lives saved by adjuvant chemotherapy, providing strong rationale to pursue efforts in early detection.

The clinical context of early detection of lung cancer

To demonstrate utility in improving lung cancer detection, biomarkers must address clinical situations encountered by practitioners. Two pressing clinical needs are to identify: 1) biomarkers that address the risk of developing lung cancer in an asymptomatic population; or 2) biomarkers that are diagnostic in nature, to distinguish malignant nodules from benign ones identified by imaging methods.

Biomarkers for lung cancer risk can be used to stratify subjects based on the likelihood that a lung tumor may develop. Since chest CT suffers from low sensitivity among those who have never smoked, low-specificity (high false positive rate) and high-cost risk markers have the potential to improve early detection by selecting those who may benefit from additional radiographic screening, thus subjecting fewer patients to unneeded radiation exposure. Several models to predict an individual's risk of developing lung cancer have been developed for stratifying their need for CT

[9–14]. Mathematical models integrating clinical, physiological, imaging and biological variables are now proposed for evaluating risk for lung cancer in clinical practice [9, 10, 12, 14, 15]. This field has made tremendous progress, and prediction models are being proposed for implementation in selecting populations for screening and or chemoprevention trials. Identifying robust risk biomarkers for developing lung cancer will better define the at-risk population, decrease the number of screening CTs performed and, ultimately, limit the harm from discovering false positive nodules.

Diagnostic biomarkers that can distinguish a benign from a malignant nodule would be of great value to pulmonary oncologists. Depending on geographic location, as many as 30% of indeterminate pulmonary nodules, when surgically resected, are found to be benign [16]. Similar numbers were reported in the NLST, where 24% of patients who underwent a diagnostic operation for a suspicious nodule had benign disease [8]. These cases illustrate the need for biomarker testing to limit the frequency of futile surgical intervention for a benign nodule.

Current guidelines recommend providers to use models to assist with determining the probability of whether a nodule identified by CT scan is malignant, requiring surgical removal [17–19]. As the technology of low-dose CT for lung cancer screening evolves with ever increasing resolution, the predictive models will hopefully benefit from an orthogonal criterion (whose results are independent and additive to those derived from imaging and other clinical or epidemiologic information) provided by biomarkers to assist the clinical provider in predicting which patients have an aggressive lung cancer.

We recently validated a blood-based proteomic signature for diagnosis of lung cancer, and demonstrated that it may improve upon the clinical and imaging assessment of indeterminate lung nodules [20]. As better biomarkers are discovered and developed, the chief goals for their utility should keep this clinical need in perspective, to assist not only in ruling out those individuals without malignancy, but also to help identifying those with a malignant nodule amenable to surgical resection and the possibility of a cure.

Current status of early detection biomarkers for lung cancer

Here, we will cover the most recent advances regarding molecular biomarkers for risk assessment and diagnosis of lung cancer, and discuss the clinical utility and limitations of different approaches. The biomarkers are first classified on the types of specimens needed for their identification – either tissue-based (Table 14.1) or biofluid-based markers. The biofluid-based biomarkers are further subclassified into blood-based (Table 14.2), sputum, exhaled breath condensate and peripheral blood cells (Table 14.3).

The phases of biomarker development are listed according to the classification system used by the Early Detection Research Network (EDRN) [21]. This paradigm was designed for early detection biomarkers in the context of screening, and may not apply to the phases of development of diagnostic biomarkers. The tables also include efforts to integrate biomarkers in models of risk prediction or diagnosis. The validation sets reported in the tables correspond to attempts to test biomarkers (or signatures) in an independent population [2].

Tissue-based biomarkers

Investigators have employed a variety of technologies to interrogate a spectrum of molecular aberrations associated with lung cancer. Important insights pointing towards key molecular events of lung cancer tumorigenesis have resulted, including:

mapping the genomic loci associated with high risk of developing lung cancer; hypermethylation of key tumor suppressor genes [22–26]; regions of chromosomal amplification or deletion [27, 28]; transcriptomic changes [29–32]; altered expression of micro RNAs [33]; and the proteomic signatures of invasive [34,35] and pre-invasive lesions of lung tissue [36,37]. This discovery work has culminated in the genome cancer atlas effort recently reported for lung adenocarcinoma [38, 39] and squamous cell carcinoma [40,41].

Several research groups have investigated genetic and proteomic alterations in surrogate tissues, such as bronchial brushings and biopsies, to determine the probability of having lung cancer [26–28, 37, 42] – see Table 14.1. These markers, obtained from the airways through bronchoscopy, may complement CT imaging to provide additional information when evaluating individuals at high risk for lung cancer. Another potential widely available tissue source to identify biomarkers is surgical pathology specimens, archived as formalin fixed paraffin-embedded (FFPE) blocks. These tissue blocks are amenable to profile certain genomic and proteomic aberrations in tumors. Investigations of this nature include promoter hypermethylation [43] and microRNA expression [44], which can be successfully extracted as candidate biomarkers.

MicroRNAs (miRNAs) are a class of small noncoding RNA genes that function in several cellular processes, such as the regulation of gene expression, regulation of mRNA stability, and regulation of translation of mRNA. Often, miRNAs are abnormally expressed in multiple types of cancer [45,46], and exhibit a tissue or pathologic expression pattern [46,47] that offers promise for clinical application [48]. Because microRNAs are relatively small, and can be well preserved in formalin-fixed tissue, they can easily be extracted and analyzed in routinely processed biopsy or surgical specimens [49]. Differences in microRNA expression have been reported between squamous cell carcinoma and adenocarcinoma in lung cancer [33], and similar results have been found in other cancers [47,48,50]. The current trend towards utilizing FFPE specimens takes advantage of the increased availability of clinical samples with which to do biomarker discovery and validation, thereby increasing the statistical power and generalization of results [51, 52].

Table 14.1 Characteristics and performance of most recent tissue-based candidate biomarkers for the early detection of lung cancer (data organized by year of publication and type of marker considered).

References	Specimens	Type of marker	Analytes	Clinical Purpose	# markers	Pathological subtype	Assay platform	Preclinical Samples	BM Dev. Phase	Training set	Validation set	Sensitivity	Specificity	AUC
Halling, 2006 [27]	Bronchial Specimens	DNA	5p15, 7p12 (EGFR), 8q24 (C-MYC), CEP6	Diagnosis	4	NSCLC	FISH + Cytology	n/a	I	n/a	137	61-75*	83-100*	n/a
Massion, 2009 [28]	Bronchial biopsies	DNA	TP63, MYC, CEP3, CEP6 + sputum cytology + demographics	Diagnosis	4	NSCLC	FISH	n/a	II	n/a	70	n/a	n/a	92.6
Feng, 2008 [43]	Tumors and normal tissues	DNA methylation	RARB, BVES, CDKN2A, KCNH5, RASSF1, CDH13, RUNX, CDH1	Diagnosis	8	NSCLC	Methylation array	n/a	I	49	n/a	n/a	n/a	n/a
Anglim, 2008 [23]	Tumors and normal tissues	DNA methylation	GDNF, MTHFR, OPCML, TNFRSF25, TCF21, PAX8, PTPRN2 and PITX2	Diagnosis	8	SCC	Methylation array	n/a	I	43	n/a	95.6*	95.6*	n/a
Schmidt, 2010 [26]	Bronchial aspirates	DNA methylation	SHOX2	Diagnosis	1	NSCLC	PCR	n/a	II	n/a	523	68	95	86
Richards, 2011 [25]	Tumors and normal tissues	DNA methylation	TCF21	Diagnosis	1	NSCLC	PCR	n/a	II	42	63	76	98*	n/a
Spira, 2007 [12]	airway epithelium	mRNA	gene expression signature	Diagnosis	80	NSCLC	Affy array	n/a	II	77	52	80	84	n/a
Beane, 2008 [29]	airway epithelium	mRNA	gene expression signature + clinical factors	Diagnosis	80	NSCLC & SCLC	Affy array	n/a	II	76	62	100	91	97

Reference	Sample	Type	Markers	Application	No.	Cancer	Method		BM Dev Phase					AUC
Kim, 2007 [136]	Tumors and normal tissues	mRNA	CBLC, CYP24A1, ALDH3A1, AKR1B10, S100P, PLUNC, LOC147	Diagnosis	7	NSCLC	q RT-PCR	n/a	II	32	36**	n/a	n/a	n/a
Blomquist, 2009 [31]	Tumors and normal tissues	mRNA	CAT, CEBPG, E2F1, ERCC4, ERCC5, GPX1, GPX3, GSTM3, GSTP1, GSTT1, GSTZ1, MGST1, SOD1, XRCC1	Diagnosis	14	NSCLC	RT-PCR	n/a	II	n/a	49:40	n/a	n/a	82-87
Rahman, 2011 [37]	Bronchial biopsies	MALDI signature	TMLS4, ACBP, CSTA, cyto C, MIF, ubiquitin, ACBP, Des-ubiquitin	Diagnosis	9	NSCLC	MALDI MS	n/a	II	51	60	66	88	77
Bediaga, 2013 [64]	Biopsies	miRNA	Let-7i, miR-183, miR-27b, miR34a, miR450a, miR577, miR-9, miR96	Diagnosis	8	NSCLC	qRT-PCR	n/a	II	40	40:47	97.5	96.3	99

Abbreviations. AUC = area under the curve, FISH = fluorescence in situ hybridization, MALDI-MS = matrix-assisted laser desorption/ionization mass spectrometry, miRNA = microRNA, NSCLC = non-small cell lung cancer, SCC = squamous cell carcinoma, SCLC = small cell lung cancer, RT-PCR = reverse transcriptase polymerase chain reaction.- q-PCR = quantitative (real time PCR), lung cancer, SNP = single nucleotide polymorphism, SCC = squamous cell carcinoma, Note* = values derived from training set only; ** = validation and training sets overlap; BM Dev Phase = Biomarker Development Phase, n/a = not available.

The molecular changes associated with progression from normal to malignant tissue may lead to the discovery of markers detectable in blood or other biofluids. Because biomarkers released by tumors will be diluted in other body fluids, they are often diluted out with molecules from other organ sources, equating biomarker discovery with trying to find a needle in the haystack. Their discovery first in tissue samples facilitates analyzing their presence and quantitation in other biofluids. Limited access to early stage tumor tissue samples, tumor heterogeneity, the complex scope of changes found at genomic and proteomic levels, and the low abundance of potential biomarkers from small numbers of cells at early stage cancers, pose the most difficult challenges that translational researchers face when attempting to discover these biomarker candidates.

The feasibility of using tissue-based biomarkers is highly dependent on the availability of sufficient numbers and quality specimens, and the robustness of the assay offered. FFPE samples are preferred by scientists, because they are so widely available, but molecular analysis from these samples remains more challenging. Obtaining specimens through non-invasive diagnostic approaches is preferred, as it may take additional time to refine an airway epithelium-based biomarker whose source is further away from the primary site of the tumor. For example, the development of surrogate biomarkers of early stage lung cancer from tissues in the field of cancerization (bronchial brushings or biopsies) may require testing in more proximal and less invasive samples (e.g. nasal epithelium) [53]. This is usually less of a problem for prognostic or predictive biomarkers of response to therapy, because tumor samples will be generally available for analysis.

Although molecular analysis of lung tumor tissues holds great promise for revolutionizing our understanding of the disease development and progression, tissue-based biomarkers from the bronchial airway have significant limitations, such as population representativeness, specimen availability, and relative invasiveness of the procedure required to obtain the samples. Nevertheless, if the tissue-based markers can be translated into finding the same or related markers in more accessible sampling sites, this can help guide the development of biofluids-based early detection strategies.

Biofluids-based markers

The underlying premise of biomarkers that can be detected in biofluids is that tumor cells synthesize molecules not found in normal tissues, and these molecules are then released or secreted by the cell to the extracellular environment. Biofluid-based detection strategies are an attractive approach for screening, primarily because specimens can be obtained non-invasively. In principle, lung cancer biomarkers might be found in peripheral blood and its components (circulating cells, plasma, and serum), exhaled breath condensate (EBC), urine, and sputum. The variety of discoverable markers includes genomic DNA and its methylated footprints, overexpressed mRNA, microRNA, proteins, or metabolites that are released into the extracellular microenvironment by normal cellular processes, or by necrosis of tumor cells. Therefore, detection of biomarkers in biofluids is an attractive approach to take for ultimate translation into the clinic [54].

Blood-based markers

Blood is a complex and dynamic medium, whose components can reflect various physiological or pathological states of an individual. Detectable markers of the blood have been investigated by many methods, and include multiple elements such as circulating tumor cells, cell-free DNA and RNA, proteins, peptides, autoantibodies, and metabolites [55]. Tumor-derived aberrations in genomic DNA have been found in blood, including DNA methylation [56, 57], DNA amplification, and gene expression [58] from lung cancer patients (Table 14.2).

microRNAs

Recently, microRNAs have been identified in the blood of lung cancer patients [59, 60]. To confirm if miRNA profiles can be used to predict lung tumor development, diagnosis or prognosis, an extensive microRNA profiling was performed at the time of diagnosis by spiral CT in paired lung tumor and normal lung tissue along with miRNA detected in plasma collected from the patients. In two independent cohorts of patients a 15 microRNA panel from plasma identified subjects at high risk of developing lung cancer with 80% sensitivity and 90% specificity [61, 62]. This panel was subsequently validated in an independent study of over 900 subjects [62]. Another study

Table 14.2 Characteristics and performance of most recent blood-based candidate biomarkers for the early detection of lung cancer. (data organized by year of publication, specimen type and type of marker considered).

References	Specimens	Type of marker	Analyte	Clinical Purpose	# markers	Pathological subtype	Assay platform	Preclinical Samples	BM Dev. Phase	Training set	Validation set	Sensitivity	Specificity	AUC
Zhong, 2006 [79]	Serum	AutoAB	phage peptide clones	Diagnosis	5	Lung cancer	ELISA	n/a	II	46	56	91*	91*	99*
Chapman, 2008 [84]	Serum	AutoAB	p53, cmyc, HER2, NY-ESO-1, CAGE, MUC1, GBU4-5	Diagnosis	7	Lung cancer	ELISA	n/a	I	154	n/a	n/a	n/a	n/a
Qiu, 2008 [85]	Serum	AutoAB	annexin I, 14-3-3 theta, LAMR1	Diagnosis	3	NSCLC	Protein-array	170	III		170	51	82	73
Wu, 2010 [83]	Serum	AutoAB	phage peptide clones	Diagnosis	6	NSCLC	ELISA	n/a	II	20	180	92	92	96
Farlow, 2010 [86]	Serum	AutoAB	LMPDH, PGAM1, ubiquillin, ANXA1, ANXA2, HSP70-9B	Diagnosis	6	NSCLC	ELISA	n/a	II	196	n/a	94.8*	91.1*	96.4*
Boyle, 2010 [137]	Serum	AutoAB	p53, NY-ESO-1, CAGE, GBU4-5, Annexin 1 and SOX2	Diagnosis	6	NSCLC	ELISA	n/a	II	241	255	32	91	64
Greenberg, 2007 [56]	Serum	DNA methylation	S-Adenosylmethionine	Diagnosis	1	Lung cancer	HPLC	n/a	I	68	n/a	92-100*	91-97*	94-99*
Begum, 2011 [57]	Serum	DNA methylation	APC, CDH1, MGMT, DCC, RASSF1A, AIM	Diagnosis	6	NSCLC	q-PCR	n/a	II	32-639	106	84	57	n/a
Chen, 2011 [138]	Serum	micro RNA	micro RNA signature	Diagnosis	10	NSCLC	qRT-PCR	n/a	II	310	310	93	90	97
Bianchi, 2011 [63]	Serum	micro RNA	miRNA signature	Diagnosis	34	NSCLC	qRT-PCR	n/a	II	64	64	71	90	89
Kulpa, 2002 [139]	Serum	Protein	CEA, CYFRA 21-1, SCC-Ag, NSE	Diagnosis	4	SCC	ELISA	n/a	II		420	20-62	95	71-90

(continued)

Table 14.2 (Continued)

References	Specimens	Type of marker	Analyte	Clinical Purpose	# markers	Pathological subtype	Assay platform	Preclinical Samples	BM Dev. Phase	Training set	Validation set	Sensitivity	Specificity	AUC
Patz, 2007 [67]	Serum	Protein	CEA, RBP4, hAAT, SCCA	Diagnosis	4	Lung cancer	ELISA	n/a	II	100	97	78	75	n/a
Takano, 2009 [140]	Serum	Protein	Nectin-4	Diagnosis	1	NSCLC	ELISA	n/a	II		295	54	98	n/a
Yildiz, 2007 [68]	Serum	Protein	MALDI MS signature	Diagnosis	7	NSCLC	MALDI MS	n/a	II	185	106	58	85.7	82
Pecot, 2012 [20]	Serum	Protein	Model: MALDI MS signature + clinical and imaging data	Diagnosis	7	Indeterm. Lung nodule	MALDI MS	n/a	II		100	n/a	n/a	72
Diamandis, 2011 [141]	Serum	Protein	Pentraxin-3	Diagnosis	1	Lung cancer	ELISA	n/a	I		426	37-48	80-90	60-74
Ostroff, 2010 [142]	Serum	Aptamers	cadherin-1, CD30 ligand, endostatin, HSP90a, LRIG3, MIP-4, pleiotrophin, PRKCI, RGM-C, SCF-sR, sL-selectin, and YES	Diagnosis	6	NSCLC	Aptamers	n/a	II	985	341	89	83	90
Zhong, 2005 [143]	Plasma	AutoAB	TAA signature	Diagnosis	5	NSCLC	Protein microarray	5	I	81	n/a	90*	95*	n/a
Kneip, 2011 [144]	Plasma	DNA Methylation	SHOX2	Diagnosis	1	NSCLC	qPCR	n/a	II	40	371	60	90	78
Shen, 2010 [145]	Plasma	micro RNA	miRNA-21, -126, -210, 486-5p	Diagnosis	4	NSCLC	qRT-PCR	n/a	II	28	87	86	97	93
Wei, 2011 [146]	Plasma	micro RNA	miRNA-21	Diagnosis	1	NSCLC	qRT-PCR	n/a	I	93	n/a	76*	70*	77.5*

Taguchi, 2011 [147]	Plasma	Protein, 2 panels	EGFR, SFTPB, WFDC2, ANGPTL3, ANXA1, YWHAQ Lmr1	Diagnosis	7	NSLCL	ELISA	52	III		n/a	n/a	n/a	89
Boeri, 2011 [61]	Plasma/ tissues	micro RNA	miRNA signature	Diagnosis	13	Lung cancer	miRNA array & RT-PCR	n/a	II	19	22	75	100	88
Boeri, 2011 [61]	Plasma/ tissues	micro RNA	miRNA signature	Diagnosis	15	Lung cancer	miRNA array & RT-PCR	25	III	20	25	80	90	85
Sin, 2013 [75]	Plasma	Protein	Pro-surfactant protein B	Diagnosis	1	NSCLC	ELISA	61	II	2,485	182	n/a	n/a	68.3
Shiels, 2013 [76]	Serum	Protein	CRP, SAA, sTNFRII, IL-1RA, IL-7, TGF-A, ENA 87/CXCL5, BCA-1/CXCL13, TARC/CCL17	Risk	11	Lung cancer	Luminex	n/a (526)	I	1,118	n/a	n/a	n/a	n/a
Han, 2013 [74]	Plasma	Protein	Osteopontin	Diagnosis	1	NSCLC	ELISA	n/a	I	103	n/a	62.3	76.0	63.8
Wang, 2013 [148]	Serum	Protein	CEA, CA19-9, NSE, CYFRA21-1	Diagnosis	4	Lung Cancer	Immunoassay	n/a	I	350	n/a	90.2	75.6	n/a
Cazzoli, 2013 [66]	Exosomes	miRNA	miR-151a-5p, miR-30a-3p, miR-200b-5p, miR-629, miR-100, miR-154-3p	Diagnosis – Nodule discrimination	6	Adenocarcinoma vs granuloma	qRT-PCR	n/a	II	30	105	97.5	72.0	90.8
Ajona, 2013 [73]	Plasma	Protein	C4d fragment	Diagnosis/ Prognosis	1	Lung Cancer	ELISA	n/a	II	100	129	n/a	n/a	78.2

(continued)

Table 14.2 (Continued)

References	Specimens	Type of marker	Analyte	Clinical Purpose	# markers	Pathological subtype	Assay platform	Preclinical Samples	BM Dev. Phase	Training set	Validation set	Sensitivity	Specificity	AUC
Li 2013 [149]	Plasma	Protein	LRP1, BGH3, COIA1, TETN, TSP1, ALDOA, GRP78, ISLR, FRIL, LG3BP, PRDX1, FIBA, GSLG1	Diagnosis – Nodule discrimination	13	Lung Cancer	MS-MRM	n/a	II	143	104	n/n	n/a	n/a
Sozzi 2014 [62]	Plasma	miRNA	microRNA signature classifier	Diagnosis	n/a	Lung Cancer	qRT-PCR	n/a	I	939	n/a	87	81	n/a

Abbreviations. AutoAB = autoantibody, AUC = area under the curve, ADC = adenocarcinoma, ELISA = enzyme linked immunosorbant assay, FISH = fluorescence in situ hybridization, HPLC = high performance liquid chromatography, MALDI-MS = matrix-assisted laser desorption/ionization mass spectrometry, miRNA = microRNA, NSCLC = non-small cell lung cancer, SCC+ squamous cell carcinoma, RT-PCR = reverse transcriptase polymerase chain reaction, q-PCR = quantitative (real time PCR), SNP = single nucleotide polymorphism, SCC = squamous cell carcinoma, TAA = tumor associated antigen, Note* = values derived from training set only; ** = validation and training sets overlap; BM Dev Phase = Biomarker Development Phase, n/a = not available.

reported that a panel of 34 serum miRNAs, could uniquely identify patients with early stage non-small cell lung carcinomas (NSCLCs) in a population of asymptomatic high-risk individuals with 80% accuracy [63]. Additional studies have been recently published examining miRNAs from biopsy material [64], bronchial epithelial brushings [65], and circulating exosomes [66]. These results suggest that miRNAs may be effective molecular predictors of lung cancer development and aggressiveness. Certainly these provocative results require validation by other groups as their use has significant clinical implications for lung cancer management.

Proteomic profiles
Recent proteomic studies have focused on rapid proteomic profiling in serum or plasma. Matrix-assisted laser desorption ionization time-of-flight mass spectrometry (MALDI TOF MS) patterns have been used by several groups to identify proteins or peptide fragments that correlate with early disease stage. Patz and colleagues were able to identify four serum proteins (transferrin, retinol-binding protein, antitrypsin and haptoglobin) that discriminate between NSCLC and controls [67]. Several other groups, including ours [68], have reported blood protein profiles that distinguish patients with various cancers from control subjects [69–71]. Recently, our group and another laboratory have separately validated proteomic signatures in two prospective cohorts of patients with lung nodules, suggesting that it may provide added value to the clinical assessment of indeterminate lung nodules [20,72]. In addition to proteomic profiling, many laboratories have identified individual proteins found in blood that could potentially be incorporated into larger biomarker panels, in attempts to achieve the necessary sensitivity and specificity for a clinically useful diagnostic test [73–75]. Acute phase reactants and inflammation markers have also been investigated as potential proteomic markers of risk for lung cancer [76].

Autoantibodies
Another promising development in the blood biomarkers field is the discovery of autoantibodies directed against tumor proteins. Alterations of the protein production in cancer cells, by overexpression, mutations, misfolding, truncation, proteolytic degradation, or aberrant post-translational modifications (glycosylation in particular), might render these molecules susceptible to immune responses [77]. Autoantibodies generated against these tumor-associated antigens (TAA) can be amplified by the immune system during very early phases of cancer progression, making them attractive candidates for early detection of cancer or markers of cancer risk.

Many TAAs have been identified in patient sera in several immunologic diseases and malignancies using high throughput screening platforms, such as cDNA expression libraries, phage display, and protein/peptide microarrays [78]. For example, three separate groups identified potential immunoreactive peptides for autoantibodies, using a T7-based phage library to screen sera of patients with NSCLC [79–81]. Taking this same approach, Chen *et al.* identified and validated ubiquilin 1 as a potential autoantibody target in early stage lung adenocarinomas [82]. More recently, Wu *et al.* reported the identification of six peptide clones discriminatory of NSCLC, although only one protein has been confirmed [83].

Recent improvements in blood fractionation techniques and liquid chromatography have led to the identification of several other autoantibodies [54]. Autoantibodies against known lung cancer-associated proteins, such as p53, c-Myc, HER2, MUC1, CAGE, GBU4-5, NY-ESO-1 [84] or annexin I, 14-3-3 theta, and LAMAR1 [85], or IMPDH, PGAM1 and ANXA2 [86], have been reported as independent signatures. These autoantibody studies are particularly provocative, because the immune system may act as a beacon warning of an impending cancer, well prior to any clinical manifestations of lung cancer.

Circulating tumor cells (CTCs)
The ability to capture and study CTCs from blood is an emerging and exciting development, carrying the potential to become a non-invasive tool for early detection and diagnosis of cancer, measuring response to therapy, and possibly offering a window into understanding cancer progression and metastasis [87–94]. CTCs originate from a malignancy, and circulate freely in the peripheral blood, but their numbers are quite low, so sensitive approaches

must be taken to identify them. CTCs are usually captured by immobilized antiepithelial-cell-adhesion-molecule (EpCAM) antibodies on either chip or bead platforms [95, 96]. Since this technology is still in the early phases, development of additional cell surface markers should continue to improve specificity for isolation of CTCs.

Circulating DNA (ctDNA)

Detection methods for circulating DNA have been developing rapidly to assess cancer burden non-invasively [97–100]. A deep sequencing approach called CAPP-seq was found to detect ctDNA in all advanced stage disease, and in about 50% of stage 1 disease with outstanding specificity [101]. We can anticipate that this type of technology will improve and, if proven useful in early stage disease, could detect and monitor diverse malignancies and greatly facilitate disease management.

Peripheral mononuclear lymphocytes (PMNLs)

While it does not seem intuitive that cancer biomarkers can be found associated with circulating white blood cells, several lines of evidence suggest otherwise. Several laboratories have published reports suggesting that transcriptomic profiles of PMNLs from cancer patients is influenced by the presence of lung tumors, and may offer diagnostic potential [102]. The RNA profiles of PMNLs before and after surgical removal of the tumor may also provide important prognostic indicators for recurrence [103]. It is feasible that, if these results can be validated in other cohorts and laboratories, PMNLs may serve as a surrogate for cancer detection.

Another exciting development along these lines is the potential use of PMNLs to determine an individual's risk for lung cancer in heavy smokers. DNA repair is an important process for limiting gene mutations, one of the primary molecular events leading to cancer initiation and progression. It can be surmised that an individual's ability to repair DNA could be correlated with their risk for developing cancer. Since heavy smokers introduce large quantities of mutagenic compounds into their airway throughout much of their life, DNA repair efficiency is a critical factor to minimize mutational insults to the lung and airways.

The laboratory of Livneh has investigated whether activities of several DNA repair enzymes

in PMNLs can be used as surrogate markers to determine a subject's risk for developing lung cancer. The initial studies for the first enzyme tested (8-oxoguanine glycosylase or OGG1) proved promising. People with a heavy smoking history and relatively low OGG1 activity in their PMNLs showed up an to 20-fold higher odds ratio of developing lung cancer than matched individuals with higher OGG1 activity, or nonsmokers with low OGG1 activity [104]. Subsequently these studies have been extended to include additional DNA repair enzymes with promising results [105, 106]. These results suggest it may be feasible to stratify smokers on their risk for developing lung and other upper aerodigestive cancers, thus indicating which subjects need particularly stringent monitoring.

In summary, peripheral blood offers a rich medium for identifying cancer-specific markers, ranging from small molecules such as microRNAs to whole cells. Perhaps the greatest opportunity for developing a minimally invasive diagnostic test of lung cancer is to exploit this biofluid. However, several challenges pose significant hurdles in bringing blood-based biomarkers to clinical use. The high level of proteomic complexity of blood, the low levels of tumor markers released into circulation at early stage disease, and the lack of sensitive, reproducible, and high throughput verification modalities, all contribute to the difficulties encountered with these prospects for peripheral blood. New and innovative fractionation techniques, more sensitive and specific detection reagents, and well validated assays, should enhance our chances of successfully identifying blood-based biomarkers.

Exhaled breath condensate

Exhaled breath condensate (EBC) can readily be obtained non-invasively and, because its contents are derived directly from the airway, it should hypothetically contain components that are released by lung tumors. The analysis of volatile organic compounds (VOCs) correlated with lung cancer may provide a novel means to for the identification of diagnostic cancer biomarkers. This approach is particularly attractive, since large volumes of EBC can be readily and inexpensively collected [107, 108]. The underlying rationale of this approach is predicated on the realization that altered gene expression in tumors often leads to peroxidation of the cell membrane, resulting in the emission of VOCs [108].

Several recent studies have combined gas chromatography with mass spectrometry (GC-MS) for the analysis of VOCs [109–113] and chemical nanoarray [114]. Other studies have searched for volatile polypeptides present in EBC as potential biomarkers for lung cancer [115]. These intriguing findings lend credence to the feasibility of exploiting EBC for identifying molecular signatures to detect lung cancer non-invasively. To translate this type of technology into the clinic, standardization of collection devices and proof of analytical specificity for such tests are still needed.

Because GC-MS is not a convenient technology to use in the clinic, several groups have tried developing more simplified platforms to detect VOCs in breath. Array-based sensors can use different methods of VOC detection, including quartz crystal microbalance, gold/platinum nanoparticles, carbon nanotube-based sensors, conducting polymer composites, and colorimetric array sensors [116]. The major disadvantage of array-based sensors is that the chemical identities of the VOCs detected cannot be determined but, rather, they respond to functionally reactive groups on the VOCs and, thus, require a considerable amount of training and standardization for use as a diagnostic test. The advantage of these sensors is that they are inexpensive to manufacture, simple to use, and sensitive to detect compounds of low abundance. It will be interesting to see if any of these array-based sensors show diagnostic performance worthy of routine use in the clinic. Early studies in the development of these arrays have been promising for diagnosing lung cancer in EBC [117, 118].

Sputum

Chronic exposure to cigarette smoke induces increased airway secretion of glycoproteins, and shedding of inflammatory and exfoliated epithelial cells from the bronchial walls. Because sputum is easily inducible in current and former smokers, many laboratories have sought to interrogate its molecular and cellular constituents for diagnostic purposes on lung cancer [22]. Although diagnosis of lung cancer by sputum cytology shows low sensitivity [119], combining cytology with genetic abnormalities significantly improves

diagnostic accuracy. Deletions of a variety of genes [49], chromosomal aneusomy [120,121], and altered patterns of DNA methylation [122, 123], have been identified as genomic aberrations that confer diagnostic value for diagnosis of lung cancer (Table 14.3). Furthermore, combining pulmonary function measurements with genomic aneuploidy significantly improves risk prediction of lung cancer [124]. Despite these positive findings, more extensive validation of these markers remains to demonstrate the clinical value of these tests.

Urine

Urine is another easily accessible body fluid that can be collected without discomfort. Unlike sputum and EBC, urine suffers from not having direct exposure to the airway, where the lung has immediate access. However, it can be considered to be in a similar category to blood, where certain classes of small molecules can enter circulation from the tumor and be excreted via filtration through the kidney.

Some recent proof of principle studies for detecting biomarkers of lung cancer in urine have been attempted with mass spectrometry [125]. In animal models for lung cancer, certain VOCs were identified [126], and these studies are recently being extended to in lung cancer patients [116, 127]. Metabolites of polycyclic aromatic hydrocarbons and tobacco smoke [128] found in urine have been examined as biomarkers for risk of developing lung cancer. As was described for detection of VOCs in exhaled breath, colorimetric array-based sensors are also being tested for biomarker signature detection in urine samples, where the diagnostic performance may be close to that observed in EBC (P. Mazzone & P. Rhodes, private communication).

Current challenges in improving lung cancer diagnosis

The chief clinical needs in diagnosing early stage lung cancer, when intervention is effective at reducing death and morbidity, is to identify biomarkers that stratify individuals based on their level of risk for developing lung cancer, and biomarkers that can distinguish benign and malignant lung nodules identified by CT. Where CT imaging reveals a suspicious pulmonary nodule in a

Table 14.3 Characteristics and performance of most recent sputum, EBC, peripheral blood cells candidate biomarkers for the early detection of lung cancer (data organized by year of publication, specimen type and type of marker considered).

References	Specimens	Type of marker	Analyte	Clinical Purpose	# markers	Pathological subtype	Assay platform	Preclinical Samples	BM Dev. Phase	Training set	Validation set	Sensitivity	Specificity	AUC
Palmisano, 2000 [150]	Sputum	DNA methylation	p16, MGMT	Diagnosis	2	SCC	PCR	11	III	144	n/a	n/a	n/a	n/a
Belinsky, 2002 [123]	Sputum	DNA methylation	p16, MGMT, DAP, RASSF1A	Diagnosis	4	NSCLC	PCR	n/a	I	141	n/a	n/a	n/a	n/a
Garcia, 2004 [120]	Sputum	DNA	Chromosomal aneusomy + cytology	Diagnosis	4	Lung cancer	FISH + Cytology	36	III	66	n/a	83*	80*	n/a
Li, 2007 [49]	Sputum	DNA	HYAL2, FHIT, SFTPC	Diagnosis	3	NSCLC	FISH	n/a	I	102	n/a	76*	92*	n/a
Yu, 2010 [151]	Sputum	micro RNA	miR-21, miR-486, miR-375, miR-200b	Diagnosis	4	NSCLC	qRT-PCR	n/a	II	72	122	70	80	84
Showe, 2009 [58]	Peripheral blood cells	mRNA	gene expression signature	Diagnosis	29	NSCLC	cDNA-array	n/a	II	228	55	76	82	n/a
Tanaka, 2009 [152]	Peripheral blood cells	CTC	Circulating tumor cells (CTCs)	Diagnosis	1	NSCLC	Cell search-system	n/a	I	150	n/a	30*	88*	60*
Sevilya, 2014 [106]	Peripheral blood cells	DNA repair activities	OGG, MPE, APE1	Risk	3	Lung Cancer	Enzymatic assays	n/a	I	192	n/a	n/a	n/a	n/a
Philips, 1999 [109]	EBC	VOCs	VOCs signature	Diagnosis	22	NSCLC	GC-MS	n/a	I	108	n/a	100*	81*	n/a
Bajtarevic, 2009 [111]	EBC	VOCs	VOCs signature	Diagnosis	50	Lung cancer	GC-MS	n/a	I	96	n/a	52-80*	100*	n/a
Gessner, 2010 [115]	EBC	Protein	VEGF, bFGF, ANG,TNF-alpha, IL-8	Diagnosis	5	NSCLC	ELISA	n/a	I	192	74	n/a	n/a	99-100
Mazzone, 2012 [118]	EBC	VOC	VOCs signature	Diagnosis	n/a	ADC, SCC	Colorimetric sensor array	n/a	II	143	229	80 (ADC), 91 (SCC)	86 (ADC), 73 (SCC)	82 (ADC), 85 (SCC)
Gessner, 2010 [115]	EBC	Protein	VEGF, bFGF, ANG,TNF-alpha, IL-8	Diagnosis	5	NSCLC	ELISA	n/a	I	74	74	n/a	n/a	99-100
Mazzone, 2012 [118]	EBC	VOC	VOCs signature	Diagnosis	n/a	ADC, SCC	Colorimetric sensor array	n/a	II	143	229	80 (ADC), 91 (SCC)	86 (ADC), 73 (SCC)	82 (ADC), 85 (SCC)

Abbreviations. AutoAB = autoantibody, AUC = area under the curve, ADC = adenocarcinoma, EBC = exhaled breath condensate, CTCs = circulating tumor cells, ELISA = enzyme linked immunosorbent assay, FISH = fluorescence in situ hybridization, GC-MS = gas chromatography mass spectrometry, miRNA = microRNA, NSCLC = non-small cell lung cancer, q-PCR = quantitative (real time PCR), SCLC = small cell lung cancer, SNP = single nucleotide polymorphism, SCC = squamous cell carcinoma, VOCs = volatile organic compounds. Note* = values derived from training set only; ** = validation and training sets overlap; BM Dev Phase = Biomarker Development Phase. n/a = not available.

patient, predictive models for assessing malignancy have been developed by Cummings [129], Gurney [130], Swensen [131], Gould [17], and McWilliams [18]. However, these models suffer from relatively poor accuracy; unfortunately, their ability to predict a malignancy is not sufficient to adequately select patients for surgery [16]. Although these models include parameters such as patient age, smoking status, duration and intensity of smoking, cancer history, gender, race, asbestos exposure, COPD/emphysema, and pulmonary nodule characteristics by CT (size, shape, density, and location), the inclusion of biomarkers during this assessment may provide complementary data to improve the accuracy of these models in predicting malignancy.

Recently, gene expression profiles in cytologically normal large airway epithelium sampled during bronchoscopy [29], or serum proteomic profiles in patients presenting with pulmonary nodules [20], have been explored as molecular signatures that might improve the diagnostic accuracy of these models. Unfortunately, these initial attempts have shown little clinical utility. Despite these initial setbacks, it is likely that the future development of predictive models will incorporate the currently identified predictors and newly identified molecular biomarkers [132].

Although intense efforts by many laboratories taking different "omics" approaches has yielded a large number of candidate diagnostic biomarkers, few have progressed to the level of FDA approval [133]. Insufficient rigor in the discovery, development and validation of these markers is a common criticism. The disappointingly meager pace of biomarker discovery and validation is attributed to several fundamental factors. The failure to deliver on an effective diagnostic test can partially be explained by the fact that most discovery approaches are neither reliable nor efficient. Discovery efforts that do not follow the recommended PRoBE study design [134] are already likely flawed at the outset, due to inherent bias in the samples being analyzed, or underlying populations being non-representative due to limitations of specimen availability. Further, our analytical technologies may still suffer from the ability to detect low-level markers released by small numbers of tumor cells against a background of high-abundance molecular species in complex media

such as blood. It is likely that low-abundance molecules in biofluids will prove to be the most promising cancer biomarkers. As a result, the best candidate biomarkers are probably missed during the discovery.

Additional limitations in progressing biomarkers forward are the capacity to verify and analytically validate existing candidate markers in a high-throughput manner. The lack of quality specific recognition reagents, such as antibodies, and techniques to reassign identification of biomarkers in tissue specimens to quantification in blood, remain as significant road blocks. The possibility exists that clinically beneficial biomarkers have already been identified, but their validation has still not been achieved. Contributing to this demise in discovery efforts is the realization that the reproducibility of much of the biomarker data to date has been flawed because of poor study design (e.g., studies lacking a nested case-control design, as recommended by PRoBE [134]), model over-fitting, and the lack of validation with samples independent from those where discovery occurred.

Furthermore, after a list of candidate biomarkers is compiled, a trustworthy set of guidelines is still needed to select those candidates that are most promising to clinically test for validation, and that will complement each other to achieve maximum sensitivity and specificity. Evolving technology, low-abundance biomarkers, difficulties in carrying out prospective studies, and low incidence of a heterogeneous disease, all combine to account for the most significant obstacles in developing biomarker based early diagnostic tests for lung cancer.

Conclusions and future clinical perspectives

The molecular analysis of a variety of biospecimens has allowed the discovery of candidate biomarkers, consequently leading to the identification of novel proteins that may play important roles in lung cancer progression. Many of these newly identified candidate biomarkers have arisen from the high volume of data produced from varied high-throughput biochemical analyses of clinical material. Thus far, none of the published biomarkers of risk, or for lung cancer diagnosis, are suitable for clinical use, and few have moved to phase III of biomarker development.

Lung cancer is recognized as a complex and heterogeneous disease, not only at the biochemical level, but also at the tissue, organism, and population level. There is a great need for incorporating findings from multiple discovery platforms into a framework that can improve our level of understanding of this disease. The continual goal of this field is to develop a biofluids-based molecular test to improve the selection of high risk individuals for CT screening, to distinguish malignant from benign lesions in patients with indeterminate pulmonary nodules, and to diagnose patients with particularly aggressive cancer. The clinical benefit of successful biomarker tests will result in significant reductions in mortality and notable cost-savings to the healthcare system.

Acknowledgment

We would like to acknowledge the following funding source for support of this work: National Institutes of Health (U01CA152662 and RO1 CA102353) awarded to PPM, Veterans Health Administration (VA-CDA2) awarded to ELG. A Vanderbilt Clinical and Translational Research Scholars Award awarded to MCA. We would like to thank Mr. William Alborn for his insightful comments and suggestions. We thank Judith Roberts from the Vanderbilt Tumor Registry for her help in providing data to support the estimates of lives saved from adjuvant chemotherapy in the US.

References

1. Jemal A, Bray F, Center MM, Ferlay J, Ward E, Forman D (2011). Global cancer statistics. *CA: A Cancer Journal for Clinicians* **61**, 69–90.

2. Brenner DE, Normolle DP (2007). Biomarkers for cancer risk, early detection, and prognosis: the validation conundrum. *Cancer Epidemiology, Biomarkers & Prevention* **16**, 1918–20.

3. Jemal A, Center MM, DeSantis C, Ward EM (2010). Global patterns of cancer incidence and mortality rates and trends. *Cancer Epidemiology, Biomarkers & Prevention* **19**, 1893–907.

4. Hoffman PC, Mauer AM, Vokes EE (2000). Lung cancer. *The Lancet* **355**, 479–85.

5. Fontana RS, Sanderson DR, Taylor WF, Woolner LB, Miller WE, Muhm JR, et al. (1984). Early lung cancer detection: results of the initial (prevalence) radiologic and cytologic screening in the Mayo Clinic study. *American Review of Respiratory Disease* **130**, 561–5.

6. Stitik FP, Tockman MS (1978). Radiographic screening in the early detection of lung cancer. *Radiologic Clinics of North America* **16**, 347–66.

7. Henschke CI, McCauley DI, Yankelevitz DF, Naidich DP, McGuinness G, Miettinen OS, et al. (1999). Early Lung Cancer Action Project: overall design and findings from baseline screening. *The Lancet* **354**, 99–105.

8. Aberle DR, Adams AM, Berg CD, Black WC, Clapp JD, Fagerstrom RM, et al. (2011). Reduced lung-cancer mortality with low-dose computed tomographic screening. *New England Journal of Medicine* **365**, 395–409.

9. Bach PB, Kattan MW, Thornquist MD, Kris MG, Tate RC, Barnett MJ, et al. 2003 (). Variations in lung cancer risk among smokers. *Journal of the National Cancer Institute* **95**, 470–8.

10. Cassidy A, Myles JP, van Tongeren M, Page RD, Liloglou T, Duffy SW, et al. (2008). The LLP risk model: an individual risk prediction model for lung cancer. *British Journal of Cancer* **98**, 270–6.

11. Peto R, Darby S, Deo H, Silcocks P, Whitley E, Doll R (2000). Smoking, smoking cessation, and lung cancer in the UK since 1950: combination of national statistics with two case-control studies. *BMJ* **321**, 323–9.

12. Spitz MR, Hong WK, Amos CI, Wu X, Schabath MB, Dong Q, et al. (2007). A risk model for prediction of lung cancer. *Journal of the National Cancer Institute* **99**, 715–26.

13. D'Amelio AM, Jr., Cassidy A, Asomaning K, Raji OY, Duffy SW, Field JK, et al. (2010). Comparison of discriminatory power and accuracy of three lung cancer risk models. *British Journal of Cancer* **103**, 423–9.

14. Tammemagi MC, Katki HA, Hocking WG, Church TR, Caporaso N, Kvale PA, et al. (2013). Selection criteria for lung-cancer screening. *New England Journal of Medicine* **368**, 728–36.

15. Maisonneuve P, Bagnardi V, Bellomi M, Spaggiari L, Pelosi G, Rampinelli C, et al. (2011). Lung cancer risk prediction to select smokers for screening CT – a model based on the Italian COSMOS trial. *Cancer Prevention Research (Philadelphia)* **4**, 1778–89.

16. Isbell JM, Deppen S, Putnam JB, Jr., Nesbitt JC, Lambright ES, Dawes A, et al. (2011). Existing general population models inaccurately predict lung cancer risk in patients referred for surgical evaluation. *Annals of Thoracic Surgery* **91**, 227–33; discussion 33.

17. Gould MK, Ananth L, Barnett PG (2007). A clinical model to estimate the pretest probability of lung

cancer in patients with solitary pulmonary nodules. *Chest* **131**, 383–8.

18. McWilliams A, Tammemagi MC, Mayo JR, Roberts H, Liu G, Soghrati K, *et al.* (2013). Probability of cancer in pulmonary nodules detected on first screening CT. *New England Journal of Medicine* **369**, 910–9.

19. Gould MK, Donington J, Lynch WR, Mazzone PJ, Midthun DE, Naidich DP, *et al.* (2013). Evaluation of individuals with pulmonary nodules: when is it lung cancer? Diagnosis and management of lung cancer, 3rd ed: American College of Chest Physicians evidence-based clinical practice guidelines. *Chest* **143**, e93S–120S.

20. Pecot CV, Li M, Zhang XJ, Rajanbabu R, Calitri C, Bungum A, *et al.* (2012). Added value of a serum proteomic signature in the diagnostic evaluation of lung nodules. *Cancer Epidemiology, Biomarkers & Prevention* **21**, 786–92.

21. Pepe MS, Etzioni R, Feng Z, Potter JD, Thompson ML, Thornquist M, *et al.* (2001). Phases of biomarker development for early detection of cancer. *Journal of the National Cancer Institute* **93**, 1054–61.

22. Belinsky SA (2004). Gene-promoter hypermethylation as a biomarker in lung cancer. *Nature Reviews Cancer* **4**, 707–17.

23. Anglim PP, Galler JS, Koss MN, Hagen JA, Turla S, Campan M, *et al.* (2008). Identification of a panel of sensitive and specific DNA methylation markers for squamous cell lung cancer. *Molecular Cancer* **7**, 62.

24. Castro MA, Dal-Pizzol F, Zdanov S, Soares M, Muller CB, Lopes FM, *et al.* (2010). CFL1 expression levels as a prognostic and drug resistance marker in nonsmall cell lung cancer. *Cancer* **116**, 3645–55.

25. Richards KL, Zhang B, Sun M, Dong W, Churchill J, Bachinski LL, *et al.* (2011). Methylation of the candidate biomarker TCF21 is very frequent across a spectrum of early-stage nonsmall cell lung cancers. *Cancer* **117**, 606–17.

26. Schmidt B, Liebenberg V, Dietrich D, Schlegel T, Kneip C, Seegebarth A, *et al.* (2010). SHOX2 DNA methylation is a biomarker for the diagnosis of lung cancer based on bronchial aspirates. *BMC Cancer* **10**, 600.

27. Halling KC, Rickman OB, Kipp BR, Harwood AR, Doerr CH, Jett JR (2006). A comparison of cytology and fluorescence in situ hybridization for the detection of lung cancer in bronchoscopic specimens. *Chest* **130**, 694–701.

28. Massion PP, Zou Y, Uner H, Kiatsimkul P, Wolf HJ, Baron AE, *et al.* (2009). Recurrent genomic gains in preinvasive lesions as a biomarker of risk for lung cancer. *PloS One* **4**, e5611.

29. Beane J, Sebastiani P, Whitfield TH, Steiling K, Dumas Y-M, Lenburg ME, *et al.* (2008). A Prediction Model for Lung Cancer Diagnosis that Integrates Genomic and Clinical Features. *Cancer Prevention Research* **1940-6207**.CAPR-08-0011.

30. Beer DG, Kardia SL, Huang CC, Giordano TJ, Levin AM, Misek DE, *et al.* (2002). Gene-expression profiles predict survival of patients with lung adenocarcinoma. *Nature Medicine* **8**, 816–24.

31. Blomquist T, Crawford EL, Mullins D, Yoon Y, Hernandez DA, Khuder S, *et al.* (2009). Pattern of antioxidant and DNA repair gene expression in normal airway epithelium associated with lung cancer diagnosis. *Cancer Research* **69**, 8629–35.

32. Wilkerson MD, Yin X, Hoadley KA, Liu Y, Hayward MC, Cabanski CR, *et al.* (2010). Lung squamous cell carcinoma mRNA expression subtypes are reproducible, clinically important, and correspond to normal cell types. *Clinical Cancer Research* **16**, 4864–75.

33. Yanaihara N, Caplen N, Bowman E, Seike M, Kumamoto K, Yi M, *et al.* (2006). Unique microRNA molecular profiles in lung cancer diagnosis and prognosis. *Cancer Cell* **9**, 189–98.

34. Yanagisawa K, Shyr Y, Xu BJ, Massion PP, Larsen PH, White BC, *et al.* (2003). Proteomic patterns of tumour subsets in non-small-cell lung cancer. *The Lancet* **362**, 433–9.

35. Yanagisawa K, Tomida S, Shimada Y, Yatabe Y, Mitsudomi T, Takahashi T (2007). A 25-signal proteomic signature and outcome for patients with resected non-small-cell lung cancer. *Journal of the National Cancer Institute* **99**, 858–67.

36. Rahman SM, Shyr Y, Yildiz PB, Gonzalez AL, Li H, Zhang X, *et al.* (2005). Proteomic patterns of preinvasive bronchial lesions. *American Journal of Respiratory and Critical Care Medicine* **172**, 1556–62.

37. Rahman SM, Gonzalez AL, Li M, Seeley EH, Zimmerman LJ, Zhang XJ, *et al.* (2011). Lung cancer diagnosis from proteomic analysis of preinvasive lesions. *Cancer Research* **71**, 3009–17.

38. Ding L, Getz G, Wheeler DA, Mardis ER, McLellan MD, Cibulskis K, *et al.* (2008). Somatic mutations affect key pathways in lung adenocarcinoma. *Nature* **455**, 1069–75.

39. (2014) Comprehensive molecular profiling of lung adenocarcinoma. *Nature* **511**, 543–50.

40. Abazeed ME, Adams DJ, Hurov KE, Tamayo P, Creighton CJ, Sonkin D, *et al.* (2013). Integrative radio-genomic profiling of squamous cell lung cancer. *Cancer Research* **3**(20), 6289–98.

41. Kim Y, Hammerman PS, Kim J, Yoon JA, Lee Y, Sun JM, *et al.* (2014). Integrative and comparative genomic analysis of lung squamous cell carcinomas in East Asian patients. *Journal of Clinical Oncology* **32**, 121–8.

42. Spira A, Beane JE, Shah V, Steiling K, Liu G, Schembri F, *et al.* (2007). Airway epithelial gene expression in the diagnostic evaluation of smokers with suspect lung cancer. *Nature Medicine* **13**, 361–6.

43. Feng H, Shuda M, Chang Y, Moore PS (2008). Clonal integration of a polyomavirus in human Merkel cell carcinoma. *Science* **319**, 1096–100.

44. Lebanony D, Benjamin H, Gilad S, Ezagouri M, Dov A, Ashkenazi K, *et al.* (2009). Diagnostic assay based on hsa-miR-205 expression distinguishes squamous from nonsquamous non-small-cell lung carcinoma. *Journal of Clinical Oncology* **27**, 2030–7.

45. Volinia S, Calin GA, Liu CG, Ambs S, Cimmino A, Petrocca F, *et al.* (2006). A microRNA expression signature of human solid tumors defines cancer gene targets. *Proceedings of the National Academy of Sciences of the United States of America* **103**, 2257–61.

46. Lu J, Getz G, Miska EA, Alvarez-Saavedra E, Lamb J, Peck D, *et al.* (2005). MicroRNA expression profiles classify human cancers. *Nature* **435**, 834–8.

47. Roldo C, Missiaglia E, Hagan JP, Falconi M, Capelli P, Bersani S, *et al.* (2006). MicroRNA expression abnormalities in pancreatic endocrine and acinar tumors are associated with distinctive pathologic features and clinical behavior. *Journal of Clinical Oncology* **24**, 4677–84.

48. Rosenfeld N, Aharonov R, Meiri E, Rosenwald S, Spector Y, Zepeniuk M, *et al.* (2008). MicroRNAs accurately identify cancer tissue origin. *Nature Biotechnology* **26**, 462–9.

49. Li R, Todd NW, Qiu Q, Fan T, Zhao RY, Rodgers WH, *et al.* (2007). Genetic deletions in sputum as diagnostic markers for early detection of stage I non-small cell lung cancer. *Clinical Cancer Research* **13**, 482–7.

50. Feber A, Xi L, Luketich JD, Pennathur A, Landreneau RJ, Wu M, *et al.* (2008). MicroRNA expression profiles of esophageal cancer. *Journal of Thoracic and Cardiovascular Surgery* **135**, 255–60; discussion 60.

51. Hui A, How C, Ito E, Liu FF (2011). Micro-RNAs as diagnostic or prognostic markers in human epithelial malignancies. *BMC Cancer* **11**, 500.

52. Tam S, de Borja R, Tsao MS, McPherson JD (2014). Robust global microRNA expression profiling using next-generation sequencing technologies. *Laboratory Investigation* **94**, 350–8.

53. Zhang X, Sebastiani P, Liu G, Schembri F, Dumas YM, Langer EM, *et al.* (2010). Similarities and differences between smoking-related gene expression in nasal and bronchial epithelium. *Physiological Genomics* **41**, 1–8.

54. Hanash SM, Pitteri SJ, Faca VM (2008). Mining the plasma proteome for cancer biomarkers. *Nature* **452**, 571–9.

55. Duarte IF, Rocha CM, Gil AM (2013). Metabolic profiling of biofluids: potential in lung cancer screening and diagnosis. *Expert Review of Molecular Diagnostics* **13**, 737–48.

56. Greenberg AK, Rimal B, Felner K, Zafar S, Hung J, Eylers E, *et al.* (2007). S-adenosylmethionine as a biomarker for the early detection of lung cancer. *Chest* **132**, 1247–52.

57. Begum S, Brait M, Dasgupta S, Ostrow KL, Zahurak M, Carvalho AL, *et al.* (2011). An epigenetic marker panel for detection of lung cancer using cell-free serum DNA. *Clinical Cancer Research* **17**, 4494–503.

58. Showe MK, Vachani A, Kossenkov AV, Yousef M, Nichols C, Nikonova EV, *et al.* (2009). Gene expression profiles in peripheral blood mononuclear cells can distinguish patients with non-small cell lung cancer from patients with nonmalignant lung disease. *Cancer Research* **69**, 9202–10.

59. Lai CY, Yu SL, Hsieh MH, Chen CH, Chen HY, Wen CC, *et al.* (2011). MicroRNA expression aberration as potential peripheral blood biomarkers for schizophrenia. *PloS One* **6**, e21635.

60. Li S, Zhu J, Zhang W, Chen Y, Zhang K, Popescu LM, *et al.* (2011). Signature microRNA expression profile of essential hypertension and its novel link to human cytomegalovirus infection. *Circulation* **124**, 175–84.

61. Boeri M, Verri C, Conte D, Roz L, Modena P, Facchinetti F, *et al.* (2011). MicroRNA signatures in tissues and plasma predict development and prognosis of computed tomography detected lung cancer. *Proceedings of the National Academy of Sciences of the United States of America* **108**, 3713–8.

62. Sozzi G, Boeri M, Rossi M, Verri C, Suatoni P, Bravi F, *et al.* (2014). Clinical utility of a plasma-based miRNA signature classifier within computed tomography lung cancer screening: a correlative MILD trial study. *Journal of Clinical Oncology* **32**, 768–73.

63. Bianchi F, Nicassio F, Marzi M, Belloni E, Dall'olio V, Bernard L, *et al.* (2011). A serum circulating miRNA diagnostic test to identify asymptomatic high-risk individuals with early stage lung cancer. *EMBO Molecular Medicine* **3**, 495–503.

64. Bediaga NG, Davies MP, Acha-Sagredo A, Hyde R, Raji OY, Page R, *et al.* (2013). A microRNA-based prediction algorithm for diagnosis of non-small lung cell carcinoma in minimal biopsy material. *British Journal of Cancer* **109**, 2404–11.

65. Perdomo C, Campbell JD, Gerrein J, Tellez CS, Garrison CB, Walser TC, *et al.* (2013). MicroRNA 4423 is a primate-specific regulator of airway epithelial cell differentiation and lung carcinogenesis. *Proceedings of the National Academy of Sciences of the United States of America* **110**, 18946–51.

66. Cazzoli R, Buttitta F, Di Nicola M, Malatesta S, Marchetti A, Rom WN, *et al.* (2013). microRNAs

derived from circulating exosomes as noninvasive biomarkers for screening and diagnosing lung cancer. *Journal of Thoracic Oncology* **8**, 1156–62.

67. Patz EF, Jr., Campa MJ, Gottlin EB, Kusmartseva I, Guan XR, Herndon JE, 2nd (2007). Panel of serum biomarkers for the diagnosis of lung cancer. *Journal of Clinical Oncology* **25**, 5578–83.

68. Yildiz PB, Shyr Y, Rahman JS, Wardwell NR, Zimmerman LJ, Shakhtour B, *et al.* (2007). Diagnostic accuracy of MALDI mass spectrometric analysis of unfractionated serum in lung cancer. *Journal of Thoracic Oncology* **2**, 893–901.

69. Ocak S, Chaurand P, Massion PP (2009). Mass spectrometry-based proteomic profiling of lung cancer. *Proceedings of the American Thoracic Society* **6**, 159–70.

70. Wang WJ, Tao Z, Gu W, Sun LH (2013). Clinical observations on the association between diagnosis of lung cancer and serum tumor markers in combination. *Asian Pacific Journal of Cancer Prevention* **14**, 4369–71.

71. Shevchenko VE, Kovalev SV, Arnotskaya NE, Zborovskaya IB, Akhmedov BB, Polotskii BE, *et al.* (2013). Human blood plasma proteome mapping for search of potential markers of the lung squamous cell carcinoma. *European Journal of Mass Spectrometry* **19**, 123–33.

72. Li T, Kung HJ, Mack PC, Gandara DR (2013). Genotyping and genomic profiling of non-small-cell lung cancer: implications for current and future therapies. *Journal of Clinical Oncology* **31**, 1039–49.

73. Ajona D, Pajares MJ, Corrales L, Perez-Gracia JL, Agorreta J, Lozano MD, *et al.* (2013). Investigation of complement activation product c4d as a diagnostic and prognostic biomarker for lung cancer. *Journal of the National Cancer Institute* **105**, 1385–93.

74. Han SS, Lee SJ, Kim WJ, Ryu DR, Won JY, Park S, *et al.* (2013). Plasma osteopontin is a useful diagnostic biomarker for advanced non-small cell lung cancer. *Tuberculosis and Respiratory Diseases* **75**, 104–10.

75. Sin DD, Tammemagi CM, Lam S, Barnett MJ, Duan X, Tam A, *et al.* (2013). Pro-surfactant protein B as a biomarker for lung cancer prediction. *Journal of Clinical Oncology* **31**, 4536–43.

76. Shiels MS, Pfeiffer RM, Hildesheim A, Engels EA, Kemp TJ, Park JH, *et al.* (2013). Circulating inflammation markers and prospective risk for lung cancer. *Journal of the National Cancer Institute* **105**, 1871–80.

77. Caron M, Choquet-Kastylevsky G, Joubert-Caron R (2007). Cancer immunomics using autoantibody signatures for biomarker discovery. *Molecular & Cellular Proteomics* **6**, 1115–22.

78. Feng Z, Prentice R, Srivastava S (2004). Research issues and strategies for genomic and proteomic biomarker discovery and validation: a statistical perspective. *Pharmacogenomics* **5**, 709–19.

79. Zhong L, Coe SP, Stromberg AJ, Khattar NH, Jett JR, Hirschowitz EA (2006). Profiling tumor-associated antibodies for early detection of non-small cell lung cancer. *Journal of Thoracic Oncology* **1**, 513–9.

80. Khattar NH, Coe-Atkinson SP, Stromberg AJ, Jett JR, Hirschowitz EA (2010). Lung cancer-associated auto-antibodies measured using seven amino acid peptides in a diagnostic blood test for lung cancer. *Cancer Biology & Therapy* **10**(3), 267–272.

81. Pedchenko T, Mernaugh R, Parekh D, Li M, Massion PP (2013). Early detection of NSCLC with scFv selected against IgM autoantibody. *PloS One* **8**, e60934.

82. Chen HY, Yu SL, Chen CH, Chang GC, Chen CY, Yuan A, *et al.* (2007). A five-gene signature and clinical outcome in non-small-cell lung cancer. *New England Journal of Medicine* **356**, 11–20.

83. Wu ST, Ouyang Z, Olah TV, Jemal M (2011). A strategy for liquid chromatography/tandem mass spectrometry based quantitation of pegylated protein drugs in plasma using plasma protein precipitation with water-miscible organic solvents and subsequent trypsin digestion to generate surrogate peptides for detection. *Rapid Communications in Mass Spectrometry* **25**, 281–90.

84. Chapman CJ, Murray A, McElveen JE, Sahin U, Luxemburger U, Tureci O, *et al.* (2008). Autoantibodies in lung cancer: possibilities for early detection and subsequent cure. *Thorax* **63**, 228–33.

85. Qiu J, Choi G, Li L, Wang H, Pitteri SJ, Pereira-Faca SR, *et al.* (2008). Occurrence of autoantibodies to annexin I, 14-3-3 theta and LAMR1 in prediagnostic lung cancer sera. *Journal of Clinical Oncology* **26**, 5060–6.

86. Farlow EC, Vercillo MS, Coon JS, Basu S, Kim AW, Faber LP, *et al.* (2010). A multi-analyte serum test for the detection of non-small cell lung cancer. *British Journal of Cancer* **103**, 1221–8.

87. Stahel RA, Mabry M, Skarin AT, Speak J, Bernal SD (1985). Detection of bone marrow metastasis in small-cell lung cancer by monoclonal antibody. *Journal of Clinical Oncology* **3**, 455–61.

88. Peck K, Sher YP, Shih JY, Roffler SR, Wu CW, Yang PC (1998). Detection and quantitation of circulating cancer cells in the peripheral blood of lung cancer patients. *Cancer Research* **58**, 2761–5.

89. Pachmann K, Camara O, Kavallaris A, Schneider U, Schunemann S, Hoffken K (2005). Quantification of the response of circulating epithelial cells to neodadjuvant treatment for breast cancer: a new tool for therapy monitoring. *Breast Cancer Research* **7**, R975–9.

90. Pachmann K, Heiss P, Demel U, Tilz G (2001). Detection and quantification of small numbers of circulating tumour cells in peripheral blood using laser

scanning cytometer (LSC). *Clinical Chemistry and Laboratory Medicine* **39**, 811–7.

91. Rolle A, Gunzel R, Pachmann U, Willen B, Hoffken K, Pachmann K (2005). Increase in number of circulating disseminated epithelial cells after surgery for non-small cell lung cancer monitored by MAINTRAC(R) is a predictor for relapse: A preliminary report. *World Journal of Surgical Oncology* **3**, 18.

92. Hodgkinson CL, Morrow CJ, Li Y, Metcalf RL, Rothwell DG, Trapani F, et al. (2014). Tumorigenicity and genetic profiling of circulating tumor cells in small-cell lung cancer. *Nature Medicine* **20**(8), 897–903.

93. Naito T, Tanaka F, Ono A, Yoneda K, Takahashi T, Murakami H, et al. (2012). Prognostic impact of circulating tumor cells in patients with small cell lung cancer. *Journal of Thoracic Oncology* **7**, 512–9.

94. Hou JM, Krebs MG, Lancashire L, Sloane R, Backen A, Swain RK, et al. (2012). Clinical significance and molecular characteristics of circulating tumor cells and circulating tumor microemboli in patients with small-cell lung cancer. *Journal of Clinical Oncology* **30**, 525–32.

95. Nagrath S, Sequist LV, Maheswaran S, Bell DW, Irimia D, Ulkus L, et al. (2007). Isolation of rare circulating tumour cells in cancer patients by microchip technology. *Nature* **450**, 1235–9.

96. Wu C, Hao H, Li L, Zhou X, Guo Z, Zhang L, et al. (2009). Preliminary investigation of the clinical significance of detecting circulating tumor cells enriched from lung cancer patients. *Journal of Thoracic Oncology* **4**, 30–6.

97. Taly V, Pekin D, Benhaim L, Kotsopoulos SK, Le Corre D, Li X, et al. (2013). Multiplex picodroplet digital PCR to detect KRAS mutations in circulating DNA from the plasma of colorectal cancer patients. *Clinical chemistry* **59**, 1722–31.

98. Bettegowda C, Sausen M, Leary RJ, Kinde I, Wang Y, Agrawal N, et al. (2014). Detection of circulating tumor DNA in early- and late-stage human malignancies. *Science Translational Medicine* **6**, 224ra24.

99. Diehl F, Schmidt K, Choti MA, Romans K, Goodman S, Li M, et al. (2008). Circulating mutant DNA to assess tumor dynamics. *Nature Medicine* **14**, 985–90.

100. Murtaza M, Dawson SJ, Tsui DW, Gale D, Forshew T, Piskorz AM, et al. (2013). Non-invasive analysis of acquired resistance to cancer therapy by sequencing of plasma DNA. *Nature* **497**, 108–12.

101. Newman AM, Bratman SV, To J, Wynne JF, Eclov NC, Modlin LA, et al. (2014). An ultrasensitive method for quantitating circulating tumor DNA with broad patient coverage. *Nature Medicine* **20**, 548–54.

102. Bloom CI, Graham CM, Berry MP, Rozakeas F, Redford PS, Wang Y, et al. (2013). Transcriptional blood signatures distinguish pulmonary tuberculosis, pulmonary sarcoidosis, pneumonias and lung cancers. *PloS One* **8**, e70630.

103. Kossenkov AV, Dawany N, Evans TL, Kucharczuk JC, Albelda SM, Showe LC, et al. (2012). Peripheral immune cell gene expression predicts survival of patients with non-small cell lung cancer. *PloS One* **7**, e34392.

104. Paz-Elizur T, Krupsky M, Blumenstein S, Elinger D, Schechtman E, Livneh Z (2003). DNA repair activity for oxidative damage and risk of lung cancer. *Journal of the National Cancer Institute* **95**, 1312–9.

105. Leitner-Dagan Y, Sevilya Z, Pinchev M, Kramer R, Elinger D, Roisman LC, et al. (2012). N-methylpurine DNA glycosylase and OGG1 DNA repair activities: opposite associations with lung cancer risk. *Journal of the National Cancer Institute* **104**, 1765–9.

106. Sevilya Z, Leitner-Dagan Y, Pinchev M, Kremer R, Elinger D, Rennert HS, et al. (2014). Low integrated DNA repair score and lung cancer risk. *Cancer Prevention Research (Philadelphia)* **7**, 398–406.

107. Backlund MG, Amann JM, Johnson DH (2008). Novel strategies for the treatment of lung cancer: modulation of eicosanoids. *Journal of Clinical Oncology* **26**, 825–7.

108. Mazzone PJ (2008). Analysis of volatile organic compounds in the exhaled breath for the diagnosis of lung cancer. *Journal of Thoracic Oncology* **3**, 774–80.

109. Phillips A, Lawrence G (1999). Resection rates in lung cancer. *Thorax* **54**, 374–5.

110. Fuchs P, Loeseken C, Schubert JK, Miekisch W (2010). Breath gas aldehydes as biomarkers of lung cancer. *International Journal of Cancer* **126**, 2663–70.

111. Bajtarevic A, Ager C, Pienz M, Klieber M, Schwarz K, Ligor M, et al. (2009). Noninvasive detection of lung cancer by analysis of exhaled breath. *BMC Cancer* **9**, 348.

112. Ligor M, Ligor T, Bajtarevic A, Ager C, Pienz M, Klieber M, et al. (2009). Determination of volatile organic compounds in exhaled breath of patients with lung cancer using solid phase microextraction and gas chromatography mass spectrometry. *Clinical Chemistry and Laboratory Medicine* **47**, 550–60.

113. Mazzone PJ, Hammel J, Dweik R, Na J, Czich C, Laskowski D, et al. (2007). Diagnosis of lung cancer by the analysis of exhaled breath with a colorimetric sensor array. *Thorax* **62**, 565–8.

114. Peled N, Hakim M, Bunn PA, Jr., Miller YE, Kennedy TC, Mattei J, et al. (2012). Non-invasive breath analysis of pulmonary nodules. *Journal of Thoracic Oncology* **7**, 1528–33.

115. Gessner C, Rechner B, Hammerschmidt S, Kuhn H, Hoheisel G, Sack U, et al. (2010). Angiogenic markers in breath condensate identify non-small cell lung cancer. *Lung Cancer* **68**, 177–84.

116. Queralto N, Berliner AN, Goldsmith B, Martino R, Rhodes P, Lim SH (2014). Detecting cancer by breath volatile organic compound analysis: a review of array-based sensors. *Journal of Breath Research* **8**, 027112.

117. Peng G, Hakim M, Broza YY, Billan S, Abdah-Bortnyak R, Kuten A, *et al.* (2010). Detection of lung, breast, colorectal, and prostate cancers from exhaled breath using a single array of nanosensors. *British Journal of Cancer* **103**, 542–51.

118. Mazzone PJ, Wang XF, Xu Y, Mekhail T, Beukemann MC, Na J, *et al.* (2012). Exhaled breath analysis with a colorimetric sensor array for the identification and characterization of lung cancer. *Journal of Thoracic Oncology* **7**, 137–42.

119. Melamed MR (2000). Lung cancer screening results in the National Cancer Institute New York study. *Cancer* **89**, 2356–62.

120. Varella-Garcia M, Kittelson J, Schulte AP, Vu KO, Wolf HJ, Zeng C, *et al.* (2004). Multi-target interphase fluorescence in situ hybridization assay increases sensitivity of sputum cytology as a predictor of lung cancer. *Cancer Detection and Prevention* **28**, 244–51.

121. Katz RL, Zaidi TM, Fernandez RL, Zhang J, He W, Acosta C, *et al.* (2008). Automated detection of genetic abnormalities combined with cytology in sputum is a sensitive predictor of lung cancer. *Modern Pathology* **21**, 950–60.

122. Palmisano WA, Divine KK, Saccomanno G, Gilliland FD, Baylin SB, Herman JG, *et al.* (2000). Predicting lung cancer by detecting aberrant promoter methylation in sputum. *Cancer Research* **60**, 5954–8.

123. Belinsky SA, Palmisano WA, Gilliland FD, Crooks LA, Divine KK, Winters SA, *et al.* (2002). Aberrant promoter methylation in bronchial epithelium and sputum from current and former smokers. *Cancer Research* **62**, 2370–7.

124. Tammemagi MC, Lam SC, McWilliams AM, Sin DD (2011). Incremental value of pulmonary function and sputum DNA image cytometry in lung cancer risk prediction. *Cancer Prevention Research (Philadelphia)* **4**, 552–61.

125. M'Koma AE, Blum DL, Norris JL, Koyama T, Billheimer D, Motley S, *et al.* (2007). Detection of pre-neoplastic and neoplastic prostate disease by MALDI profiling of urine. *Biochemical and Biophysical Research Communications* **353**, 829–34.

126. Matsumura K, Opiekun M, Oka H, Vachani A, Albelda SM, Yamazaki K, *et al.* (2010). Urinary volatile compounds as biomarkers for lung cancer: a proof of principle study using odor signatures in mouse models of lung cancer. *PloS One* **5**, e8819.

127. Li Y, Zhang Y, Qiu F, Qiu Z (2011). Proteomic identification of exosomal LRG1: a potential urinary biomarker for detecting NSCLC. *Electrophoresis* **32**, 1976–83.

128. Yuan JM, Butler LM, Gao YT, Murphy SE, Carmella SG, Wang R, *et al.* (2014). Urinary metabolites of a polycyclic aromatic hydrocarbon and volatile organic compounds in relation to lung cancer development in lifelong never smokers in the Shanghai Cohort Study. *Carcinogenesis* **35**, 339–45.

129. Cummings SR, Lillington GA, Richard RJ (1986). Managing solitary pulmonary nodules. The choice of strategy is a "close call". *American Review of Respiratory Disease* **134**, 453–60.

130. Gurney JW, Lyddon DM, McKay JA (1993). Determining the likelihood of malignancy in solitary pulmonary nodules with Bayesian analysis. *Part II. Application. Radiology* **186**, 415–22.

131. Swensen SJ, Silverstein MD, Ilstrup DM, Schleck CD, Edell ES (1997). The probability of malignancy in solitary pulmonary nodules. Application to small radiologically indeterminate nodules. *Archives of Internal Medicine* **157**, 849–55.

132. Moons KG, Altman DG, Vergouwe Y, Royston P (2009). Prognosis and prognostic research: application and impact of prognostic models in clinical practice. *BMJ* **338**, b606.

133. Anderson JE, Hansen LL, Mooren FC, Post M, Hug H, Zuse A, *et al.* (2006). Methods and biomarkers for the diagnosis and prognosis of cancer and other diseases: towards personalized medicine. *Drug Resistance Updates* **9**, 198–210.

134. Pepe MS, Feng Z, Janes H, Bossuyt PM, Potter JD (2008). Pivotal evaluation of the accuracy of a biomarker used for classification or prediction: standards for study design. *Journal of the National Cancer Institute* **100**, 1432–8.

135. Hassanein M, Rahman JS, Chaurand P, Massion PP (2011). Advances in proteomic strategies toward the early detection of lung cancer. *Proceedings of the American Thoracic Society* **8**, 183–8.

136. Kim B, Lee HJ, Choi HY, Shin Y, Nam S, Seo G, *et al.* (2007). Clinical validity of the lung cancer biomarkers identified by bioinformatics analysis of public expression data. *Cancer Research* **67**, 7431–8.

137. Boyle P, Chapman CJ, Holdenrieder S, Murray A, Robertson C, Wood WC, *et al.* (2011). Clinical validation of an autoantibody test for lung cancer. *Annals of Oncology* **22**, 383–9.

138. Chen X, Hu Z, Wang W, Ba Y, Ma L, Zhang C, *et al.* (2012). Identification of ten serum microRNAs from a genome-wide serum microRNA expression profile as novel noninvasive biomarkers for nonsmall cell lung cancer diagnosis. *International Journal of Cancer* **130**, 1620–8.

139. Kulpa J, Wojcik E, Reinfuss M, Kolodziejski L (2002). Carcinoembryonic antigen, squamous cell carcinoma antigen, CYFRA 21-1, and neuron-specific enolase in squamous cell lung cancer patients. *Clinical Chemistry* **48**, 1931–7.

140. Takano A, Ishikawa N, Nishino R, Masuda K, Yasui W, Inai K, *et al.* (2009). Identification of nectin-4 oncoprotein as a diagnostic and therapeutic target for lung cancer. *Cancer Research* **69**, 6694–703.

141. Diamandis EP, Goodglick L, Planque C, Thornquist MD (2011). Pentraxin-3 is a novel biomarker of lung carcinoma. *Clinical Cancer Research* **17**, 2395–9.

142. Ostroff RM, Bigbee WL, Franklin W, Gold L, Mehan M, Miller YE, *et al.* (2010). Unlocking biomarker discovery: large scale application of aptamer proteomic technology for early detection of lung cancer. *PloS One* **5**, e15003.

143. Zhong L, Hidalgo GE, Stromberg AJ, Khattar NH, Jett JR, Hirschowitz EA (2005). Using protein microarray as a diagnostic assay for non-small cell lung cancer. *American Journal of Respiratory and Critical Care Medicine* **172**, 1308–14.

144. Kneip C, Schmidt B, Seegebarth A, Weickmann S, Fleischhacker M, Liebenberg V, *et al.* (2011). SHOX2 DNA methylation is a biomarker for the diagnosis of lung cancer in plasma. *Journal of Thoracic Oncology* **6**, 1632–8.

145. Shen J, Todd NW, Zhang H, Yu L, Lingxiao X, Mei Y, *et al.* (2011). Plasma microRNAs as potential biomarkers for non-small-cell lung cancer. *Laboratory Investigation* **91**, 579–87.

146. Wei J, Gao W, Zhu CJ, Liu YQ, Mei Z, Cheng T, *et al.* (2011). Identification of plasma microRNA-21 as a biomarker for early detection and chemosensitivity of non-small cell lung cancer. *Chinese Journal of Cancer* **30**, 407–14.

147. Taguchi A, Politi K, Pitteri SJ, Lockwood WW, Faca VM, Kelly-Spratt K, *et al.* (2011). Lung cancer signatures in plasma based on proteome profiling of mouse tumor models. *Cancer Cell* **20**, 289–99.

148. Wang P, Piao Y, Zhang X, Li W, Hao X (2013). The concentration of CYFRA 21-1, NSE and CEA in cerebro-spinal fluid can be useful indicators for diagnosis of meningeal carcinomatosis of lung cancer. *Cancer Biomarkers : Section A of Disease Markers* **13**, 123–30.

149. Li XJ, Hayward C, Fong PY, Dominguez M, Hunsucker SW, Lee LW, *et al.* (2013). A blood-based proteomic classifier for the molecular characterization of pulmonary nodules. *Science Translational Medicine* **5**, 207ra142.

150. Palmisano WA, Crume KP, Grimes MJ, Winters SA, Toyota M, Esteller M, *et al.* (2003). Aberrant promoter methylation of the transcription factor genes PAX5 alpha and beta in human cancers. *Cancer Research* **63**, 4620–5.

151. Yu L, Todd NW, Xing L, Xie Y, Zhang H, Liu Z, *et al.* (2010). Early detection of lung adenocarcinoma in sputum by a panel of microRNA markers. *International Journal of Cancer* **127**, 2870–8.

152. Tanaka F, Yoneda K, Kondo N, Hashimoto M, Takuwa T, Matsumoto S, *et al.* (2009). Circulating tumor cell as a diagnostic marker in primary lung cancer. *Clinical Cancer Research* **15**, 6980–6.

CHAPTER 15

Commonalities in Lung Cancer and COPD

Malgorzata Wojtowicz and Eva Szabo

Lung and Upper Aerodigestive Cancer Research Group, Division of Cancer Prevention, National Cancer Institute, National Institutes of Health, Bethesda, MD, USA

Introduction

Despite significant efforts, lung cancer and chronic obstructive pulmonary disease (COPD) remain leading causes of significant morbidity and mortality in the United States and worldwide. Both are believed to result from the combined effect of environmental exposure to cigarette smoke and genetic predisposition [1, 2]. It is estimated that approximately 20 million Americans have COPD, which caused approximately 140 000 deaths in 2010 and is the third leading cause of death in the USA [3]. In 2014, over 224 000 new cases, and almost 160 000 deaths from lung cancer, were projected to occur in the US [4] while, globally, more than 1.37 million deaths take place every year [5]. Although improved, current lung cancer therapies only achieve approximately 17% overall five-year survival, maintaining lung cancer as a leading cause of cancer death [6].

In spite of high levels of public awareness of tobacco-related health risks, and declining smoking rates, an estimated 43.8 million Americans still actively smoked in 2011 [7]. In the developing world, smoking rates continue to rise, especially in China and India, where additional significant environmental risk exists in air pollution resulting from burning of biomass fuels [8, 9] – see http://www.cdc.gov/tobacco/data_statistics/sgr/2004/index.htm.

Although smoking cessation reduces the incidence of lung cancer and COPD, the risks of both diseases in former smokers remains elevated for years following successful quitting, when compared to those who have never smoked (roughly equal proportions of lung cancers are being diagnosed in former smokers and current smokers; ≈40–45% each) [10]. This is believed to be due, at least in part, to the persistent molecular damage in the airway epithelium of smokers, which does not return to normal for decades following cessation of smoking [11, 12].

Additionally, although smoking accounts for the majority (80–90%) of all lung cancers and COPD, genetic components also modify susceptibility to both conditions, since only a subset of smokers develops either COPD (20–30%) or lung cancer (10–15%) [3, 13]. Furthermore, around 10% of new lung cancers in men and 20% in women occur in lifetime never-smokers [14]. Similarly, although published prevalence estimates vary greatly, it has been estimated that, worldwide, as many as 25–45% of patients with COPD have never smoked, with other causes such as biomass fuel, outdoor air pollution, occupational exposure to dust and gases, history of pulmonary tuberculosis, chronic asthma, poor socioeconomic status, etc. posing a risk [15]. Therefore, despite significant global efforts, COPD and lung cancer will remain major health concerns worldwide for many decades to come,

Biomarkers in Cancer Screening and Early Detection, First Edition. Edited by Sudhir Srivastava.
© 2017 John Wiley & Sons, Inc. Published 2017 by John Wiley & Sons, Inc.

demanding intense and continuous research in this field.

Natural history of COPD and lung cancer

Chronic obstructive lung disease (COPD)

The Global Initiative on Chronic Obstructive Lung Disease (GOLD) defines COPD as a preventable and treatable disease which is characterized by air-flow limitation that is not fully reversible. COPD is usually progressive and is associated with an enhanced chronic inflammatory response to noxious particles or gases [16]. It results in small airway remodeling, increased mucus production, airway ciliary malfunction, and the loss of alveolar elastic recoil due to destruction of alveolar walls.

Typically, COPD is divided into two major pathophysiologic components:

1 chronic bronchitis – obstructive airway disease (airflow obstruction) resulting from narrowing of bronchi; and
2 emphysema – alveolar destruction from alveolar obliteration [17].

COPD is highly heterogeneous with significant variability within the two components and most patients having varying degrees of contribution from each component. Therefore, defining the COPD phenotype in each individual requires assessment of both elements, traditionally by combining history of exposure, symptoms, and physical exam with results of pulmonary function tests (PFTs) and chest computed tomography (CT; for radiologic evidence of emphysema). Abnormal pulmonary function (specifically, the ratio of forced expiratory volume in one second (FEV1) and the forced vital capacity (FVC); FEV1/FVC) is a major criterion for diagnosis of COPD and for defining disease severity (GOLD classification system).

The natural course of COPD includes periods of stability interrupted by episodes of acute exacerbations [18]. General management of COPD includes emphases on smoking cessation, pulmonary rehabilitation and use of long-acting inhaled beta-agonists, anticholinergics and glucocorticoids. COPD exacerbation requiring hospitalization is associated with increased 30-day rate of death from any cause by 4–30%. Declining lung function is also a strong predictor of COPD-related morbidity and mortality, with many other factors influencing the outcome as well.

The risk of death increases with increasing GOLD stage (in multivariate analysis, risks of death by GOLD stage are: GOLD 1 – Hazard Ratio (HR) = 1.2, 95% Confidence Intervals(CI), 1.01–1.4; GOLD 2 – HR = 1.6, 95%CI, 1.4–2.0; GOLD 3 – HR = 2.7, 95%CI, 2.1–3.5) [19]. Accumulating data provide strong evidence for COPD to be an inflammatory disease, not only locally in the lungs, but also systemically. This systemic chronic inflammation is thought to be, at least in part, implicated in pathogenesis of co-morbid conditions frequently seen in COPD – especially cardiovascular disease and its complications [17, 20].

Lung cancer

Lung cancer is a heterogeneous group of diseases that have historically been divided into two major categories based on the differences in biology, therapy and prognosis. These are:

1 small cell lung cancer (SCLC) which constitutes ~10–15% of all lung cancers, is of neuroendocrine cell origin, and has quick clinical growth with early dissemination; and
2 non-small cell lung cancer (NSCLC) which accounts for the majority (≥85%) of all lung cancers, is of epithelial cell origin and is further subdivided (based on histology) into:

  a squamous cell cancer (SCC, ~40% of NSCLC);
  b adenocarcinoma (ADC; ~50% of NSCLC); and
  c other less common histologies including large cell carcinoma [21].

SCLCs and NSCLC-SCCs tend to arise in more proximal airways (central lung) and are more strongly associated with cigarette smoking than adenocarcinomas, which usually arise in more distal airways (peripheral lung). Lung adenocarcinoma is currently the most frequently diagnosed type of lung cancer in never-smokers as well as in smokers, with continuously rising trends [22]. In this chapter we will focus primarily on NSCLC.

NSCLC is potentially curable if diagnosed at an early stage (five-year survival for stage I = 45–65%) [23]. Surgical resection is the main therapeutic strategy in early disease with some role for adjuvant chemotherapy and/or radiation in specific cases [23, 24]. Locally advanced tumors are usually treated with combined chemotherapy and radiation. Metastatic disease is generally considered to be incurable (five-year survival 1–2%) [25], and the goal of treatment, typically with systemic therapy (chemotherapy, molecular targeted agents, immunotherapy), is lengthened survival and symptom palliation.

Recent advances in the understanding of lung cancer genomes and signaling pathways have resulted in the development of new, more effective targeted therapies. However, responses to these agents, even when significant, are of limited duration. The newest promising treatment strategy is immunotherapy with checkpoint blockade, but more work is needed to better define its role in the treatment armamentarium of lung cancer.

Therefore, early lung cancer detection is one important strategy for improved outcome. Although the majority of lung cancers are diagnosed clinically at an advanced stage (approximately 70% present with locally advanced or metastatic disease), screening with CT shifts the detection to an earlier stage and the National Lung Cancer Screening Trial (NLST) [26] demonstrated a 20% relative reduction in mortality from lung cancer with the use of three annual low-dose helical CT scans when compared with standard chest X-ray. The US Centers for Medicare and Medicaid Services (CMS) announced recently [27] approval of coverage for lung cancer screening of high risk individuals using low-dose CT. Although not without its challenges with regard to overdiagnosis and implementation at a population level, this represents an important step in reducing deaths from lung cancer.

Potential link between COPD and lung cancer

With the goal of developing successful strategies to prevent lung cancer, intensive research is attempting to better understand the early steps of lung carcinogenesis. One of these efforts is to investigate the molecular links between COPD and lung cancer. A growing body of evidence supports a direct link between COPD and lung cancer, independent of smoking. Approximately 50–70% of lung cancer patients have some spirometric evidence of COPD and COPD is a major independent risk factor for lung cancer [28–30]. Specifically, airflow limitation has been shown to be an independent risk factor for lung cancer among smokers [31], with different stages of COPD conferring different lung cancer risks. Mild-to-moderate COPD raises this risk by threefold within ten years, while severely reduced airflow elevates lung cancer risk tenfold [32]. Even mild reduction in airflow (as defined by FEV1 at 90% of the predicted value) has been linked to higher lung cancer risk [30]. CT-defined emphysema, even when controlled for airflow obstruction, has also been reported to be independently related to higher lung cancer risk [29, 33] and mortality [34].

Similarly, ongoing studies are examining whether analogous links exist in those who have never smoked. In a large prospectively followed cohort of lifelong non-smokers, Turner *et al.* reported that emphysema, and the combined endpoint of emphysema and chronic bronchitis, were significantly associated with mortality from lung cancer (HR = 1.66, 95%CI, 1.06–2.59; HR = 2.44, 95%CI, 1.22–4.90, respectively) [35]. Although no association was seen with chronic bronchitis alone, there was some suggestion that chronic bronchitis may be more strongly associated with lung cancer in men (HR = 1.59, 95%CI, 0.95–2.66) than in women (HR = 0.82, 95%CI, 0.58 = 1.16; *p* for interaction of 0.04).

Thus, there appears to be independent relationship between COPD and lung cancer although the nature of the association is poorly understood (Figure 15.1). The importance of understanding this interplay resulted in an NIH initiative aimed at fostering integrated research between the COPD and lung cancer research communities, to investigate common pathogenetic mechanisms responsible for the two diseases [36]. Below, we discuss the state of the science in ongoing research in this field which, among others, focuses on discovery of clinically relevant biomarkers to predict COPD development, COPD progression, and risks of developing lung cancer in individuals with COPD. Although there are no specific biomarkers

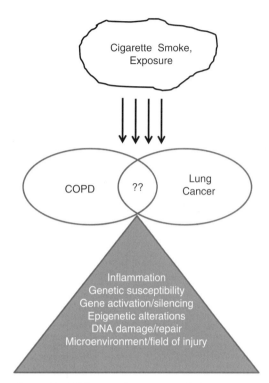

Figure 15.1 Link between lung cancer and COPD. Pathogenetic mechanisms responsible for the lung cancer-COPD association are poorly understood. Biomarkers common to both disease processes fall into many categories, but all require further validation. For a color version of this figure please see color plate section.

responses involving quiescent stem cells entering the cell cycle in an attempt to repair injury). The repair phase involves high DNA replicative activity, with high sensitivity to mutagenic damage from inflammatory mediators (e.g., reactive oxygen species) and/or environmental carcinogens (cigarette smoke, pollutants, etc). Although the majority of genetically damaged cells are eliminated, some cells will escape by accumulating additional genetic and epigenetic damage with each injury-repair cycle.

The immune system has the ability to eliminate such "cancer-prone cells" through the process called immunosurveillance. However, chronic inflammation induces an immune-inhibitory environment via the recruitment of a plethora of immune suppressive cells (e.g., myeloid-derived suppressor cells – MDSC, T-regulatory cells), immune inhibitory cytokines (e.g., interleukins such as IL-10, IL-6) and other mechanisms, actively suppressing this protective anti-tumoral immunity. This allows immune evasion and the escape of abnormal cells, leading to development of cancer, which is associated with additional mechanisms to effectively avoid immune recognition and elimination (reviewed in [39] and [40]).

Transcription factors STAT3 (signal transducer and activator of transcription-3) and NF-ƙB (nuclear factor of kappa light polypeptide gene enhancer in B-cells) have been identified as key effectors in molecular networks linking inflammation and carcinogenesis. STAT3, a core molecular node linking numerous oncogenic signaling pathways, has been associated with several receptors such as IL-6 (involved in inflammation), EGFR (epidermal growth factor receptor, involved in epithelial repair) and VEGF (vascular endothelial growth factor, involved in angiogenesis). STAT3 signaling supports the inflammatory state, promotion of tissue remodeling and angiogenesis, and induction of cell proliferation with suppression of apoptosis [40]. It induces tumor cells to release immunosuppressive (e.g., IL-6, IL-10) and angiogenic (e.g., VEGF) factors which, in turn, stimulate STAT3 activation in tumor-infiltrating immune cells, and lead to suppression of effective anti-tumor immunity and tumor immune evasion [41]. Of note, gene expression of STAT3 has been shown to be increased in human COPD lung tissue

yet identified and validated, the ultimate goal of these studies is to identify clinically relevant tools leading to improved diagnostic and therapeutic interventions for COPD as well as prevention of lung cancer.

Commonalities in the molecular pathogenesis of lung cancer and COPD

Inflammation

Chronic inflammation is a well-recognized hallmark of cancer and thus the inflammatory milieu of COPD could support lung carcinogenesis [37]. In general, carcinogenesis in the inflammatory microenvironment is thought to be driven by ongoing cycles of tissue injury and repair [38]. Tissue damage stimulates necrotic cell death (which, in turn, recruits inflammatory cells) and loss of tissue integrity (which induces regenerative with further increase in lung cancer, as compared with normal human lung tissue. Consequently, STAT3 may be involved in progression from COPD to lung cancer [42] and is a potential target for cancer immunotherapy [41].

NF-ƙB is another important transcription factor involved in inflammation and carcinogenesis. Protein expression of p65, a major subunit of NF-ƙB, was shown to be elevated in bronchial biopsies from "healthy" smokers and COPD patients when compared to non-smokers, and correlating with airflow obstruction [43]. Of interest, persistent STAT3 activation was reported to result in constitutive NF-ƙB activation not only in tumors, but also in tumor-infiltrating immune cells [44]. This further suggests that NF-ƙB may be a potential marker of inflammation and COPD-associated lung carcinogenesis.

Matrix-degrading proteinases are important components of inflammation with potential links to cancer. Neutrophil elastase (NE), a proteolytic enzyme in neutrophils, is a particularly important driver of emphysema formation [45], with excess levels measured in human COPD lungs. NE has also been reported to promote growth of lung tumors in a K-ras-driven mouse model of lung adenocarcinoma [46]. Mice with both K-ras mutation and knockout of NE showed a markedly lower tumor burden and longer survival than K-ras mutant mice with intact NE. NE was shown to directly induce tumor cells proliferation by degrading insulin receptor substrate-1 (IRS-1), thereby increasing the interaction between PI3K (phosphoinositide 3-kinase) and PDGFR (platelet derived growth factor receptor). This interaction was also demonstrated to occur in human lung adenocarcinomas.

Similarly, MMP-12 (matrix metalloproteinase-12), a proteinase induced mainly in macrophages and dendritic cells, is necessary for the development of smoke-induced emphysema in mice and is highly expressed in alveolar macrophages of COPD patients [47, 48]. MMP-12 can sustain the chronic inflammatory state and tissue remodeling through generation of elastin fragments which are chemotactic for inflammatory monocytes. This can contribute to persistence of airway inflammation long after cessation of smoking [49]. Interestingly, overexpression of MMP-12 in the airways leads not only to sustained inflammation and emphysema,

but also to the development of areas of adenocarcinoma via IL-6/STAT3 signaling [40, 50].

Finally, MMP-9 is a metalloproteinase produced by neutrophils and macrophages with high activity in lungs of COPD patients that correlates with the degree of airway obstruction. MMP-9 production by inflammatory cells supports tumor progression via, among others, the release of angiogenic factors triggering the "angiogenic switch" during carcinogenesis [51].

On a clinical level, repeated bacterial and viral infections, with their attendant inflammation, are well known complications of COPD. Of note, in the K-ras mouse lung carcinogenesis model, exposure to Haemophilus influenza (a frequent pathogen in COPD) caused airway inflammation and led to increased total burden of lung tumors [52]. These data indicate that, in addition to chronic inflammation, "acute-on-chronic" COPD lung inflammation contributes to lung carcinogenesis.

Overall, these findings support the notion that specific components of inflammatory signaling provide a link between COPD and tumor growth. There is a need, however, to investigate which elements of the COPD-related inflammation can be identified as potential biomarkers of COPD progression and lung cancer.

Molecular field of injury

Combined effects of cigarette smoke create large fields of injury throughout the lungs where a range of histologic preneoplastic (and overtly neoplastic) abnormalities may co-exist. Furthermore, histologically normal epithelium may already contain unique molecular alterations that could eventually give rise to cancer. This is the premise of the "field cancerization" concept which was first introduced by Slaughter *et al.* in 1953 [53] and appears also to be operational in lung carcinogenesis. Multiple independent clones with deleterious genetic mutations can populate large areas of the lung epithelium, expand regionally, and provide foci of cells which can accrue additional mutation(s) and, at some point, may reach the required level of alterations to become overtly malignant. This process of accumulation of genetic alterations causing progression from the normal cell to a cancer cell is referred to as "multistep carcinogenesis", and is well established [54]. The development of squamous cell carcinoma in particular appears to follow this pattern as evidenced by the appearance of progressive histologic changes from normal, to metaplasia, to dysplasia, to carcinoma *in situ* and finally, to invasive cancer.

Spira and colleagues have applied profiling of cytologically normal bronchial epithelium to study lung cancer and COPD and to develop biomarkers of these disease processes for the early detection of cancer [12, 55, 56]. They identified an 80-gene signature in histologically normal airway epithelium obtained at bronchoscopy that was able to distinguish smokers with and without lung cancer with ~90% sensitivity for stage I cancer [56]. In addition, the group has identified a robust 119-genes smoking-related signature in the bronchial epithelium of smokers that is able to significantly separate never or former smokers from current smokers. This signature has also been identified in the easily obtainable nasal epithelium, which is potentially a surrogate tissue for bronchial epithelium (as part of the field of molecular injury due to exposure to cigarette smoke) [12, 57]. Currently, efforts are ongoing to investigate whether distinct molecular signatures of the COPD-related oncogenic processes and pathways can be identified through airway epithelial profiling, thereby allowing for subsequent non-invasive monitoring of these processes and potential early detection of the signatures prior to the development of lung cancer.

Genetics

COPD and lung cancer are frequently cited examples of diseases resulting from gene-environment interactions. Alpha-1 antitrypsin (A1AT) deficiency is the best established genetic risk factor for development of emphysema [58]. A1AT (encoded by SERPINA1) is an inhibitor of neutrophil elastase (NE), which degrades elastin (a protein important for the lung's ability to recoil; see previous discussion of NE in the section on inflammation). Individuals who are homozygous for alleles associated with A1AT deficiency (ZZ) develop premature, severe emphysema even with minimal or no cigarette smoke exposure.

An increased risk of lung cancer has been seen in individuals who are carriers of A1AT deficiency alleles, especially the S and Z variants, across the spectrum of tobacco exposure [59]. Never-smokers who are A1AT deficiency allele carriers are at a 2.2-fold higher risk of lung cancer than non-carriers, after adjusting for age, gender and history of COPD. Smokers with a <20 pack year smoking history who are A1AT deficiency carriers have a 2.0-fold higher risk of lung cancer, while smokers with ≥20 pack-year smoking exposure have 2.3-fold greater risk than non-carriers. Additionally, a history of COPD among A1AT carriers was shown to further increase the risk of lung cancer across all groups of smokers, from 2.5- to 5.9-fold, with the largest impact on never smokers.

Conversely, both Z and S alleles of the A1AT gene as well as polymorphism in the NE gene were more common in patients with lung cancer when compared with the general population [60, 61]. This observation would suggest that imbalance between excessive NE activity and deficient A1AT inhibitory ability could be a contributing factor to the development of both COPD and lung cancer [62]. These observations are concordant with the biologic studies in NE knockout mice discussed previously, where NE deficiency reduced tumor burden and mortality in a K-ras-driven mouse model of lung carcinogenesis [46].

Evidence supporting the existence of a common familial predisposition to lung cancer and COPD, independent of smoking, has been known for a long time [63]. However, only recently has it been reported that individuals with a family history of lung cancer are at 2–3 fold higher risk of developing lung malignancy (after adjusting for cigarette smoking) as compared to the general population [64, 65]. Several linkage studies focusing on genes involved in lung function and COPD, as well as candidate susceptibility genes involved in COPD and lung cancer, have identified markers on chromosome 6q for lung cancer and abnormal lung function and on chromosome 12 for lung cancer, COPD and lung function [65, 66]. This is in addition to many other candidate susceptibility genes involved in detoxification, immune regulation, matrix remodeling, DNA repair, cellular proliferation and tumor suppression, all of which, theoretically, could have mechanistic roles in the genesis of both lung cancer and COPD.

Genetic mapping studies have distinguished several single nucleotide polymorphisms (SNPs) which were associated with both lung cancer and

COPD. Many of these SNPs are located in candidate gene families such as proteinases (e.g., ADAM19), detoxifying enzymes (e.g., GSTM1) and inflammatory cytokines (1q21-23 (CRP, IL-6R)). More recently reported genome-wide association studies (GWAS) for lung cancer, lung function and COPD have identified several chromosomal regions and candidate genes that are thought to impact both smoking behavior and lung carcinogenesis. Interestingly, several of these genetic loci associated with lung cancer and/or COPD appear to have overlapping functions in the development of both lung cancer and COPD (reviewed in [67–69]).

Genetic associations for lung cancer and COPD that are of particular interest include the locus on the long arm of chromosome 15 (15q25) that maps to CHRNA3 and CHRNA5 (nicotinic α receptor subunits 3 and 5), which encode nicotinic acetylcholine (Ach) receptors [70]. The 15q25 gene has been shown to be associated with susceptibility to both lung cancer and COPD [71]. In addition, both CHRNA3 and CHRNA5 are also associated with cigarette smoke consumption and nicotine dependence [72].

Other genes involved in pathogenesis of COPD and lung cancer include Hedgehog interacting protein (HHIP) and family with sequence similarity 13 member A (FAM13A). Both the HHIP and FAM13A, initially associated with reduced risk of COPD [73], have also been independently associated with reduced risk of lung cancer [74, 75]. As reviewed by Young *et al.* [67], genes identified by these studies would suggest that overlapping genetic susceptibility for COPD and lung cancer could be mediated via receptors expressed on the bronchial epithelium that are involved in molecular pathways underlying both diseases.

HHIP is expressed on bronchial epithelium and modulates epithelial repair, smoke-induced epithelial-mesenchymal transition, and cigarette smoke induced oncogenic transformation of bronchial epithelial cells [76]. FAM13A, which is also expressed on the bronchial epithelium, has been shown to possess Rho GTPase activating protein (Rho-GAP) activity which would suggest both anti-inflammatory and tumor-suppressor function even though little is known of the true function of this protein [77]. Although these genetic associations and their biological effects require further study, these data support the hypothesis that COPD and lung cancer are directly linked at the molecular genetic level and suggest that the response of the airway epithelium to smoking likely has a critical role in both processes.

Epigenetic modifications

Epigenetic modifications are functionally relevant changes that alter gene expression and cell function without changes in DNA sequence. They include DNA methylation and post-translational modification of histones (e.g., acetylation, methylation, phosphorylation), which control chromatin structure and remodeling that determine subsequent transcriptional outcomes of the cell. The major epigenetic modifications involved in lung cancer include DNA regional (promoter) hypermethylation (usually leading to gene silencing), DNA global hypomethylation, post-translational modification of histones, miRNA expression, and miRNA silencing by DNA hypermethylation. Epigenetic modifications could represent another link between COPD and lung cancer through commonalities in methylation features and subsequent changes in genes expression resulting from exposure to cigarette smoke or air pollution.

DNA hypermethylation is the most extensively studied epigenetic event in lung cancer and is implicated in altered expression of a number of oncogenes and tumor suppressor genes related to this disease as well as genes involved in DNA repair, apoptosis, cell adhesion, and other critical cellular processes [78]. Among the most frequently hypermethylated genes in NSCLC are p16^{INK4a}, RAS associated domain family member 1 (RASSF1A), O-6-methylguanine-DNA methyltransferase (MGMT), and death associated protein kinase (DAPK). p16^{INK4a} is a tumor suppressor of particular interest, due to its role in cell cycle progression and its frequent promoter hypermethylation in many cancers. p16^{INK4a} methylation has been shown to be associated with poor prognosis after diagnosis of NSCLC [79]. Additionally, methylation of p16^{INK4a} is an early event in lung carcinogenesis and can be detected in sputum of COPD patients even before the clinical diagnosis of lung cancer [80]. Similarly, a recent study comparing lung cancer patients with and without COPD demonstrated significantly increased levels of methylation of IL-12Rβ2 and Wif-1 in cancer patients with COPD as compared with those without COPD [81].

While these data are tantalizing, methylation markers have not yet emerged as sensitive and specific biomarkers of lung cancer, and even less is known about methylation in COPD (recently reviewed in [82]). However, with the advent of high-throughput technologies, it will now be possible to interrogate the entire methylome in both lung cancer and COPD to identify possible overlap.

The past decade has witnessed a growing interest in miRNAs, which are small (18–24 nucleotide) noncoding endogenous regulatory RNAs that regulate gene expression at the post-translational level. miRNAs have been shown to be involved in the pathogenesis of several diseases and are involved in many important biological processes such as development, differentiation, proliferation and apoptosis [83]. Expression patterns of miRNAs often change in disease states and, therefore, unique miRNA expression profiles can be identified in various conditions and could potentially serve as disease specific biomarkers.

Animal studies have described miRNA alterations throughout all stages of lung carcinogenesis in response to cigarette smoke. Importantly, these changes could be efficiently reversed by chemopreventive agents [84]. Similar dysregulation in patterns of miRNA expression was observed in human bronchial epithelium from smokers when compared with never-smokers. One of these miRNAs, miR-218, which is strongly downregulated by smoking, was able to regulate the airway epithelial gene expression response to cigarette smoke, supporting a role for miRNAs in regulating host response to environmental toxins [85].

Early studies have begun to identify common miRNA dysregulation in COPD and lung cancer. Molina-Pinelo et al. examined miRNA expression in bronchoalveolar lavage fluid from patients with lung adenocarcinoma, COPD, both diseases, or controls [86]. Only three miRNAs – miR15b, miR486-3p, and miR425 – were found upregulated in both lung cancer and COPD (independently in each disease as well as when both were present in the same patient). miR15b was also overexpressed in lung tissue from COPD patients, suggesting that miR15b may have a role in the genesis of both COPD and lung cancer [87].

The let-7 family is of particular interest in lung cancer, where reduced let-7 expression was significantly associated with shortened survival [88]. In addition, loss of let-7 function has been shown to enhance lung tumor formation in vivo, suggesting that reduced expression of let-7 may play a role in the pathogenesis of lung cancer. Exogenous delivery of let-7 to established tumors in mouse models of NSCLC led to significant reduction in tumor burden, indicating potential therapeutic usefulness of let-7 [89].

Intriguingly, two studies have also identified dysregulation of let-7 family members in COPD patients. One small study examined miRNA expression in sputum from current smokers with or without COPD and from healthy non-smokers and found reduced let-7c expression associated with COPD [90]. A second small study found decreased let-7a expression in exhaled breath condensate from patients with COPD [91]. Although all of these studies are still preliminary and are focused on different types of biospecimens, they suggest that specific miRNAs may be similarly dysregulated in both lung cancer and COPD and, thus, should be investigated as potential biomarkers of these diseases. The stability of miRNAs and the potential to identify them from non-invasively obtained specimens such as blood or sputum offers the promise of identifying high risk individuals and early disease detection.

Challenges and future directions

Historically, lung cancer and COPD have been studied by investigators from different segments of the research community. The increasing recognition of commonalities between these two diseases and the potential benefit of recognizing both diseases early is spurring efforts to understand common mechanisms and identify at-risk populations. However, the complexity of disease phenotypes and molecular subtypes, each with potentially different pathogenetic mechanisms, complicates the identification of biomarkers that would be useful as targets for disease prevention or for early detection. The lack of suitable preclinical models (e.g., mouse models) that adequately recapitulate both lung cancer and COPD simultaneously is but one barrier to progress. The difficulty in obtaining human lung tissues from early phases of development of lung cancer and COPD is yet another challenge.

Much work needs to be done to understand the complex mechanisms governing the interaction between lung cancer and COPD. Ongoing studies are using high-throughput technologies to decipher molecular abnormalities in the at-risk field and in surrogate tissues, ranging from bronchoscopic brushings and lavage fluid to blood, nasal epithelium, and sputum. Assay development with adaptation to easily obtained fluids/biospecimens needs to proceed concurrently with these studies. Novel tissue culture models, such as bronchial epithelial cells grown at the air-liquid interface, need further development.

It is critical to collect and carefully annotate appropriate tissues from individuals whose COPD and lung cancer are well characterized. As new insights (such as the role of immunotherapy in lung cancer treatment or the role of the microbiome in disease causation) occur, they need to inform the study of lung cancer and COPD. Finally, and perhaps most important, there is a critical need to form interdisciplinary collaborations that bring together diverse areas of expertise. Data from these multiple areas of study will guide the development of novel biomarkers to define populations at risk, development of tools to calculate risk, and identification of targets for therapeutic and preventive interventions for both COPD and lung cancer.

References

1. Talikka M, Sierro N, Ivanov NV, Chaudhary N, Peck MJ, Hoeng J, et al. (2012). Genomic impact of cigarette smoke, with application to three smoking-related diseases. *Critical Reviews in Toxicology* **42**(10), 877–89.

2. Yang IA, Relan V, Wright CM, Davidson MR, Sriram KB, Savarimuthu Francis SM, et al. (2011). Common pathogenic mechanisms and pathways in the development of COPD and lung *Cancer Expert Opinion on Therapeutic Targets* **15**(4), 439–56.

3. U.S. Department of Health and Human Services (2014). *The Health Consequences of Smoking – 50 Years of Progress; A Report of the Surgeon General.*

4. American Cancer Society (2015). *Cancer Facts & Figures 2014.* Atlanta: American Cancer Society; 2014.

5. World Health Organization – International Agency for Research on Cancer (2015). *Estimated Cancer Incidence, Mortality and Prevalence Worldwide in 2012.* Lung Cancer GLOBOCAN 2012.

6. Siegel R, Naishadham D, Jemal A (2013). Cancer Statistics, 2013. *CA: A Cancer Journal for Clinicians* **63**(1), 11–30.

7. Centers for Disease Control and Prevention (2015). *Current Cigarette Smoking Among Adults – United States 2011, 2012.*

8. WHO – World Health Organization (2013). *Review of Evidence on Health Aspects of Air Pollution – REVIHAAP Project.*

9. World Health Organization (2008). *WHO Report On The Global Tobacco Epidemic.*

10. Peto R, Darby S, Deo H, Silcocks P, Whitley E, Doll R (2000). Smoking, smoking cessation, and lung cancer in the UK since 1950: combination of national statistics with two case-control studies. *BMJ* **321**(7257), 323–9.

11. Wistuba, II, Lam S, Behrens C, Virmani AK, Fong KM, LeRiche J, et al. (1997). Molecular damage in the bronchial epithelium of current and former smokers. *Journal of the National Cancer Institute* **89**(18), 1366–73.

12. Spira A, Beane J, Shah V, Liu G, Schembri F, Yang X, et al. (2004). Effects of cigarette smoke on the human airway epithelial cell transcriptome. *Proceedings of the National Academy of Sciences of the United States of America* **101**(27), 10143–8.

13. Lokke A, Lange P, Scharling H, Fabricius P, Vestbo J (2006). Developing COPD: a 25 year follow up study of the general population. *Thorax* **61**(11), 935–9.

14. Scagliotti GV, Longo M, Novello S (2009). Nonsmall cell lung cancer in never smokers. *Current Opinion in Oncology* **21**(2), 99–104.

15. Salvi SS, Barnes PJ (2009). Chronic obstructive pulmonary disease in non-smokers. *The Lancet* **374**(9691), 733–43.

16. Global Initiative for Chronic Obstructive Lung Disease (2013). *Global Strategy for the Diagnosis, Management, and Prevention of Chronic Obstructive Pulmonary Disease.*

17. Mannino DM, Watt G, Hole D, Gillis C, Hart C, McConnachie A, et al. (2006). The natural history of chronic obstructive pulmonary disease. *European Respiratory Journal* **27**(3), 627–43.

18. Evensen AE (2010). Management of COPD exacerbations. *American Family Physician* **81**(5), 607–13.

19. Mannino DM, Buist AS, Petty TL, Enright PL, Redd SC (2003). Lung function and mortality in the United States: data from the First National Health and Nutrition Examination Survey follow up study. *Thorax* **58**(5), 388–93.

20. Sin DD, Man SF (2003). Why are patients with chronic obstructive pulmonary disease at increased risk of

cardiovascular diseases? The potential role of systemic inflammation in chronic obstructive pulmonary disease. *Circulation* **107**(11), 1514–9.

21. Chen Z, Fillmore CM, Hammerman PS, Kim CF, Wong KK (2014). Non-small-cell lung cancers: a heterogeneous set of diseases. *Nature Reviews Cancer* **14**(8), 535–46.

22. Lewis DR, Check DP, Caporaso NE, Travis WD, Devesa SS (2014). US lung cancer trends by histologic type. *Cancer Sep* 15;**120**(18), 2883–92.

23. National Comprehensive Cancer Network (2015). Clinical Practice Guidelines in Oncology, V 4.2015.

24. Molina JR, Yang P, Cassivi SD, Schild SE, Adjei AA (2008). Non-small cell lung cancer: epidemiology, risk factors, treatment, and survivorship. *Mayo Clinic Proceedings* **83**(5), 584–94.

25. Cetin K, Ettinger DS, Hei YJ, O'Malley CD (2011). Survival by histologic subtype in stage IV nonsmall cell lung cancer based on data from the Surveillance, Epidemiology and End Results Program. *Clinical Epidemiology* **3**, 139–48.

26. National Lung Screening Trial Research Team, Aberle DR, Adams AM, Berg CD, Black WC, Clapp JD, *et al.* (2011). Reduced lung-cancer mortality with low-dose computed tomographic screening. *New England Journal of Medicine* **365**(5), 395–409.

27. The Centers for Medicare & Medicaid Services (CMS) (2014). *Screening for Lung Cancer with Low Dose Computed Tomography (LDCT).*

28. Young RP, Hopkins RJ, Christmas T, Black PN, Metcalf P, Gamble GD (2009). COPD prevalence is increased in lung cancer, independent of age, sex and smoking history. *European Respiratory Journal* **34**(2), 380–6.

29. Wilson DO, Weissfeld JL, Balkan A, Schragin JG, Fuhrman CR, Fisher SN, *et al.* (2008). Association of radiographic emphysema and airflow obstruction with lung Cancer. *American Journal of Respiratory and Critical Care Medicine* **178**(7), 738–44.

30. Calabro E, Randi G, La Vecchia C, Sverzellati N, Marchiano A, Villani M, *et al.* (2010). Lung function predicts lung cancer risk in smokers: a tool for targeting screening programmes. *European Respiratory Journal* **35**(1), 146–51.

31. Wasswa-Kintu S, Gan WQ, Man SF, Pare PD, Sin DD (2005). Relationship between reduced forced expiratory volume in one second and the risk of lung cancer: a systematic review and meta-analysis. *Thorax* **60**(7), 570–5.

32. Mannino DM, Aguayo SM, Petty TL, Redd SC (2003). Low lung function and incident lung cancer in the United States: data From the First National Health and Nutrition Examination Survey follow-up. *Archives of Internal Medicine* **163**(12), 1475–80.

33. de Torres JP, Bastarrika G, Wisnivesky JP, Alcaide AB, Campo A, Seijo LM, *et al.* (2007). Assessing the

relationship between lung cancer risk and emphysema detected on low-dose CT of the chest. *Chest* **132**(6), 1932–8.

34. Zulueta JJ, Wisnivesky JP, Henschke CI, Yip R, Farooqi AO, McCauley DI, *et al.* (2012). Emphysema scores predict death from COPD and lung *Cancer Chest* **141**(5), 1216–23.

35. Turner MC, Chen Y, Krewski D, Calle EE, Thun MJ (2007). Chronic obstructive pulmonary disease is associated with lung cancer mortality in a prospective study of never smokers. *American Journal of Respiratory and Critical Care Medicine* **176**(3), 285–90.

36. Punturieri A, Szabo E, Croxton TL, Shapiro SD, Dubinett SM (2009). Lung cancer and chronic obstructive pulmonary disease: needs and opportunities for integrated research. *Journal of the National Cancer Institute* **101**(8), 554–9.

37. Hanahan D, Weinberg RA (2011). Hallmarks of cancer: the next generation. *Cell* **144**(5), 646–74.

38. Vakkila J, Lotze MT (2004). Inflammation and necrosis promote tumour growth. *Nature Reviews Immunology* **4**(8), 641–8.

39. Mittal D, Gubin MM, Schreiber RD, Smyth MJ (2014). New insights into cancer immunoediting and its three component phases – elimination, equilibrium and escape. *Current Opinion in Immunology* **27**, 16–25.

40. Vermaelen K, Brusselle G (2013). Exposing a deadly alliance: novel insights into the biological links between COPD and lung Cancer. *Pulmonary Pharmacology and Therapeutics* **26**(5), 544–54.

41. Yu H, Kortylewski M, Pardoll D (2007). Crosstalk between cancer and immune cells: role of STAT3 in the tumour microenvironment. *Nature Reviews Immunology* **7**(1), 41–51.

42. Qu P, Roberts J, Li Y, Albrecht M, Cummings OW, Eble JN, *et al.* (2009). Stat3 downstream genes serve as biomarkers in human lung carcinomas and chronic obstructive pulmonary disease. *Lung Cancer* **63**(3), 341–7.

43. Di Stefano A, Caramori G, Oates T, Capelli A, Lusuardi M, Gnemmi I, *et al.* (2002). Increased expression of nuclear factor-kappaB in bronchial biopsies from smokers and patients with COPD. *European Respiratory Journal* **20**(3), 556–63.

44. Lee H, Herrmann A, Deng JH, Kujawski M, Niu G, Li Z, *et al.* (2009). Persistently activated Stat3 maintains constitutive NF-kappaB activity in tumors. *Cancer Cell* **15**(4), 283–93.

45. Sandhaus RA, Turino G (2013). Neutrophil elastase-mediated lung disease. *COPD* **10** Suppl 1, 60–3.

46. Houghton AM, Rzymkiewicz DM, Ji H, Gregory AD, Egea EE, Metz HE, *et al.* (2010). Neutrophil

elastase-mediated degradation of IRS-1 accelerates lung tumor growth. *Nature Medicine* **16**(2), 219–23.

47. Bracke K, Cataldo D, Maes T, Gueders M, Noel A, Foidart JM, *et al.* (2005). Matrix metalloproteinase-12 and cathepsin D expression in pulmonary macrophages and dendritic cells of cigarette smoke-exposed mice. *International Archives of Allergy and Immunology* **138**(2), 169–79.

48. Molet S, Belleguic C, Lena H, Germain N, Bertrand CP, Shapiro SD, *et al.* (2005). Increase in macrophage elastase (MMP-12) in lungs from patients with chronic obstructive pulmonary disease. *Inflammation Research* **54**(1), 31–6.

49. Houghton AM, Quintero PA, Perkins DL, Kobayashi DK, Kelley DG, Marconcini LA, *et al.* (2006). Elastin fragments drive disease progression in a murine model of emphysema. *The Journal of Clinical Investigation* **116**(3), 753–9.

50. Qu P, Du H, Wang X, Yan C (2009). Matrix metalloproteinase 12 overexpression in lung epithelial cells plays a key role in emphysema to lung bronchioalveolar adenocarcinoma transition. *Cancer Research* **69**(18), 7252–61.

51. Bergers G, Brekken R, McMahon G, Vu TH, Itoh T, Tamaki K, *et al.* (2000). Matrix metalloproteinase-9 triggers the angiogenic switch during carcinogenesis. *Nature Cell Biology* **2**(10), 737–44.

52. Moghaddam SJ, Li H, Cho SN, Dishop MK, Wistuba, II, Ji L, *et al.* (2009). Promotion of lung carcinogenesis by chronic obstructive pulmonary disease-like airway inflammation in a K-ras-induced mouse model. *American Journal of Respiratory Cell and Molecular Biology* **40**(4), 443–53.

53. Slaughter DP, Southwick HW, Smejkal W (1953). Field cancerization in oral stratified squamous epithelium; clinical implications of multicentric origin. *Cancer* **6**(5), 963–8.

54. Fearon ER, Vogelstein B (1990). A genetic model for colorectal tumorigenesis. *Cell* **61**(5), 759–67.

55. Spira A, Beane J, Pinto-Plata V, Kadar A, Liu G, Shah V, *et al.* (2004). Gene expression profiling of human lung tissue from smokers with severe emphysema. *American Journal of Respiratory Cell and Molecular Biology* **31**(6), 601–10.

56. Spira A, Beane JE, Shah V, Steiling K, Liu G, Schembri F, *et al.* (2007). Airway epithelial gene expression in the diagnostic evaluation of smokers with suspect lung cancer *Nature Medicine* **13**(3), 361–6.

57. Sridhar S, Schembri F, Zeskind J, Shah V, Gustafson AM, Steiling K, *et al.* (2008). Smoking-induced gene expression changes in the bronchial airway are reflected in nasal and buccal epithelium. *BMC Genomics* **9**, 259.

58. Foreman MG, Campos M, Celedon JC (2012). Genes and chronic obstructive pulmonary disease. *The Medical Clinics of North America* **96**(4), 699–711.

59. Yang P, Sun Z, Krowka MJ, Aubry MC, Bamlet WR, Wampfler JA, *et al.* (2008). Alpha1-antitrypsin deficiency carriers, tobacco smoke, chronic obstructive pulmonary disease, and lung cancer risk. *Archives of Internal Medicine* **168**(10), 1097–103.

60. Yang P, Wentzlaff KA, Katzmann JA, Marks RS, Allen MS, Lesnick TG, *et al.* (1999). Alpha1-antitrypsin deficiency allele carriers among lung cancer patients. *Cancer epidemiology, Biomarkers & Prevention* **8**(5), 461–5.

61. Yang P, Bamlet WR, Sun Z, Ebbert JO, Aubry MC, Krowka MJ, *et al.* (2005). Alpha1-antitrypsin and neutrophil elastase imbalance and lung cancer risk. *Chest* **128**(1), 445–52.

62. Sun Z, Yang P (2004). Role of imbalance between neutrophil elastase and alpha 1-antitrypsin in cancer development and progression. *The Lancet Oncology* **5**(3), 182–90.

63. Cohen BH, Diamond EL, Graves CG, Kreiss P, Levy DA, Menkes HA, *et al.* (1977). A common familial component in lung cancer and chronic obstructive pulmonary disease. *The Lancet* **2**(8037), 523–6.

64. Cote ML, Kardia SL, Wenzlaff AS, Ruckdeschel JC, Schwartz AG (2005). Risk of lung cancer among white and black relatives of individuals with early-onset lung cancer. *JAMA* **293**(24), 3036–42.

65. Schwartz AG, Ruckdeschel JC (2006). Familial lung cancer: genetic susceptibility and relationship to chronic obstructive pulmonary disease. *American Journal of Respiratory and Critical Care Medicine* **173**(1), 16–22.

66. Bailey-Wilson JE, Amos CI, Pinney SM, Petersen GM, de Andrade M, Wiest JS, *et al.* (2004). A major lung cancer susceptibility locus maps to chromosome 6q23-25. *American Journal of Human Genetics* **75**(3), 460–74.

67. Young RP, Hopkins RJ (2011). How the genetics of lung cancer may overlap with COPD. *Respirology* **16**(7), 1047–55.

68. El-Zein RA, Young RP, Hopkins RJ, Etzel CJ (2012). Genetic predisposition to chronic obstructive pulmonary disease and/or lung cancer: important considerations when evaluating risk. *Cancer Prevention Research (Philadelphia)* **5**(4), 522–7.

69. Young RP, Hopkins RJ, Whittington CF, Hay BA, Epton MJ, Gamble GD (2011). Individual and cumulative effects of GWAS susceptibility loci in lung cancer: associations after sub-phenotyping for COPD. *PloS One* **6**(2), e16476.

70. Hung RJ, McKay JD, Gaborieau V, Boffetta P, Hashibe M, Zaridze D, *et al.* (2008). A susceptibility locus for lung cancer maps to nicotinic acetylcholine receptor subunit genes on 15q25. *Nature* **452**(7187), 633–7.

71. Young RP, Hopkins RJ, Hay BA, Epton MJ, Black PN, Gamble GD (2008). Lung cancer gene associated with COPD: triple whammy or possible confounding effect? *European Respiratory Journal* **32**(5), 1158–64.

72. Thorgeirsson TE, Geller F, Sulem P, Rafnar T, Wiste A, Magnusson KP, *et al.* (2008). A variant associated with nicotine dependence, lung cancer and peripheral arterial disease. *Nature* **452**(7187), 638–42.

73. Hancock DB, Eijgelsheim M, Wilk JB, Gharib SA, Loehr LR, Marciante KD, *et al.* (2010). Meta-analyses of genome-wide association studies identify multiple loci associated with pulmonary function. *Nature Genetics* **42**(1), 45–52.

74. Young RP, Whittington CF, Hopkins RJ, Hay BA, Epton MJ, Black PN, *et al.* (2010). Chromosome 4q31 locus in COPD is also associated with lung *Cancer European Respiratory Journal* **36**(6), 1375–82.

75. Young RP, Hopkins RJ, Hay BA, Whittington CF, Epton MJ, Gamble GD (2011). FAM13A locus in COPD is independently associated with lung cancer – evidence of a molecular genetic link between COPD and lung cancer. *Application of Clinical Genetics* **4**, 1–10.

76. Watkins DN, Berman DM, Burkholder SG, Wang B, Beachy PA, Baylin SB (2003). Hedgehog signalling within airway epithelial progenitors and in small-cell lung cancer. *Nature* **422**(6929), 313–7.

77. Kandpal RP (2006). Rho GTPase activating proteins in cancer phenotypes. *Current Protein & Peptide Science* **7**(4), 355–65.

78. Belinsky SA (2015). Unmasking the lung cancer epigenome. *Annual Review of Physiology* **77**, 453–74.

79. Toyooka S, Suzuki M, Maruyama R, Toyooka KO, Tsukuda K, Fukuyama Y, *et al.* (2004). The relationship between aberrant methylation and survival in non-small-cell lung cancers. *British Journal of Cancer* **91**(4), 771–4.

80. Belinsky SA, Klinge DM, Dekker JD, Smith MW, Bocklage TJ, Gilliland FD, *et al.* (2005). Gene promoter methylation in plasma and sputum increases with lung cancer risk. *Clinical Cancer Research* **11**(18), 6505–11.

81. Suzuki M, Wada H, Yoshino M, Tian L, Shigematsu H, Suzuki H, *et al.* (2010). Molecular characterization of chronic obstructive pulmonary disease-related non-small cell lung cancer through aberrant methylation and alterations of EGFR signaling. *Annals of Surgical Oncology* **17**(3), 878–88.

82. Kabesch M, Adcock IM (2012). Epigenetics in asthma and COPD. *Biochimie* **94**(11), 2231–41.

83. Grosshans H, Filipowicz W (2008). Molecular biology: the expanding world of small RNAs. *Nature* **451**(7177), 414–6.

84. Izzotti A, Larghero P, Balansky R, Pfeffer U, Steele VE, De Flora S (2011). Interplay between histopathological alterations, cigarette smoke and chemopreventive agents in defining microRNA profiles in mouse lung. *Mutation Research* **717**(1–2), 17–24.

85. Schembri F, Sridhar S, Perdomo C, Gustafson AM, Zhang X, Ergun A, *et al.* (2009). MicroRNAs as modulators of smoking-induced gene expression changes in human airway epithelium. *Proceedings of the National Academy of Sciences of the United States of America* **106**(7), 2319–24.

86. Molina-Pinelo S, Pastor MD, Suarez R, Romero-Romero B, Gonzalez De la Pena M, Salinas A, *et al.* (2014). MicroRNA clusters: dysregulation in lung adenocarcinoma and COPD. *European Respiratory Journal* **43**(6), 1740–9.

87. Ezzie ME, Crawford M, Cho JH, Orellana R, Zhang S, Gelinas R, *et al.* (2012). Gene expression networks in COPD: microRNA and mRNA regulation. *Thorax* **67**(2), 122–31.

88. Takamizawa J, Konishi H, Yanagisawa K, Tomida S, Osada H, Endoh H, *et al.* (2004). Reduced expression of the let-7 microRNAs in human lung cancers in association with shortened postoperative survival. *Cancer Research* **64**(11), 3753–6.

89. Trang P, Medina PP, Wiggins JF, Ruffino L, Kelnar K, Omotola M, *et al.* (2010). Regression of murine lung tumors by the let-7 microRNA. *Oncogene*. **29**(11), 1580–7.

90. Van Pottelberge GR, Mestdagh P, Bracke KR, Thas O, van Durme YM, Joos GF, *et al.* (2011). MicroRNA expression in induced sputum of smokers and patients with chronic obstructive pulmonary disease. *American Journal of Respiratory and Critical Care Medicine* **183**(7), 898–906.

91. Pinkerton M, Chinchilli V, Banta E, Craig T, August A, Bascom R, *et al.* (2013). Differential expression of microRNAs in exhaled breath condensates of patients with asthma, patients with chronic obstructive pulmonary disease, and healthy adults. *Journal of Allergy and Clinical Immunology* **132**(1), 217–9.

CHAPTER 16

Prostate Cancer

Jacob Kagan,[1] Ian M Thompson,[2] and Daniel W Chan[3,4]

[1] Division of Cancer Prevention, National Cancer Institute, Bethesda, MD, USA

[2] CHRISTUS Santa Rosa Medical Center, San Antonio, TX, USA

[3] Department of Pathology, Johns Hopkins University School of Medicine, Baltimore, MD, USA

[4] Center for Biomarker Discovery and Translation, Johns Hopkins Medical Institutions, Baltimore, MD, USA

Introduction

Prostate cancer (PCa) is the most frequently diagnosed cancer and the second leading cause of death due to cancer among American men. In 2014 it was estimated that 233 000 US men were diagnosed with prostate cancer, and approximately 29 480 died from this disease [1]. The prevalence and death due to prostate cancer among African-American men is the highest in the world. African-Americans have a 1.6-fold increased chance of being diagnosed with prostate cancer and a 2.5-fold greater chance of dying from it, compared with Caucasian or Hispanic/Latino American men [2, 3]. On the other hand, the prevalence of prostate cancer among Asian men is 50% lower than among Caucasian men [3, 4]. About 60% of all prostate cancers are detected in men at age 66 or older, and 97% occurs in men at 50 or older; diagnosis before age 40 is rare [2, 3].

Prostate cancer is a heterogeneous and frequently multifocal cancer, and its development is primarily driven by androgen receptor (AR) signaling [5, 6]. Large prostate tumors are frequently the result of mergers of multiple smaller tumors [7]. Distinct tumor foci may display striking differences in grade, molecular markers, and DNA ploidy [8]. The most important pathologic prognostic marker for prostate cancer on biopsy is Gleason grade [9].

Biomarker-based screening, detection, diagnosis, prognosis, as well as prostate cancer management, were revolutionized with the introduction of prostate specific antigen (PSA) (also known as human kallikrein 3, KLK3) as a serum biomarker [10–12]. Since the introduction of PSA screening in the early 1990s, the number of incident cases has doubled, and the mortality rate has declined by 44% [13,14]. Interestingly, more than half of the detected cancers by PSA screening are organ-confined, are non-aggressive, and are unlikely to progress to life-threatening aggressive cancer [15–19].

The lifetime risk of developing prostate cancer among American men is approximately 1 in 6, and the mortality risk is 1 in 35 [20]. These observations suggest that PSA screening will lead to the discovery of a large number of low-grade, low-stage indolent prostate cancers, which are unlikely to progress to the level of invasive or metastatic disease. Such an "insignificant tumor" is frequently defined as a prostate organ-confined tumor with a volume of <0.5 cm^3 and a Gleason score of 6 or less (no pattern 4 or 5) at prostatectomy [21]. Criteria for an insignificant tumor on prostate biopsy were proposed by Epstein, and include the following criteria: (1) stage T1c, (2) PSA density <0.15 ng/ml/gm, (3) Gleason score = 6 (with no pattern 4 or 5), and (4) tumor detected in fewer than three cores, with no core having more than 50% of tumor involvement [22,23].

However, these criteria are not validated and are imperfect, as about 30% of patients meeting

Biomarkers in Cancer Screening and Early Detection, First Edition. Edited by Sudhir Srivastava.
© 2017 John Wiley & Sons, Inc. Published 2017 by John Wiley & Sons, Inc.

these criteria are ultimately proved to have unfavorable pathologic findings at radical prostatectomy [17, 18, 24]. The development of an accurate tool for determining the presence of an insignificant tumor could help clinicians better manage patients with these common findings, potentially managing patients with active surveillance, and avoiding the potentially-morbid side effects of surgery or radiation [25–28]. Equally important will be the development and validation of biomarkers that will identify high-risk tumors, in which treatment may reduce mortality from the disease.

While the classification of hematopoietic malignances is well established, and is primarily based on specific genetic alterations, such as chromosomal rearrangements (e.g., bcr-abl rearrangement is the hallmark of chronic myeloid leukemia [CML]). Similar rearrangement were reported only in very small proportions of epithelial cancers. Recent advances in bioinformatics, molecular genetics, and DNA and RNA sequencing technologies, has led to the discovery of new genetic rearrangements, especially in prostate cancer [29–32]. Approximately 50% of all prostate cancers harbor genetic rearrangements which generate fusion transcripts, especially with member of the ETS (Avian erythroblastosis virus E26 homolog family members) oncogenes. ETS genetic rearrangements frequently place ETS oncogenic transcription factors under the control of androgen regulated promoters (Figure 16.1) [32].

Other recurrent genetic alterations involve androgen receptor (AR) gene amplifications [33, 34] or mutations [35], which are primarily detected in castration resistant metastatic tumors, or the loss of phosphatase and tensin homolog (PTEN)/mutated in multiple advanced cancer (MMAC1), which is tightly linked to aberrant activation of phosphatidylinositide 3-kinase [PI3K] pathway [36–39]. Additional alterations in gene copy number and point mutations were recently detected through extensive sequencing efforts of prostate cancers, including castration-resistant prostate cancers [40–43]. These studies identified frequent mutation in SPOP (≈13%), which were mutually exclusive from ETS gene fusions and were highly correlated with CHD1 allelic losses, and mutations in FOXA1 (≈4%); MED12 (≈5%) and MAGI-2 (≈5%). Mutations in AURKA were detected in 40% of neuroendocrine prostate cancers [44]. Although promising, the diagnostic and or prognostic value of these potential markers must be further studied and validated. The following review will focus on current Food and Drug Administration (FDA) approved and Laboratory Developed Tests (LDT) (CLIA regulated) for prostate cancer.

US Food and Drug Administration (FDA) approved/cleared clinical diagnostic tests

The US FDA is responsible for protecting the public health by assuring the safety, efficacy and security of human and veterinary drugs, biological products, medical devices, the USA food

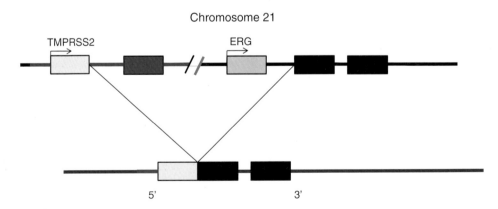

Figure 16.1 Example of a genomic rearrangement on chromosome 21 that juxtaposed an androgen responsive promoter and a noncoding exon of the TMPRSS2 gene to an ETS gene family member, ERG. The rearrangement caused the aberrant expression of the ERG proto-oncogene. For a color version of this figure please see color plate section.

supply, cosmetics, and products that emit radiation. Among others, the FDA regulates diagnostic and prognostic tests, including tests based on cancer biomarkers. The importance of FDA-approved/cleared tests is that they guarantee that both the analytical and clinical performance of the test have been critically evaluated and approved for a specific intended use. The requirements for analytical performance of biomarker tests include precision, trueness, specificity, interference, and carryover. The requirements for appropriate clinical performance include diagnostic accuracy, area under the curve (AUC) by receiver-operating characteristic (ROC) analysis, and positive and negative predictive values (PPV and NPV, respectively). An FDA approved test, which is always limited to a specific intended use, sets a standard for what is a clinically acceptable test, and is more likely to be reimbursed by the insurance companies [45].

[-2]proPSA and the *Phi* index

To improve the clinical utility of PSA for early detection and risk assessment, investigators developed different approaches including detection of molecular forms of PSA, PSA density, PSA velocity, age-adjusted PSA range, multi-parametric analysis using artificial neural networks, and a variety of other models [46–48]. Interestingly, men diagnosed with prostate cancer had a lower percentage of free PSA and a higher percentage of protease inhibitors, alpha 1-antichymotrypsin bound PSA [49, 50]. These differences were the basis of development of commercial assays for free PSA (fPSA) and complex PSA [51, 52].

Despite the fact that free PSA improves on total PSA in detection of cancer in the range of 4–10 ng/mL of total PSA, its utility is limited by the fact that it consists of several isoforms that are produced either by the prostate cancer or by regions of the prostate gland with benign prostatic hyperplasia [53]. The proenzyme PSA (proPSA) is a form of a fPSA that is highly associated with prostate cancer and is primarily detected in the peripheral zone of the prostate and in blood [53, 54]. It contains a seven-amino acid leader peptide, and is enzymatically inactive. Conversion of proPSA to enzymatically active PSA occurs through cleavage of the leader peptide by enzymes, such as human kallikrein 2 and trypsin. proPSA forms, with

varying lengths of leader peptides, are detected in blood, including [-2]proPSA, which is a stable form resistant to enzymatic cleavage and activation to mature PSA [53, 55].

An automated blood based assay for [-2]proPSA has been developed by Beckman-Coulter, Inc., and has received the Food and Drug Administration (FDA), as well as the European Union regulatory approvals. The Beckman-Coulter, Inc., Prostate Health index, *Phi*, is indicated for use in men with elevated PSA in the range of 4–10 ng/mL, which usually triggers a biopsy test for cancer. The *Phi* test is a mathematical combination of total PSA, fPSA and [-2]proPSA according to the formula [-2]proPSA/fPSA$\times\sqrt{tPSA}$.

Recent studies indicate that the *Phi* test may be useful in prostate cancer detection, to decrease unnecessary biopsy in men 50 years old or older with a PSA range between 2–10 ng/ml and negative digital rectal examination (DRE) [56, 57]. Also recently, the National Cancer Institute (NCI) Early Detection Research Network (EDRN) validated the utility of %[-2]proPSA in two blinded multicenter studies (retrospective and prospective) [58,59].

%[-2]proPSA showed potential utility in the range of 2–10 ng/mL of total PSA, and a multivariate model showed a significant improvement (AUC, 0.76) over individual PSA forms ($P < 0.01$ to <0.0001). At 80% sensitivity, the specificity of %[-2]proPSA (44.9%; 95% CI, 38.4–51.5%) was significantly higher than PSA (30.8%; 95% CI, 24.9–37.1%) and relatively higher than %fPSA (34.6%; 95% CI, 28.5–41.4%). %[-2]proPSA increased with increasing Gleason score ($P < 0.001$). and was higher in aggressive cancers ($P = 0.03$) [59].

A meta-analysis, based on recent publications, determined that the sensitivity for the detection of prostate cancer was 90% for %[-2]proPSA and *Phi*, while the pooled specificity was 32.5% (95% CI 30.6–34.5) and 31.6% (95% CI 29.2–34.0) for %[-2]proPSA and *Phi*, respectively. The measurement of %[-2]proPSA improves the accuracy of prostate cancer detection, in comparison with PSA or %fPSA [57].

The observations that higher [-2]proPSA and %[-2]proPSA values were highly associated with significant disease (based on Epstein criteria [60] as well as recent reports [61,62]), demonstrated that

%[-2]proPSA and [-2]proPSA/%fPSA could distinguish between Gleason sum <7 and =7 cancers, and also between organ confined and non-organ confined disease. This suggests that these assays may improve the detection of aggressive prostate cancers.

Prostate Cancer Antigen 3 (PCA3)

Prostate cancer antigen 3 (PCA3) (also known as differential display code 3 [DD3]) is a prostate-specific gene that has been detected in over 90% of prostate cancers (PCa) [63, 64]. PCA3, a non-coding gene, is significantly overexpressed in cancer tissues versus benign tissues. Clinically, PCA3 mRNA is detectable in the urine and prostatic fluid of men with PCa [64, 65]. PCA3 mRNA expression was found to be independent of prostate volume and serum PSA, but was higher in patients who had larger, more aggressive tumors.

Hologic/GenProbe Co. developed a urine assay, Progensa, which obtained FDA approval in 2012. The intended use is for diagnosis of men who are suspected to have prostate cancer, based on rising PSA and/or digital rectal exam (DRE), and have one or more negative biopsies. In this clinical application, the PCA3 test may reduce the number of unnecessary repeat biopsies. The assay measures the relative abundance of PCA3 and PSA mRNA expression using qRT-PCR amplification (PCA3 score) in post-DRE urine. A score of = 25 is associated with decreased probability of having prostate cancer [66–68]. It is important to note that lowering the PCA3 score cut-off to 10 from 35 reduced the number of false-positives by 35.4%, while false-negatives increased by only 5.6% [66]

Ploussard et al. [69] published a repeat analysis of a previously published multi-center study [70], which compared the performance characteristics of PCA3 with that of free/total PSA ratio (low free/total PSA ratio is associated with an increased specificity for prostate cancer detection) in a cohort of more than 300 men, who had a previous negative biopsy and total serum PSA levels between 2.5–10.0 ng/ml (the PSA diagnostic "gray zone" for detection of aggressive cancer). PCA3 score had a superior specificity and predictive values, but inferior sensitivity, compared with PSA. Interestingly, PCA3 score did not correlate with prostate volume or Gleason score but, on the other hand, the free/total PSA ratio correlated with prostate volume, age and stage.

An extensive review of 11 PCA3 clinical studies, six of which were multi-center studies, with 2737 men was published by Vlaeminick-Guillem et al. [67]. The AUC values ranged from 0.66–0.75; sensitivity ranged between 53–69%, with specificity ranging between 71–83%. For patients who had a previous negative biopsy- the average sensitivity was 52.6% and the average specificity was 71.6%; the resulting average PPV was ≈40%, and NPV was 80%.

Overall, the PCA3 urine-based assay improves prostate cancer diagnosis, especially in identifying patients who may benefit from a repeat biopsy. However, it does not improve the detection of aggressive cancers. Further expected improvements will include the development of a panel or panels of cancer specific biomarkers (for more specific diagnostic and prognostic tests), based on recent discoveries of recurrent cancer fusion transcripts (TMPRSS2-ERG, TMPRSS2-ETV1) [30, 71–74]; recurrent mutations (SPOP, FOXA1, MED12) [41]; differentially expressing coding and noncoding genes (SPINK1, AGR2, SChLAP1); and tissue based markers such as PSA isoforms.

Clinical Laboratory Improvement Amendments (CLIA) and Laboratory Developed Test (LDT)

The Centers for Medicare & Medicaid Services (CMS) regulates all laboratory testing (except research) performed on humans in the USA, through the Clinical Laboratory Improvement Amendments (CLIA). The objective of the CLIA program is to ensure quality laboratory testing, especially for Laboratory Developed Tests (LDTs) that are not approved by FDA. The FDA defines a Laboratory Developed Test as an *in vitro* diagnostic test that is manufactured by, and used within, a *single* laboratory (i.e. a laboratory with a single CLIA certificate) (LDTs are also sometimes called in-house developed tests, or "home brew" tests).

Although a CLIA test must meet certain analytical performance criteria, these requirements are not as rigorous as those required for an FDA approved test/assay. The major disadvantage might stem from the fact that there might be greater variability in performance of such an assay between different CLIA laboratories. The analytical validation is limited, however, to the specific conditions, staff, equipment and patient population of the particular laboratory, so the findings of these laboratory-specific analytical validation are not meaningful outside of the laboratory that did the analysis. Furthermore, the laboratory's analytical validation of LDTs is reviewed during its routine biennial survey – after the laboratory has already started testing. While some of the LDTs have gone through extensive validation, for others there may be limited published data.

For a more detailed discussion of the issues related to CLIA vs FDA approved clinical diagnostics for prostate cancer, readers are encouraged to read a recent review by Sartori and Chan [75].

TMPRSS2-ERG

Prostate cancer research was revolutionized by the discovery of frequent recurrent genetic rearrangements that result in the generation of fusion transcripts, such as TMPRSS2-ERG [29]. Further investigation revealed that this rearrangement was one of many prostate cancer genetic rearrangements that produced gene fusions that juxtaposed the promoter region of androgen-regulated genes – most frequently the TMPRSS2 (transmembrane protease inhibitor 2) – with transcription factors of the ETS (erythroblastosis virus E26 transforming sequence) family of oncogenic transcription factors [29, 30, 32, 76, 77]. Genetic rearrangements occur in ≈50% of all prostate cancers, with TMPRSS2-ERG rearrangement being by far the most frequent (>90% of all rearrangements) [32, 76, 77].

ERG is not expressed in normal prostatic tissue, and is detected only in high-grade prostatic intraepithelial neoplasia (HGPIN) and prostate tumors [78, 79]. As a biomarker, TMPRSS2-ERG fusion has a low sensitivity (37%), but high specificity (93%) and a PPV of 94%. Despite the high specificity, it is important to note that most prostate cancer patients have multiple foci which contribute to tumor heterogeneity. This diagnostic problem can be dealt with by including additional biomarkers as a panel for detection and diagnosis [80–82].

The association of tumor aggressiveness and the expression of TMPRSS2-ERG fusion transcripts, or the detection of truncated ERG proteins, have been assessed in several studies. Leyten et al., examined 1180 prostatectomy specimens, finding TMPRSSE-ERG expression in 49%. There was a significant correlation between TMPRSS2-ERG expression and high stage tumor ($P < 0.01$). However, there were insignificant correlations with Gleason score ($P = 0.58$), lethality ($P = 0.99$), and biochemical reoccurrence ($P = 0.60$) [82].

Despite extensive efforts by many laboratories to identify the prognostic value of ERG in prostate cancer carcinogenesis, its clinical significance remains controversial [78, 83]. Minner et al., analyzed ERG alterations by immunohistochemistry and FISH, using tissue microarray containing samples from more than 2800 prostate cancers with clinical outcomes. ERG expression did not correlate with clinical outcome and the tumor phenotype in early cancers that had not been hormonally treated. Additional markers tested included AMACR, Annexin A3, Bcl2, CD10, ALCAM, chromogranin A, epidermal growth factor receptor (EGFR), HER2, mTOR, p53, and synaptophysin status and there were significant differences found in their expression in a very small number of cases. The most striking difference was found for AR expression, which was markedly higher in ERG-positive cancers.

In vitro studies showed ERG-dependent impairment of AR-mediated transcriptional activity. The marked difference in AR levels between ERG-positive and -negative cancers supports a systematic difference in potential response to hormonal therapy, as previously observed in clinical trials [84]

Recently, an EDRN laboratory at the University of Michigan Health System developed the Mi-Prostate Score (MiPS), which is based on urine tests for PCA3 from Progensa, TMPRSS2-ERG, and serum PSA levels, to produce a risk assessment score for prostate cancer aggressiveness. MiPS was validated on approximately 2000 urine specimens, and is available as a CLIA test [80, 82, 85].

Oncotype Dx

The Oncotype DX Prostate Cancer Assay is based on differential expression of multiple cancer-related genes in prostate cancer. The assay was developed to assess risk for cancer progression, using formalin-fixed, paraffin-embedded (FFPE) biopsy specimens. As little as 20 ng mRNA can be used. The assay measures expression of 12 cancer-related genes, including genes associated with the androgen pathway (AZGP1, KLK2, SRD5A2, and FAM13C); cellular organization (FLNC, GSN, TPM2 and GSTM2); proliferation (TPX2); and reactive stroma gene response (BGN, COL1A1 and SFRP4). Five reference genes include ARF, ATP5E, CLTC, GPS1, and PGK1. These reference genes were selected because of their low inter-patient variability, independence of clinical outcome, and their robust analytical performance. In addition, the reference genes are used for normalization, and to control sources of variability such as fixation, RNA fragmentation, tissue quality, reagents quality, instrumentation, including pipetting of liquids, and input of RNA. An algorithm based on reference genes and normalized expression of the 12 cancer-related genes is used to calculate the Genomic Prostate Score(GPS) [86]. The Oncotype DX assay was recently validated in a study on 413 men [87].

Prolaris Score

Prolaris Score is a LDT offered by Myriad Genetics, Inc. The intended use is identification of patients who are likely to progress to aggressive disease among patients with organ-confined disease. The test is based on gene expression of a panel of 46 different genes, including 31 cell cycle progression (CCP) genes and 15 housekeeping genes. The signature was developed and tested using two independent retrospective cohorts – the first based on 366 US men who had undergone radical prostatectomy, and the second based on 337 UK men with clinically localized prostate cancer, diagnosed by a transurethral resection (TURP) [88]. Additional studies confirmed that the level of gene expression correlates with tumor aggressiveness, and suggested that the CCP score could serve as a prognostic marker [87,89–92].

Prostarix

Metabolon, Inc. recently announced a new LDT, Prostarix, which is offered through Bostwick CLIA laboratories. The intended use is to assist clinicians in identifying patients who need a biopsy or repeat biopsy, and had a moderate level of PSA and negative DRE. The test is performed on patient's urine sediment, and is based on a proprietary metabolomics signature, including sarcosine (also known as N-methylglycine), which was previously reported by the University of Michigan EDRN laboratory and Metabolon as differentially expressed in aggressive and metastatic prostate cancer [93].

In a recent study by the Metabolon group, McDunn et al., analyzed prostatectomy specimens from 331 prostate tumor and 178 cancer-free prostate tissues. Gas chromatography-mass spectrometry and ultrahigh performance liquid chromatography-tandem mass spectrometry (LC/MS-MS) were used to identify significantly altered metabolite profiles between cancer and cancer-free prostate tissues. Aggressive disease was associated with high abundance of some metabolites, while normal prostatic tissue highly expressed citrate and polyamines. The addition of certain metabolites to a multiparametric nomogram improved prediction of organ confined tumors (AUC from 0.53 to 0.62) and five-year recurrence (AUC from 0.53 to 0.64) [94]. Despite these promising early results, further independent validation is necessary.

4K Score

4K Score is a LDT offered by OPKO, Inc., and is based on the quantitative detection of a panel of four Kallikreins in the blood. Kallikreins are serine proteases – enzymes that cleave peptide bonds in proteins, and they participate in a number of physiological functions, including blood pressure and semen liquefaction. The 4K panel includes the following: Kallikreins; total PSA; free PSA; intact PSA; and Kallikrein-related peptide 2 (hK2) [95–99]. OPKO developed an algorithm that combines the blood test results with clinical data (age, positive or negative DRE, and data on prior negative biopsy) to a score which is used to estimate the probability of finding a high-grade, Gleason score = 7 prostate cancer on biopsy.

A recent study suggested that the 4K Score could be used to distinguish between insignificant and aggressive prostate tumors and reduce unnecessary biopsies. Interestingly, Vickers et al., reported that a 20% risk of prostate cancer as a threshold for biopsy would have reduced the number of biopsies by 57%, while missing 20% of the low-grade and 7.5% of the high-grade cancers [95]. The AUC for 4K Score improved the AUC from 0.68 for total PSA to 0.83 with the 4K Score for the prediction of PCa at biopsy [99].

Except for hK2, the 4K score is very similar to the Beckman-Coulter Prostate Health Index, *Phi*, which was approved by the FDA and was discussed at length earlier in this chapter [56, 57, 95, 97, 99].

References

1. Siegel R, Naishadham D, Jemal A (2013). Cancer statistics, 2013. *CA: A Cancer Journal for Clinicians* **63**, 11–30.

2. Kamangar F, Dores GM, Anderson WF (2006). Patterns of cancer incidence, mortality, and prevalence across five continents: defining priorities to reduce cancer disparities in different geographic regions of the world. *Journal of Clinical Oncology* **24**, 2137–2150.

3. Martin DN, Starks AM, Ambs S (2013). Biological determinants of health disparities in prostate cancer. *Current Opinion in Oncology* **25**, 235–241.

4. Clegg LX, Li FP, Hankey BF, Chu K, Edwards BK (2002). Cancer survival among US whites and minorities: a SEER (Surveillance, Epidemiology, and End Results) Program population-based study. *Archives of Internal Medicine* **162**, 1985–1993.

5. Tomlins SA, Rubin MA, Chinnaiyan AM (2006). Integrative biology of prostate cancer progression. *Annual Review of Pathology* **1**, 243–271.

6. Tamburrino L, Salvianti F, Marchiani S, *et al.* (2012). Androgen receptor (AR) expression in prostate cancer and progression of the tumor: Lessons from cell lines, animal models and human specimens. *Steroids* **77**, 996–1001.

7. Miller GJ, Cygan JM (1994). Morphology of prostate cancer: the effects of multifocality on histological grade, tumor volume and capsule penetration. *Journal of Urology* **152**, 1709–1713.

8. Karavitakis M, Ahmed HU, Abel PD, Hazell S, Winkler MH (2011). Tumor focality in prostate cancer: implications for focal therapy. *Nature Reviews Clinical Oncology* **8**, 48–55.

9. Epstein JI, Allsbrook WC, Jr., Amin MB, Egevad LL (2005). The 2005 International Society of Urological Pathology (ISUP) Consensus Conference on Gleason Grading of Prostatic Carcinoma. *American Journal of Surgical Pathology* **29**, 1228–1242.

10. Stamey TA, Yang N, Hay AR, McNeal JE, Freiha FS, Redwine E (1987). Prostate-specific antigen as a serum marker for adenocarcinoma of the prostate. *New England Journal of Medicine* **317**, 909–916.

11. Catalona WJ, Smith DS, Ratliff TL, *et al.* (1991). Measurement of prostate-specific antigen in serum as a screening test for prostate cancer. *New England Journal of Medicine* **324**, 1156–1161.

12. Chan DW, Bruzek DJ, Oesterling JE, Rock RC, Walsh PC (1987). Prostate-specific antigen as a marker for prostatic cancer: a monoclonal and a polyclonal immunoassay compared. *Clinical Chemistry* **33**, 1916–1920.

13. Siegel R, Naishadham D, Jemal A (2012). Cancer statistics, 2012. *CA: A Cancer Journal for Clinicians* **62**, 10–29.

14. Etzioni R, Gulati R, Cooperberg MR, Penson DM, Weiss NS, Thompson IM (2013). Limitations of basing screening policies on screening trials: The US Preventive Services Task Force and Prostate Cancer Screening. *Medical Care* **51**, 295–300.

15. Draisma G, Etzioni R, Tsodikov A, *et al.* (2009). Lead time and overdiagnosis in prostate-specific antigen screening: importance of methods and context. *Journal of the National Cancer Institute* **101**, 374–383.

16. Welch HG, Black WC (2010). Overdiagnosis in cancer. *Journal of the National Cancer Institute* **102**, 605–613.

17. Drazer MW, Huo D, Schonberg MA, Razmaria A, Eggener SE (2011). Population-based patterns and predictors of prostate-specific antigen screening among older men in the United States. *Journal of Clinical Oncology* **29**, 1736–1743.

18. Etzioni R, Penson DF, Legler JM, *et al.* (2002). Overdiagnosis due to prostate-specific antigen screening: lessons from U.S. prostate cancer incidence trends. *Journal of the National Cancer Institute* **94**, 981–990.

19. McGregor M, Hanley JA, Boivin JF, McLean RG (1998). Screening for prostate cancer: estimating the magnitude of overdetection. *Canadian Medical Association Journal* **159**, 1368–1372.

20. Wolf AM, Wender RC, Etzioni RB, *et al.* (2010). American Cancer Society guideline for the early detection of prostate cancer: update 2010. *CA: A Cancer Journal for Clinicians* **60**, 70–98.

21. Noguchi M, Stamey TA, McNeal JE, Yemoto CM (2001). Relationship between systematic biopsies and histological features of 222 radical prostatectomy specimens: lack of prediction of tumor significance for men with nonpalpable prostate cancer. *Journal of Urology* **166**, 104–109; discussion 109–110.

22. Epstein JI, Sanderson H, Carter HB, Scharfstein DO (2005). Utility of saturation biopsy to predict insignificant cancer at radical prostatectomy. *Urology* **66**, 356–360.

23. Ploussard G, Epstein JI, Montironi R, *et al.* (2011). The contemporary concept of significant versus insignificant prostate cancer. *European Urology* **60**, 291–303.

24. Kassouf W, Nakanishi H, Ochiai A, Babaian KN, Troncoso P, Babaian RJ (2007). Effect of prostate volume on tumor grade in patients undergoing radical prostatectomy in the era of extended prostatic biopsies. *Journal of Urology* **178**, 111–114.

25. Thompson IM, Klotz L (2010). Active surveillance for prostate cancer. *JAMA* **304**, 2411–2412.

26. Ochiai A, Troncoso P, Chen ME, Lloreta J, Babaian RJ (2005). The relationship between tumor volume and the number of positive cores in men undergoing multisite extended biopsy: implication for expectant management. *Journal of Urology* **174**, 2164–2168, discussion 2168.

27. Ganz PA, Barry JM, Burke W, *et al.* (2012). National Institutes of Health State-of-the-Science Conference: role of active surveillance in the management of men with localized prostate cancer. *Annals of Internal Medicine* **156**, 591–595.

28. Lucia MS, Darke AK, Goodman PJ, *et al.* (2008). Pathologic characteristics of cancers detected in The Prostate Cancer Prevention Trial: implications for prostate cancer detection and chemoprevention. *Cancer Prevention Research (Philadelphia)* **1**, 167–173.

29. Tomlins SA, Rhodes DR, Perner S, *et al.* (2005). Recurrent fusion of TMPRSS2 and ETS transcription factor genes in prostate cancer. *Science* **310**, 644–648.

30. Tomlins SA, Laxman B, Dhanasekaran SM, *et al.* (2007). Distinct classes of chromosomal rearrangements create oncogenic ETS gene fusions in prostate cancer. *Nature* **448**, 595–599.

31. Helgeson BE, Tomlins SA, Shah N, *et al.* (2008). Characterization of TMPRSS2:ETV5 and SLC45A3:ETV5 gene fusions in prostate cancer. *Cancer Research* **68**, 73–80.

32. Kumar-Sinha C, Tomlins SA, Chinnaiyan AM (2008). Recurrent gene fusions in prostate cancer. *Nature Reviews Cancer* **8**, 497–511.

33. Visakorpi T, Hyytinen E, Koivisto P, *et al.* (1995). *In vivo* amplification of the androgen receptor gene and progression of human prostate cancer. *Nature Genetics* **9**, 401–406.

34. Linja MJ, Savinainen KJ, Saramaki OR, Tammela TL, Vessella RL, Visakorpi T (2001). Amplification and overexpression of androgen receptor gene in hormone-refractory prostate cancer. *Cancer Research* **61**, 3550–3555.

35. Taplin ME, Bubley GJ, Shuster TD, *et al.* (1995). Mutation of the androgen-receptor gene in metastatic androgen-independent prostate cancer. *New England Journal of Medicine* **332**, 1393–1398.

36. Li J, Yen C, Liaw D, *et al.* (1997). PTEN, a putative protein tyrosine phosphatase gene mutated in human brain, breast, and prostate cancer. *Science* **275**, 1943–1947.

37. Steck PA, Pershouse MA, Jasser SA, *et al.* (1997). Identification of a candidate tumour suppressor gene, MMAC1, at chromosome 10q23.3 that is mutated in multiple advanced cancers. *Nature Genetics* **15**, 356–362.

38. Cairns P, Okami K, Halachmi S, *et al.* (1997). Frequent inactivation of PTEN/MMAC1 in primary prostate cancer. *Cancer Research* **57**, 4997–5000.

39. Carver BS, Tran J, Gopalan A, *et al.* (2009). Aberrant ERG expression cooperates with loss of PTEN to promote cancer progression in the prostate. *Nature Genetics* **41**, 619–624.

40. Grasso CS, Wu YM, Robinson DR, *et al.* (2012). The mutational landscape of lethal castration-resistant prostate cancer. *Nature* **487**, 239–243.

41. Barbieri CE, Baca SC, Lawrence MS, *et al.* (2012). Exome sequencing identifies recurrent SPOP, FOXA1 and MED12 mutations in prostate cancer. *Nature Genetics* **44**, 685–689.

42. Barbieri CE, Demichelis F, Rubin MA (2012). Molecular genetics of prostate cancer: emerging appreciation of genetic complexity. *Histopathology* **60**, 187–198.

43. Berger MF, Lawrence MS, Demichelis F, *et al.* (2011). The genomic complexity of primary human prostate cancer. *Nature* **470**, 214–220.

44. Beltran H, Rickman DS, Park K, *et al.* (2011). Molecular characterization of neuroendocrine prostate cancer and identification of new drug targets. *Cancer Discovery* **1**, 487–495.

45. Fuzery AK, Levin J, Chan MM, Chan DW (2013). Translation of proteomic biomarkers into FDA approved cancer diagnostics: issues and challenges. *Clinical Proteomics* **10**, 13.

46. Makarov DV, Loeb S, Getzenberg RH, Partin AW (2009). Biomarkers for prostate cancer. *Annual Review of Medicine* **60**, 139–151.

47. Thompson IM, Ankerst DP (2007). Prostate-specific antigen in the early detection of prostate cancer. *Canadian Medical Association Journal* **176**, 1853–1858.

48. Stephan C, Cammann H, Meyer HA, Lein M, Jung K (2007). PSA and new biomarkers within multivariate models to improve early detection of prostate cancer. *Cancer Letters* **249**, 18–29.

49. Lilja H, Christensson A, Dahlen U, *et al.* (1991). Prostate-specific antigen in serum occurs predominantly in complex with alpha 1-antichymotrypsin. *Clinical Chemistry* **37**, 1618–1625.

50. Stenman UH, Leinonen J, Alfthan H, Rannikko S, Tuhkanen K, Alfthan O (1991). A complex between prostate-specific antigen and alpha 1-antichymotrypsin is the major form of prostate-specific antigen in serum of patients with prostatic cancer: assay of the complex improves clinical sensitivity for cancer. *Cancer Research* **51**, 222–226.

51. Catalona WJ, Partin AW, Slawin KM, *et al.* (1998). Use of the percentage of free prostate-specific antigen to enhance differentiation of prostate cancer from benign prostatic disease: a prospective multicenter clinical trial. *JAMA* **279**, 1542–1547.

52. Partin AW, Brawer MK, Bartsch G, *et al.* (2003). Complexed prostate specific antigen improves specificity for

prostate cancer detection: results of a prospective multi-center clinical trial. *Journal of Urology* **170**, 1787–1791.

53. Mikolajczyk SD, Marker KM, Millar LS, *et al.* (2001). A truncated precursor form of prostate-specific antigen is a more specific serum marker of prostate cancer. *Cancer Research* **61**, 6958–6963.

54. Mikolajczyk SD, Millar LS, Marker KM, *et al.* (2000). Seminal plasma contains "BPSA," a molecular form of prostate-specific antigen that is associated with benign prostatic hyperplasia. *Prostate* **45**, 271–276.

55. Mikolajczyk SD, Marks LS, Partin AW, Rittenhouse HG (2002). Free prostate-specific antigen in serum is becoming more complex. *Urology* **59**, 797–802.

56. Catalona WJ, Partin AW, Sanda MG, *et al.* (2011). A multicenter study of [-2]pro-prostate specific antigen combined with prostate specific antigen and free prostate specific antigen for prostate cancer detection in the 2.0 to 10.0 ng/ml prostate specific antigen range. *Journal of Urology* **185**, 1650–1655.

57. Filella X, Gimenez N (2013). Evaluation of [-2] proPSA and Prostate Health Index (phi) for the detection of prostate cancer: a systematic review and meta-analysis. *Clinical Chemistry and Laboratory Medicine* **51**, 729–739.

58. Sokoll LJ, Wang Y, Feng Z, *et al.* (2008). [-2]proenzyme prostate specific antigen for prostate cancer detection: a national cancer institute early detection research network validation study. *Journal of Urology* **180**, 539–543; discussion 543.

59. Sokoll LJ, Sanda MG, Feng Z, *et al.* (2010). A prospective, multicenter, National Cancer Institute Early Detection Research Network study of [-2]proPSA: improving prostate cancer detection and correlating with cancer aggressiveness. *Cancer Epidemiology, Biomarkers & Prevention* **19**, 1193–1200.

60. Epstein JI, Walsh PC, Carmichael M, Brendler CB (1994). Pathologic and clinical findings to predict tumor extent of nonpalpable (stage T1c) prostate cancer. *JAMA* **271**, 368–374.

61. Stephan C, Kahrs AM, Cammann H, *et al.* (2009). A [-2]proPSA-based artificial neural network significantly improves differentiation between prostate cancer and benign prostatic diseases. *Prostate* **69**, 198–207.

62. Makarov DV, Isharwal S, Sokoll LJ, *et al.* (2009). Pro-prostate-specific antigen measurements in serum and tissue are associated with treatment necessity among men enrolled in expectant management for prostate cancer. *Clinical Cancer Research* **15**, 7316–7321.

63. Bussemakers MJ, van Bokhoven A, Verhaegh GW, *et al.* (1999). DD3: a new prostate-specific gene, highly overexpressed in prostate cancer. *Cancer Research* **59**, 5975–5979.

64. de Kok JB, Verhaegh GW, Roelofs RW, *et al.* (2002). DD3(PCA3), a very sensitive and specific marker to detect prostate tumors. *Cancer Research* **62**, 2695–2698.

65. Hessels D, Klein Gunnewiek JM, van Oort I, *et al.* (2003). DD3(PCA3)-based molecular urine analysis for the diagnosis of prostate cancer. *European Urology* **44**, 8–15; discussion 15–16.

66. Crawford ED, Rove KO, Trabulsi EJ, *et al.* (2012). Diagnostic performance of PCA3 to detect prostate cancer in men with increased prostate specific antigen: a prospective study of 1,962 cases. *Journal of Urology* **188**, 1726–1731.

67. Vlaeminck-Guillem V, Ruffion A, Andre J, Devonec M, Paparel P (2010). Urinary prostate cancer 3 test: toward the age of reason? *Urology* **75**, 447–453.

68. Auprich M, Bjartell A, Chun FK, *et al.* (2011). Contemporary role of prostate cancer antigen 3 in the management of prostate cancer. *European Urology* **60**, 1045–1054.

69. Ploussard G, Haese A, Van Poppel H, *et al.* (2010). The prostate cancer gene 3 (PCA3) urine test in men with previous negative biopsies: does free-to-total prostate-specific antigen ratio influence the performance of the PCA3 score in predicting positive biopsies? *BJU International* **106**, 1143–1147.

70. Haese A, de la Taille A, van Poppel H, *et al.* (2008). Clinical utility of the PCA3 urine assay in European men scheduled for repeat biopsy. *European Urology* **54**, 1081–1088.

71. Prensner JR, Rubin MA, Wei JT, Chinnaiyan AM (2012). Beyond PSA: the next generation of prostate cancer biomarkers. *Science Translational Medicine* **4**, 127rv123.

72. Mehra R, Han B, Tomlins SA, *et al.* (2007). Heterogeneity of TMPRSS2 gene rearrangements in multifocal prostate adenocarcinoma: molecular evidence for an independent group of diseases. *Cancer Research* **67**, 7991–7995.

73. Sun C, Dobi A, Mohamed A, *et al.* (2008). TMPRSS2-ERG fusion, a common genomic alteration in prostate cancer activates C-MYC and abrogates prostate epithelial differentiation. *Oncogene* **27**, 5348–5353.

74. Braun M, Goltz D, Shaikhibrahim Z, *et al.* (2012). ERG protein expression and genomic rearrangement status in primary and metastatic prostate cancer – a comparative study of two monoclonal antibodies. *Prostate Cancer and Prostatic Diseases* **15**, 165–169.

75. Sartori DA, Chan DW (2014). Biomarkers in prostate cancer: what's new? *Current Opinion in Oncology* **26**, 259–264.

76. Svensson MA, LaFargue CJ, MacDonald TY, *et al.* (2011). Testing mutual exclusivity of ETS rearranged prostate cancer. *Laboratory Investigation* **91**, 404–412.

77. Rubin MA, Maher CA, Chinnaiyan AM (2011). Common gene rearrangements in prostate cancer. *Journal of Clinical Oncology* **29**, 3659–3668.

78. Rosen P, Sesterhenn IA, Brassell SA, McLeod DG, Srivastava S, Dobi A (2012). Clinical potential of the ERG oncoprotein in prostate cancer. *Nature Reviews Urology* **9**, 131–137.

79. Sreenath TL, Dobi A, Petrovics G, Srivastava S (2011). Oncogenic activation of ERG: A predominant mechanism in prostate cancer. *Journal of Carcinogenesis* **10**, 37.

80. Salami SS, Schmidt F, Laxman B, *et al.* (2013). Combining urinary detection of TMPRSS2:ERG and PCA3 with serum PSA to predict diagnosis of prostate cancer. *Urologic Oncology* **31**, 566–571.

81. Tomlins SA, Aubin SM, Siddiqui J, *et al.* (2011). Urine TMPRSS2:ERG fusion transcript stratifies prostate cancer risk in men with elevated serum PSA. *Science Translational Medicine* **3**, 94ra72.

82. Leyten GH, Hessels D, Jannink SA, *et al.* (2014). Prospective multicentre evaluation of PCA3 and TMPRSS2-ERG gene fusions as diagnostic and prognostic urinary biomarkers for prostate cancer. *European Urology* **65**, 534–542.

83. Clark JP, Cooper CS (2009). ETS gene fusions in prostate cancer. *Nature Reviews Urology* **6**, 429–439.

84. Minner S, Enodien M, Sirma H, *et al.* (2011). ERG status is unrelated to PSA recurrence in radically operated prostate cancer in the absence of antihormonal therapy. *Clinical Cancer Research* **17**, 5878–5888.

85. Cornu JN, Cancel-Tassin G, Egrot C, Gaffory C, Haab F, Cussenot O (2013). Urine TMPRSS2:ERG fusion transcript integrated with PCA3 score, genotyping, and biological features are correlated to the results of prostatic biopsies in men at risk of prostate cancer. *Prostate* **73**, 242–249.

86. Knezevic D, Goddard AD, Natraj N, *et al.* (2013). Analytical validation of the Oncotype DX prostate cancer assay – a clinical RT-PCR assay optimized for prostate needle biopsies. *BMC Genomics* **14**, 690.

87. Cooperberg MR, Simko JP, Cowan JE, *et al.* (2013). Validation of a cell-cycle progression gene panel to improve risk stratification in a contemporary prostatectomy cohort. *Journal of Clinical Oncology* **31**, 1428–1434.

88. Cuzick J, Swanson GP, Fisher G, *et al.* (2011). Prognostic value of an RNA expression signature derived from cell cycle proliferation genes in patients with prostate cancer: a retrospective study. *Lancet Oncology* **12**, 245–255.

89. Cuzick J, Berney DM, Fisher G, *et al.* (2012). Prognostic value of a cell cycle progression signature for prostate cancer death in a conservatively managed needle biopsy cohort. *British Journal of Cancer* **106**, 1095–1099.

90. Freedland SJ, Gerber L, Reid J, *et al.* (2013). Prognostic utility of cell cycle progression score in men with prostate cancer after primary external beam radiation therapy. *International Journal of Radiation Oncology • Biology • Physics* **86**, 848–853.

91. Arsov C, Jankowiak F, Hiester A, *et al.* (2014). Prognostic value of a cell-cycle progression score in men with prostate cancer managed with active surveillance after MRI-guided prostate biopsy – a pilot study. *Anticancer Research* **34**, 2459–2466.

92. Shore N, Concepcion R, Saltzstein D, *et al.* (2014). Clinical utility of a biopsy-based cell cycle gene expression assay in localized prostate cancer. *Current Medical Research and Opinion* **30**, 547–553.

93. Sreekumar A, Poisson LM, Rajendiran TM, *et al.* (2009). Metabolomic profiles delineate potential role for sarcosine in prostate cancer progression. *Nature* **457**, 910–914.

94. McDunn JE, Li Z, Adam KP, *et al.* (2013). Metabolomic signatures of aggressive prostate cancer. *Prostate* **73**, 1547–1560.

95. Vickers AJ, Cronin AM, Aus G, *et al.* (2008). A panel of kallikrein markers can reduce unnecessary biopsy for prostate cancer: data from the European Randomized Study of Prostate Cancer Screening in Goteborg, Sweden. *BMC Medicine* **6**, 19.

96. Benchikh A, Savage C, Cronin A, *et al.* (2010). A panel of kallikrein markers can predict outcome of prostate biopsy following clinical work-up: an independent validation study from the European Randomized Study of Prostate Cancer screening, France. *BMC Cancer* **10**, 635.

97. Gupta A, Roobol MJ, Savage CJ, *et al.* (2010). A four-kallikrein panel for the prediction of repeat prostate biopsy: data from the European Randomized Study of Prostate Cancer screening in Rotterdam, Netherlands. *British Journal of Cancer* **103**, 708–714.

98. Voigt JD, Zappala SM, Vaughan ED, Wein AJ (2014). The Kallikrein Panel for prostate cancer screening: its economic impact. *Prostate* **74**, 250–259.

99. Carlsson S, Maschino A, Schroder F, *et al.* (2013). Predictive value of four kallikrein markers for pathologically insignificant compared with aggressive prostate cancer in radical prostatectomy specimens: results from the European Randomized Study of Screening for Prostate Cancer section Rotterdam. *European Urology* **64**, 693–699.

PART III

Biomarkers, Screening and Precision Health: Implications for Public Health

CHAPTER 17

Improving the Clinical Validity of Biomarker Research in Cancer Detection

David F Ransohoff

Department of Medicine, Lineberger Comprehensive Cancer Center, University of North Carolina at Chapel Hill, Chapel Hill, NC, USA

Background, purpose and organization

A Holy Grail goal in cancer-screening research has been to develop a non-invasive biomarker for cancer diagnosis, like a blood-based test for cancer screening. Historically, however, the field has been characterized by strong claims in research papers and news reports that are followed by disappointment when results are not reproduced in "validation" studies. While cycles of hope and disappointment may be expected in any field of research, such cycles' magnitude seems especially dramatic in this field. By understanding the concept of "clinical validity", and how it applies to research about markers for cancer screening, it may be possible to derive practical lessons that can moderate these cycles and improve the process of this kind of research.

A first step is to distinguish the term "clinical validity" from other terms that sound similar and may cause confusion. Next is to examine promising marker study results that were not reproducible, in order to derive practical lessons to improve the reliability and efficiency of research about molecular markers for diagnosis [1,2].

Distinguishing clinical validity from analytical validity and clinical utility

The term clinical validity must first be differentiated from analytical validity and clinical utility, in order to allow appropriate focus on specific kinds of research questions and their design issues. The three terms, though related, each involve different questions and designs, with their own distinct "threats" to validity. A clear consideration of these three terms is provided by the Evaluation of Genomic Applications in Practice and Prevention (EGAPP) [3] work, and has been used by others [4,5].

- *Analytical validity* refers to "… the technical performance of the test" [3] and whether it measures what it is supposed to measure – for example, whether a PSA test measures the analyte that is claimed.
- *Clinical validity* refers to "… the strength of the association between a [test result] and [the] disorder of interest" [3]. If the marker measures what is claimed (analytic validity), then clinical validity asks "does doing that measurement provide

Biomarkers in Cancer Screening and Early Detection, First Edition. Edited by Sudhir Srivastava.
© 2017 John Wiley & Sons, Inc. Published 2017 by John Wiley & Sons, Inc.

"discrimination" – namely, the "ability to diagnose a disorder, assess susceptibility or risk, or provide information on prognosis or variation in drug response" [3]?

- *Clinical utility* refers to whether that discrimination, when combined with "change(d) patient management decisions…(can) improve net health outcomes" [3].

The three terms are related in the sense that research about a subsequent term may depend on valid or reproducible research about the previous term. That is: first, a test should measure what it claims to measure; second, conducting that measurement should allow discrimination of clinically important groups (e.g. discrimination of persons with or without a diagnosis); and third, that discrimination, when combined with an intervention, should lead to a beneficial outcome.

A focus on clinical validity might look narrow, but is important for several reasons. First, many studies in the field of marker research address clinical validity, while clinical utility is less often studied, because it generally requires conducting an expensive cumbersome randomized controlled clinical trial (RCT). Second, studies of clinical validity are particularly difficult because they are "observational," meaning the causal agent cannot be randomly assigned to two otherwise equal groups. Randomization is a powerful tool to avoid bias, but it cannot be done in a study of clinical validity of a marker, because it is not possible to randomly assign disease status, in order to learn a disease's effect on a biomarker [6]. Last, many studies in which strong promise has been followed by disappointment are about clinical validity. For these reasons, clinical validity research warrants focused discussion.

Internal validity and external validity

Any study conducting a comparison – such as studies about clinical validity, analytic validity, or clinical utility – involves two types of "validity" (internal and external) that affect what the results of the comparison mean:

- *Internal validity* refers to whether the comparison within the study is fair, or is biased in some systematic way. For example, if cancer subjects are older than controls, then a distorted comparison,

with erroneously positive results, might be due to that systematic difference, rather than being due to the presence of cancer.

- *External validity* refers to whether the results of the comparison generalize beyond (external to) those in the study. For example, if cancer subjects have advanced disease, then results might not be generalizable to persons with early disease.

While these examples are simple, and may sound easy to avoid, or at least to recognize, in reality the sources of bias are numerous and difficult; furthermore, any one bias can be fatal, if it is responsible for a study's substantially erroneous result [6]. Internal validity will be the primary focus of this essay, because it is a particularly knotty challenge in observational research like that used to study clinical validity.

Past lessons: CEA blood test for colon cancer

The kinds of problems that can occur – and how lessons may be learned from considering problems – are illustrated by an early example about a promising biomarker for cancer screening. The carcinoembryonic antigen (CEA) blood test was claimed, in initial reports, to have almost 100% sensitivity and specificity for colorectal cancer (CRC) [7]. Strong promise and extensive press coverage provided the foundation for a costly prospective study, sponsored by the National Cancer Institute of Canada and the American Cancer Society, to "validate" the initial findings. The results of that study, however, and others, showed much lower sensitivity than had been initially reported [8].

The reason the CEA test did not "validate" in this expensive late-stage study was because subjects in the initial discovery research had advanced cancer [7], while subjects in the later validation study had less extensive disease, or a different "spectrum" [9] – a problem of external validity – in which sensitivity was lower. Lessons from the CEA experience helped establish the field of methodology to evaluate the design and conduct of studies of diagnostic tests [9].

Recent lessons: proteomics blood tests for ovarian cancer

The recent history of claims for blood tests to detect ovarian cancer provide additional lessons to improve the reliability and efficiency of research about clinical validity of molecular markers.

Initial promising claims

A major initial report about a serum-based proteomics test for ovarian cancer received intense attention, not only because of the claimed discrimination of nearly 100% sensitivity and specificity, but also because there was no other good screening test available for ovarian cancer. In this setting, a successful test would have provided a long-awaited advance. The approach described in an article in the *Lancet* in 2002 involved analysis of wave peaks generated by a mass spectrometer using SELDI (surface-enhanced laser desorption/ionization) technology [10]. Among patients with and without ovarian cancer, including early stage, mass spectrometry patterns were analyzed using an "iterative searching algorithm" to find patterns that would identify persons with and without ovarian cancer. Analytes were not identified specifically; rather, patterns of peaks were considered to contain the information that produced discrimination. A training set of bloods from persons with and without ovarian cancer was used to develop the mathematical analysis algorithm, while a validation set, totally independent of the group used in training, was used to assess whether the assay that had been developed in training could discriminate.

The discrimination reported was eventually thought by observers to have been due to a problem of internal validity, in which signal or bias was "hardwired" into the comparison. By analyzing raw data that the study authors had posted on the Web (a credit to the investigators' thoroughness of reporting), it appeared that the mass spectrometer analyses of cancers and controls had been done on different days [11–14]. Because the spectrometer machine's output signal "wandered" over time, and had to be adjusted each day, it was possible that the "discrimination" – or high sensitivity and specificity – was due to a spurious difference related to the sample run-date, not to cancer.

In 2008, a different blood-based proteomics assay was reported to have nearly 100% sensitivity and specificity for ovarian cancer [15]. In this assay, six specific analytes were measured. The major potential problem again appeared to be one of internal validity: cancer subjects had come from a group of women with pelvic masses that, at later scheduled surgery, were determined to be malignant or not. The comparison group of non-cancer subjects came from women seen in a screening clinic in a different setting. One suggested explanation for discrimination was that, because the analytes being examined included "stress proteins," patients with masses might, because of stress, have been systematically different from the comparison subjects from a screening clinic [16]. These alternate explanations for the discrimination found were not discussed in interpretation of the original manuscript [15], nor in the publicity and press releases surrounding the publication of data.

Later promising claims lead to an NCI study to assess clinical validity

By 2008, there were at least five major claims about blood tests for early detection of ovarian cancer, but no assay had been evaluated in a blinded validation of early cancer subjects. When several investigators requested use of the National Cancer Institute's (NCI) blood specimens banked during the course of a major NCI study of cancer screening, NCI decided to develop a blinded "validation" study to assess the several competing claims. The primary goal would be to learn whether any of the assay panels "validated" – that is, whether it successfully discriminated OvCa vs normal better than CA125, the current test.

NCI's study to assess clinical validity

The specimens collected during the course of a RCT had special strengths to assess clinical validity – strengths that have lessons for how to design and conduct marker research in the future. The original study (called PLCO) had been organized in the 1990s, to assess the clinical utility of different screening modalities to reduce mortality for four cancers: PSA screening (and treatment) for prostate cancer (P); chest x-ray (and treatment) for lung cancer (L); sigmoidoscopy screening (and treatment) for colo-rectal cancer (C); and CA125 screening (and treatment) for ovarian cancer (O) [17].

Within this RCT, then, a study of clinical validity was later "designed" after the RCT had completed all data collection. What made such a study feasible was that PLCO investigators had decided, soon after the RCT was begun, to add, or piggyback, collection of a "biospecimen repository" onto the RCT infrastructure [17]. While such a repository was not required to address the study's primary goal of assessing outcomes and clinical utility, it was thought that adding specimens might be useful at some later point for studies about etiology or diagnosis. The biorepository included cancer tissue as well as blood specimens (including plasma and serum), periodically collected from some subjects in routine follow-up visits prior to the diagnosis of cancer. With this background, in 2008, NCI designed a study whose goal was to assess the clinical validity of the assays that investigators had already developed [18].

Design and conduct

The study designed within PLCO is called a "validation" study in this essay, although other adjectives might be used like "confirmation" or "replication". Any of the terms suggests an assessment of strength or validity, as demonstrated by a blinded test of a pre-stated hypothesis.

The study design used in PLCO was suitable to evaluate clinical validity because of the way that blood specimens were collected (they were collected frequently, and were stored blind as to whether subjects had symptoms or the outcome of cancer), and because of the way that outcome was followed equally intensely in all subjects, so that the true state (presence or absence of cancer) could be known. Even though no specific study question about clinical validity had been thought of or planned when specimens began to be collected, the design and conduct happened to provide for equal assessment of the true state among persons being followed, and equal handling of bloods, regarding collection methods and storage. Among people who eventually became cases, bloods drawn before diagnosis (e.g., within a year prior to diagnosis) could be used to assess markers at a time when a person was considered asymptomatic, or at least not symptomatic enough to have provoked an independent visit to a clinician. Matched controls could be selected. The design utilized basically reflects the nested case-control design described by Pepe [19] and others [1, 2], that minimizes spurious differences (bias) between the compared groups.

The primary analysis was a blinded validation, or hypothesis test, of each investigative group's pre-specified and locked-down assay. Each group used the same blinded specimens from PLCO to perform its assay, and sent results to NCI for unblinding.

Results

The results were that no assay did better than CA125 [18].

Following this result, each investigative group was then invited to design and conduct a new discovery and validation study, utilizing specimens that had been part of the initial "validation" study but were still blinded. NCI staff unblinded roughly half the specimens for further discovery, to identify new markers. The specimens remaining, still blinded to the investigator teams, could then be used in a next step to validate markers found in that discovery [18]. The results were that no highly discriminatory new markers were identified.

While it was bad news that no blood test worked better than CA125, the good news was that this set of studies demonstrated the usefulness of a biorepository that was strongly unbiased because it had been piggybacked on to an RCT infrastructure. This case control study, nested within a cohort [19], could be used to address different questions of clinical validity, including both in validation (of pre-stated hypothesis or assay) and then in discovery (development of a new assay) and its validation [1, 2].

Thinking big: using banked specimens in both discovery and validation

The PLCO experience provides lessons about how to develop more efficient and reliable research processes, to assure and assess the clinical validity of diagnostic markers. Using already-banked specimens can provide material for both validation and discovery, if design and conduct of specimen-collection happens to be strong. The key requirement is that enough blood specimens (or other fluids/sample) be collected prior and near to the time of diagnosis of early cancer.

Imagine what might be done if "enough" specimens were available, so that they were not considered a "precious resource", as they generally are now. Imagine that almost unlimited numbers and volumes of specimens from cohort studies like PLCO were available. Suppose that tens or hundreds of thousands of people were followed over time, in a cohort in which blood, urine, saliva, or other fluids were collected in large volumes, and in which people were followed regularly to outcomes of early cancer. Such a biospecimen repository could provide strongly-unbiased comparisons using the nested case-control approach. The design and conduct would provide for strong external validity, because specimens would come from subjects with early and asymptomatic cancer. The design and conduct would provide strong internal validity, because specimens are collected and handled equally before diagnosis. A biorespository large enough could be used in both discovery and validation.

Logistically, of course, this effort would be huge, because many thousands of people would need to be followed for years to accumulate enough "outcomes" of cancer, which is (at least in absolute terms) a low-incidence disease. The PLCO repository cost millions of dollars, and has required much work to create and maintain. Nevertheless, imagining what might be done illustrates a feature of diagnostic marker research that makes it fundamentally different from drug development research. It is possible, in studying diagnostic markers, to collect specimens in advance of actually having a specific test to test; one can analyze banked specimens, using nested case-control approaches [1, 2, 19]. In drug trials, in contrast, it is impossible to do this kind of "retrospective" research with banked specimens, because the drug is an intervention that must be administered prospectively.

In a study of diagnostic markers, the study can be designed and conducted in advance, as long as the outcome is known, and specimens can be collected near to the time of the diagnosis of the outcome. To set up the cohort requires anticipating the type of analyte, protein or DNA for example, to arrange proper specimen collection, spinning, storage, and so on. At this time, there is substantial demand for such high-quality specimens that have been collected during the course of RCTs like PLCO and the Women's Health Initiative.

Practical issues I: how validity "gets in" to a study (design and conduct) and is measured (interpretation and reporting)

How are details of validity, like those discussed above, applied in a practical way? How does validity get "into" a study, and how is validity measured?

The examples above describe how investigators' decisions about design and conduct – what was done – determine what the "validity" of a study is. How a study's validity is measured then depends on investigators' decisions about interpretation and reporting. All four steps comprise a kind of package that determines validity in the eyes of observer, such as another investigator, a reviewer, or a policymaker.

Design

Design refers to how the study was planned, particularly with regard to threats to validity. If a study is planned "prospectively" (i.e. before data are collected), then an investigator can anticipate – and design – a study to avoid potential biases, like randomization (when it can be done), or blinding, or providing equally intense follow-up to the compared groups. On the other hand, if a study is done "retrospectively," meaning the study was done after data were collected (for example, by using previously-banked specimens), then no attention may have been provided to "design" when the specimens were collected.

In a "convenience sample", there typically may be no "design" in what was conducted or done. This means an investigator considering use of convenience samples will want to consider, as early as possible, what the design and conduct of the study were that produced those specimens. Even if no design or conduct was planned, the details of "what was done" critically affect validity, and will have to be reported in a research article. If the design and conduct that were done incurred fatal flaws or biases in the fundamental comparison, then the investigator may want to think hard about whether doing analyses in such study are worth the effort in the first place. A general lack of attention to the consequences of design and conduct has led to major problems in this field [6, 20].

The problem for the investigator is that, when the time comes to do interpreting and reporting, the fact of "no design" and "no attention to conduct" may reveal problems, including fatal ones, that affect the interpretation of the results. It is possible in some circumstances, though, that design and conduct, in retrospect, may have avoided problems; this method is discussed regarding the PRoBE approach or nested case-control design discussed elsewhere [1, 2, 19, 20].

Conduct

Conduct refers to how features of design were actually executed in the study that was done. For example, if blinding was intended, but the blind was broken, then that feature of conduct would need to be considered for its possible impact on interpretation and reporting of results.

Interpretation

After a study is completed, the investigator must interpret results and draw conclusions. If, for example, blinding was compromised, then an investigator would report, in interpretation, the possible impact on "validity." Whether that impact is significant depends on how extensive the unblinding was, and on whether the outcome being measured was subjective and, thus, could be measured in a biased manner. Or, if the intended comparison is cancer vs normal but the cancer subjects are older and the normals are younger, the potential importance of that "threat to validity" should be discussed.

Reporting

Reporting detail has two purposes. One is to allow other scientists to reproduce the study design and conduct, and to see whether they can obtain the same results. Another is to allow readers to judge, even if they do not plan to reproduce the study, how well the study results may be relied on – for example, to base other research or to base policy.

In order for these two purposes to be accomplished, it is necessary for investigators to report sufficient detail for outsiders to judge. To reach that goal, reporting standards have been developed for many different kinds of research, now including studies of diagnostic markers or clinical validity. It is important to understand from the outset, however, that reporting detail does not *make* a study strong. An investigator should not think, "If I report details of design and conduct according to a reporting guideline, then any problems can be 'accounted for' in analysis to produce a strong reproducible result." The problem is that what is done (design and conduct) is done, and nothing can change that. The goal of reporting what has been done is to let others see enough detail to determine whether what was done supports the conclusions that have been drawn.

Role of standards for reporting

Standards for reporting were developed first for RCTs in the CONSORT (Consolidated standards of reporting clinical trials) standards [21], because the experimental method used in RCTs is well understood, and because RCTs are so heavily relied on to answer certain questions. Following the development of reporting standards for RCTs, standards have been developed for studies of diagnostic tests (STARD) [22, 23] and of prognosis (REMARK) [24, 25]. The field of reporting guidelines has itself become a somewhat large field (EQUATOR) [26, 27].

Even though reporting standards prescribe details of design and conduct that should be reported, they do not prescribe precisely what design and conduct should be, because that level of prescription would be too complicated and difficult. Judging design and conduct is work left to peer reviewers; the goal of reporting standards is simply to provide them enough detail to judge.

With this explanation of reporting guidelines' role, it should be clear that reporting guidelines must not be regarded as some perfunctory checklist to be addressed after the study is done. Rather, they should be regarded as guides to be considered in the earliest parts of planning design and conduct, so that, when the time comes to "report," the details being reported will pass the judgment of a knowledgeable reviewer.

Practical issues II: how "valid" does a study need to be? And "when" or at what stage or phase is validity important – early (discovery) or late ("validation")?

How valid does a study need to be? On one hand, avoiding bias in design and conduct can be cumbersome and expensive, and an investigator may, in early discovery research, be tempted to think, "Assessing validity can wait until later." The problem is that if early shortcuts lead to erroneous conclusions, then later effort risks being wasted, if it is built on a weak foundation. A "validation" study does not *make* a research strong or reproducible; it simply assesses the strength of what was supposedly "discovered" in earlier research.

Principles

Several principles may help guide investigators' decisions about "how valid does a study need to be?" Perhaps an overarching principle is to be "fair to the data," whether they are weak or strong, and to not fool yourself or others. Fundamental principles of science apply in this situation, just as they were described by top scientists in physics a generation ago. Albert Einstein said, "The right to search for truth implies also a duty; one must not conceal any part of what one has recognized to be true." Similarly, Richard Feynman said, "[I]f you're doing an experiment, you should report everything that might make it invalid… other causes that could possibly explain your results…. Details that could throw doubt on your interpretation must be given, if you know them" [28]. It is part of the scientist's job, these scientific greats are telling us, to contemplate and describe – in interpretation and reporting – whatever limitations there may have been in design and conduct.

The point here is not that a study must be perfect. No research is perfect or can be expected to be. "Perfect" really *is* the enemy of good. The point is that whatever is done must be interpreted and reported fairly. It would be hoped that an author is not penalized for reporting weaknesses in a research report (or a grant proposal). Another point is that an investigator should perhaps not even report a study with flaws or biases so large that they are likely to be "fatal." Deciding exactly what is fatal involves scientific judgment of investigators, reviewers, and editors. In the meantime, it can sometimes seem, both in published research and in submitted manuscripts, that some investigators are paying almost no attention to these kinds of issues.

Importance

The critical importance of internal validity and avoiding bias is indicated by how the potential bias of baseline inequality is handled in design, conduct, and reporting of a RCT. RCTs, of course, are the gold standard for providing strong or valid conclusions, because their design makes it relatively easy to avoid bias compared to other study designs. In a RCT, randomization is part of design and conduct, and – although randomization almost always works – the results of randomization are typically expected to be reported in detail, commonly as "Table 1" in the published report of a RCT (for example, showing each group's age, gender, severity of disease, and other features at baseline).

The purpose of detailed reporting is to learn whether features unequally distributed between compared groups might explain a difference in study results. Even though randomization almost always works to produce equivalent groups, baseline equality is considered so critical that the results of randomization are expected to be reported. Randomization works not only to assure equality of the known variables described in "Table 1", but it also should equalize potentially important variables that cannot be measured, or are not known. In contrast, in an observational study baseline equality is similarly important – indeed, more important, because randomization cannot be done to make the compared groups otherwise equal. Yet, "other possible differences between the compared groups that might explain the observed results" may not be described at all, or only in scant detail.

Challenge of addressing bias in observational research

Complicating the challenge of addressing threats to internal validity is that the "research architecture" of studies of diagnostic tests can be complex to consider, even for research methodologists. While those details go far beyond this discussion, the flavor of the challenge involved is illustrated by examining how leading methodologists discuss the issues [29–33]. One source [34] cautions "how complicated just the basic strategy of comparison may be in assessing diagnostic accuracy: 'general design' can involve '(1) a survey of the total study population, (2) a case-referent approach, or (3) a test-based enrolment'. Further, even basic approaches to data collection may vary dramatically: 'The direction of the data should generally be prospective, but ambispective and retrospective approaches are some- times appropriate'. The complexity of these choices makes [RCT] research seem simple and almost pedestrian" [1]. The recent focus on the nested case-control design [19] has helped clarify a design approach that may help avoid bias in studies about clinical validity of diagnostic tests.

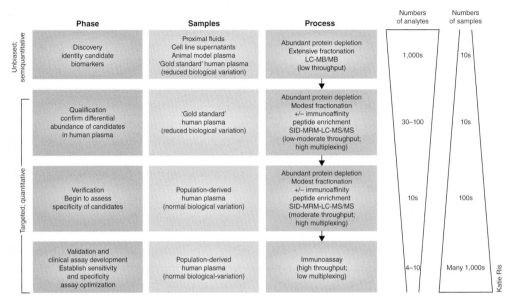

Figure 17.1 In this figure, illustrating process flow for development of biomarker candidates, the word "validation" appears in the bottom row in the fourth "phase." In phases 2 and 3, the concept of validity (i.e., "how valid is the study result") is relevant, even if the word "validation" is not used. For a color version of this figure please see color plate section.

Confusion caused by terminology: the "validation study"

The term "validation" can itself cause confusion, in discussing "where" validity is important, because the word "validation" is commonly used to refer to one kind of study – late-stage research – thus, perhaps, suggesting that considerations of "validity" can wait until some late time (see Figure 17.1) In a formulation by Rifai *et al.*, the fourth phase is named "validation" [35] and, as indicated in row 4, it deals with specimens from blood or plasma. On the other hand, as shown in Figure 17.1, research studies in rows 2 and 3 – in the process of discovery and development – also address discrimination or clinical validity, where the generic issue of "validity" is also clearly important. Again, if the design and conduct in early studies are weak, then results will not "validate" later. The overall point is that the generic issue of "validity" – design, conduct, interpretation, and reporting – has importance at every stage of research.

The question about "where is validity important" can also be considered in light of a widely-used system of "phases" of research about molecular markers for cancer. In this formulation, five phases are prescribed, comprising over 20 questions that may be addressed in the process of marker development [36]. However, the formulation does not discuss, for any of the studies prescribed, details of study design and conduct, and how to avoid problems of bias in internal validity [1]. In an essay of nearly 6000 words, the word "validity" is used once, while the word bias, referring to systematic difference between groups, is not used at all. For any of the studies proposed to achieve "validity" and avoid bias, then, an investigator must look elsewhere. Investigators knowledgeable about methods of clinical research will understand this limitation, but investigators in fields of basic biology or technology may be unfamiliar with the need to look elsewhere for details of study design and conduct in order to provide "validity." [37].

"Validity" of discovery research

If weak discovery is a major explanation for the cycles of hope and disappointment in the last ten years, then discovery research needs stronger design and conduct, so that its promises have a greater chance of being validated. As stated by one observer, "We need to turn conventional wisdom on its head", and use precious specimens far earlier than we currently do (Z. Feng, personal communication). The main idea, then, is that "validity" is important at any stage of research, even if that stage is not called "validation".

Lessons for the future

In summary, lessons from the past 15 years may help point the way to improve the reliability and efficiency of marker research.

1 **Clinical validity is addressed in research design, conduct, interpretation, and reporting**

   Validity or strength *comes from* design and conduct – what was done in the study. Interpretation (investigators' judgments) and reporting (investigators' description of details of design, conduct, and interpretation) produce what other scientists and observers then learn about what was done. All four features – design, conduct, interpretation and reporting – are critical in creating and measuring validity.

2 **Specimens are the product of a "study"; that study has design and conduct, whether or not specimen-collection was ever thought of as a "study"**

   Specimens cannot be considered independent of their provenance. Rather, they must be considered the product of some study, whose design and conduct will eventually be reported and interpreted. If a design is so weak (for example in "convenience samples") that it threatens the validity of the fundamental comparison, then investigators should consider – by thinking about what they will eventually have to report and interpret – whether it is even worth doing the "study" in the first place.

3 **Weak discovery is a major problem in assessing the clinical validity of much current research about molecular markers for cancer screening**

   A major rate limiting step in studies of clinical validity of molecular markers for cancer diagnosis has been weak early discovery that produces findings that do not "validate" in later validation studies. If discovery is "weak," then the result of a "validation study" will be simply to show that discovery was weak. This means that what we call "discovery" research must be made stronger, by better design and conduct, and must be described fairly in interpretation and reporting, so that observers understand the strengths

and weaknesses. Saving effort to assure "validity" until the end may be, overall, an inefficient strategy in marker development, to the extent that building on a weak foundation leads to wasted effort. Similarly, the use of "phases" does not assure the "strength" of a study in any phase. The utilization of "high-quality" – or strongly unbiased – specimens in discovery would be a change from much past practice and approach, where the most precious specimens may be saved for last.

4 **Sources of specimens for strongly unbiased comparison**

   A rate-limiting step in recent research about clinical validity of molecular markers for cancer screening has been not having sufficient specimens that are products of strongly unbiased studies and can provide strong comparisons [20]. Specimens from existing cohorts, like PLCO, WHI, and CARET, are indeed "precious" for use in validation, much less in earlier stages like discovery. Precious specimens might be made less precious – and more useful – by collecting and banking many more specimens "in advance" (i.e., in advance of knowing exactly which analyte is being assessed). In other words, it may be possible to "cultivate cohorts" that already exist, including in ongoing RCTs (as was done in PLCO), in observational cohort research studies, and within practice settings like HMOs, that have the strong features of study design and conduct that are required to reliably answer questions about the clinical validity of molecular markers in screening [38].

References

1. Ransohoff DF (2007). How to improve reliability and efficiency of research about molecular markers: roles of phases, guidelines, and study design. *Journal of Clinical Epidemiology* **60**(12), 1205–1219.

2. Ransohoff DF (2007). Response to commentary. *Journal of Clinical Epidemiology* **60**(12), 1226–1228.

3. Teutsch SM, Bradley LA, Palomaki GE, Haddow JE, Piper M, Calonge N, *et al.* (2009). The Evaluation of Genomic Applications in Practice and Prevention (EGAPP) Initiative: Methods of the EGAPP Working Group. *Genetics in Medicine* **11**(1), 3–14.

4. Micheel C, Nass SJ, Omenn GS, eds (2012). *Evolution of Translational Omics: Lessons Learned and the Path Forward*. Washington, DC: Committee on the Review of

Omics-Based Tests for Predicting Patient Outcomes in Clinical Trials; Board on Health Care Services; Board on Health Sciences Policy; Institute of Medicine.

5. Hayes DF, Allen J, Compton C, Gustavsen G, Leonard DG, McCormack R, et al. (2013). Breaking a vicious cycle. *Science Translational Medicine* 5(196), 196cm6.

6. Ransohoff DF (2005). Bias as a threat to the validity of cancer molecular-marker research. *Nature Reviews Cancer* 5(2), 142–149.

7. Thomson DM, Krupey J, Freedman SO, Gold P (1969). The radioimmunoassay of circulating carcinoembryonic antigen of the human digestive system. *Proceedings of the National Academy of Sciences of the United States of America* 64(1), 161–167.

8. Miller AB (1974). The joint National Cancer Institute of Canada-American Cancer Society study of a test for carcinoembryonic antigen (CEA). *Cancer* 34(3), suppl, 932–935.

9. Ransohoff DF, Feinstein AR (1978). Problems of spectrum and bias in evaluating the efficacy of diagnostic tests. *New England Journal of Medicine* 299(17), 926–930.

10. Petricoin EF, Ardekani AM, Hitt BA, Levine PJ, Fusaro VA, Steinberg SM, et al. (2002). Use of proteomic patterns in serum to identify ovarian cancer. *The Lancet* 359(9306), 572–577.

11. Baggerly KA, Coombes KR, Morris JS (2005). Bias, randomization, and ovarian proteomic data: a reply to "Producers and consumers". *Cancer Informatics* 1, 9–14.

12. Baggerly KA, Morris JS, Edmonson SR, Coombes KR (2005). Signal in noise: evaluating reported reproducibility of serum proteomic tests for ovarian cancer. *Journal of the National Cancer Institute* 97(4), 307–309.

13. Baggerly KA, Morris JS, Coombes KR (2004). Reproducibility of SELDI-TOF protein patterns in serum: comparing datasets from different experiments. *Bioinformatics* 20, 777–785.

14. Liotta LA, Lowenthal M, Mehta A, Conrads TP, Veenstra TD, Fishman DA, et al. (2005). Importance of communication between producers and consumers of publicly available experimental data. *Journal of the National Cancer Institute* 97(4), 310–314.

15. Visintin I, Feng Z, Longton G, Ward DC, Alvero AB, Lai Y, et al. (2008). Diagnostic markers for early detection of ovarian cancer. *Clinical Cancer Research* 14(4), 1065–1072.

16. McIntosh M, Anderson G, Drescher C, Hanash S, Urban N, Brown P, et al. (2008). Ovarian cancer early detection claims are biased. *Clinical Cancer Research* 14(22), 7574.

17. Prorok PC, Andriole GL, Bresalier RS, Buys SS, Chia D, Crawford ED, et al. (2000). Design of the Prostate, Lung, Colorectal and Ovarian (PLCO) Cancer Screening Trial. *Controlled Clinical Trials* 21(6 Suppl), 273S–309S.

18. Zhu CS, Pinsky PF, Cramer DW, Ransohoff DF, Hartge P, Pfeiffer RM, et al. (2011). A framework for evaluating biomarkers for early detection: validation of biomarker panels for ovarian cancer. *Cancer Prevention Research (Philadelphia)* 4(3), 375–383.

19. Pepe MS, Feng Z, Janes H, Bossuyt PM, Potter JD (2008). Pivotal evaluation of the accuracy of a biomarker used for classification or prediction: standards for study design. *Journal of the National Cancer Institute* 100(20), 1432–1438.

20. Ransohoff DF, Gourlay ML (2010). Sources of bias in specimens for research about molecular markers for cancer. *Journal of Clinical Oncology* 28(4), 698–704.

21. Rennie D (1996). How to report randomized controlled trials. The CONSORT statement. *JAMA* 276(8), 649.

22. Bossuyt PM, Reitsma JB, Bruns DE, Gatsonis CA, Glasziou PP, Irwig LM, et al. (2003). Towards complete and accurate reporting of studies of diagnostic accuracy: The STARD Initiative. *Annals of Internal Medicine* 138(1), 40–44.

23. Bossuyt PM, Reitsma JB, Bruns DE, Gatsonis CA, Glasziou PP, Irwig LM, et al. (2003). The STARD statement for reporting studies of diagnostic accuracy: explanation and elaboration. *Annals of Internal Medicine* 138(1), W1–12.

24. Altman DG, McShane LM, Sauerbrei W, Taube SE (2012). Reporting recommendations for tumor marker prognostic studies (REMARK): explanation and elaboration. *BMC Medicine* 10, 51.

25. McShane LM, Altman DG, Sauerbrei W, Taube SE, Gion M, Clark GM (2005). Reporting recommendations for tumor marker prognostic studies (REMARK). *Journal of the National Cancer Institute* 97(16), 1180–1184.

26. Altman DG, Simera I, Hoey J, Moher D, Schulz K (2008). EQUATOR: reporting guidelines for health research. *The Lancet* 371(9619), 1149–1150.

27. Simera I, Altman DG (2009). Writing a research article that is "fit for purpose": EQUATOR Network and reporting guidelines. *Evidence-Based Medicine* 14(5), 132–134.

28. Feynman RP (1974). Cargo cult science. *Engineering and Science* (June), 10–13.

29. Knottnerus JA, van Weel C (2002). General introduction: evaluation of diagnostic procedures. In: Knottnerus JA (ed). *The evidence base of clinical diagnosis*, pp. 1–17. London: BMJ Books.

30. Buntinx F, Knottnerus JA (2006). Are we at the start of a new era in diagnostic research? *Journal of Clinical Epidemiology* 59(4), 325–326.

31. Knottnerus JA, Muris JW (2002). Assessment of the accuracy of diagnostic tests: the cross-sectional study. In: Knottnerus JA (ed). *The evidence base of clinical diagnosis*, pp. 39–59. London: BMJ Books.

32. Sackett DL, Haynes RB (2002). The architecture of diagnostic research. In: Knottnerus JA (ed). *The evidence base of clinical diagnosis*, pp.19–38. London: BMJ Books.

33. Feng Z, Yasui Y, McLerran D, Adam B-L, Semmes J (2005). Statistical design and analytical strategies for discovery of disease-specific protein patterns (Chapter 18). In: Srivastava S (ed). *Informatics in proteomics*, 367–389: Marcell Dekker.

34. Knottnerus JA, Muris JW ()2003. Assessment of the accuracy of diagnostic tests: the cross-sectional study. *Journal of Clinical Epidemiology* **56**(11), 1118–1128.

35. Rifai N, Gillette MA, Carr SA (2006). Protein biomarker discovery and validation: the long and uncertain path to clinical utility. *Nature Biotechnology* **24**(8), 971–983.

36. Sullivan Pepe M, Etzioni R, Feng Z, Potter JD, Thompson ML, Thornquist M, *et al.* (2001). Phases of biomarker development for early detection of cancer. *Journal of the National Cancer Institute* **93**(14), 1054–1061.

37. Ransohoff DF (2004). Rules of evidence for cancer molecular-marker discovery and validation. *Nature Reviews Cancer* **4**(4), 309–314.

38. Ransohoff DF (2013). Cultivating cohort studies for observational translational research. *Cancer Epidemiology, Biomarkers & Prevention* **22**(4), 481–484.

CHAPTER 18

Cancer Overdiagnosis, Ramifications and Research Strategies

Barbara K Dunn[1] and Barnett S Kramer[2]

[1]National Cancer Institute, Division of Cancer Prevention, Chemoprevention Agent Development Research Group, Bethesda, MD, USA

[2]National Cancer Institute, Division of Cancer Prevention, Bethesda, MD, USA

What is overdiagnosis?

Screening for specific cancers is routinely carried out with the intent of detecting lesions at a stage that is early enough to improve the chances of a cure and reduce the morbidity of treatment. However, along with these potential benefits, a number of harms may ensue from screening. As with all medicine, the overall goal in screening is to optimize the balance between the benefits and harms, in order to make informed decisions regarding its implementation. The purpose of this chapter is to explore the nature and consequences of one of the key harms that can result from screening for early detection of cancer: overdiagnosis.

The first requirement for overdiagnosis is the existence of a substantial reservoir of subclinical or occult disease that would elude detection in the absence of an intentional search [1, 2]. The second requirement is the use of tests or examinations capable of tapping into that reservoir of indolent lesions. With the technological focus on increasingly sensitive screening tests, many lesions are detectable that pose no threat of morbidity or early death to the individual [3]. These "overdiagnoses", or "pseudodisease" [1,4], have been "overdetected" [5] and would never have been clinically

meaningful [6]. The marketing of "whole body scans", or "virtual physical exams", which also reveal asymptomatic lesions, is an example [7,8]. The ability to detect progressively smaller lesions brings these into the scope of cancer [1], broadening the definition of disease and increasing the number of healthy people labeled as having cancer [9].

Histopathological diagnosis offers a snapshot, not a dynamic picture, of a lesion's natural history. This is a crude surrogate for tumor behavior, since similarly appearing lesions are biologically heterogeneous (Figure 18.1). While some screen-detected cancers have lethal potential, others are very slowly progressive or are non-progressive. In randomized clinical trials (RCTs), the percentage of overdiagnoses among cancers detected by screening shows wide variation, depending on the cancer site, the stages defined as cancer (e.g. invasive +/− *in situ*), screening modality, and study methods [4, 5]. In addition, overdiagnoses must be distinguished from false positive screening tests. Patients with false positive diagnoses will not be treated for cancer. Patients with overdiagnoses usually are.

Some cancer screening tests lead to the diagnosis of non-invasive "pre-malignant" lesions such as carcinoma *in situ* [10]. Diagnosis of pre-cancers

Biomarkers in Cancer Screening and Early Detection, First Edition. Edited by Sudhir Srivastava.
© 2017 John Wiley & Sons, Inc. Published 2017 by John Wiley & Sons, Inc.

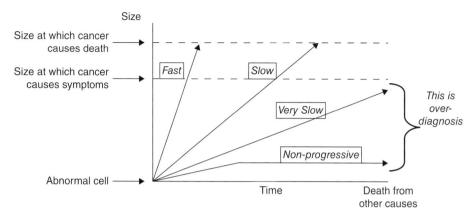

Figure 18.1 The heterogeneity of cancer progression is reflected in the variation in growth rate of similarly appearing cancers. Growth rate contributes to whether, and when, an occult cancer within the preclinical reservoir becomes clinically symptomatic within the individual's lifetime. For a color version of this figure please see color plate section.

poses a logistical challenge since, at present, we cannot distinguish lesions destined to become invasive and progress to metastases from those that remain "benign", or progress so slowly that they pose no danger during the individual's lifetime. Yet premalignancies are routinely treated, in some cases with therapy as aggressive as that used for documented invasive lesions.

Evidence that a reservoir of subclinical disease, both non-invasive and invasive, exists for certain cancers (prostate, breast, thyroid) comes from autopsy studies, as well as incidental findings from surgeries for other disease sites [2, 11–14]. The size and natural history of the reservoir of latent asymptomatic lesions affects the balance of benefits, and harms of any given screening test (Figures 18.1, 18.2). As illustrated in Figure 18.2, many currently available screening tests detect slow-growing tumors out of proportion to the fast-growing ones. This is because slow-growing tumors remain in the asymptomatic state longer, offering more opportunity for detection before they become symptomatic. This phenomenon is known as "length-biased sampling." Overdiagnosis is an extreme form of length-time bias [3, 14, 15].

Population-level data supporting the overdiagnosis

Overdiagnosis can be discerned from population level data by examining cancer incidence and mortality trends. A rise in new diagnoses, especially

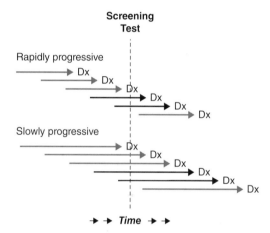

Figure 18.2 Periodic screening selectively detects slowly progressing cancers. Many of these might never have become clinically symptomatic and are, therefore, overdiagnoses. For a color version of this figure please see color plate section.

early-stage disease, that parallels increases in screening, suggests that the excess is due primarily to the institution of a periodic screening program, as seen with breast cancer through the 1980s and 1990s [3, 16] (Figure 18.3).

If the screening program were simply pulling late-stage cancers out of the future into the present as early-stage cancers then, eventually, the incidence of late-stage cancer and cancer deaths should decline by an equivalent amount [14] (Figures 18.4, 18.5). Flat mortality trends, despite increased incidence, in concert with dissemination of a

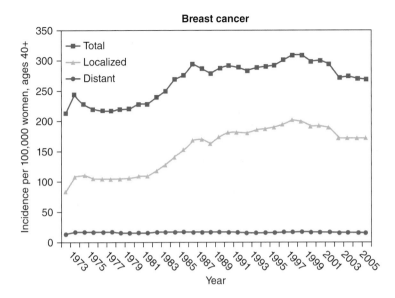

Figure 18.3 Incidence of localized breast cancer increases in parallel with increasing use of mammographic screening during the 1980s and 1990s. Distant disease remains constant, suggesting overdiagnosis. Adapted from [3]. For a color version of this figure please see color plate section.

screening test, suggest overdiagnosis. Successful therapy is unlikely to account for this entire cancer/mortality differential since, for this to be the case, the rate of improvement in treatment would have to match exactly the increase in true disease burden [4]. Decreasing mortality trends suggest effectiveness of screening or advances in effective therapy, but the relative contribution of the effects may be difficult to sort out.

Evidence for overdiagnosis from screening at individual disease sites

Analysis of trends in screening versus incidence, stage at diagnosis and mortality strongly suggest that overdiagnosis has been on the rise for a number of cancers.

Neuroblastoma

Neuroblastoma offers a classic example of extreme overdiagnosis, due to aggressive screening programs. This tumor of the sympathetic nervous system generally presents as a mass in the neck, chest, abdomen or pelvis in infants and toddlers [17]. Because fewer than 50% of cases are localized in an unscreened population, and many advanced tumors relapse after aggressive chemotherapy, screening for early detection seemed to offer promise for management of this disease.

The ease of screening, involving quantitation of the urinary catecholamine metabolites vanillylmandelic and homovanillic acid produced by neuroblastomas, led to adoption of these analyses as part of the standard evaluation of infants in Japan in 1984 [18]. The rates of diagnosis in Japan increased substantially, with age-standardized incidence rates for neuroblastoma in children younger than 15 years ranging from 7.5 to $9.1/10^6$ prior to 1985, in contrast to $19.5/10^6$ following the introduction of screening [19].

A population-based study in Osaka, Japan showed that incidence rates increased from 1970–84 (7.5 cases/10^6 children) to 1985–94 ($20.5/10^6$), the period of screening, whereas mortality rates remained stable ($4.3/10^6$) [18], strongly suggesting overdiagnosis. The increase in incidence was fully attributable to screening, since the incidence of clinically detected neuroblastomas (missed by screening) remained stable throughout the program. Studies in other countries yielded similar results. In Japan, the screening program was subsequently discontinued.

Breast cancer

Estimates of overdiagnosis with mammographic screening vary widely, ranging from less than 1% to nearly 50%, depending on the study methods and the denominator used (entire population eligible for screening; population actually screened; cancers

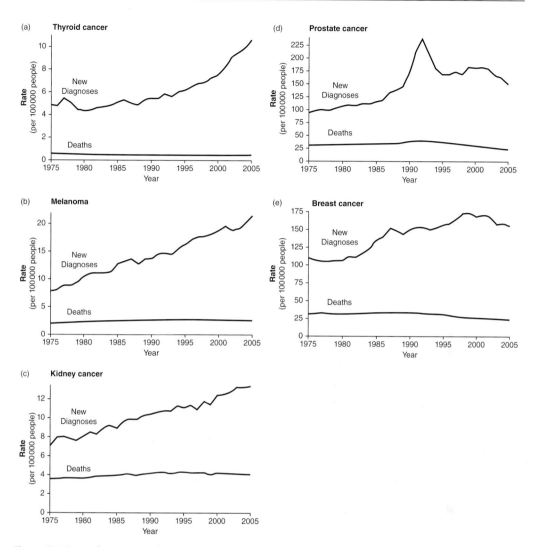

Figure 18.4 Rates of new cancer diagnoses are juxtaposed against cancer deaths for five different cancer types. Data are from the Surveillance, Epidemiology, and End Results (SEER) for years 1975 to 2005. Adapted from [4].

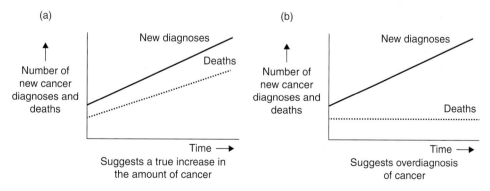

Figure 18.5 Two distinct relationships between new cancer diagnoses and cancer deaths are suggestive of true cancers versus overdiagnosed cancers. Adapted from [4].

among those screened), and depending upon whether *in situ* lesions are included [10, 16, 20]. A recent analysis examined trends in breast cancer incidence (invasive and *in situ*) from 1976 to 2008 in women 40 years of age or older, using the US Surveillance Epidemiology and End Results (SEER) data [16], encompassing eras before and after institution of mammographic screening in the US. A doubling of early-stage breast cancer cases detected each year (112 to 234 cases per 100 000 women) was seen, with a concomitant reduction in rate of late stages of only 8% (102 to 94 cases per 100 000 women) in the same time period, suggesting that only eight of these additional 122 early-stage cancers would have progressed to a late-stage cancer. The small observed reduction in late-stage cancers was restricted to locally advanced cancers, with metastatic disease showing virtually no decrease in rate. The authors estimated that 31% of all breast cancers diagnosed reflected overdiagnoses, with breast cancer having been overdiagnosed in 1.3 million US women in the past three decades [16].

Lung cancer

The Mayo Lung Project, one of the first lung cancer screening trials, provides evidence that screening can even lead to overdiagnosis of cancers generally felt to be highly lethal [21]. This RCT of 9211 male cigarette smokers, comparing standard chest X-rays (CXRs) plus sputum cytology to usual care, showed that lung cancer mortality was equivalent in the two arms. However, there was a persistent excess of cases in the screening arm during a 16-year follow-up period – 585 versus 500, suggesting overdiagnosis.

The randomized Prostate, Lung, Colorectal, and Ovarian (PLCO) Cancer Screening Trial similarly showed no reduction in lung cancer mortality using CXR, compared with usual care [22,23]. The 53 454 high-risk participants (due to a history of heavy smoking) enrolled in the US National Cancer Institute's National Lung Screening Trial (NLST) were randomized to undergo three annual screenings with Low Dose/Helical Computed Tomography (LDCT) ($n = 26\,722$) or single-view posteroanterior CXR ($n = 26\,732$) [24]. There is preliminary evidence, based on tumor doubling times of lung cancers detected by low-dose helical CT scans in a cohort study, that some tumors may be

overdiagnosed [25]. However, better evidence regarding whether LDCT is associated with overdiagnosis should come from ongoing analyses of randomized trials.

Prostate cancer

Since its introduction as a common screening test in the 1980s [26], routine prostate specific antigen (PSA) testing of healthy men has detected large numbers of prostate cancers from a reservoir of latent disease that would otherwise have remained undiscovered during their lifetime. The existence of this compartment of clinically occult disease is supported by incidental findings of prostate cancer, both in autopsy studies as well as radical cystoprostatectomy specimens [15,27]. This observation, together with the increasing proportion of tumors with low-risk features (clinically localized, stage T1c-T2a, Gleason score $\leq$ 6, PSA < 10 ng/ml)[1] supports the indolent nature of much of screen-detected disease [15].

Several large screening trials give insight into the impact of PSA screening on overdiagnosis. In the 76 693 men in the PLCO trial, the annual screening relative to the observation group showed a 22% increased prostate cancer incidence at seven years median follow-up [28], and a 12% relative increase at 13 years follow-up [29]. Yet, prostate cancer mortality did not differ significantly between the two arms at either follow-up analysis (7 years: 2.0 deaths/10 000 person-years with screening versus 1.7 deaths/10 000 person-years with observation, RR = 1.13; 95% CI, 0.75–1.70 [28]; 13 years: 3.7 deaths/10 000 person-years with screening versus 3.4 deaths/10 000 person-years with observation, RR = 1.09, CI = 0.87–1.36 [29]).

The European Study of Screening for Prostate Cancer (ERSPC) trial [30,31] included 162 387 men in the core 55–69 year age group, who were randomized to be offered screening every four years at most of the trial's European centers, versus usual care. A 71% increased incidence of prostate cancer was observed with screening versus usual care [30]. At nine years median follow-up, death due to prostate cancer or prostate cancer-related interventions in the screening, compared with the control group, showed a RR = 0.80 (95% CI = 0.65–0.98; $p = 0.04$), a small but significant absolute reduction of 0.71 prostate-cancer death/1000 men [30].

At 11 years median follow-up, RR = 0.79 (95% CI = 0.68–0.91; p = 0.0001) for prostate cancer-related death in the screening versus control group, there was an absolute reduction of 0.10 death/1000 men [31]. The inconsistency of the ERSPC's findings of a significant 20% (9 years) and 21% (11 years) risk reduction in the rate of prostate cancer-associated death with PSA-based screening versus the PLCO trial's findings may be due to the considerable differences in the study designs of the two trials.

Based in part on the clear evidence of overdiagnosis and resulting overtreatment, along with uncertain evidence of benefits, the US Preventive Services Task Force (USPSTF) issued a recommendation against routine prostate cancer screening in 2012 [32].

Thyroid cancer

The incidence of thyroid cancer has been increasing since at least 1973 among both women and men in every racial/ethnic group (except American Indian and Alaska Native men) in the US and internationally [33–35]. The increase is limited to the most common histologic type, papillary cancer, representing 80–85% of all thyroid cancers [33]. Although rising rates have been seen for all stages, the greatest increase has been in localized disease and in small cancers [34, 35]. Papillary thyroid cancers are known for their slow-growing behavior. Coincident with increased incidence, thyroid cancer-specific mortality remained stable [33, 34]. This disjoint between rising incidence (particularly of small cancers) and stable mortality rates is consistent with overdiagnosis.

Unlike the previous examples of cancers detected early as a result of directed, widespread implementation of new screening modalities, thyroid cancer is generally detected following palpation of a thyroid nodule on a routine physical exam (up to 21% are detectable by palpation) [36]. Such nodules are common, and are generally followed by ultrasound of the neck as a first-line diagnostic procedure, and then by fine needle aspiration cytology or increasingly invasive procedures to establish definitively the presence of malignancy [33, 36].

Cancer of the kidney and renal pelvis

The incidence of kidney cancer has also risen steadily in the US in recent decades [37], likely due to increased use of abdominal diagnostic imaging procedures such as computed tomography (CT) scanning, magnetic resonance imaging (MRI), and ultrasound even though there are no general screening programs for kidney cancer [38, 39]. Although apparent for all stages in a 1973 to 1998 analysis of SEER data, localized kidney cancer incidence increased more than regional and distant disease in this time period [37], and also from 1999 through 2008 [34]. Whole-body scans, a form of non-targeted screening that extends from the thorax to the pelvis, have also contributed to the up-tick in cases of tumors of the kidney and renal pelvis [8].

Melanoma

Population trends suggest a large measure of overdiagnosis of cutaneous melanoma [40–42]. There have been increased numbers of biopsies which were compounded, in the 1970s and 1980s, by changes in the pathologic criteria for diagnosing melanoma [40]. The heavy emphasis on screening for skin cancer by international public health recommendations, despite lack of evidence from RCTs, set the stage for overdiagnosis [43]. Furthermore, in a study of melanoma trends from 1986 to 2001, not only was the rising incidence of melanoma shown to correlate with increases in the average biopsy rate in the same period, but also the additional cases were limited to early-stage cancer, with mortality remaining stable [44]. Again, the disjoint between incidence/biopsy rate and stable mortality suggests overdiagnosis, explained by "increased diagnostic scrutiny and not an increase in the true incidence of disease" [44].

Overdiagnosis of non-invasive, premalignant lesions

Periodic screening of healthy individuals has resulted in increased numbers of pathologically non-invasive (i.e., pre-malignant) lesions, leaving in question whether, left alone, these would progress to invasive cancers that have potential to metastasize and kill. Routine mammographic screening starting in the 1980s led to a marked increase in detected cases of ductal carcinoma *in situ* (DCIS) [45]. It is likely that less than 50% of DCIS lesions go on to become invasive or metastasize, yet this pathologically non-invasive lesion is generally approached medically as if it is as life-threatening as invasive breast cancer [46], resulting in surgery, radiation and tamoxifen. In addition, the label "DCIS" – specifically, inclusion of the word "carcinoma" in its name – leads many patients to perceive themselves as "cancer patients" [47]. The anxiety attendant on this label can precipitate psychological, social and economic sequelae that compound the harms associated with physical overtreatment.

Barrett's esophagus (BE) is another non-invasive lesion that is often viewed as "pre-malignant". However, BE progresses to cancer – specifically esophageal adenocarcinoma (EA) – in only a small percent of cases, with 90–95% of patients with BE dying of unrelated causes, and the majority of EA cases occurring in patients with no prior diagnosis of BE [48]. Clearly, BE represents a situation of overdiagnosis of a pre-malignant lesion which only rarely is destined to progress to a symptomatic and lethal cancer.

Why does overdiagnosis matter and what can we do about it?

A diagnosis of "cancer" changes a person's life. The person has now become a patient with a dreaded disease [1, 49]. Physically debilitating diagnostic and therapeutic interventions are instituted as "logical" sequelae of the diagnosis. A myriad of negative psychosocial, quality-of-life and practical consequences ensue [50]. Anxiety, stress, and even suicide may increase following a diagnosis. Personal expenditures mount, there is discrimination regarding health and life insurance, and unemployment and even personal bankruptcy may also occur.

The notion that early detection necessarily improves outcomes is intuitive, resonating with patients, the public and health professionals [14, 50]. As far back as 1861, British physician Horace Dobell advanced regular health examinations as "the only means by which to reach the evil and to obtain the good" [3]. In the US, public health messages encouraging early detection rose to the forefront in the early 1900s, ultimately leading to the formation of what is now the American Cancer Society [51].

The strategy has been to inculcate a sense of vulnerability to cancer, and then offer hope [50,52]. The uncritical acceptance of screening has been called "a system without negative feedback." [53] Strong positive reinforcement is generated with each decision to screen for cancer, regardless of the outcome. If the screen is negative, the patient and the physician, reassured by the result, are pleased. If the screen is positive, both are grateful for early detection, irrespective of the nature of the discovered lesion and its downstream sequelae. Even overdiagnosis and overtreatment lead to a cycle of positive feedback [2, 53]. Evidence-based screening guidelines, such as those put forth by the USPSTF, have met with hostility from patients and physicians, who find them to be counterintuitive [14].

In 2012, the US National Cancer Institute convened a group of experts to consider remedies to the overdiagnosis-overtreatment conundrum [54]. A first suggestion was to revise nomenclature, reserving "cancer" or "carcinoma" for lesions likely to progress if untreated. This trend is already evident in terms like "cervical intraepithelial neoplasia" and "epithelial tumors of low malignant potential" for ovary. Similarly, an NIH State-of-the-Science Conference in 2009 proposed removing "carcinoma" from "DCIS" [55]. One suggestion is that lesions determined to be low-risk or indolent based on molecular analyses should be reclassified as "IDLE" (InDolent Lesion of Epithelial origin) [54]. Closely allied to lesion labeling that more accurately reflects tumor behavior is a proposal to reduce overdiagnosis by raising the threshold for calling a finding "abnormal" for call-back following radiologic or other technologic assessment [1, 4, 56].

"Companion diagnostics" [54] must accompany the changes in cancer terminology, so that tumor labels are tightly linked to the underlying biological behavior of the lesion. At the root of companion diagnostics is molecular profiling of tumors, to enable overdiagnoses to be distinguished from aggressive cancers [57, 58]. This discriminatory ability would facilitate appropriate targeting of therapeutic interventions to lesions destined to grow and metastasize. Lesions molecularly characterized as indolent – "overdiagnosed" – could avoid "overtreatment" and be managed by surveillance or less aggressive interventions. Already, early-stage estrogen receptor-positive breast cancers are being categorized into prognostic levels by molecular signatures based on the Oncotype DX® (Genomic Health) test [59]. The Oncotype DX "recurrence score" guides decisions as to whether adjuvant chemotherapy should be administered.

The development of increasingly accurate models of cancer risk is critical, in order to better define cohorts to which validated screening modalities are targeted. This should increase the likelihood that a "positive" screening outcome is meaningful. Established risk factors for some common cancers have informed the design of screening and prevention trials with high-risk cohorts, based on our current state of knowledge [60–62]. Women at increased breast cancer risk have been identified, based on Gail model risk factors [63]. Men at increased risk of prostate cancer may be identified, based on family history of the disease and African-American race [64]. Efforts to refine risk models for specific cancers are ongoing [32, 63, 65, 66], incorporating newer information, such as mammographic density [67] and genetic variants derived from genome-wide association studies (GWAS) for breast cancer [68].

The patient, especially, must be brought into the conversation. The complexity of decision-making with respect to being screened for cancer, and what to do if "abnormalities" are discovered, can be overwhelming. The prospective RCTs that underlie screening recommendations are conducted at a population, not an individual, level. The outcomes are couched in probabilities or risks. A key challenge in communicating screening recommendations to patients is to make the connection between such probabilistic results and the individual in front of the physician in the clinic. A deeper understanding of this critical distinction requires that we educate patients and the public at large on how "to work with probabilities and changes in probabilities" [69].

The conundrum posed by screen-detected diagnoses is that there is currently no way to determine which are overdiagnoses at the time of screening [4]. Overtreatment and associated adverse sequelae can only be reduced by improving our ability to distinguish overdiagnoses from aggressive cancers detected by cancer screens, based on their respective molecular profiles. In addition to the cancer cells themselves, the tumor microenvironment undergoes changes – for example, compromises in its immune and vascular components – that promote carcinogenesis. A better understanding of the relationship of tumor aggressiveness to the state of the microenvironment should also assist in identifying overdiagnoses. Technological inroads into identifying genomic signatures that characterize cancers and pre-cancers already offer tools for making decisions about therapy in specific cancer presentations [59]. Comparable approaches to seeking associations between prognoses and the molecular features of screen-detected tumors should facilitate identification of lesions that are overdiagnoses and do not require aggressive interventions.

This discussion of overdiagnosis is not intended to debunk the potential value of screening for preclinical cancers with the goal of catching cancers early, in order to optimize treatment outcomes. The purpose is, rather, to emphasize the need for balanced messages to convey that overdiagnosis and resulting overtreatment are not rare, in an era of increasingly sensitive screening tests. We need to develop refined approaches that delve within the reservoir of pre-cancers to distinguish indolent (i.e., overdiagnosed) lesions from clinically meaningful cancers requiring treatment. The overall goal is not to discourage screening tests of proven efficacy but, rather, to maximize the benefits of those screening tests that have proven efficacy, and to minimize their harms [50].

References

1. Moynihan R, Doust J, Henry D (2012). Preventing overdiagnosis: how to stop harming the healthy. *BMJ* **344**, e3502.

2. Klotz L (2012). Cancer overdiagnosis and overtreatment. *Current Opinion in Urology* **22**, 203–9.

3. Croswell JM, Ransohoff DF, Kramer BS (2010). Principles of cancer screening: lessons from history and study design issues. *Seminars in Oncology* **37**, 202–15.

4. Welch HG, Black WC (2010). Overdiagnosis in cancer. *Journal of the National Cancer Institute* **102**, 605–13.

5. Draisma G, Boer R, Otto SJ, *et al.* (2003). Lead times and overdetection due to prostate-specific antigen screening: estimates from the European Randomized Study of Screening for Prostate Cancer. *Journal of the National Cancer Institute* **95**, 868–78.

6. Klotz L (2013). Prostate cancer overdiagnosis and overtreatment. *Current Opinion in Endocrinology, Diabetes, and Obesity* **20**, 204–9.

7. Orme NM, Fletcher JG, Siddiki HA, *et al.* (2010). Incidental findings in imaging research: evaluating incidence, benefit, and burden. *Archives of Internal Medicine* **170**, 1525–32.

8. Fenton JJ, Weiss NS (2004). Screening computed tomography: will it result in overdiagnosis of renal carcinoma? *Cancer* **100**, 986–90.

9. Schwartz LM, Woloshin S (1999). Changing disease definitions: implications for disease prevalence. Analysis of the Third National Health and Nutrition Examination Survey, 1988–1994. *Effective Clinical Practice* **2**, 76–85.

10. Nelson HD, Tyne K, Naik A, Bougatsos C, Chan BK, Humphrey L (2009). Screening for breast cancer: an update for the U.S. *Preventive Services Task Force. Annals of Internal Medicine* **151**, 727–37, W237–42.

11. Welch HG, Black WC (1997). Using autopsy series to estimate the disease "reservoir" for ductal carcinoma *in situ* of the breast: how much more breast cancer can we find? *Annals of Internal Medicine* **127**, 1023–8.

12. Stamatiou K, Alevizos A, Agapitos E, Sofras F (2006). Incidence of impalpable carcinoma of the prostate and of non-malignant and precarcinomatous lesions in Greek male population: an autopsy study. *Prostate* **66**, 1319–28.

13. Damiano R, Di Lorenzo G, Cantiello F, *et al.* (2007). Clinicopathologic features of prostate adenocarcinoma incidentally discovered at the time of radical cystectomy: an evidence-based analysis. *European Urology* **52**, 648–57.

14. Kramer BS, Croswell JM (2009). Cancer screening: the clash of science and intuition. *Annual Review of Medicine* **60**, 125–37.

15. Sandhu GS, Andriole GL (2012). Overdiagnosis of prostate cancer. J Natl Cancer Inst Monogr; 2012, 146–51.

16. Bleyer A, Welch HG (2012). Effect of three decades of screening mammography on breast-cancer incidence. *New England Journal of Medicine* **367**, 1998–2005.

17. Maris JM. Recent advances in neuroblastoma (2010). *New England Journal of Medicine* **362**, 2202–11.

18. Ajiki W, Tsukuma H, Oshima A, Kawa K (1998). Effects of mass screening for neuroblastoma on incidence, mortality, and survival rates in Osaka, Japan. Cancer Causes Control;9, 631–6.

19. Bessho F (1996). Effects of mass screening on age-specific incidence of neuroblastoma. *International Journal of Cancer* **67**, 520–2.

20. Kalager M, Adami HO, Bretthauer M, Tamimi RM (2012). Overdiagnosis of invasive breast cancer due to mammography screening: results from the Norwegian screening program. *Annals of Internal Medicine* **156**, 491–9.

21. Marcus PM, Bergstralh EJ, Zweig MH, Harris A, Offord KP, Fontana RS (2006). Extended lung cancer incidence follow-up in the Mayo Lung Project and overdiagnosis. *Journal of the National Cancer Institute* **98**, 748–56.

22. Oken MM, Hocking WG, Kvale PA, *et al.* (2011). Screening by chest radiograph and lung cancer mortality: the Prostate, Lung, Colorectal, and Ovarian (PLCO) randomized trial. *JAMA* **306**, 1865–73.

23. Hocking WG, Hu P, Oken MM, *et al.* (2010). Lung cancer screening in the randomized Prostate, Lung, Colorectal, and Ovarian (PLCO) Cancer Screening Trial. *Journal of the National Cancer Institute* **102**, 722–31.

24. Aberle DR, Adams AM, Berg CD, *et al.* (2011). Reduced lung-cancer mortality with low-dose computed tomographic screening. *New England Journal of Medicine* **365**, 395–409.

25. Veronesi G, Maisonneuve P, Bellomi M, *et al.* (2012). Estimating overdiagnosis in low-dose computed tomography screening for lung cancer: a cohort study. *Annals of Internal Medicine* **157**, 776–84.

26. Catalona WJ, Smith DS, Ratliff TL, *et al.* (1991). Measurement of prostate-specific antigen in serum as a screening test for prostate cancer. *New England Journal of Medicine* **324**, 1156–61.

27. Pettus JA, Al-Ahmadie H, Barocas DA, *et al.* (2008). Risk assessment of prostatic pathology in patients undergoing radical cystoprostatectomy. *European Urology* **53**, 370–5.

28. Andriole GL, Crawford ED, Grubb RL, 3rd, *et al.* (2009). Mortality results from a randomized prostate-cancer screening trial. *New England Journal of Medicine* **360**, 1310–9.

29. Andriole GL, Crawford ED, Grubb RL, 3rd, *et al.* (2012). Prostate Cancer Screening in the Randomized Prostate, Lung, Colorectal, and Ovarian Cancer Screening Trial: Mortality Results after 13 Years of Follow-up. *Journal of the National Cancer Institute* **104**, 125–32.

30. Schroder FH, Hugosson J, Roobol MJ, *et al.* (2009). Screening and prostate-cancer mortality in a randomized European study. *New England Journal of Medicine* **360**, 1320–8.

31. Schroder FH, Hugosson J, Roobol MJ, *et al.* (2012). Prostate-cancer mortality at 11 years of follow-up. *New England Journal of Medicine* **366**, 981–90.

32. Moyer VA (2012). Screening for prostate cancer: U.S. Preventive Services Task Force recommendation statement. *Annals of Internal Medicine* **157**, 120–34.

33. Davies L, Welch HG (2006). Increasing incidence of thyroid cancer in the United States, 1973–2002. *JAMA* **295**, 2164–7.

34. Simard EP, Ward EM, Siegel R, Jemal A (2012). Cancers with increasing incidence trends in the United States: 1999 through 2008. *CA: A Cancer Journal for Clinicians* **62**, 118–28.

35. Hakala T, Kellokumpu-Lehtinen P, Kholova I, Holli K, Huhtala H, Sand J (2012). Rising incidence of small size papillary thyroid cancers with no change in disease-specific survival in finnish thyroid cancer patients. *Scandinavian Journal of Surgery* **101**, 301–6.

36. Pacini F, Castagna MG, Brilli L, Pentheroudakis G (2012). Thyroid cancer: ESMO Clinical Practice Guidelines for diagnosis, treatment and follow-up. *Annals of Oncology* **23** Suppl 7, vii110–9.

37. Hock LM, Lynch J, Balaji KC (2002). Increasing incidence of all stages of kidney cancer in the last 2 decades in the United States: an analysis of surveillance, epidemiology and end results program data. *Journal of Urology* **167**, 57–60.

38. Mitchell TL, Pippin JJ, Devers SM, *et al.* (2000). Incidental detection of preclinical renal tumors with electron beam computed tomography: report of 26 consecutive operated patients. *Journal of Computer Assisted Tomography* **24**, 843–5.

39. Hara AK, Johnson CD, MacCarty RL, Welch TJ (2000). Incidental extracolonic findings at CT colonography. *Radiology* **215**, 353–7.

40. Weyers W (2012). The 'epidemic' of melanoma between under- and overdiagnosis. *Journal of Cutaneous Pathology* **39**, 9–16.

41. Koh HK (1991). Cutaneous melanoma. *New England Journal of Medicine* **325**, 171–82.

42. Glusac EJ (2012). The melanoma 'epidemic': lessons from prostate cancer. *Journal of Cutaneous Pathology* **39**, 17–20.

43. Wolff T, Tai E, Miller T (2009). Screening for skin cancer: an update of the evidence for the U.S. Preventive Services Task Force. *Annals of Internal Medicine* **150**, 194–8.

44. Welch HG, Woloshin S, Schwartz LM (2005). Skin biopsy rates and incidence of melanoma: population based ecological study. *BMJ* **331**, 481.

45. Ernster VL, Barclay J (1997). Increases in ductal carcinoma in situ (DCIS) of the breast in relation to mammography: a dilemma. *Journal of the National Cancer Institute. Monographs* 151–6.

46. Ganz PA (2010). Quality-of-life issues in patients with ductal carcinoma *in situ*. *Journal of the National Cancer Institute. Monographs* **2010**, 218–22.

47. Veronesi U, Zurrida S, Goldhirsch A, Rotmensz N, Viale G (2009). Breast cancer classification: time for a change. *Journal of Clinical Oncology* **27**, 2427–8.

48. Reid BJ, Li X, Galipeau PC, Vaughan TL (2010). Barrett's oesophagus and oesophageal adenocarcinoma:

time for a new synthesis. *Nature Reviews Cancer* **10**, 87–101.

49. Welch HG, Schwartz LM, Woloshin S (2011). *Overdiagnosed. Making People Sick in the Pursuit of Health.* Boston, Massachusetts: Beacon Press.

50. Dunn BK, Srivastava S, Kramer BS (2013). The word "cancer": how language can corrupt thought. *BMJ* **347**, f5328.

51. Cantor D (2007). Introduction: cancer control and prevention in the twentieth century. *Bulletin of the History of Medicine* **81**, 1–38.

52. Woloshin S, Schwartz LM, Black WC, Kramer BS (2012). Cancer screening campaigns – getting past uninformative persuasion. *New England Journal of Medicine* **367**, 1677–9.

53. Ransohoff DF, McNaughton Collins M, Fowler FJ (2002). Why is prostate cancer screening so common. when the evidence is so uncertain? A system without negative feedback. *American Journal of Medicine* **113**, 663–7.

54. Esserman LJ, Thompson IM, Reid B (2013). Overdiagnosis and Overtreatment in Cancer: An Opportunity for Improvement. *JAMA* **310**, 797–8.

55. NIH State-of-the-Science Conference (2009): *Diagnosis and Management of Ductal Carcinoma in Situ (DCIS)*. September 22–24 (Accessed August 21, 2013, at http://consensus.nih.gov/2009/dcis.htm).

56. Smith-Bindman R, Chu PW, Miglioretti DL, *et al.* (2003). Comparison of screening mammography in the United States and the United kingdom. *JAMA* **290**, 2129–37.

57. Crispo A, Barba M, D'Aiuto G, *et al.* (2013). Molecular profiles of screen detected vs. symptomatic breast cancer and their impact on survival: results from a clinical series. *BMC Cancer* **13**, 15–25.

58. Domingo L, Blanch J, Servitja S, *et al.* (2013). Aggressiveness features and outcomes of true interval cancers: comparison between screen-detected and symptom-detected cancers. *European Journal of Cancer Prevention* **22**, 21–8.

59. Paik S, Shak S, Tang G, *et al.* (2004). A multigene assay to predict recurrence of tamoxifen-treated, node-negative breast cancer. *New England Journal of Medicine* **351**, 2817–26.

60. Gohagan JK, Prorok PC, Hayes RB, Kramer BS (2000). The Prostate, Lung, Colorectal and Ovarian (PLCO) Cancer Screening Trial of the National Cancer Institute: history, organization, and status. *Controlled Clinical Trials* **21**, 251S–72S.

61. Fisher B, Costantino JP, Wickerham DL, *et al.* (1998). Tamoxifen for prevention of breast cancer: report of the National Surgical Adjuvant Breast and Bowel Project P-1 Study. *Journal of the National Cancer Institute* **90**, 1371–88.

62. Thompson IM, Goodman PJ, Tangen CM, *et al.* (2003). The influence of finasteride on the development of prostate cancer. *New England Journal of Medicine* **349**, 215–24.

63. Gail MH, Brinton LA, Byar DP, *et al.* (1989). Projecting individualized probabilities of developing breast cancer for white females who are being examined annually. *Journal of the National Cancer Institute* **81**, 1879–86.

64. Zhu X, Albertsen PC, Andriole GL, Roobol MJ, Schroder FH, Vickers AJ (2012). Risk-Based Prostate Cancer Screening. *European Urology* **61**, 652–61.

65. Tyrer J, Duffy SW, Cuzick J (2004). A breast cancer prediction model incorporating familial and personal risk factors. *Statistics in Medicine* **23**, 1111–30.

66. Tammemagi MC, Katki HA, Hocking WG, *et al.* (2013). Selection criteria for lung-cancer screening. *New England Journal of Medicine* **368**, 728–36.

67. Chen J, Pee D, Ayyagari R, *et al.* (2006). Projecting absolute invasive breast cancer risk in white women with a model that includes mammographic density. *Journal of the National Cancer Institute* **98**, 1215–26.

68. Wacholder S, Hartge P, Prentice R, *et al.* (2010). Performance of common genetic variants in breast-cancer risk models. *New England Journal of Medicine* **362**, 986–93.

69. Woloshin S, Schwartz LM, Welch HG (2007). The effectiveness of a primer to help people understand risk: two randomized trials in distinct populations. *Annals of Internal Medicine* **146**, 256–65.

CHAPTER 19

Predictive Markers and Driver Genes From Treatment Trials: Potential Utility For Early Diagnosis

Brian S Sorg, Sarfraz Memon, Kelly Y Kim, Aniruddha Ganguly, Tracy Lively, James Tricoli, Magdalena Thurin, Lokesh Agrawal, Tawnya C McKee, Barbara A Conley, and J Milburn Jessup

Cancer Diagnosis Program, Division of Cancer Treatment and Diagnosis, Bethesda, MD, USA

All of the authors are employees of the US Federal Government and declare that they do not have financial conflicts of interest.

Introduction

A biomarker is a "characteristic that is objectively measured and evaluated as an indicator of normal biological processes, pathogenic processes, or pharmacologic responses to a therapeutic intervention" [1]. As reviewed by Poste *et al.* [2], there are five types of markers used in clinical trials. Pharmacokinetic markers assess the absorption, distribution, metabolism, and excretion of a drug or agent, while pharmacodynamic markers measure whether an agent interacts with its intended target. These markers are important in early-phase trials, are not used for medical decision-making, and do not need to be performed in a clinical laboratory. In contrast, the other three markers (pharmacogenomics, prognostic and predictive) are often used for medical decision-making and, therefore, need to be performed in an appropriately certified clinical laboratory.

Pharmacogenomic markers are inherited in the germ line, typically involve single nucleotide polymorphisms (SNPs) or variants with more than one nucleotide, and identify the risk of organ-based toxicities or altered metabolism and/or responses to therapeutic agents. Prognostic markers are associated with survival or other clinical endpoints *independently* of any specific treatment. In contrast, predictive markers predict the response to a *specific therapy*, and identify individual patients who are more likely to respond to a particular drug. Once molecular alterations are identified, then patients whose tumors contain those alterations are candidates for therapy.

We will focus in this chapter primarily on mutations in driver genes that are also predictive markers in current clinical trials and might be useful for early diagnosis, if they may be detected with minimally invasive technologies. This will entail, first, a broad listing of predictive markers, followed by

Biomarkers in Cancer Screening and Early Detection, First Edition. Edited by Sudhir Srivastava.
© 2017 John Wiley & Sons, Inc. Published 2017 by John Wiley & Sons, Inc.

a brief discussion of minimally invasive technologies that may be applicable to early diagnosis, and then to review the current status of genetic alterations that are predictive markers, may be useful for early diagnosis, and are derived from The Cancer Genome Atlas (TCGA) studies of over 3000 tumors [3]. This review suggests how driver genes and therapeutic predictive markers may be integrated into a screening program for cancer prior to the development of clinical symptoms.

Common predictive markers

Predictive markers have different levels of importance for treatment trials, because they may be integral (essential for the performance of the trial), integrated (performed in all or a predefined subset of patients in a trial, or to test a prespecified hypothesis), or research (hypothesis generating) markers. We will focus on those predictive markers that result from genetic alteration during carcinogenesis, because those markers are the ones that may be detected by minimally invasive, but sensitive, sequencing technologies. However, it is important to realize that important integral predictive markers are not always the result of somatic mutation, but may involve the altered expression of otherwise normal hormones and other proteins or biological substances.

As can be seen (Table 19.1), a number of these markers predict either a direct response within a patient's tumor, or suggest a treatment approach that is likely to yield improved clinical outcome. A survey of predictive markers in NCI-supported trials suggests that considerable research and development of new agents has focused on the RAS/RAF/MAPK and PI3K-AKT/PTEN pathways (Figure 19.1). This is because these two pathways control cell proliferation and survival, either directly or through cross-talk with other pathways, such as the Insulin Growth Factor (IGF) pathway, which is important in many malignancies. Description of such cross-talk, and even the other pathways involved, is beyond the scope of this review.

Minimally invasive technologies

Following the introduction of polymerase chain reaction (PCR) techniques to measure mutations in

such genes as *APC*, *KRAS* and *TP53* in various body fluids in the 1990s (reviewed in Burchill and Selby [4] and Sidransky [5]), it became clear that assessment of DNA, or even RNA, in plasma or serum was possible, especially with the finding by Diehl *et al.* [6] that an emulsion-based digital PCR technique enabled estimation of the number of copies of a gene in the circulation, and even the fraction of copies that are mutated. Diehl *et al.* [6] found that not only did patients with advanced cancer have circulating DNA with mutated *APC*, but 60% of early stage I and II colorectal carcinoma patients also had detectable mutant *APC* in their plasma DNA, albeit at a level that was about one-tenth of the levels in advanced disease patients. This supported the finding that patients with cancer generally have as much as two- to five-fold more circulating cell free DNA (cfDNA) in plasma or serum [7–13] than patients without cancer, even in patients with early stage disease [11].

Zhang *et al.* [13] performed a meta-analysis of cfDNA, as a screening assay for lung cancer, which suggested that elevation of circulating cfDNA had an accuracy of 88% for a cancer diagnosis. Of course, cfDNA may also be increased in plasma or serum by inflammation, trauma and other conditions that cause tissue degradation [14–19]. As detailed below, the cfDNA levels may be elevated in patients without cancer beyond those expected for patients with cancer, but identification of mutated DNA enables detection of cancer prior to symptoms. Patient history, as well as standard tumor markers, may also clarify whether other conditions cause an elevation in cfDNA. While most of this cfDNA is degraded to fairly small sizes, it is similar to the DNA that is obtained from formalin-fixed paraffin-embedded tissues, which is now being analyzed by next generation sequencing [20,21]. Thus, a strategy for screening patients with cancer in a general low-risk population may be to screen for patients with high cfDNA levels, and then to do more extensive studies to identify mutations within those patients.

Mutational landscape of driver genes in cancer

In an overview of the implications of the current state of mutational analysis of cancers presented

Table 19.1 Predictive markers currently in use either as part of standard treatment or under clinical investigation.

Breast carcinoma			
Marker	*Alteration*	*Clinical use*	*Current development status*
Estrogen receptor (ER)	Expression	Targeted therapy, therapeutic decision-making	Standard treatment
Progesterone receptor (PR)	Expression	Targeted therapy, therapeutic decision-making	Standard treatment
HER2	Expression	Targeted therapy, therapeutic decision-making	Standard treatment
MAPK	mutation	Targeted therapy	Investigational
Colorectal carcinoma			
Marker	*Alteration*	*Clinical use*	*Current development status*
KRAS	mutation	Resistance to anti-EGFR therapy	Standard treatment
BRAF	mutation	Resistance to anti-EGFR therapy	Investigational
PI3KCA	mutation	Resistance to anti-EGFR therapy	Investigational
PTEN	expression	Resistance to anti-EGFR therapy	Investigational
Melanoma			
Marker	*Alteration*	*Clinical use*	*Current development status*
BRAF	mutation	Targeted therapy	Standard treatment
NRAS	mutation	Therapeutic decision-making	Investigational
PIK3CA	mutation	Therapeutic decision-making	Investigation
Ovarian carcinoma			
Marker	*Alteration*	*Clinical use*	*Current development status*
c-KIT and PDGFR	mutation	Targeted therapy	Investigational
CA125	expression	Therapeutic decision-making	Standard treatment
TP53	mutation	Diagnosis	Standard treatment
Non-small cell lung cancer			
Marker	*Alteration*	*Clinical use*	*Current development status*
EGFR	mutation	Targeted therapy	Standard treatment
KRAS	mutation	Therapeutic decision-making	Investigational
EML-ALK	fusion gene	Targeted therapy	Standard treatment
Head and neck cancer			
Marker	*Alteration*	*Clinical use*	*Current development status*
HPV and p16	Protein/gene expression	Therapeutic decision-making	Investigational
Prostate			
Marker	*Alteration*	*Clinical use*	*Current development status*
Testosterone	Hormone expression	Therapeutic decision-making, targeted therapy	Standard treatment
Synaptophysin	Protein expression	Therapeutic decision-making	Standard treatment
Prostate-Specific Antigen (PSA)	Protein expression	Therapeutic decision-making	
TMPRSS2-ETS	fusion gene	Therapeutic decision-making	Investigational
Hepatocellular carcinoma			
Marker	*Alteration*	*Clinical use*	*Current development status*
Alpha-fetoprotein (α-fetoprotein, AFP)	Protein expression	Therapeutic decision-making	Standard treatment
EGFR	Protein expression	Therapeutic decision-making	Investigational

(continued)

Table 19.1 (Continued)

Glioblastoma			
Marker	Alteration	Clinical use	Current development status
MGMT (06-methylguanine-DNAMT3A	Gene expression	Therapeutic decision-making	Standard treatment
IDH1/2	mutation	Targeted therapy	Investigational
EGFR	Protein expression	Therapeutic decision-making	Investigational
Myeloproliferative diseases			
Marker	Alteration	Clinical use	Current development status
JAK2	Mutation	Targeted therapy	Standard treatment
PDGFR	Fusion gene	Targeted therapy	Investigational
FLT3	mutation	Targeted therapy	Investigational
Cereblon	Gene expression	Targeted therapy	Investigational
Bruton tyrosine kinase	Gene expression	Targeted therapy	Investigational
Chronic lymphocytic leukemia (CLL)			
Marker	Alteration	Clinical use	Current development status
IgVH	Mutation, fusion gene	Therapeutic decision-making	Investigational
17p deletion	Cytogenetics	Therapeutic decision-making	Standard treatment
13q deletion	Cytogenetics	Therapeutic decision-making	Standard treatment
11q deletion	Cytogenetics	Therapeutic decision-making	Standard treatment
Notch1	Mutation	Therapeutic decision-making	Investigational
SF3B1	Mutation	Therapeutic decision-making	Investigational
CD38	Protein expression	Targeted therapy, therapeutic decision-making	Investigational

Marker – the name of marker, whether it is a gene, protein or cytogenetic marker,

Alteration – refers to the type of change sought in a marker: mutation indicates that an alteration in the DNA (commonly) or RNA sequence is assayed; fusion gene indicates that the marker is part of a translocation where the DNA sequence of the fusion is assayed; expression indicates that the protein or gene transcript or hormone is measured.

Clinical use – indicates whether the marker is used for targeted therapy (directed to the marker itself) or for therapeutic decision-making (marker used in deciding what treatment to give a patient – treatment generally does not target marker directly).

Current development status – refers to whether marker is accepted into standard clinical practice (standard treatment) or is under development as a marker in clinical trials (investigational).

by Vogelstein and colleagues [22], several 'facts' appeared to emerge from present DNA sequencing studies, as well as earlier studies based on the development of colorectal carcinoma [23]:

1 most mutations in cancers occur stochastically during aging, or in response to genetic stressors (e.g., UV light for cutaneous melanoma, or cigarette smoking for lung cancer);

2 most mutations, therefore, occur during the preneoplastic growth phase;

3 only a few mutations are drivers, each of these drivers confers only a small growth advantage

for the malignancy [24], and metastasis may not require specific additional gene mutations, since even normal cells placed in abnormal tissue sites may form colonies [25].

Other alterations that may also be measured in tumors are promoter methylation, amplifications/deletions, or other copy number changes that may involve not only genes, but also whole chromosomes (aneuploidy), as well as chromosome translocations (e.g., BCR-ABL in chronic myelogenous leukemia). The important point is the concept that most somatic mutations in cancers are present

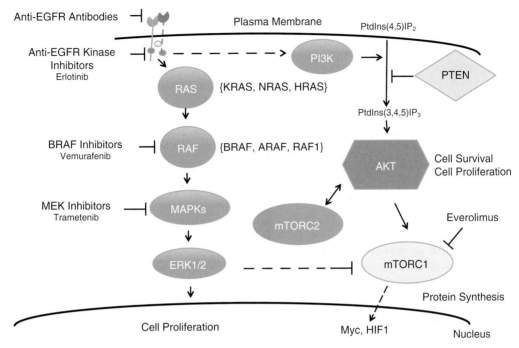

Figure 19.1 Predictive markers in human cancers. The common markers are depicted that are the targets of specific therapies, as indicated by the (⊣). The dashed brown receptor kinase indicates a mutation in the receptor that may cause constitutive activation of that receptor with consequent activation of the downstream molecules.

While EGFR is depicted, other receptors, such as the Insulin Growth Factor Receptor (IGFR), the Platelet Derived Growth Factor Receptor (PDGFR), and so on, may also be activated by mutation or even fusion with other genes. Arrows denote stimulation of the molecular marker. For a color version of this figure please see color plate section.

at the time of diagnosis. Vogelstein *et al.* [22] put forth the concept that, since mutation in *TP53* is the most frequently mutated gene in cancer, its loss of the ability to initiate apoptosis during DNA damage enables the cancer cell to survive the otherwise deleterious effect of many translocations and somatic mutations. A summary of the number of driver gene mutations in common cancers suggests that:

1 There are ≈ 125 driver genes, with 71 tumor suppressors and 54 oncogenes.
2 Common cancers contain on average only between 1 and 8 driver oncogene and/or tumor suppressor genes.

The implication of these findings is that if preneoplastic or early malignant lesions release DNA or protein into the circulation or other body fluids, then it should be possible, with current and

evolving technologies, to identify these mutations to indicate the presence of cancer.

The Pan-Cancer analysis project of TCGA [3] analyzed 3281 cancers across 12 common sites that included bladder urothelial carcinoma, breast invasive carcinoma, colon and rectum adenocarcinoma, Glioblastoma multiformae, head and neck squamous cell carcinoma, kidney renal clear-cell carcinoma, acute myeloid leukemia, lung adenocarcinoma, lung squamous cell carcinoma, ovarian serous cystadenocarcinoma, and uterine corpus endometrioid. The formal analysis [26] identified what it called 127 significantly mutated genes, similar to those Vogelstein *et al.* [22] reported. In addition, these authors assessed the frequency of variant alleles in tumors of the 12 disease types that are similar to what Vogelstein *et al.* [22] termed the trunks of cancers, or the early appearing drivers.

By concentrating on those genes with mutations that have a greater than median variant allele fraction (VAF), one might be able to screen for cancer by testing for driver mutations whose expression in cfDNA is likely to be high enough to be able to be detected across common cancers. Using this approach with data from the Pan-Cancer Analysis (Supplementary Table 11b) [26], there are 41 genes whose VAF is greater than the median in at least one of the 12 disease types (Table 19.2). These genes might be useful for early screening if there was a way to easily screen for those patients where the prevalence of cancer may be increased, over that of the general population that does not have an inherited cancer syndrome.

What are the predictive markers that are most likely to be useful for early diagnosis?

As suggested by Vogelstein *et al.* [22] and the Pan-Cancer Analysis [26], there are several pathways that have commonly activated driver mutations, so that they are primary targets for therapy and have a high median VAF. Since the postulate is that most cancers will have evolved with the primary driver mutations established in the cancer by the time of diagnosis, it is reasonable to theorize that searching for the common driver mutations in body fluids such as blood may aid in the early diagnosis of cancer. The following sections describe candidates that could be used for early detection, based on driver mutations/predictive markers in the pathways of *PI3K/AKT/PTEN* and *RAS/RAF/MAPK/AKT* and then individual genes *TP53, c-KIT, IDH1/2,* and *DNMT3A*. There are a number of other driver genes that are potential candidates (Table 19.2) but, with the exception of *TP53*, the following genes are targets for drugs in current clinical trials that predict response to therapy, so that identification of mutation in these genes may also suggest a possible treatment.

The *PI3K/AKT/PTEN* pathway

Defects in this pathway appear to be important for resistance to inhibition of the erb-B family members, such as inhibition of Epidermal Growth Factor Receptor (*EGFR, erb-B1*) or *HER-2* (erb-B2),

as well the ligands for the erb-B receptors such as neuregulin. Defects in this signaling pathway are very common in breast cancer [27]. Loss of PTEN expression and mutational activation of *PI3K/AKT* appear to be a frequent mechanism of acquired resistance to anti-HER2 agents [28]. The results of phase II/III clinical trials of small-molecule inhibitors of mTOR are very promising in breast cancer [29].

Activating mutations in *PI3K* and/or loss of PTEN expression constitutively activate the *PI3K/AKT* pathway, and have been associated with lack of response to anti-EGFR therapy in the *KRAS* wild type Colorectal Carcinoma (CRC) [30]. The *PI3KCA* gene encodes the p110 alpha catalytic subunit of PI3K. Somatic mutations in *PI3KCA* have been identified in 10–20% of CRC, and are associated with proximal location, MSI and *KRAS* mutation. The majority of these activating mutations map to exon 9 (codons 542 and 545 in the helical domain) and exon 20 (codon 1047 in the kinase domain). PTEN activity may also be lost, due to a number of mechanisms including mutations, deletion, and promoter methylation [31]. Retrospective analyses suggest that non-responders to anti-EGFR therapy can be identified by alterations in *KRAS, BRAF, PIK3CA,* and *PTEN,* and that patients who are "quadruple negative" for these mutations and alterations may have the highest probability of response to anti-EGFR therapies [30, 31].

Genetic alterations in the *PI3K/AKT* pathway in melanoma are not as prevalent as in the MAPK pathway alterations, but large genetic diversity affects this pathway. Although activating mutations in *PI3K* are rare, expression of downstream effectors, including PTEN and AKT, is altered in a subset of melanomas [32]. Allelic loss or altered expression through epigenetic silencing or mutations of PTEN comprises 20% and 40% of melanomas, respectively. *PTEN* loss leads to activation of AKT, which acts as a regulator of another downstream effector, mTOR pathway, and inhibitors of AKT and mTOR are being explored in the clinic.

Murtaza *et al.* [33] were able to sequence *PIK3CA* mutations in plasma cfDNA, as were Higgins *et al.* [34]. This provides the proof of principle that somatic mutations in the PI3K/AKT/PTEN pathway may be detected. Recent studies have also

Table 19.2 Most common driver genes in the pan-cancer analysis in the 12 disease sites in TCGA.

Gene	Primary site(s)								
ACVR1B	CRC								
AKT1	Breast								
ARID1A	NSCLC-Sq	Endometrium							
BAP1	RCC								
CBFB	Breast								
CCND1	Endometrium								
CTCF	Breast								
CTNNB1	CRC								
DNMT3A	AML								
EPHA3	NSCLC-Sq								
FGFR2	Endometrium								
FGFR3	Bladder								
FOXA2	Endometrium								
IDH1	AML	GBM							
IDH2	AML	GBM							
KEAP1	NSCLC-Sq	NSCLC-Ad							
KIT	AML								
KRAS	NSCLC-Ad	CRC							
MAP2K	Breast	NSCLC-Ad							
MLL2	Bladder								
NCOR1	Breast								
NOTCH1	NSCLC-Sq								
NSD1	H & N								
PBRM1	RCC								
PIK3CA	Endometrium	Breast	CRC	NSCLC-Ad	NASCLC-Sq				
PPP2R1A	Endometrium								
PTEN	NSCLC-Sq	Endometrium	CRC						
RAD21	AML								
RB1	Bladder	Breast	NSCLC-Sq						
RPL22	Endometrium								
RUNX1	AML								
SMAD4	CRC								
SMC3	AML								
SOX17	Endometrium								
SPOP	Endometrium								
STK11	NSCLC-Ad								
TBX3	Breast								
TP53	Bladder	Breast	NSCLC-Ad	CRC	AML	H&N	RCC	NSCLC-Sq	Endometrium
U2AF1	AML								
VHL	RCC								
WT1	AML								

3281 different leukemias or solid tumors were sequenced by investigators in TCGA [26] and the 127 most common drivers identified within the 12 disease types studied. Since there was overlap among the disease sites, these 41 genes are the most common drivers, and are tabulated along with their most commonly associated organ in which they are activated. Many of these genes are also predictive markers (Table 19.1), and are in **bold**.

All tumors are carcinomas unless otherwise specified:

AML – Acute myelogenous leukemia

NSCLC-Sq – Non-small cell lung carcinoma – squamous

NSCLC-Ad – Non-small cell lung carcinoma – adenocarcinoma

CRC – Colorectal carcinoma

H & N – Head and neck squamous cell carcinoma

RCC – Renal cell carcinoma (including clear cell)

begun to mine cfDNA for promoter methylation [35–37], as well as copy number changes in cfDNA [21] that may identify loss of expression, such as occurs with PTEN.

The *RAS/RAF/MAPK/ERK* pathway

KRAS

KRAS belongs to a family of genes that includes *KRAS, HRAS* and *NRAS*, which encode small 21 kD guanosine triphosphate (GTP)/guanosine diphosphate (GDP) binding proteins that transmit extracellular signals from transmembrane tyrosinase kinase receptors (e.g., EGFR) to the nucleus. Mutations in *KRAS* lead to constitutively active GTP-bound protein, which activates *BRAF* and the downstream MAPK signaling pathway. Point mutations in *KRAS* occur most frequently in exon 2 (codons 12, 13), which accounts for 95% of all mutations. Other mutations in exon 3 (codon 61), and exon 4 (codon 146) occur less frequently, accounting for 5% of all mutation type [38].

Activating mutations in codon 12, 13 or 61 of the *KRAS* gene are present in approximately 40% of CRCs, and are associated with resistance to the anti-EGFR antibodies cetuximab and panitumumab [39, 40]. Patients with wild type *KRAS*, treated with cetuximab, resulted in significantly improved overall survival and progression-free survival, whereas patients whose tumors harbor mutations in *KRAS* gene do not respond.

KRAS is also mutated in up to 30% of NSCLC adenocarcinoma cases, and blocks the effects of many targeted agents, as identified by TCGA. Mutations in *KRAS* adenocarcinomas of the lung appear to be independent of mutations in *EGFR* [41], and therefore may not have the same impact in EGFR inhibitor resistance as they do in CRC. However, their presence may still be a useful diagnostic tool for lung cancer.

KRAS mutations occur in other cancers, especially in pancreatic carcinoma, where up to 95% of cancer may contain a *KRAS* mutation [42].

BRAF

KRAS mutational status analysis is insufficient for predicting the efficacy of anti-EGFR therapy in CRC, as only 20% of *KRAS* wild type patients will respond to anti-EGFR antibody therapy. Analyzing mutations in factors downstream of *KRAS*, like the serine/threonine kinase *BRAF*, is important in CRC, as mutations in *BRAF* may also cause resistance to treatment with an anti-EGFR agent [30,43]. Mutations in *BRAF* lead to constitutive activation of the *RAS/RAF/MAPK/ERK* pathway, and explains much of the lack of response to anti-EGFR therapy [44]. A key mutation in exon 15 of *BRAF* (nucleotide 1799T >A) changes amino acid valine to glutamate (V600E), a substitution that constitutively activates the *MAPK* signaling pathway. The *BRAF* V600E mutation is present in 5–10% of CRC patients, and is mutually exclusive of *KRAS* mutation [45]. Dual treatment with an inhibitor of BRAF or an inhibitor of MAPK, another kinase downstream of BRAF, is currently being tested in trials where BRAF mutations are important, such as CRC [46].

BRAF is mutated in over half of melanomas. The most common mutation in melanoma occurs in exon 15, just as in CRC, and results in a valine-to-glutamate substitution at codon 600 (BRAF V600E) in 85% of tumors harboring mutated *BRAF*. Other, less frequent, mutations (V600K, V600D) also occur in codon 600 in another 15–20% of melanoma patients. Vemurafenib was the first agent to provide clinical regression of advanced melanoma, but only in those patients whose tumors harbor mutated *BRAF* [47]. *BRAF* is mutated in ≈ 5% of NSCLC [41] as well.

NRAS

Treatment with BRAF inhibitors often causes a relatively short response in melanoma patients who develop resistance to treatment that is based on increased activity of kinases that either are downstream of *BRAF*, or increase the activity of the other RAFs (ARAF or c-RAF) as *BRAF* is inhibited [48]. In addition, approximately 20% of cutaneous melanoma patients have an activating mutation in *NRAS*, whereas mutations of the other RAS genes, such as *HRAS* and *KRAS*, are rare [49]. The most common *NRAS* mutations affect residues in exon 1 (codon 12) or 2 (codon 60 and 61), and they are mutually exclusive with activating V600E mutations. Attempts to directly target *NRAS* have not been successful, but *NRAS* activates both the

PI3K/AKT/PTEN and *RAS/RAF/MAPK/ERK* pathways. This leads to targeting the MAPK kinases MAP2K1 and MAP2K2 with trametinib, either as a single agent or in combination with BRAF inhibitors. Somatic mutations in *MAPK1* or *2* are present in approximately 10% of melanomas, and may render *MAPK1/2*-mutated tumors susceptible to targeted therapy [50]. Thus, while MEK inhibitors target *BRAF*-mutant disease, they may also be effective in other malignancies that harbor RAS mutations, or other RAF mutations that increase the general activity of the *MAPK* pathway.

As proof of principle for detecting *KRAS* and *BRAF* mutations in cfDNA, Taly *et al.* [51] used digital PCR to study *KRAS* mutations in patients with CRC. They found that 19 of 50 primary CRCs contained a *KRAS* mutation in codons 12 or 13. Plasma cfDNA contained the same mutation in 14 of the 19 patients while one sample contained a different mutation, and four did not demonstrate a *KRAS* mutation. In addition, two samples from patients who initially were considered to have wild type *KRAS* had mutated *KRAS* in plasma cfDNA. Subsequent deeper analysis of these two tumors confirmed a low allelic fraction of the same mutant *KRAS*. In addition, all five patients whose tumors contained mutant *BRAF* also had the same mutation in plasma cfDNA.

Mouliere *et al.* [52] made a similar finding in a small set of CRC samples after establishing their assay in a preclinical model. Using an allele-specific PCR reaction on cfDNA from a set of 38 patients, the investigators identified mutant *KRAS* alleles at mean fractions of 8% in Stage II/III, and 22% in Stage IV patients. On a per patient basis, there were five patients with stage II/III disease, and one had an allele fraction greater than 10%, with the other four greater than 5%.

Another use for the detection of *KRAS* and *BRAF* mutations in cfDNA is to predict response to anti-EGFR antibody therapy. Spindler *et al.* [53] studied the levels of circulating plasma cfDNA and the levels of *KRAS* and *BRAF* in 108 advanced CRC patients who received cetuximab and irinotecan. Thirty-two of 41 patients (78%) whose tumors contained KRAS mutations also had detectable mutant KRAS in their plasma. There was good correlation for the allele fraction in tumor and plasma cfDNA. Interestingly, patients with an allele

fraction of *KRAS* mutation in the highest quartile did not respond to treatment, whereas the patients in the lower three quartiles had a 42% response rate.

Finally, Maire *et al.* [54] have studied the use of *KRAS* mutation in serum cfDNA and serum CA19-9 levels, to distinguish pancreatic carcinoma from chronic pancreatitis. This is a common problem and is often difficult to distinguish with circulating markers [55]. Maire *et al.* [54] studied 47 carcinomas and 31 chronic pancreatitis patients and found:
1 there was no difference between the level of cfDNA in the two groups; and
2 there were *KRAS* mutations in the sera of 22 patients (47%) with pancreatic carcinoma, and four of the chronic pancreatitics (13%).

When the serum *KRAS* mutations were combined with CA19-9 levels, the sensitivity, specificity, positive and negative predictive values were 98, 77, 87 and 96%. Taken together, these results with *KRAS* and *BRAF* detection in cfDNA provide a proof of principle for using analysis of cfDNA and specific targeted mutations. While the data are largely collected in patients with advanced disease, there is enough data to suggest that such studies may be useful for early detection.

TP53

TP53 is the most commonly mutated gene in all cancers (Table 19.2). It would be helpful, for early diagnosis to detect mutations in *TP53* in plasma or serum cfDNA, if driver mutations may complement predictive markers for early detection. Forshew *et al.* [20] developed tagged amplicon deep sequencing (TAM-seq) to study mutations in *TP53* in plasma cfDNA at allele frequencies as low as 2%, with high sensitivity and specificity, in a patient with advanced high-grade serous ovarian carcinoma. These authors demonstrated that this TAM-seq approach could be used to follow the course of disease in different patients while undergoing treatment, and that the levels of *TP53* mutation in cfDNA paralleled the response of CA125, as well as a competing digital PCR treatment. The authors concluded that TAM-seq was a sensitive and specific assay that not only could detect mutations in *TP53*, but also others in *PTEN* and *EGFR*, with a high throughput deep sequencing workflow. With adaptation, this assay may be sensitive enough to be used for early detection strategies.

A set of screening trials provides further support for using mutations in *TP53* and plasma or serum cfDNA levels for early diagnosis. First, Hainaut and colleagues have studied patients with chronic Hepatitis C viral (HCV) or Hepatitis B virus (HBV) infection, which is associated with the development of both hepatocellular carcinoma and Non-Hodgkin Lymphoma (NHL). In addition, these patients are exposed to aflatoxin, which is associated with specific mutations in *TP53* (p.R249S). In an early case control study of 348 controls, 98 cirrhotics and 186 HCC patients in The Gambia, the R249S mutation in TP53 was found in the plasma cfDNA of 3.5% of controls, 15.4% of cirrhotics and 39.8% of HCC patients [56]. cfDNA levels were higher in patients with hepatocellular carcinoma than in HCV or hepatitis B virus (HBV) carriers or serologically negative controls [57].

Further, analysis of cfDNA from 255 patients identified the *TP53* serine-249 mutation in 5% of the patients' cfDNA, where the expected mutation rate in HCC tumor biopsies was 10%. A year later, these investigators demonstrated in a smaller case control study of NHL, confirmed elevated serum cfDNA in NHL patients, compared with controls, as well as a spectrum of mutations in 30% of the NHL patients in exons 5–9 of *TP53* [58]. In addition, this group [59] developed a mass spectrometry assay that was more sensitive for the R249S *TP53* mutation, and which is now being used to support epidemiologic studies of the interaction between aflatoxin, HBV, and HCV in the carcinogenesis of HCC [60]. Combined, these studies provide a proof of principle that mutation in *TP53*, the most common driver gene, may be useful in an early diagnosis strategy.

c-KIT

While activating *BRAF* and RAS activating mutations are common in cutaneous melanoma, a much smaller subset of melanomas that arise in mucosal, acral and chronic sun damage skin demonstrate alterations in the c-*KIT* receptor tyrosine, which do not coincide with BRAF and NRAS mutations. The vast majority of c-*KIT*-activating point mutations are in exon 11, and may activate both the

RAS/RAF/MAPK/ERK and *PI3K/AKT/PTEN* pathways. Amplification and over-expression of the c-*KIT* gene are also common alterations in these subtypes of melanoma. These mutations and alterations are considered targetable, and trials have been initiated to evaluate imatinib and other KIT inhibitors, such as sunitinib, sorafenib, nilotinib, masatinib and desatinib. Assessment of specific *KIT* mutations as predictive markers for targeted therapy is critical for patients' selection and use Fluorescence In Situ Hybridization (FISH), as well as PCR and sequencing, to identify patients who may benefit from KIT inhibitors [61].

c-*Kit* mutations have also been identified in AML, with an overall incidence of 17% for mutations and internal tandem duplications leading to kinase activation [62]. The highest frequency of alterations occurs in 25–30% of the core binding factor subtype of AML [63]. To date it is not clear that investigators have published on studies involving detection of c-*KIT* in cfDNA.

IDH1/2

Parsons *et al.* [64] performed an unbiased genomic analysis of glioblastoma multiforme (GBM) and found, among other observations, that 12% of their sample had mutations in *IDH1*. Further examination suggested that these mutations were present in secondary GBMs, which are ≈ 5% of the total GBM population. These results also suggested that mutation in *IDH1* was a relatively late event. Subsequently, Yan *et al.* [65] studied 939 glioblastomas, and found that 17% had mutations in *IDH1* at amino acid R132. In addition, since *IDH2* is quite homologous, an analysis of the analogous residue R172 revealed another nine somatic mutations. Neither gene had mutations at other residues, and both mutations reduced enzymatic activity in these GBM patients. Also, patients whose tumors harbored a mutated *IDH1* or *IDH2* had a more favorable prognosis than patients with wild type IDH1 or IDH2, and generally had grade I or II GBM.

Noushmehr *et al.* [66] also confirmed that *IDH1* mutations were associated with a Cpg-Island methylator phenotype, and occurred in younger patients with lower grade lesions and who also had better clinical outcomes. Thus, *IDH1* or *IDH2* mutation is a favorable prognostic marker, and is now being assessed as a possible target for therapy.

A similar unbiased genomic analysis of AML has also been performed and reported by Mardis et al. [67], who found that 16% of AML contained a mutation in *IDH1*, often in otherwise cytogenetically normal AML. These investigators did not identify a significant prognostic effect of IDH1 mutation. In contrast, Marcucci et al. [68] found a 33% incidence of *IDH* mutations in cytogenetically normal AML, with 14% in IDH1 and 19% in IDH2. In this study from one of the Cooperative Oncology Groups, *IDH1*-mutated patients had shorter survival rates when their mutation was associated with young age, and either *NPM1* mutation or *FLT3*-internal tandem duplication negative, than in higher risk patients with wild *IDH1* and *IDH2*. Thus, mutations in *IDH1* at the R132 residue or in *IDH2* at the R172 or R132 residues may be useful markers for identification for early diagnosis.

DNMT3A

The Pan Cancer Analysis also found that one of the critical mutations was in *DNMT3A*, primarily in AML (Table 19.2). Gaidzik et al. [69] found that mutations in *DNMT3A* occurred in 21% of 1770 young adult patients with AML. In addition, mutations in *DNMT3A* were associated with cytogenetically normal AML, *NPM1* mutations, *FLT3*-Internal Tandem Duplications and *IDH1/2* mutations. Mutations in *DNMT3A* were not associated with clinical outcome. Renneville et al. [70] found similar associations with other mutations but, in this study, mutations in *DNMT3A* were an independent adverse prognostic factor for poor overall survival.

Shivarov et al. [71] performed a meta-analysis of *DNMT3A* mutations in AML that confirmed that *DNMT3A* mutations were associated with significant decreased overall and relapse-free survival. Kim et al. [72] performed an initial survey of mutations in *DNMT3A* across a number of cancers, and found that mutations in *DNMT3A* were present in only AML (9.4%), ALL (1.4%) and non-small cell lung cancer (2%). They [72] also examined different cancers for loss of heterozygosity (LOH), and found LOH in 16% of leukemias, 48% of Non-Hodgkin lymphoma, 18% of lung, 24% of gastric, 19% of colorectal and 21% of breast cancer, but only 1% of prostate cancer. Thus, LOH is a critical component of the alteration of *DNMT3A* activity and its effect on epigenetic regulation of gene expression. However, LOH may be harder to assess in cfDNA than detection of mutations, although Heitzer et al. [21] have been able to perform copy number variation in cfDNA.

Summary

This chapter covers driver mutations that are currently considered to be important therapeutic targets, as well as several genes that are also frequently mutated in human cancer. These driver genes and predictive markers may be useful in strategies for the early detection of cancer since, as Vogelstein et al. [22] postulate, most important driver/predictive marker mutations occur by the time of diagnosis of the cancer. Such a screening strategy may focus on the detection of elevations in cfDNA first, and then the potential application of further analysis for copy number, promoter methylation or somatic mutations in the cfDNA. As sequencing becomes cheaper, and deep sequencing becomes available, it is possible that detection of important somatic mutations at even low allelic fractions in plasma may be measured.

The problem of dilution of DNA from tumors into plasma or serum by normal DNA, especially in conditions of trauma or acute or chronic inflammation, is a major problem. We do not discuss the role of circulating tumor cells, because they are well covered elsewhere, and often are not detectable as intact cells, except in advanced stages of cancer. Coumans et al. [73] described this in a modeling paper, where they estimated that in small (tumor diameter of 2.7 mm) there will be only 9 ± 6 cells per liter of blood, or 0.067 cells per 7.5 ml of blood, for the FDA approved CellSearch assay! Folkman et al. [74] described that solid tumors are dormant until they are vascularized, which usually occurs around a diameter of 2–3 mm. Once vascularization is achieved, then the release of cells and cell components may occur into the bloodstream. Since the detection of cfDNA may be more sensitive than current technologies to detect intact cells, it may be possible that the evaluation of cfDNA may be more likely to detect cancer in early stage disease than it is through evaluation of intact circulating tumor cells.

This chapter also does not describe the use of micro-RNAs as an early diagnosis marker, although they clearly can be measured in plasma [75]. This is because most significant micro-RNAs, such as let-7f, are decreased during neoplastic transformation, since most have an inhibitory role in gene regulation and it is hard to define markers whose expression decreases in disease states.

To make sure that cfDNA and the analysis of genetic alterations within it is adequately studied, there must be rigorous attention paid to standardization of technology and pre-analytic factors. The various studies presented here are generally small studies that appear to use different techniques for measuring plasma or serum cfDNA, let alone the methods to detect somatic mutations. It is critical that these technologies be optimized in such a way that enhances reproducibility and applicability. Hopefully, this may then lead to cost-effective strategies for the application of driver gene/predictive marker mutation into successful strategies for early diagnosis.

References

1. Atkinson AJ Jr., Colburn WA, DeGruttola VG, et al. (2007). Biomarkers and surrogate endpoints: preferred definitions and conceptual framework. *Clinical Pharmacology & Therapeutics* **69**, 89–95.
2. Poste G, Carbone DP, Parkinson DR, et al. (2012). Leveling the playing field: bringing development of biomarkers and molecular diagnostics up to the standards for drug development. *Clinical Cancer Research* **18**, 1515–23.
3. Cancer Genome Atlas Research Network, Weinstein JN, Collisson EA, Mills GB, Shaw KR, Ozenberger BA, Ellrott K, Shmulevich I, Sander C, Stuart JM (2013). The Cancer Genome Atlas Pan-Cancer analysis project. *Nature Genetics* **45**, 1113–20.
4. Burchill SA, Selby PJ (2000). Molecular detection of low-level disease in patients with cancer. *Journal of Pathology* **190**, 6–14.
5. Sidransky D (2002). Emerging molecular markers of cancer. *Nature Reviews Cancer* **2**, 210–9.
6. Diehl F, Li M, Dressman D, et al. (2005). Detection and quantification of mutations in the plasma of patients with colorectal tumors. *Proceedings of the National Academy of Sciences of the United States of America* **102**, 16368–73.
7. Mouliere F, Thierry AR (2012). The importance of examining the proportion of circulating DNA originating from tumor, microenvironment and normal cells in colorectal cancer patients. *Expert Opinion on Biological Therapy* **12** Suppl 1, S209–15.
8. Schwarzenbach H, Hoon DS, Pantel K (2011). Cell-free nucleic acids as biomarkers in cancer patients. *Nature Reviews Cancer* **11**, 426–37.
9. Mussolin L, Burnelli R, Pillon M, et al. (2013). Plasma cell-free DNA in paediatric lymphomas. *Journal of Cancer* **4**, 323–9.
10. Catarino R, Coelho A, Araújo A, et al. (2012). Circulating DNA: diagnostic tool and predictive marker for overall survival of NSCLC patients. *PLoS One* **7**, e38559.
11. Flamini E, Mercatali L, Nanni O, et al. (2006). Free DNA and carcinoembryonic antigen serum levels: an important combination for diagnosis of colorectal cancer. *Clinical Cancer Research* **12**, 6985–8.
12. Gormally E, Caboux E, Vineis P, Hainaut P (2007). Circulating free DNA in plasma or serum as biomarker of carcinogenesis: Practical aspects and biological significance. *Mutation Research* **635**, 105–117.
13. Zhang R, Shao F, Wu X, Ying K (2010). Value of quantitative analysis of circulating cell free DNA as a screening tool for lung cancer: a meta-analysis. *Lung Cancer* **69**, 225–31.
14. Nakahira K, Kyung SY, Rogers AJ, et al. (2013). Circulating mitochondrial DNA in patients in the ICU as a marker of mortality: derivation and validation. *PLoS Medicine* **10**, e1001577.
15. Arnalich F, Maldifassi MC, Ciria E, et al. (2013). Plasma levels of mitochondrial and nuclear DNA in patients with massive pulmonary embolism in the emergency department: a prospective cohort study. *Critical Care* **17**, R90.]
16. Macher H, Egea-Guerrero JJ, Revuelto-Rey J, et al. (2012). Role of early cell-free DNA levels decrease as a predictive marker of fatal outcome after severe traumatic brain injury. *Clinica Chimica Acta* **414**, 12–7.
17. Huttunen R, Kuparinen T, Jylhävä J, et al. (2011). Fatal outcome in bacteremia is characterized by high plasma cell free DNA concentration and apoptotic DNA fragmentation: a prospective cohort study. *PLoS One* **6**, e21700.
18. Swarup V, Srivastava AK, Padma MV, Rajeswari MR (2011). Quantification of circulating plasma DNA in Friedreich's ataxia and spinocerebellar ataxia types 2 and 12. *DNA and Cell Biology* **30**, 389–94.
19. El Tarhouny SA, Hadhoud KM, Ebrahem MM, Al Azizi NM (2010). Assessment of cell-free DNA with microvascular complication of type II diabetes mellitus, using PCR and ELISA. *Nucleosides, Nucleotides and Nucleic Acids* **29**, 228–36.

20. Forshew T, Murtaza M, Parkinson C, *et al.* (2012). Non-invasive identification and monitoring of cancer mutations by targeted deep sequencing of plasma DNA. *Science Translational Medicine* **4**, 136ra68.

21. Heitzer E, Ulz P, Belic J, Gutschi S, *et al.* (2013). Tumor-associated copy number changes in the circulation of patients with prostate cancer identified through whole-genome sequencing. *Genome Medicine* **5**, 30.

22. Vogelstein B, Papadopoulos N, Velculescu VE, *et al.* (2013). Cancer genome landscapes. *Science* **339**, 1546–58.

23. Fearon ER, Vogelstein B (1990). A genetic model for colorectal tumorigenesis. *Cell* **61**, 759–67.

24. Bozic I, Antal T, Ohtsuki H, *et al.* (2010). Accumulation of driver and passenger mutations during tumor progression. *Proceedings of the National Academy of Sciences of the United States of America* **107**, 18545–50.

25. Komori J, Boone L, DeWard A, *et al.* (2012). The mouse lymph node as an ectopic transplantation site for multiple tissues. *Nature Biotechnology* **30**, 976–83.

26. Kandoth C, McLellan MD, Vandin F, *et al.* (2013). Mutational landscape and significance across 12 major cancer types. *Nature* **502**, 333–9.

27. Lauring J, Park BH, Wolff AC (2013). The phosphoinositide-3-kinase-Akt-mTOR pathway as a therapeutic target in breast cancer. *Journal of the National Comprehensive Cancer Network* **11**, 670–8.

28. Chandarlapaty S, Sakr RA, Giri D, *et al.* (2012). Frequent mutational activation of the PI3K-AKT pathway in trastuzumab-resistant breast cancer. *Clinical Cancer Research* **18**, 6784–91.

29. Baselga J, Campone M, Piccart M, *et al.* (2012). Everolimus in postmenopausal hormone-receptor-positive advanced breast cancer. *New England Journal of Medicine* **366**, 520–9.

30. De Roock W, Claes B, Bernasconi D *et al.* (2010). Effects of KRAS, BRAF, NRAS, and PIK3CA mutations on the efficacy of cetuximab plus chemotherapy in chemotherapy-refractory metastatic colorectal cancer: a retrospective consortium analysis. *Lancet Oncology* **11**, 753–762.

31. Loupakis F, Pollina L, Stasi I, *et al.* (2009). PTEN expression and KRAS mutations on primary tumors and metastases in the prediction of benefit from cetuximab plus irinotecan for patients with metastatic colorectal cancer. *Journal of Clinical Oncology* **27**, 2622–2629.

32. Stahl JM, Sharma A, Cheung M *et al.* (2004). Deregulated Akt3 activity promotes development of malignant melanoma. *Cancer Research* **64**, 7002–7010.

33. Murtaza M, Dawson SJ, Tsui DW, *et al.* (2013). Non-invasive analysis of acquired resistance to cancer therapy by sequencing of plasma DNA. *Nature* **497**, 108–12.

34. Higgins MJ, Jelovac D, Barnathan E, *et al.* (2012). Detection of tumor PIK3CA status in metastatic breast cancer using peripheral blood. *Clinical Cancer Research* **18**, 3462–9.

35. Kwee S, Song MA, Cheng I, *et al.* (2012). Measurement of circulating cell-free DNA in relation to 18F-fluorocholine PET/CT imaging in chemotherapy-treated advanced prostate cancer. *Clinical and Translational Science* **5**, 65–70.

36. Lefebure B, Charbonnier F, Di Fiore F, *et al.* (2010). Prognostic value of circulating mutant DNA in unresectable metastatic colorectal cancer. *Annals of Surgery* **251**, 275–80.

37. Frattini M, Gallino G, Signoroni S, *et al.* (2008). Quantitative and qualitative characterization of plasma DNA identifies primary and recurrent colorectal cancer. *Cancer Letters* **263**, 170–81.

38. Schubbert S, Shannon K, Bollag G (2007). Hyperactive Ras in developmental disorders and cancer. *Nature Reviews Cancer* **7**, 295–308.

39. Amado RG, Wolf M, Peeters M *et al.* (2008). Wild-type KRAS is required for panitumumab efficacy in patients with metastatic colorectal cancer. *Journal of Clinical Oncology* **26**, 1626–1634.

40. Karapetis CS, Khambata-Ford S, Jonker DJ *et al.* (2008). K-ras mutations and benefit from cetuximab in advanced colorectal cancer. *New England Journal of Medicine* **359**, 1757–1765.

41. Pao W, Girard N (2011). New driver mutations in non-small-cell lung cancer. *Lancet Oncology* **12**, 175–80.

42. Almoguera C, Shibata D, Forrester K, *et al.* (1988). Most human carcinomas of the exocrine pancreas contain mutant c-K-ras genes. *Cell* **53**, 549–54.

43. Lochhead P, Kuchiba A, Imamura Y, *et al.* (2013). Microsatellite instability and BRAF mutation testing in colorectal cancer prognostication. *Journal of the National Cancer Institute* **105**, 1151–6.

44. Di Nicolantonio F, Martini M, Molinari F *et al.* (2008). Wild-type BRAF is required for response to panitumumab or cetuximab in metastatic colorectal cancer. *Journal of Clinical Oncology* **26**, 5705–5712.

45. Frattini M, Balestra D, Suardi S, *et al.* (2004). Different genetic features associated with colon and rectal carcinogenesis. *Clinical Cancer Research* **10**, 4015–4021.

46. Prahallad A, Sun C, Huang S, *et al.* (2012). Unresponsiveness of colon cancer to BRAF(V600E) inhibition through feedback activation of EGFR. *Nature* **483**, 100–103.

47. Flaherty KT, Puzanov I, Kim KB, *et al.* (2010). Inhibition of mutated, activated BRAF in metastatic melanoma. *New England Journal of Medicine* **363**, 809–819.

48. Sullivan RJ, Flaherty KT (2013). Resistance to BRAF-targeted therapy in melanoma. *European Journal of Cancer* **49**, 1297–304.

49. Jakob JA, Bassett RL, Jr., Ng CS, *et al.* (2012). NRAS mutation status is an independent prognostic factor in metastatic melanoma. *Cancer* **118**, 4014–4023.

50. Nikolaev SI, Rimoldi D, Iseli C *et al.* (2011). Exome sequencing identifies recurrent somatic MAP2K1 and MAP2K2 mutations in melanoma. *Nature Genetics* **44**, 133–139.

51. Taly V, Pekin D, Benhaim L, *et al.* (2013). Multiplex Picodroplet Digital PCR to Detect KRAS Mutations in Circulating DNA from the Plasma of Colorectal Cancer Patients. *Clinical Chemistry* **59**, 1722–31.

52. Mouliere F, El Messaoudi S, Gongora C, *et al.* (2013). Circulating Cell-Free DNA from Colorectal Cancer Patients May Reveal High KRAS or BRAF Mutation Load. *Translational Oncology* **6**, 319–28.

53. Spindler KL, Pallisgaard N, Vogelius I, Jakobsen A (2012). Quantitative cell-free DNA, KRAS, and BRAF mutations in plasma from patients with metastatic colorectal cancer during treatment with cetuximab and irinotecan. *Clinical Cancer Research* **18**, 1177–85.

54. Maire F, Micard S, Hammel P, *et al.* (2002). Differential diagnosis between chronic pancreatitis and pancreatic cancer: value of the detection of KRAS2 mutations in circulating DNA. *British Journal of Cancer* **87**, 551–4.

55. Klomp HJ, Zernial O, Flachmann S, Wellstein A, Juhl H (2002). Significance of the expression of the growth factor pleiotrophin in pancreatic cancer patients. *Clinical Cancer Research* **8**, 823–7.

56. Kirk GD, Lesi OA, Mendy M, *et al.* (2005). 249(ser) TP53 mutation in plasma DNA, hepatitis B viral infection, and risk of hepatocellular carcinoma. *Oncogene* **24**, 5858–67.

57. Hosny G, Farahat N, Tayel H, Hainaut P (2008). Ser-249 TP53 and CTNNB1 mutations in circulating free DNA of Egyptian patients with hepatocellular carcinoma versus chronic liver diseases. *Cancer Letters* **264**, 201–8.

58. Hosny G, Farahat N, Hainaut P (2009). TP53 mutations in circulating free DNA from Egyptian patients with non-Hodgkin's lymphoma. *Cancer Letters* **275**, 234–9.

59. Lleonart ME, Kirk GD, Villar S, *et al.* (2005). Quantitative analysis of plasma TP53 249Ser-mutated DNA by electrospray ionization mass spectrometry. *Cancer Epidemiology, Biomarkers & Prevention* **14**, 2956–62.

60. Villar S, Le Roux-Goglin E, Gouas DA, *et al.* (2011). Seasonal variation in TP53 R249S-mutated serum DNA with aflatoxin exposure and hepatitis B virus infection. *Environmental Health Perspectives* **119**, 1635–40

61. Carvajal RD, Antonescu CR, Wolchok JD *et al.* (2011). KIT as a therapeutic target in metastatic melanoma. *JAMA* **305**, 2327–2334.

62. Malaise M, Steinbach D, Corbacioglu S (2009). Clinical implications of c-Kit mutations in acute myelogenous leukemia. *Current Hematologic Malignancy Reports* **4**, 77–82.

63. Paschka P (2008). Core binding factor acute myeloid leukemia. *Seminars in Oncology* **35**, 410–417.

64. Parsons DW, Jones S, Zhang X (2008). An integrated genomic analysis of human glioblastoma multiforme. *Science* **321**, 1807–12.

65. Yan H, Parsons DW, Jin G, *et al.* (2009). IDH1 and IDH2 mutations in gliomas. *New England Journal of Medicine* **360**, 765–73.

66. Noushmehr H, Weisenberger DJ, Diefes K, *et al.* (2010). Identification of a CpG island methylator phenotype that defines a distinct subgroup of glioma. *Cancer Cell* **17**, 510–22.

67. Mardis ER, Ding L, Dooling DJ, *et al.* (2009). Recurring mutations found by sequencing an acute myeloid leukemia genome. *New England Journal of Medicine* **361**, 1058–66.

68. Marcucci G, Maharry K, Wu YZ, *et al.* (2010). IDH1 and IDH2 gene mutations identify novel molecular subsets within de novo cytogenetically normal acute myeloid leukemia: a Cancer and Leukemia Group B study. *Journal of Clinical Oncology* **28**, 2348–55.

69. Gaidzik VI, Schlenk RF, Paschka P, *et al.* (2013). Clinical impact of DNMT3A mutations in younger adult patients with acute myeloid leukemia: results of the AML Study Group (AMLSG). *Blood* **121**, 4769–77.

70. Renneville A, Boissel N, Nibourel O, *et al.* (2012). Prognostic significance of DNA methyltransferase 3A mutations in cytogenetically normal acute myeloid leukemia: a study by the Acute Leukemia French Association. *Leukemia* **26**, 1247–54.

71. Shivarov V, Gueorguieva R, Stoimenov A, Tiu R (2013). DNMT3A mutation is a poor prognosis biomarker in AML: results of a meta-analysis of 4500 AML patients. *Leukemia Research* **37**, 1445–50.

72. Kim MS, Kim YR, Yoo NJ, Lee SH (2013). Mutational analysis of DNMT3A gene in acute leukemias and common solid cancers. *APMIS* **121**, 85–94.

73. Coumans FA, Siesling S, Terstappen LW (2013). Detection of cancer before distant metastasis. *BMC Cancer* **13**(1), 283.

74. Folkman J, Merler E, Abernathy C, Williams G (1971). Isolation of a tumor factor responsible for angiogenesis. *Journal of Experimental Medicine* **133**, 275–88.

75. Zheng H, Zhang L, Zhao Y, *et al.* (2013). Plasma miRNAs as Diagnostic and Prognostic Biomarkers for Ovarian Cancer. *PLoS One* **8**(11), e77853.

CHAPTER 20

Statistical Consideration in Predictive and Prognostic Markers

Fei Ye and Yu Shyr

Department of Biostatistics, Vanderbilt University School of Medicine, Nashville, TN, USA

Introduction

It is well recognized that cancer is a complex group of diseases, with many subtypes and considerable inter-individual variability in susceptibility and prognosis. The National Cancer Institute defines a biomarker as "a biological molecule found in blood, other body fluids, or tissues that is a sign of a normal or abnormal process or of a condition or disease." A biomarker may be objectively measured and evaluated as an indicator in risk assessment, diagnosis, prognosis and treatment predictions, pharmacodynamics and pharmacokinetics, monitoring treatment responses, and predicting recurrence. In cancer research, biomarkers are used in three primary ways: diagnostic, prognostic, and predictive.

In this chapter, we will focus on markers that forecast future states – namely, prognostic and predictive biomarkers. By definition, a prognostic biomarker provides information on the likely cancer outcome, regardless of therapy, while a predictive biomarker provides information on the likely benefit from a particular treatment. Understanding predictive and prognostic factors, and more accurately predicting cancer outcomes and response to treatment, would not only benefit survivors and health care providers, but also have a major impact on public health policy development. Despite a large body of work in cancer biomarker identification and the great potential for its use in precision medicine (sometimes referred as "personalized medicine"), few biomarkers have been robustly validated. The relative lack of robust statistical analysis, and the heterogeneity of cancer patients and experimental protocols, platforms, and designs, pose challenges to the discovery and validation of clinically relevant and reproducible biomarkers.

In oncology, studies in breast cancer have pioneered biomarker research. Established predictive and prognostic biomarkers in breast cancer include estrogen receptor (ER), progesterone receptor (PR), human epidermal growth factor receptor 2 (HER2) for prognosis and treatment predictions, as well as BRCA1 and BRCA2 for risk assessment. The marker of proliferation Ki67 has recently emerged as an important marker, due to several applications in neoadjuvant therapy, in addition to its prognostic value.

Several prediction tools and models developed for breast cancer prognosis now include biomarker predictors. Adjuvant!, the most widely used prediction tool in the USA, uses US Surveillance, Epidemiology, & End Results registry data to provide individual prediction of ten-year survival and relapse. Predictors used in Adjuvant! Standard Version 8.0 include age, tumor size, lymph node involvement, tumor grade, and estrogen receptor ER [1–10].

Biomarkers in Cancer Screening and Early Detection, First Edition. Edited by Sudhir Srivastava.
© 2017 John Wiley & Sons, Inc. Published 2017 by John Wiley & Sons, Inc.

Two other versions of Adjuvant! are available or are in development:

1 *Adjuvant! After 5 Years of Tamoxifen.* This is designed for decision-making for ER- and/or progesterone receptor (PR)-positive post-menopausal patients, after completion of five years of adjuvant tamoxifen.

2 *Adjuvant! Genomic Version 7.0.* This is for patients with node-negative, ER-positive early breast cancer for whom genomic information is available.

Adjuvant! Standard Version 9.0, which is still under development, plans to include human epi-dermal growth factor receptor 2 (HER2) status as a predictor, and trastuzumab as a treatment option [1].

Outside the US, the Nottingham prognostic index (NPI) is a well-known tool used to predict breast cancer prognosis [11–16]. This index was originally developed based on tumor size, grade, and lymph node status [21, 22]. The utility of the addition of biomarkers to the index (e.g., ER and PR or HER2 status) has been evaluated [17–22]. In addition, UK investigators have developed PREDICT, based on cancer registry data, to predict survival for patients with early breast cancer in the UK [1, 23, 24]. Biomarkers currently included in PREDICT are ER, HER2, and Ki67 status.

Over the last decade, it has been increasingly rec-ognized that breast cancer is a group of molecularly heterogeneous diseases that goes beyond the sub-types typically defined by ER, PR, and HER2 status [25], and that the molecular profile of tumors deter-mines their biological behavior and responses to treatment. In 2000, Perou *et al.* first proposed clas-sifying breast cancer into four intrinsic tumor sub-types, based on gene expression profiles – namely, luminal A (ER+ and/or PR+, HER2-), luminal B (ER+ and/or PR+, HER2+), HER2-enriched (ER-, PR-, HER2+), and basal-like (ER-/PR-/HER2- (i.e., triple negative breast cancer), plus cytokeratin (CK) 5/6+) [26–31]. Subtype-specific biomarkers have been drawing more attention in recent years. Qui-escin sulfydryl oxidase 1 (QSOX1), for example, was reported to be predictive for luminal cancers [32].

Apart from breast cancer, the number of val-idated prognostic and predictive biomarkers remains rather sparse. Examples include elevated levels of metallopeptidase inhibitor 1 (TIMP1), a marker associated with more aggressive forms of multiple myeloma [33]; a mutation in exon 11 of the proto-oncogene c-KIT, a marker indicating that a gastrointestinal stromal tumor (GIST) will likely respond to imatinibtreatment [34, 35]; and mutations in the tyrosine kinase domain of EGFR1, a marker indicating that a patient's non-small-cell lung carcinoma (NSCLC) will likely respond to gefitinib or erlotinib treatment [36, 37]. In the remaining sections, we will focus on statistical issues arising in the analysis and validation of biomarker identification and evaluation.

Biomarker identification and validation

Biomarker development originates in the drug discovery phase and leads to the clinical valida-tion stage. Clinical scientists who are interested in establishing clinical efficacy always focus on clinical difference, rather than statistical difference. Statistical significances, however, are crucial to the success of biomarker identification and validation. It has been shown that, while biological consider-ations can strengthen the case for the adoption of a biomarker, in some cases they can be misleading [38]. Therefore, it is important to understand that biology cannot substitute for the validation of biomarkers through clinical trials and statistical analyses. Statistical validation of a biomarker typically begins with an initial assessment that the marker and the outcome of interest are associated, followed by internal and external validation of the association.

Prognostic biomarkers versus predictive biomarkers

For a biomarker to be validated as prognostic, an association must be present between the status of the marker at baseline, or continuous changes in the marker over time, and a clinical end point, adjusted for the treatment effect. From a statistical standpoint, this is a relatively straightforward requirement, as it does not necessarily require any specific study design; usually, a well-designed retrospective study is sufficient. To move from the initial establishment of an association to robust val-idation, however, can sometimes prove challenging.

Validation of predictive biomarkers is not an easy task. Statistical validation of predictive biomarkers requires randomized clinical trials, where patients are divided into two or more arms – such as absent and present, or high-risk and low-risk – based on levels of the biomarker. Establishment of predictive biomarkers lays the foundation for the development of personalized treatment regimens, which may spare patients from unnecessary cancer treatment, reduce treatment-related toxicity, and also allow identification of patient subgroup(s) that are good candidates for a particular treatment, or high-risk cancer patients who would benefit from intensive follow-up programs and/or individualized lifestyle modifications. Predictive markers, however, present even greater challenges than prognostic biomarkers, both with respect to initial demonstration of an association between the outcome and the marker, and subsequent statistical validation.

Biomarker trials

Recently, due to the rapid development of advanced technologies in a number of molecular profiling areas, including proteomic profiling, metabolic analysis, genetic testing, and high-throughput deep sequencing, biomarker-adaptive design has quickly evolved, allowing for a greater degree and a broader range of precision medicine. Biomarkers have already been used in almost every stage of drug development: from compound discovery and pre-clinical studies; through each phase of clinical trials and into post-marketing evaluations; as intermediate endpoints to identify target patient populations that are most sensitive to a particular treatment (i.e., to separate good- and poor- prognosis patients); to predict patients' responses to a treatment; to replace the primary clinical outcome as a surrogate endpoint for early disease diagnosis; and to identify novel drug targets. These applications are the major contributors to the development of precision medicine.

It is of note that the selection of surrogate biomarkers in a clinical trial needs to be carefully justified, to ensure the association between biomarkers and clinical outcomes under the investigational drug. Establishing a linkage between a biomarker test and the clinical endpoint is very important in guiding therapy decisions in precision

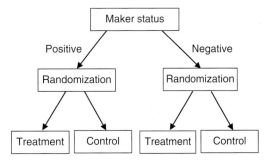

Figure 20.1 Flowchart for biomarker stratified design.

medicine, which is usually dependent on the ability to classify patients into distinct subgroups, based on their genomic or proteomic profiles.

Conventional clinical trials not involving biomarker tests only estimate the average treatment effect in the overall target population. In order to evaluate biomarker-guided treatments, several biomarker designs have been proposed, such as biomarker-stratified designs, biomarker-strategy designs, and enrichment designs. The highest level of evidence derives from trials with an "interaction" design, in which all patients are stratified by biomarker level, and then randomized to one of two treatments. In a biomarker-stratified design, patients are randomly assigned regardless of their biomarker status, but the analysis is stratified by the biomarker status, as illustrated in Figure 20.1.

The biomarker-stratified design estimates, without bias, treatment effects across biomarker-defined subgroups, by maximizing the benefits of randomization. In some cases, however, it is believed that the treatment may benefit only patients of certain biomarker-defined subgroups, so therefore, the use of biomarker-stratified design may not be ethical. In this situation, the biomarker enrichment design can be used as an alternative to estimate the treatment effect among patients of certain biomarker status. Initially, biomarker profiles are obtained from all participating patients but, based on these profiles, only patients who are believed to benefit from the treatment will remain in the trial, as is displayed in Figure 20.2.

Another biomarker design is the biomarker-strategy design. In this design, patients are randomly assigned either to a biomarker-guided arm,

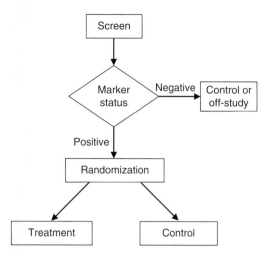

Figure 20.2 Flowchart for biomarker enrichment design.

or to a control arm that is not biomarker-based. Within the biomarker-guided arm, biomarker-positive patients are assigned to the investigational treatment, and biomarker-negative patients, together with patients in the control arm, are given the standard treatment. A diagram of the study's design is given in Figure 20.3.

A drawback of the biomarker-strategy design is that the observed treatment effect may be diluted by having overlapping on-treatment assignments between the treatment arm and the control arm, consequently reducing the trial's statistical power. Additionally, it may not be easy to interpret a significant observed treatment effect, because it may be either that the biomarker is useful in guiding

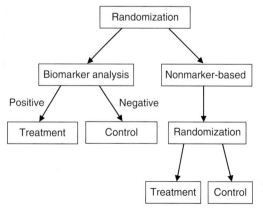

Figure 20.3 Flowchart for biomarker strategy design.

the personalized regimen, or that one treatment is simply more effective than the other, regardless of the biomarker status [39].

Model development

The strategy for the identification of a prognostic or predictive biomarker should involve the following ten steps:

1 Choose an appropriate model, based on the nature of the outcome variable (continuous, categorical, ordinal, or time-to-event), the type of censoring in the case of time-to-event data, and the correlation structure between observations.

2 Assess the pattern of missing data and, when appropriate, perform imputation to maximize the use of partial information on a subject [40, 41].

3 Decide on the allowable complexity of the model (i.e., the number of predictors), based on the overfitting-corrected R^2 and calibration diagnositcs.

4 Ensure the model will only include factors that are independently associated with the outcome; reduce collinearity in the variables (if detected), by transforming the information matrix to a correlation form, or grouping highly correlated variables.

5 Check linearity assumptions, and use spline regression models, to estimate nonlinear associations between the continuous predictors and the outcome.

6 Check additivity assumptions and incorporate pre-specified clinically motivated interactions between two independent variables, such as combined effects of a biomarker and a known clinical factor, and compare models with and without the interaction terms (e.g., using likelihood ratio tests).

7 Check to see if there are overly influential observations, and evaluate the need for truncating the range of highly skewed variables or making other pre-fitting transformations.

8 Check distributional assumptions and consider a different model, if necessary.

9 Graphically interpret the model, using partial effect plots and nomograms.

10 Assess model fit (check constant variance assumptions, normality assumptions, correlation patterns, etc.).

Regularized least squares regression models

When the goal is to identify a panel of biomarkers simultaneously, instead of a single biomarker, LASSO (least absolute shrinkage and selection operator) [42], a technique for L1-norm regularization, has been widely used for variable selection and dimension reduction in recent years, especially for $p > N$ problems (N: sample size; p: number of features). In order to produce parsimonious, interpretable models, LASSO minimizes the ordinary sum of squared errors with a bound on the sum of the absolute values of the coefficients. The LASSO method has its limitations:

1 when faced with a group of highly correlated features, the lasso will select only one predictor; and
2 the lasso can select at most N predictors.

A recently proposed generalization of the lasso and LARS is called the elastic net [43]. This method provides variable selection in the $p \gg N$ case, without being limited by the sample size. It improves performance in the case of highly correlated predictor variables (where the lasso is dominated by ridge regression), and improves selection when groups of predictors are highly correlated. The basic idea of the elastic net is to combine the ridge regression and lasso penalties. In the naive elastic net, a convex combination of L1- and L2- norms of the regression coefficients is constrained. The naive elastic net parameter estimates are obtained via the constrained minimization:

$$\hat{\beta}_{nEN} = \arg \min_{\beta} \sum_{i=1}^{N} (y_i - \beta_j' x_i)^2 \text{ subject to } (1 - \alpha)$$

$$\times \sum_{j=1}^{p} |\beta_j| + \alpha \sum_{j=1}^{p} \beta_j^2 \le t \text{ for some } t.$$

A modified procedure proposed by the same authors uses rescaling to avoiding overshrinking, while preserving the advantageous properties the elastic net. This is given by:

$$\hat{\beta}_{nEN} = \arg \min_{\beta} \beta' \left(\frac{X'X + \lambda_2 I}{1 + \lambda_2} \right) \beta - 2y'X\beta$$

$$+ \lambda_1 \sum_{j=1}^{p} |\beta_j|$$

If prediction is the goal, the LASSO may be preferred, because it selects only one representative predictor from highly correlated groups. An example is the use of LASSO-penalized logistic regression in case-control disease gene mapping with a large number of SNPs as candidate predictors [44]. However, if interpretation is the goal, the elastic net may be preferred, because it will include all the important predictors in a highly correlated group. For example, Zou and Hastie suggest the elastic net as a useful method in the analysis of microarray data, where the inclusion of highly correlated groups of predictors is preferred, because these groups are biologically meaningful and are valuable for further investigations.

Model validation and evaluation

Statistical validation techniques can be divided into two types: external and internal. Internal validation aims to correct for potential overfitting and to estimate the model's likely performance on a new sample. The most popular methods are bootstrap [45, 46] and cross-validation. Cross-validation is a simple and intuitive approach that provides a nearly unbiased estimate of the future error. The bootstrap is commonly believed to be more biased than cross-validation, but to have lower variance. Efron and Tibshirani showed that .632+ bootstrap (the number .632 comes from the probability that an observation is in a bootstrap sample, that is $1 - 1/e$.) substantially outperforms cross-validation in their simulation study [45].

However, it is worth noting that validation techniques including both bootstrap methods and cross-validation methods require the estimators to be smooth functions, whereas variable selection/dimension reduction techniques such as LASSO and elastic nets, have discontinuous first derivatives and may, therefore, produce substantial bias. This is an important issue related to model selection, and it does not yet have a well-defined and researched solution. The entire model-building procedure, instead of the final model, can be internally validated using the .632+ bootstrap method for the evaluation and correction of potential optimism in the performance of the predictive model, by balancing the bias and variance in the prediction error. Steps 5–8 in Section 20.2.3 can be repeated for each bootstrap replicate, to the extent needed.

The accuracy of the model predictions should be evaluated, both in terms of how well the model separates individuals who develop the outcome from those who do not (discrimination), and how close are the predicted risks to the actual observed risks (calibration). Model discrimination can be evaluated by calculating the area under the receiver-operator-characteristic (ROC) curve (AUC; also known as c statistic [47]), calculated for the outcome variables, such as disease-specific and overall deaths at five years post-diagnosis.

The ROC curve plots sensitivity against 1-specificity at different predicted risk thresholds, in which observed and model-based estimated five-year overall survival within deciles of risk score are compared. The added predictive value of a particular predictor can be evaluated by comparing models with and without the predictor, with regard to c statistics and the integrated discrimination improvement. The difference in c statistics between the two models will be tested using a nonparametric Mann-Whitney U test [47], and the integrated discrimination improvement will be evaluated using a simple asymptotic Z test [48]. These two statistics will be calibrated using the same bootstrap procedures described above, and the 95% bootstrap-based confidence intervals will be calculated. Model calibration will be assessed using a simplified goodness-of-fit method for the Cox proportional hazards model [49,50]. Both Pearson and deviance residual plots will be generated to identify covariate patterns that are poorly fit by the model. The predicted benefit of a marker can be calculated as an absolute percentage survival benefit for an individual patient, by applying the relative risk reduction of a particular marker to the outcomes.

Biomarker discover: challenges and obstacles

Data torture and multiple comparison problem

As in any other type of studies, if data are manipulated enough times and in enough different ways, they can be made to prove whatever the investigator intends to prove. Data torturing is scientifically unethical, because either the data are manipulated to fit a favored hypothesis – or, as more commonly seen in biomarker studies, the investigator analyzes the data multiple times, until a significant association is found between variables, and then devises a biologically plausible hypothesis to fit the association [51]. In this case, a *post-hoc* hypothesis is generated to explain the association that may or may not be observed by chance. This kind of data manipulation is sometimes referred to as a "fishing expedition" – one never knows what one will find.

Data torturing is especially problematic in biomarker studies for the following three reasons:

1 Biomarker studies often generate high-throughput genomic or proteomic data. In this case, hundreds, thousands, or even more independent tests are performed, and the investigator can find significant results even when none exist, simply by making multiple comparisons. Several statistical methods developed to correct for the multiple testing problem generally require a more stringent level of significance to be observed, in order for an individual comparison to be significant, so as to compensate for the inflated overall type I error rate based on the number of inferences being made. Commonly applied methods for biomarker studies include the Bonferroni correction, in which the p-values are multiplied by the number of comparisons, and some other less conservative procedures that give control of the family-wise error rate (FWER) [52–54], or methods that give control of the false discovery rate (FDR) [55, 56]. It is important to distinguish between the FWER and the FDR. The FWER is defined as the probability of rejecting at least one null hypothesis when all null hypotheses are true; and the FDR is defined as the expected proportion of falsely rejected hypotheses among all rejected hypotheses. Therefore, FDR is equivalent to the FWER only when all null hypotheses are true, but is smaller otherwise. Differences between the FDR and the FWER become larger as the number of tests increases and/or the number of true null hypotheses decreases. For this reason, studies designed to screen large numbers of biomarkers usually control for the FDR instead of FWER, since the latter can be too conservative.

2 When the biomarker is a continuous variable by nature, some data torturers take advantage of the lack of a well-established cutoff point in biomarker studies by performing the same

analysis with various cutoff points, to categorize the variable and select the point that produces the most significant results. This will lead to overestimation of the true effects, and a low reproducibility in subsequent validation studies. It should be noted that the presence of a dose-response relation is evidence that the reported effect is genuine, not the result of arbitrary classification [51].

3 When a pre-specified null hypothesis cannot be rejected, some investigators will perform a number of *ad hoc* analyses – possibly dozens or hundreds – such as subgroup analyses defined by arbitrarily chosen cutoffs of a biomarker, or different combinations of a panel of markers, in the hopes of finding some associations that were statistically significant, and choose to only report on these significant associations. The more subgroups created, the higher chance for the investigator to find associations that are statistically significant if not appropriately adjusted for multiple comparisons, as discussed above.

Statistical power

Of major importance in clinical trials involving biomarker predictors is the ability to predict individual patient outcome or endpoints using biomarkers efficiently and accurately. The power of a biomarker for the prediction of responses to cancer therapies, however, can be limited by two facts.

First, specific responses may be driven by multiple markers and interactions among the markers. This motivates researchers to discover combinations of gene expression and genomic variation data (such as gene signatures) that, together, are useful in drug response prediction (see Section 20.2.4). However, the study power in situations where multiple biomarkers are tested is not always well defined, regardless of how the false discoveries are controlled for multiplicity and, as a consequence, they may lead to seriously incorrect inferences. It is, therefore, important to establish the definition of study power: is it the probability of finding at least one true marker? Is it the probability of finding all true markers? Or is it the true discovery rate over all found markers?

Second, some biomarkers, such as gene expression, may have very small effect sizes on outcome measures, especially after adjusting for known clinical predictors. On the other hand, studies using biomarkers as the surrogate outcome can have dramatically inflated type I error rate, when the treatment has no effect on the true endpoint but does have an effect on the biomarker substitute. Furthermore, without knowing the strength and direction of the relationship between the surrogate outcome and the definitive outcome over time, incorrect inferences may be drawn from a study using biomarkers as the sole surrogate endpoint for the clinical outcome of interest [57]. Therefore, it is usually a better approach to use biomarkers as predictors of the primary endpoint, instead of a surrogate endpoint.

In addition to larger scale Phase II and Phase III trials, it has become increasingly popular for Phase I trials of targeted agents to open enriched expansion cohorts based on biomarker profiles, once the recommended phase II dose has been reached, with the hope of gaining insight on the so-called proof-of-concept, and to acquire early hints of anti-tumor activity in patients felt to possess the greatest chance of response. Molecular profiling of tumors, using genotyping technologies for somatic mutations and gene amplifications, or selection of tumor types based on published frequencies of molecular aberrations, are examples of enrichment strategies that have been used at the end of Phase II trials or in early Phase II trials.

While some clinical investigators strongly believe that this approach will speed up the drug development path, others fear that it is too limited without sufficient scientific justification, mainly due to the limited sample size of these Phase I expansion cohorts, and consequently, low study power. It is, therefore, important to recognize the potential of a biomarker trial design to increase the chance of erroneous positive conclusions, as an inflated overall type I error rate can result in misleading, or even counter-productive, design decisions. Studies with expansion cohorts, in particular, should always include sample size justifications at the planning/design stage (i.e., *a priori* power analysis).

The power analysis of biomarker studies generally focus on demonstrating that the sensitivity and/or specificity of a biomarker is superior to some pre-specified, clinically meaningful value (e.g., sensitivity > 0.7). The focus on sensitivity and specificity is important, even if the predictive values are of greater interest (as they usually are), because predictive values are also dependent on the prevalence of the underlying disease in the target population, which is often unknown.

Reproducibility and generalizability

Even though the clinical potential of biomarker discovery seems to be high, reproducibility remains the key obstacle to biomarker discovery. Biomarkers identified by different research groups often differ greatly, and even results based on different experiments from within the same groups can be inconsistent. Hence, there is an emerging need for efficient statistical methods that will address issues of reproducibility and increase our confidence in detected markers.

When a candidate biomarker is evaluated, it is critical to examine whether the candidate biomarker improves the predictive accuracy of the best available model that incorporates existing predictors of the study disease, including both validated biomarkers and known clinical factors. Univariate analysis, such as two-sample t-test, or discrimination measures such as AUC ROC and c statistic (introduced in Section 20.2.5), is commonly used in the analysis of biomarker data. However, a clear drawback of univariate methods is that they ignore the correlations between features and, hence, disregard the multidimensional structure of the data. A more suitable strategy is to select a set of features that together explain a large amount of the variation in the data, using a multivariate model-based approach, such as the aforementioned LASSO and elastic net methods. In this case, feature selection methods try to find a small subset of features that result in the most accurate predictive model.

Unfortunately, even with the most efficient feature selection algorithms, one may identify different subsets of candidate biomarkers from the same data. Even worse, different random subsets of similar size drawn from the original data can lead to different optimal feature subsets. Moreover, the bioinformatics tools used in discovery sets often seek to overfit the data, erring on the side of not missing a potential biomarker, but resulting in sensitivities and specificities that may not be reproducible.

While there is a large body of literature describing biomarker discovery, there are dramatically fewer publications validating identified markers, among which the majority include only internal validations. This is partially due to publication bias, in the sense that analysis results of data reported for a given biomarker resulting in publication may be different from that of unpublished studies. This is obviously because positive results are much more frequently reported than negative results, particularly in biomarker studies. So, because many candidate biomarkers will not be validated, few investigators are interested in devoting effort to a project that will likely not result in publication. It should be emphasized that consistency of results reported by multiple independent studies is a key factor for assessing external validity or generalizability of findings about candidate biomarkers, and this has a major influence on implementation of biomarkers in medical practices [58].

In oncology, it is quite common to discover a biomarker among a highly heterogeneous group of patients that is significantly associated with outcome based on univariate analyses but, in reality, correlates so strongly with known clinical factors (e.g., tumor size, grade, stage) that, on multivariate analysis, it provides no independent prognostic or predictive information. It is, therefore, also important to provide clinical factors with the same opportunities as potential biomarkers to be identified as predictors of a given disease. The added predictive ability of a biomarker, as well as a clinical factor, can be evaluated as previously discussed in Section 20.2.5.

Discussion

In this chapter, we have discussed the statistical issues involved in biomarker identification and validation. As new biomarkers, especially predictive markers, are discovered, it is increasingly important that a mechanism exists by which the most promising biomarkers can be validated using external samples. In some recently developed oncology trials, a biomarker is used as the surrogate endpoint, or is used for the interim analysis, to determine the adaptive modification. This strategy has the potential to foster advances in precision medicine, by identifying patient sub-groups who are more likely to respond to a certain treatment based on their genetic profiles, in addition to their clinical characteristics.

If there is uncertainty regarding the biomarker's predictive ability for the corresponding clinical endpoint, however, the use of a biomarker surrogate may lead to difficulties both for design and for final assessment of treatments. Introduction of bias to the trial by using a biomarker surrogate is also a concern, because of such uncertainty attached; therefore, statistical adjustments are required to control the type I error rate. Additionally, in many circumstances – especially in complex diseases such as cancer – not all treatment effects can be fully accounted for by a single biomarker. The use of multiple biomarkers for one disease, however, requires a more comprehensive assessment of treatment effects.

References

1. Wishart GC, Bajdik CD, Azzato EM, *et al.* (2011). A population-based validation of the prognostic model PREDICT for early breast cancer. *European Journal of Surgical Oncology* **37**, 411–7.

2. Ravdin PM, Siminoff LA, Davis GJ, *et al.* (2001). Computer program to assist in making decisions about adjuvant therapy for women with early breast cancer. *Journal of Clinical Oncology* **19**, 980–91.

3. Olivotto IA, Bajdik CD, Ravdin PM, *et al.* (2005). Population-based validation of the prognostic model ADJUVANT! for early breast cancer. *Journal of Clinical Oncology* **23**, 2716–25.

4. Cufer T (2008). Which tools can I use in daily clinical practice to improve tailoring of treatment for breast cancer? The 2007 St Gallen guidelines and/or Adjuvant! Online. *Annals of Oncology* **19**, 41–5.

5. Huober J, Thurlimann B (2009). Adjuvant! When the new world meets the old world. *Lancet Oncology* **10**, 1028–9.

6. Schmidt M, Victor A, Bratzel D, *et al.* (2009). Long-term outcome prediction by clinicopathological risk classification algorithms in node-negative breast cancer – comparison between Adjuvant!, St Gallen, and a novel risk algorithm used in the prospective randomized Node-Negative-Breast Cancer-3 (NNBC-3) trial. *Annals of Oncology* **20**, 258–64.

7. Mook S, Schmidt MK, Rutgers EJ, *et al.* (2009). Calibration and discriminatory accuracy of prognosis calculation for breast cancer with the online Adjuvant!

program: a hospital-based retrospective cohort study. *Lancet Oncology* **10**, 1070–6.

8. Lende TH, Janssen EAM, Gudlaugsson E, *et al.* (2011). In Patients Younger Than Age 55 Years With Lymph Node-Negative Breast Cancer, Proliferation by Mitotic Activity Index Is Prognostically Superior to Adjuvant! *Journal of Clinical Oncology* **29**, 852–8.

9. Campbell HE, Taylor MA, Harris AL, Gray AM (2009). An investigation into the performance of the Adjuvant! Online prognostic programme in early breast cancer for a cohort of patients in the United Kingdom. *British Journal of Cancer* **101**, 1074–84.

10. Campbell HE, Gray AM, Harris AL, Briggs AH, Taylor MA (2010). Estimation and external validation of a new prognostic model for predicting recurrence-free survival for early breast cancer patients in the UK. *British Journal of Cancer* **103**, 776–86.

11. Haybittle JL, Blamey RW, Elston CW, *et al.* (1982). A prognostic index in primary breast cancer. *British Journal of Cancer* **45**, 361–6.

12. Todd JH, Dowle C, Williams MR, *et al.* (1987). Confirmation of a prognostic index in primary breast cancer. *British Journal of Cancer* **56**, 489–92.

13. Galea MH, Blamey RW, Elston CE, Ellis IO (1992). The Nottingham Prognostic Index in primary breast cancer. *Breast Cancer Research and Treatment* **22**, 207–19.

14. Blamey RW, Pinder SE, Ball GR, *et al.* (2007). Reading the prognosis of the individual with breast cancer. *European Journal of Cancer* **43**, 1545–7.

15. Blamey RW, Ellis IO, Pinder SE, *et al.* (2007). Survival of invasive breast cancer according to the Nottingham Prognostic Index in cases diagnosed in 1990–1999. *European Journal of Cancer* **43**, 1548–55.

16. Lundin J (2007). The Nottingham Prognostic Index – from relative to absolute risk prediction. *European Journal of Cancer* **43**, 1498–500.

17. Collett K, Skjaerven R, Maehle BO (1998). The prognostic contribution of estrogen and progesterone receptor status to a modified version of the Nottingham Prognostic Index. *Breast Cancer Research and Treatment* **48**, 1–9.

18. Sundquist M, Thorstenson S, Brudin L, Nordenskjold B (1999). Applying the Nottingham Prognostic Index to a Swedish breast cancer population South East Swedish Breast Cancer Study Group. *Breast Cancer Research and Treatment* **53**, 1–8.

19. Sauerbrei W, Hubner K, Schmoor C, Schumacher M (1997). Validation of existing and development of new prognostic classification schemes in node negative breast cancer German Breast Cancer Study Group. *Breast Cancer Research and Treatment* **42**, 149–63.

20. D'Eredita G, Giardina C, Martellotta M, Natale T, Ferrarese F (2001). Prognostic factors in breast cancer: the predictive value of the Nottingham Prognostic Index in

patients with a long-term follow-up that were treated in a single institution. *European Journal of Cancer* **37**, 591–6.

21. Balslev I, Axelsson CK, Zedeler K, Rasmussen BB, Carstensen B, Mouridsen HT (1994). The Nottingham Prognostic Index applied to 9,149 patients from the studies of the Danish Breast Cancer Cooperative Group (DBCG). *Breast Cancer Research and Treatment* **32**, 281–90.

22. Van Belle V, Van Calster B, Brouckaert O, *et al.* (2010). Qualitative assessment of the progesterone receptor and HER2 improves the Nottingham Prognostic Index up to 5 years after breast cancer diagnosis. *Journal of Clinical Oncology* **28**, 4129–34.

23. Wishart GC, Azzato EM, Greenberg DC, *et al.* (2010). PREDICT: a new UK prognostic model that predicts survival following surgery for invasive breast cancer. *Breast Cancer Research* **12**(1), published online. doi: 10.1186/bcr2464.

24. Wishart GC, Bajdik CD, Dicks E, *et al.* (2012). PREDICT Plus: development and validation of a prognostic model for early breast cancer that includes HER2. *British Journal of Cancer* **107**, 800–7.

25. Curtis C, Shah SP, Chin SF, *et al.* (2012). The genomic and transcriptomic architecture of 2,000 breast tumours reveals novel subgroups. *Nature* **486**, 346–52.

26. Bauer KR, Brown M, Cress RD, Parise CA, Caggiano V (2007). Descriptive analysis of estrogen receptor (ER)-negative, progesterone receptor (PR)-negative, and HER2-negative invasive breast cancer, the so-called triple-negative phenotype: a population-based study from the California cancer Registry. *Cancer* **109**, 1721–8.

27. Perou CM, Sorlie T, Eisen MB, *et al.* (2000). Molecular portraits of human breast tumours. *Nature* **406**, 747–52.

28. O'Brien KM, Cole SR, Tse CK, *et al.* (2010). Intrinsic breast tumor subtypes, race, and long-term survival in the Carolina Breast Cancer Study. *Clinical Cancer Research* **16**, 6100–10.

29. Carey LA, Perou CM, Livasy CA, *et al.* (2006). Race, breast cancer subtypes, and survival in the Carolina Breast Cancer Study. *JAMA* **295**, 2492–502.

30. Yang XR, Sherman ME, Rimm DL, *et al.* (2007). Differences in risk factors for breast cancer molecular subtypes in a population-based study. *Cancer Epidemiology, Biomarkers & Prevention* **16**, 439–43.

31. Spitale A, Mazzola P, Soldini D, Mazzucchelli L, Bordoni A (2009). Breast cancer classification according to immunohistochemical markers: clinicopathologic features and short-term survival analysis in a population-based study from the South of Switzerland. *Annals of Oncology* **20**, 628–35.

32. Das P, Siegers GM, Postovit LM (2013). Illuminating luminal B: QSOX1 as a subtype-specific biomarker. *Breast Cancer Research* **15**, 104.

33. Terpos E, Dimopoulos MA, Shrivastava V, *et al.* (2010). High levels of serum TIMP-1 correlate with advanced disease and predict for poor survival in patients with multiple myeloma treated with novel agents. *Leukemia Research* **34**, 399–402.

34. Demetri GD, Reichardt P, Kang YK, *et al.* (2013). Efficacy and safety of regorafenib for advanced gastrointestinal stromal tumours after failure of imatinib and sunitinib (GRID): an international, multicentre, randomised, placebo-controlled, phase 3 trial. *The Lancet* **381**, 295–302.

35. Demetri GD, van Oosterom AT, Garrett CR, *et al.* (2006). Efficacy and safety of sunitinib in patients with advanced gastrointestinal stromal tumour after failure of imatinib: a randomised controlled trial. *The Lancet* **368**, 1329–38.

36. Lynch TJ, Bell DW, Sordella R, *et al.* (2004). Activating mutations in the epidermal growth factor receptor underlying responsiveness of non-small-cell lung cancer to gefitinib. *New England Journal of Medicine* **350**, 2129–39.

37. Herbst RS, Prager D, Hermann R, *et al.* (2005). TRIBUTE: a phase III trial of erlotinib hydrochloride (OSI-774) combined with carboplatin and paclitaxel chemotherapy in advanced non-small-cell lung cancer. *Journal of Clinical Oncology* **23**, 5892–9.

38. Buyse M, Sargent DJ, Grothey A, Matheson A, de Gramont A (2010). Biomarkers and surrogate end points – the challenge of statistical validation. *Nature Reviews Clinical Oncology* **7**, 309–17.

39. Freidlin B, McShane LM, Korn EL (2010). Randomized clinical trials with biomarkers: design issues. *Journal of the National Cancer Institute* **102**, 152–60.

40. Harrell FE, Jr (2001). *Regression modeling strategies: with applications to linear models, logistic regression, and survival analysis.* Springer.

41. Resseguier N, Giorgi R, Paoletti X (2011). Sensitivity Analysis When Data Are Missing Not-at-random. *Epidemiology* **22**, 282. 10.1097/EDE.0b013e318209dec7.

42. Tibshirani R (1994). Regression Shrinkage and Selection Via the Lasso. *Journal of the Royal Statistical Society, Series B (Statistical Methodology)* **58**(1), 267–88.

43. Zou H, Hastie T (2005). Regularization and variable selection via the elastic net. *Journal of the Royal Statistical Society: Series B (Statistical Methodology)* **67**, 301–20.

44. Wu T, Chen Y, Hastie T, Sobel E, Lange K (2009). Genome-wide association analysis by lasso penalized logistic regression. *Bioinformatics* **25**, 714–21.

45. Efron B, Tibshirani R (1997). Improvements on cross-validation: The .632+ bootstrap method. *Journal of the American Statistical Association* **92**, 548–60.

46. Steyerberg EW, Harrell FE, Jr., Borsboom GJ, Eijkemans MJ, Vergouwe Y, Habbema JD (2001).

Internal validation of predictive models: efficiency of some procedures for logistic regression analysis. *Journal of Clinical Epidemiology* **54**, 774–81.

47. DeLong ER, DeLong DM, Clarke-Pearson DL (1988). Comparing the areas under two or more correlated receiver operating characteristic curves: a nonparametric approach. *Biometrics* **44**, 837–45.

48. Pencina MJ, D'Agostino RB, Sr., D'Agostino RB, Jr., Vasan RS (2008). Evaluating the added predictive ability of a new marker: from area under the ROC curve to reclassification and beyond. *Statistics in Medicine* **27**, 157–72; discussion 207–12.

49. May S, Hosmer DW (2004). A cautionary note on the use of the Gronnesby and Borgan goodness-of-fit test for the Cox proportional hazards model. *Lifetime Data Analysis* **10**, 283–91.

50. May S, Hosmer DW (1998). A simplified method of calculating an overall goodness-of-fit test for the Cox proportional hazards model. *Lifetime Data Analysis* **4**, 109–20.

51. Mills JL (1993). Data torturing. *New England Journal of Medicine* **329**, 1196–9.

52. Holm S (1979). A Simple Sequentially Rejective Multiple Test Procedure. *Scandinavian Journal of Statistics* **6**, 65–70.

53. Hochberg Y (1988). A Sharper Bonferroni Procedure for Multiple Tests of Significance. *Biometrika* **75**, 800–2.

54. Hommel G (1988). A stagewise rejective multiple test procedure based on a modified Bonferroni test. *Biometrika* **75**, 383–6.

55. Benjamini Y, Hochberg Y (1995). Controlling the False Discovery Rate: A Practical and Powerful Approach to Multiple Testing. *Journal of the Royal Statistical Society, Series B (Statistical Methodology)* **57**, 289–300.

56. Benjamini Y, Yekutieli D (2001). The Control of the False Discovery Rate in Multiple Testing under Dependency. *Annals of Statistics* **29**, 1165–88.

57. Srivastava S, Verma M, Henson DE (2001). Biomarkers for early detection of colon cancer. *Clinical Cancer Research* **7**, 1118–26.

58. Andre F, McShane LM, Michiels S, *et al.* (2011). Biomarker studies: a call for a comprehensive biomarker study registry. *Nature Reviews Clinical Oncology* **8**, 171–6.

CHAPTER 21

Clinical Validation of Molecular Biomarkers in Translational Medicine

Harry B Burke[1] and William E Grizzle[2]

[1]Biomedical Informatics and Medicine Departments, F. Edward Herbert School of Medicine, Uniformed Services University of the Health Sciences, Bethesda, MD, USA

[2]Department of Pathology, University of Alabama at Birmingham, Birmingham, AL, USA

Supported in part by the Patient Safety and Quality Academic Collaborative, a Joint Defense Health Agency, Uniformed Services University Project Pancreatic SPORE at UAB, 2P50CA101955-07, the U54 MSM/TU/UAB Comprehensive Cancer Center Partnership 2U54CA118948-06, the DOD Grants W81XWH-10-1-0543 and PC120913, the Susan G. Komen Breast Foundation, KG090969 and BCTR0600484, and the UAB Skin Disease Research Center Grant 5P30AR50948.

Translational relevance

Biomarkers are used in early detection, diagnosis, prognosis and risk assessment, in predicting responses to specific therapies, and in evaluating therapeutic/preventive approaches. Before biomarkers can be used clinically, they must be validated. However, in cancer, there are few validated biomarkers for any of the above uses. Validation is a process that is not well understood by investigators and, frequently, biomarkers are described as validated when they have only begun validation. This manuscript describes and discusses a well-defined pathway, with the steps that are necessary for validation of a biomarker for a specific use over a defined interval of time. This manuscript will aid

investigators in the validation of their biomarkers, will clarify approaches needed for validation, and will reduce the waste of resources for biomarkers that appear to be not strong enough to be validated for a specific use.

Introduction

Molecular biomarkers are required for improving the assessment of risk of disease, establishing the existence of disease, determining prognosis and treatment, and the implementing personalized medicine [1, 2], and their clinical validation is a key step in translational medicine [3–6]. Validation is a rigorous process that requires a deep understanding of molecular biomarkers and their relationship to disease, as well as an appreciation of the complexities inherent in their identification, testing, and replication [4].

In the past 20 years, there has been an exponential increase in molecular biomarker research, with thousands of new gene and protein biomarkers reported each year. At last count, there are over 500 000 papers indexed in PubMed for gene, protein, and molecular biomarkers. Although many of these papers claim to report clinically useful prognostic biomarkers, there are embarrassingly

Biomarkers in Cancer Screening and Early Detection, First Edition. Edited by Sudhir Srivastava.

© 2017 John Wiley & Sons, Inc. Published 2017 by John Wiley & Sons, Inc.

few validated cancer prognostic biomarkers [7–10]. There are many reasons for this situation [8–10], one of which is that researchers may not fully appreciate the subtleties of molecular biomarkers, and may not follow the rigorous procedures that are necessary to translate basic scientific findings to the clinic [8–10]. The result is studies replete with errors, and a literature that contains incorrect, and many times even contradictory, results [8–10]. Because biomarkers are central to translational medicine, a failure to properly understand, assess, and utilize them has prevented their use in treatment, comparative benefit analyses, and in integrating individualized patient outcomes in clinical decision-making [8–11].

The validation of molecular biomarkers has been a concern since the earliest days of molecular research. Over the last 20 years, significant problems have been noted, and recommendations regarding solving these problems have been made [12], but few of these proposals have been adopted. Pepe *et al.* [13] proposed a model for clinical validation of biomarkers for the early detection for disease, yet subsequent publications on early detection suggest that the confusion did not recede after this publication [14–17].

This manuscript proposes a straightforward, general method for validating biomarkers, to assist investigators in their validation of molecular biomarkers. Because of the inherent complexity in analyzing biomarkers and the dynamic nature of the field, commentaries and general guidelines are provided.

Validation of biomarkers

A molecular biomarker can be said to have been validated if it has been shown, in an independent prospective replication study, to predict a specific outcome in a specified patient population, reliably and accurately, over a defined time interval [1,3,4]. At a minimum, a validated biomarker consists of a set of necessary and sufficient characteristics that uniquely identify the biomarker, and includes the following:
• a detection and analysis protocol that results in high inter-laboratory agreement;

• a defined target patient population,;
• a trained statistical model (i.e., a model whose parameters have been defined by the data that contain the biomarker);
• other relevant factors and the outcome of interest; and
• a quantitative statement of the accuracy of the biomarker at predicting the outcome of interest in the target population over the specified time interval [1,4].

For the purposes of this discussion, "molecular" refers to any sub-cellular factor, including proteogenomic, transcriptional, and metabolic factors [18]. "Biomarker" refers to both individual and combinations of biological factors, including panels, patterns, profiles, pathways, and signatures that are used to predict one of three outcomes – namely, risk of disease, the existence of disease, and prognosis [1]. There are three types of prognostic biomarkers, defined in terms of their use – namely:
• natural history, which predicts the course of the disease if the patient never receives a therapy;
• therapy-specific, which predicts whether a particular therapy will benefit the patient; and
• post-therapy, which predicts that the therapy the patient received benefited the patient [4].

"Outcome" is the clinical event of interest, such as incident disease, response to therapy, recurrence, or death. Although knowledge of the biological function of a molecular biomarker can provide important basic science information, functional information is not necessary for using a biomarker to predict a clinical outcome [2].

Predictive accuracy refers to the relationship of a predicted value to a true value for each patient, across a population of patients. It has two components – discrimination (the correct ordering of the predictions) and calibration (how close the predicted value is to the true value). A very useful measure of discriminative accuracy is the receiver operating characteristic (ROC) method [19–21]. We are less interested in the calibration of the model than the correct ordering of the predictions. Poorly calibrated models can be corrected by performing a post-processor calibration [22], but there can be no recovery from the low accuracy of a model that poorly discriminates.

Table 21.1 Characteristics of validation.

Category	Stage 1	Stage 2	Stage 3
Investigator	Original	Original	Independent
Data	Retrospective or prospective	Different retrospective or prospective	Different prospective
Analysis	Any	Pre-specified	Pre-specified
Minimum model accuracy*	0.75	0.70	0.65
Reporting results	No	Qualified	Unqualified

*Minimum model accuracy is the discriminative accuracy of the statistical model that includes the biomarker, and the biomarker adds significant predictive accuracy to the model.

Three stages of validation

We propose three stages to biomarker validation:
1 identification, characterization, and evaluation;
2 data and model testing; and
3 independent prospective replication of results (Table 21.1) [4].

Each stage must be successfully completed before moving to the next stage. Prior to beginning the clinical validation process, the investigator should be satisfied that the biomarker has the potential to answer an important clinical question. In other words, does the biomarker appear to be related to the disease, does the relationship appear to be very strong, and could use of the biomarker have an impact on patient outcomes?

For diseases in which the outcomes are easily predicted, no additional biomarkers are needed and, for diseases where there is no effective treatment, biomarkers will have little clinical utility. Additionally, the investigator should consider whether the biomarker is suitable for clinical use; in other words, is it relatively easily acquired and analyzed, is the analysis reproducible across laboratories, and is the acquisition and analysis of the biomarker relatively inexpensive? Further, will the biomarker be applicable to a sufficiently large number of patients, so that its validation will make a clinical difference? Finally, the candidate biomarker should be examined in terms of whether it could add predictive accuracy when used with the current biomarkers, and whether it could eliminate one or more of the currently used biomarkers. If it neither adds predictive accuracy, nor eliminates a current biomarker, then it is probably unnecessary. If the researcher believes that the evidence suggests that all these issues will be resolved in favor of

the biomarker, then the validation process should proceed.

The validation of molecular biomarkers should progress through three stages [4]. Stage 1 has three components: identification of the biomarker; characterization of the biomarker in terms of its specimen acquisition, and analysis in its target population; and creation and evaluation of a multivariate supervised learning statistical model, to determine the predictive power of the biomarker for a specific outcome over a specified time interval.

During stage 1, the investigator learns about the biomarker, including assessing the practicality of the acquisition of the biological specimen, its accuracy in various clinical populations, trying different statistical methods, determining a threshold (cut-off point for a continuous variable) for the biomarker, and examining the effects of confounders on the biomarker's accuracy. Most of the theoretical, biological, and experimental work related to the clinical validation of a molecular biomarker occurs in the first stage, and the determination is made in this stage as to whether the biomarker is sufficiently accurate, so that it warrants proceeding to the next stage in the validation process.

Stage 2, data and model testing, takes the final results of the first stage, and attempts to implement and test them on another independent dataset from a different institution. This is an important stage, because it reveals many of the unrecognized assumptions and biases that existed in the first stage. Stage 3, replication of results, is the critical stage, since the clinical utility of the biomarker is established in this stage. Until the biomarker successfully completes the third stage, which requires an independent investigator, an independent laboratory, and independent prospectively collected patient population, there is insufficient evidence that it can be applied to an important clinical problem.

Stage 1: identification, characterization, and evaluation (ICE)

In the ICE stage, the investigator selects and assesses a biomarker. There is no restriction as to how the biomarker is discovered. One of the first steps in identifying a potential risk or diagnostic biomarker is to determine if the biomarker is expressed differentially in diseased versus nondiseased tissue. In other words, is it specific to the disease? The next step is to assess the biomarker's relationship to an outcome (i.e., risk of disease, diagnosis, or prognosis [1]). Overall, there should be some evidence that the biomarker, as measured in solid tissue or in bodily fluids, is associated with the clinical outcome.

At the completion of this stage, the biomarker should be described in sufficient detail, so that it can be unambiguously and reproducibly identified and measured by other investigators (including the acquisition, storage and analysis of the biological specimen). Its analysis is documented, a disease is specified, a clinical population relevant to the biomarker is identified, a disease-related outcome is selected, and the time interval during which the biomarker is relevant to the outcome is provided.

An example of a validated biomarker is the estrogen receptor (ER) of breast cancer [23]. ER was initially described in terms of its measurement by radioimmunoassay, the specimen of malignant tissue and controls in which it was measured, the method of data analysis, the biomarker's relevance to a population of women with nonmetastatic breast cancer, its disease-related outcome (e.g., mortality due to breast cancer), and the time interval (e.g., ten year disease-specific mortality, and better survival [24]). The presence of a certain level of ER expression in the tumor predicts that anti-hormonal therapy will be effective in reducing women's probability of a recurrence, and of dying from their breast cancer [23, 25].

Even though a single biomarker may be the primary focus of the validation, its clinical use will invariably rely on a multivariate model, because the model must contain all the predictively relevant factors, so that it can make accurate predictions [26, 27]. The goal of the model will be to contain all the independent, orthogonal predictors of the outcome. Further, the multivariate model will usually be related to an effective treatment (e.g., antihormonal therapy for ER expressing breast cancers), so that the biomarker predicts which patients will or will not respond to a specific therapy [28].

An initial approach to the analysis is to create a dataset containing patients to be analyzed for the biomarker, and to randomly split the patients into training and testing subsets. The reason to spilt the data set is because the model developed on a single dataset will always have a high accuracy when it is assessed using the exact same patients on which it was developed. This high accuracy is due to overfitting, and it reduces the model's generalizability. Therefore, the accuracy of the model should be determined on another dataset.

It should be observed that splitting the data is less than optimal, because the training and testing data are subsets of the same patient population and contain the same biases (we will discuss assessing the model's accuracy independent data sets). The training subset determines the relationship between the independent and dependent variables, and establishes that relationship in a statistical model. The test subset measures the accuracy of that trained model. For large data sets that contain many clinical (binary) events (e.g., dead/alive, recurrence/no recurrence), a fifty-fifty split is reasonable. For smaller data sets, the more important component is the correct modeling of the disease phenomena, so more data are allocated to the training subset than the testing subset. A useful heuristic for small datasets is to split the data into two-thirds to three-fourths for training, and one-fourth to one-third for testing [28].

The biomarker is modeled using an appropriate statistical method on the training dataset, and its accuracy is tested on the testing dataset. During this stage, the investigator has knowledge of each patient's outcome, and may examine the data, assess various statistical methods, add or remove biomarkers, and modify the analysis in any way. Various thresholds can be tested, and the best one selected. There are no limitations on what may be done with the data or how the results are analyzed during this stage.

The discriminative accuracy of the model that contains the biomarker as a variable is measured on the testing dataset by the receiver operating characteristic (ROC). This is a critical juncture, for it is here that investigators can take a wrong turn. There is an inclination to believe that the results obtained on the ICE testing dataset have clinical meaning. However, they do not, because the investigator has optimized the biomarker, examined and manipulated the data and the analysis, looked at the results and, through trial and error, determined the best threshold, patient population, statistical model, and outcome for the biomarker. The biomarker's accuracy on an ICE dataset is not a valid measure of biomarker's clinical utility, because this stage has the potential to produce overly optimistic and biased results. So far, the investigator does not have valid results, and neither the model nor its ROC developed in the ICE stage should be presented or published.

How to report studies of biomarkers used as prognostic factors is beyond the scope of this paper. However, other publications have addressed reporting prognostic biomarkers, including REMARK, a checklist of 20 items (truncated to 11 items by some journal editors) that can be used to determine if a study of prognostic factors should be published [27, 29, 30], and STROBE-ME [31], which provides guidance on reporting observational molecular epidemiology studies.

Focusing on an understanding of the scientific process regarding biomarker validation, which is the goal of this paper, can be more useful to an investigator than performing a study guided by whether it will meet a set of publication criteria. In other words, although problems with performing a study and problems with its publication can overlap, if the performance of a study is scientifically valid, there should be few reporting problems. However, if the study is incorrectly designed and performed, no publication guidance can save it.

Further, there are elements in some reporting approaches that may increase, rather than decrease, the quality and validity of publications on biomarkers. One example of this difficulty is the statement by Altman [27], that it is permissible to publish results after the investigator has looked at the data and used the resulting information to plan key features of the analysis to be performed using the same data. Our view is that data can only be looked at in the ICE stage, and then only with the understanding that the resulting ICE finding cannot be published.

Typically, the accuracy of a biomarker decreases as it progresses through the validation stages. At the end of the validation process, it must retain sufficient accuracy to be clinically useful. In other words, the accuracy observed in the ICE stage will almost always be higher than the final validated accuracy of the biomarker. In order to save a biomarker investigator's time and resources, we suggest the following approach. A validated biomarker should have an ROC of at least 0.70 (assuming a standard deviation of 0.05 or less) to be clinically useful [2, 32]. Experience suggests that a biomarker will lose between 0.3–0.5 of its discriminative accuracy as it progresses thorough the stages of validation. Therefore, the minimum ROC for a biomarker to move from the ICE stage to the next stage should be 0.80. The relevance of these numbers will become more apparent in the clinical utility section of this paper.

Stage 2: data and model testing (DMT)

In this stage, the investigator uses the final characterization of the biomarker and statistical model derived from the ICE stage to test the biomarker. The researcher collects a new independent patient dataset (DMT dataset) from another investigator at a different institution [33]. This includes the defined target patient population, and appropriate biological samples for the measurement of the biomarker. The biomarker characteristics were determined based on the ICE study. The investigator then tests the ICE's final statistical model on the DMT dataset of patients. The critical component of this stage is the proper application of the final methods, and results from the ICE stage to the new DMT patient population. The trained statistical model from the ICE stage can be tested *only once* on the DMT dataset.

The DMT patients are run though the predictive model, and the probability the outcome over the defined time interval is determined for each patient. The predicted outcomes are compared to the true outcomes, and the predictive accuracy of the model is determined and reported in terms of the model's

ROC on the DMT patients. The results must be sufficiently accurate to justify moving to the third stage of the validation process. In this case, the minimum ROC required to progress to the next stage is 0.75.

If the biomarker does not achieve an acceptable accuracy in the DMT stage, the investigator should determine if this failure was due to one of the following: the characterization and analysis of the biomarker; the statistical model; the characteristics of the patient population; the treatments included in the analysis; the conditions of the study; or other factors. The researcher can return to the ICE stage at any time, improve the biomarker or the model, and re-test *once* on the DMT dataset. If the researcher uses the results of the DMT stage to improve the performance of the biomarker, then another, independent patient population, must be obtained for the DMT stage (labeled DMT2 dataset).

A successful evaluation of the biomarker does not mean that it has been validated, because the same investigator who performed the ICE stage also performed its DMT stage, and the dataset was retrospectively created. At this point in the process, many unknown, and even unanticipated, sources of bias may exist that can affect the power of the biomarker and the performance of the model and, therefore, the accuracy and utility of the biomarker. For example, the investigator's method of dataset collection, biomarker analysis, and use of the statistical model are all subject to bias and error. Further, the datasets used in the first two stages are usually retrospective, and subject to all the biases inherent in retrospective studies. Positive results of the DMT stage may be reported, but the report should contain the following explicit statement: "The reported biomarker results have not been validated and the biomarker is not ready for use in clinical practice." It is important that negative results of the DMT stage should also be published [15].

Stage 3: replication of results (ROR)

Because the hallmark of science is replication, a different investigator with a prospective, independently collected dataset should replicate the results of the DMT stage. This process is similar in approach to the DMT stage. The final model from the ICE stage – the one that was successfully used in the DMT stage – is applied only *once* to the ROR dataset. The model makes its predictions for the ROR patients, and these predictions are compared to the true outcomes. If the ICE stage results were reproduced in the DMT stage, but not in the ROR stage, this suggests that either there was a bias in the datasets used in one or more of the stages of the validation process, or there were problems with the performance of the biomarker assay.

Clinical utility means that the biomarker improves the management and outcomes of patients [30]. Determining the potential clinical utility of a biomarker is a complex concept [34]. It includes, but is not limited to: the acquisition and analysis of the biomarker; the number of patients with the target disease; the severity of the target disease; the safety and efficacy of the treatment; and the accuracy of the test in predicting a therapy-specific benefit. Herein, the discussion of clinical utility is limited, and only includes the accuracy of the biomarker. A necessary requirement for clinical utility is that the biomarker is significantly more accurate than chance prediction (i.e., an ROC of 0.50). It should be noted that accuracies of at least 0.70, and a standard deviation less than 0.05, are necessary. Increasing a low ROC requires either starting with a more powerful biomarker, or reducing the variance of the predictions.

Issues related to validating biomarkers

Biomarker datasets

The datasets used for validation should include the current clinical predictive factors, the relevant confounders, and the effective treatments. They should have a sufficient number of patients and events for model stability (discussed subsequently), and the patients should be followed for a sufficient period of time, defined by the clinical problem the biomarker is addressing, so that the predictions are clinically meaningful.

Most biomarker studies are conducted using retrospective populations. These datasets have the advantages of being readily available, with relatively long periods of follow-up, thus making them quick and much less expensive to acquire and use.

The main disadvantages of retrospective data sets are:

1 They may contain biases associated with patient selection, or specimen acquisition and analysis, or treatment.
2 They usually do not contain all the relevant predictors and confounders (i.e., there can be unmeasured covariates).
3 They almost always contain heterogeneous patient populations and therapies.
4 Not all the patients may have been assessed for the candidate biomarker (i.e., appropriate biological samples may not be available).
5 The therapies are not uniformly applied across patients, resulting in a surprising number of different treatment regimens.
6 They may contain patients treated with antiquated therapies, and/or inadequate numbers of patients may have been treated with current therapies.
7 They typically contain a great deal of missing data, which can make them unsuitable for multivariate analysis.

A key issue in retrospective data is the absence of biomarker values in some of the patients. The values could be missing completely at random, but this is rarely the case [35]. Usually, a bias is at work. The investigator has a number of ways to deal with this problem, including using only the patients who have a biomarker value, imputing a central tendency biomarker value, or finding the specimens and assessing the missing biomarker value. In terms of solving the missing data problem, finding the specimens and assessing the biomarker is usually the best approach. If this is not possible, then performing multiple imputation may be a useful alternative approach [36]. In any event, if the missing biomarker values affect the validation results – for example, if there is an important bias at work in the data, it will be discovered in stage 3 by a significant decrement in accuracy. Thus, retrospective studies are not definitive evidence of the accuracy and clinical utility of a biomarker.

Prospectively collected populations avoid many of the weaknesses inherent to retrospective studies. A prospective study follows a defined population, it collects all the relevant variables and samples, it implements uniform biomarker detection methods and therapy regimens, and the patients have been followed for a pre-specified period of time. The major limitations of prospective studies are: they have entry criteria that create a relatively homogeneous patient sub-population (in part to reduce patient variability); they require extensive financial and manpower resources; and they take a long time to complete. Further, they may not be generalizable to most patients with the disease because: the patients in the study were a special sub-population; because of the study's tight clinical control; or because many patients in the real world will not receive the exact therapy offered in the trial. Due to the time and cost of prospective studies, retrospective studies are usually employed in the ICE and DMT stages, the results of which are used to justify the time and cost of a prospective replication study.

Implicit in this discussion is the knowledge that prospective datasets are usually collected to evaluate a specific therapy. Their use in the ROR stage is based on the idea that not all the patients who receive the therapy will respond, and that this differential clinical effect can be used to define the utility of the biomarker in predicting which patients will respond to the therapy (therapy-specific prognosis) and predicting which patients, after receiving the therapy, responded to it by a change in the biomarker value (post-therapy prognosis) [1].

Statistical model instability

An important consideration in building statistical models is to avoid model instability. Model instability occurs when the relationship between the independent variable and the dependent variable is not linked strongly enough in the model. The result is that the model's parameter estimates vary over too great a range. It has been suggested that, to avoid model instability, there must be at least ten events (defined subsequently) for each independent variable [37]. However, for the analysis of the predictive power of molecular biomarkers, 15–20 events for each independent variable provide a greater assurance of model stability. With this number of events, the relationship between each independent variable and the outcome can be reliably determined (to the extent that the independent variable is a strong predictor of the outcome). Alternatively, one can use the bootstrap method to test for model instability [38, 39].

Clinical events

A clinical event is defined as the least frequent clinical outcome [4]. Thus, for a binary outcome (e.g., alive or dead), whichever occurs *least* often is the event rate. The optimal event rate for the analysis of a binary outcome is 50%. As the event rate diverges from 50% toward 0% or 100%, it becomes easier to make predictions, because a model will predict that the more frequent event will always occur, and it will be correct more and more of the time. For example, in terms of percentage correct, if the event rate is 10%, the model will be correct 90% of the time if it always predicts the occurrence of the non-event.

In other words, statistical models can learn to ignore the independent variables, and "bet on the frequency" [4]. In fact, in clinical conditions with very low event rates, it is rarely possible for the independent variables to do as well as predicting the outcome as betting on the frequency. This illustrates why an analysis cannot be based on an accuracy measure such as percentage correct. The ROC adjusts for the event frequency.

Combining molecular biomarkers

Although a detailed discussion of the acquisition and analysis of molecular factors for purposes other than biomarker validation is beyond the scope of this chapter [40, 41], there are certain issues related to the validation of these biomarkers that must be addressed. One can combine molecular biomarkers under various rubrics, including panels, patterns, profiles, signatures, and pathways. The goal of combining biomarkers is usually to increase predictive power beyond that afforded by an individual molecular biomarker. There are at least two approaches to combining molecular biomarkers. One approach can be called "naïve", because it groups biomarkers using a statistical algorithm that does not use any previously known information regarding the biomarkers, or the relationships between the biomarkers. The idea is that the relationship between the biomarkers will become apparent through their statistical association.

Another approach, which can be called "functional," captures the power inherent in functionally related biomarkers, such as membership in a biological pathway that is related to the disease process. The idea is that there is prior scientific knowledge

that certain biomarkers are related to each other and to the disease, and this previous knowledge can be used to inform the statistical model. In other words, naïve groupings make use of the numerical information in the dataset, but they ignore all other information. In contrast, functional groupings use the numerical information in the dataset and, in addition, they take advantage of previous scientific knowledge regarding relationships among biomarkers.

A functional group can be any set of related biomarkers. There is no restriction on the composition of a functional group, other than it must consist of factors that are related to the disease process. The idea is that a subset of the pathway factors will be active at any one time and, thus, are predictive of the course of the disease. Furthermore, one would like to include multiple orthogonal pathways (i.e., each providing new information regarding the disease process), in order to increase predictive power further. Because of the multiplicity of molecular biomarkers that comprise a pathway, the functional approach can be an effective way to combine many related biomarkers. The biomarkers in the pathway can be integrated using partial least squares or similar dimension-reduction strategies, and the integrated biomarkers can be one variable in the multivariate statistical model. Thus, each orthogonal pathway can be represented as a variable in a multivariate model. Generally, functional groups, rather than individual biomarkers, have the greatest chance of being strongly predictive.

Sometimes investigators create a group of genes (e.g., ten genes), and claim that this is a unitary gene signature, and the genes are necessary and sufficient to be the signature for some outcome. However, when the researchers attempt to reproduce their finding in another study, instead of reproducing the entire group of significant genes, they find that only six of the genes are significantly associated with the outcome in the repeat study. They may wish to claim that the six genes are now the validated gene signature. The problem is that the researchers cannot claim that the signature is composed of ten genes, when only six of the signature genes can be reproduced, nor can they claim that the combination of six genes is a new, replicated signature. Clearly, one cannot have it both ways – one cannot claim that there is a validated gene pattern, when the pattern does not replicate completely or abandon the pattern for another pattern, yet claim that the original signature was replicated. On the other hand, in a functional group, when one claims that a related set of genes is the predictive unit of analysis, it is not expected that all the genes in the group will always be significantly over or under expressed.

One method for assessing the predictive power of a biomarker in a multivariate model is to remove the biomarker from the model, and observe a change in predictive accuracy [28]. In this approach, each variable is, in turn, removed, assessed, and returned to the model. The idea is that if the biomarker is a powerful predictor, a large decrement in accuracy will be observed when it is removed. It should be noted that this is a complex process, since it also involves issues related to collinearly and levels of analysis. Analysis levels refer to the type of units being analyzed. For example, one can posit three levels of analysis in cancer, namely, epidemiologic (e.g., age, race, etc.), anatomic and cellular (e.g., tumor size, histology, etc.), and molecular-genetic (e.g., ER, PR, HER-2 [18]).

Time denomination of the biomarker

Predictions, or the probability of the occurrence or non-occurrence of an event, must always be time denominated [1, 4]. For example, the probability of an event occurring in five years is different from the probability of that same event occurring in ten years. There are two reasons why the prediction's duration must accompany its numerical estimate. First, time itself affects the probably of the outcome. For example, it may be more difficult to make predictions in the middle of the time interval (where the interval is bounded by the index date and the end of the study). Second, the biomarker may only be related to the disease ("active") at a particular time in the disease process, rather than uniformly across the course of the disease. Thus, a biomarker may be useful in predicting an outcome at two years, but not useful in predicting the same outcome at ten years. In other words, when a biomarker makes a prediction, that prediction is only relevant for a defined population, a specific outcome, and over a specified period of time.

Finally, lifetime predictions are rarely clinically useful, because it is not clear what the duration of the patient's lifetime will be and, therefore, the time interval of the prediction is unknown.

Conclusion

If we are going to model diseases in terms of their molecular characteristics, and these models are going to drive future advances in medical care, then translational science must produce clinically validated molecular biomarkers. Unfortunately, molecular biomarkers are subtle and complex entities, and their validation is challenging. Advances in the validation of clinically useful biomarkers requires an unambiguous scientific nomenclature, clearly described and defined methods, and clinically relevant uses if the molecular biomarkers are to significantly impact medical care.

To minimize the reporting and use of biomarkers that cannot be validated, a straightforward three-stage approach to biomarker validation is described. The three stages are:

1 Biomarker identification, characterization and evaluation.
2 Data and model testing.
3 Replication of results.

This provides a scientific approach that, if followed, offers a high degree of certainty that a validated biomarker will be a true and clinically useful predictor of disease-related outcomes.

References

1. Burke HB (1994). Increasing the power of surrogate end-point biomarkers: the aggregation of predictive factors. *Journal of Cellular Biochemistry* **19S**, 278–82.
2. Burke HB (2004). Predicting prognosis and the future of the TNM staging system, *Journal of the National Cancer Institute* **96**, 1408–9.
3. Burke HB, Henson DE (1993). Criteria for prognostic factors and for an enhanced prognostic system. *Cancer* **72**, 3131–5.
4. Burke HB, Henson DE (1999). Evaluating prognostic factors. *CME Journal of Gynecologic Oncology* **4**, 244–252. (In: Ch. 13, *Prognostic Factors in Epithelial Ovarian Carcinoma* (Bōsze P, ed.))
5. Grizzle WE, Srivastava S, Manne U (2012). Translational Pathology of Neoplasia. In: Srivastava S, Grizzle WE (eds.). *Translational Pathology of Early Cancer*, pp. 7–20. IOS Press BV, Amsterdam, The Netherlands.

6. Grizzle WE, Srivastava S, Manne U (2012). The biology of incipient, pre-invasive or intraepithelial neoplasia. In: Srivastava S, Grizzle WE (eds.). *Translational Pathology of Early Cancer*, pp. 21–39. IOS Press BV, Amsterdam, The Netherlands.

7. Khleif SN, Doroshow JH, Hait WN (2010). AACR-FDA-NCI Cancer Biomarkers Collaborative. AACR-FDA-NCI Cancer Biomarkers Collaborative consensus report: advancing the use of biomarkers in cancer drug development. *Clinical Cancer Research* **16**, 3299–318.

8. McShane LM, Altman DG, Sauerbrei W (2005). Identification of clinically useful cancer prognostic factors: what are we missing? *Journal of the National Cancer Institute* **97**, 1023–5.

9. McShane LM, Altman DG, Sauerbrei W, Taube SE, Gion M, Clark GM (2006). Statistics Subcommittee of the NCI-EORTC Working Group on Cancer Diagnostics. *Experimental Oncology* **28**, 99–105.

10. Mallott S, Timmer A, Sauerbrei W, Altman DG (2010). Reporting of prognostic studies of tumor markers: a review of published articles in relation to REMARK guidelines. *British Journal of Cancer* **102**, 173–80.

11. Twomby R (2006). Identity crisis: finding, defining, and integrating biomarkers still a challenge. *Journal of the National Cancer Institute* **98**, 11–12.

12. Simon R, Altman DG (1994). Statistical aspects of prognostic factor studies in oncology. *British Journal of Cancer* **69**, 979–985.

13. Pepe MS, Etzioni R, Feng Z, Potter JD, Thompson ML, Thornquist M, *et al.* (2001). Phases of biomarker development for early detection of cancer. *Journal of the National Cancer Institute* **93**, 1054–1061.

14. Ransohoff DF (2004). Rules of evidence for cancer molecular-marker discovery and validation. *Nature Reviews* **4**, 309–314.

15. Andre F, McShane LM, Michiels S, Ransohoff DF, Altman DG, Reis-Filho JS, *et al.* (2011). Biomarker studies: a call for a comprehensive biomarker study registry. Biomarker studies: a call for a comprehensive biomarker study registry. *Nature Reviews Clinical Oncology* **8**, 171–6.

16. Pepe MS, Feng Z (2011). Improving biomarker identification with better designs and reporting. *Clinical Chemistry* **57**, 1093–5.

17. Simon R (2012). Clinical trials for predictive medicine. *Statistics in Medicine* **31**(25), 3031–40.

18. Burke HB, Hutter RVP, Henson DE (1995). Breast carcinoma. In: Hermanek P, Gospadoriwicz MK, Henson DE, Hutter RVP, Sobin LH (eds.). *UICC Prognostic factors in cancer*, pp. 165–176. Berlin: Springer-Verlag.

19. Somer RH (1962). A new asymmetric measure of association for ordinal variables. *American Sociological Review* **27**, 799–811.

20. Bamber D (1975). The area above the ordinal dominance graph and the area below the receiver operating graph. *Journal of Mathematical Psychology* **12**, 387–415.

21. Swets JA (1996). *Signal detection theory and ROC analysis in psychology and diagnostics: collected papers*. Mahwah (NJ): Lawrence Erlbaum Associates.

22. Rosen DB, Burke HB, Goodman PH (1996). *Improving prediction accuracy using a calibration postprocessor*. Proceedings of the 1996 World Congress on Neural Networks, pp.1215–1220, San Diego CA, September 15–20.

23. McGuire WL (1973). Estrogen receptors in human breast cancer. *Journal of Clinical Investigation* **52**, 73–7.

24. Hähnel R, Woodings T, Vivian AB (1979). Prognostic value of estrogen receptors in primary breast cancer. *Cancer* **44**, 671–5.

25. Ward HW (1973). Anti-oestrogen therapy for breast cancer: a trial of tamoxifen at two dose levels. *BMJ* **1**(5844), 13–14.

26. Burke HB (1998). Integrating multiple clinical tests to increase predictive accuracy. In: Hanausek M, Walaszek Z (eds.). *Methods in Molecular Biology*, Vol. XX: Tumor Marker Protocols, Chapter 1, p. 3–10. Totowa (NJ): Humana Press Inc.

27. Altman DG, McShane LM, Sauerbrei W, Taube SE (2012). Reporting recommendations for tumor marker prognostic studies (REMARK): explanation and elaboration. *BMC Medicine* **10**(51). www.biomedcentral.com/1741-7015/10/51.

28. Burke HB, Goodman PH, Rosen DB, Henson DE, Weinstein JN, Harrell FE, Jr. *et al.* (1997). Artificial neural networks improve the accuracy of cancer survival prediction. *Cancer* **79**, 857–62.

29. McShane LM, Altman DG, Sauerbrei W, Taube SE, Gion M, Clark GM (2005). Reporting recommendations for tumor marker prognostic studies. *Journal of Clinical Oncology* **23**(36), 9067–9072.

30. McShane LM, Hayes DF (2012). Publication of tumor marker research results: The necessity for complete and transparent reporting. *Journal of Clinical Oncology* **30**(34), 4223–4232.

31. Gallo V, Egger M, McCormack V, Farmer PB, Ioannidis JP, Kirsch-Volders M, *et al.* (2011). STROBE Statement. STrengthening the Reporting of OBservational studies in Epidemiology – Molecular Epidemiology (STROBE-ME): an extension of the STROBE Statement. *PLOS Medicine* **8**(10), e1001117.

32. Burke HB. Henson DE (1997). Histologic grade as a prognostic factor in breast carcinoma. *Cancer* **80**, 1703–1705.

33. Altman DG, Royston P (2000). What do we mean by validating a prognostic model. *Statistics in Medicine* **19**, 453–473.

34. Hayes DF, Bast RC, Desch CE, Fritsche H Jr, Kemeny NE, Jessup JM, *et al.* (1996). Tumor marker utility grading system: a framework to evaluate clinical utility of tumor markers. *Journal of the National Cancer Institute* **88**(20), 1456–66.

35. Little RJA, Rubin, DB (1987). *Statistical analysis with missing data*. New York: John Wiley & Sons.

36. Rosen DB, Burke HB (1997). *Applying a gaussian-bernoulli mixture model network to binary and continuous missing data in medicine*. Preliminary papers of the international workshop on artificial intelligence and statistics, pp. 429–436.

37. Harrell FE, Lee KL, Matcher DB, Reichert TA (1985). Regression models for prognostic prediction: advantages, problems, and suggested solutions. *Cancer Treatment Reports* **69**, 1071–1077.

38. Efron B (1979). Bootstrap methods: Another look at the jackknife. *Annals of Statistics* **7**, 1–26.

39. Efron B, Tibshirani RJ (1994). *Introduction to the bootstrap*. Chapman & Hall/CRC press.

40. Micheel CM, Nass SJ, Omenn GS (2012, eds.) *Evolution of translational omics: Lessons learned and the path forward*. At: www.nap.edu/catalog.php?record_id=13297. Accessed June 25, 2013.

41. Olson S, Berger AC (2012). *Genome-based diagnostics: Clarifying pathways to clinical use*. At: www.nap.edu/catalog.php?record_id=13359. Accessed June 25, 2013.

CHAPTER 22

Cancer Biomarker Assays: Performance Standards

Anna K Füzéry[1,2] *and Daniel W Chan*[3,4]

[1] Department of Laboratory Medicine and Pathology, University of Alberta, Edmonton, AB, Canada
[2] Alberta Health Services, Edmonton, AB, Canada
[3] Department of Pathology, Johns Hopkins University School of Medicine, Baltimore, MD, USA
[4] Center for Biomarker Discovery and Translation, Johns Hopkins Medical Institutions, Baltimore, MD, USA

Introduction

Tremendous efforts have been made over the past few decades to discover novel cancer biomarkers for use in clinical practice. While early work focused mostly on protein- and carbohydrate-based biomarkers, recent advances in nucleic acid technology have also led to a boom in molecular targets [1, 2]. It is becoming increasingly clear that a striking discrepancy exists between the effort directed toward biomarker discovery and the number of markers that make it into clinical practice [3–9]. One of the common difficulties in translating a novel discovery into clinical practice is a limited knowledge of performance standard requirements for clinical assays [10]. This review, which is based on a previous publication by the same authors [11], provides an introduction to such considerations, with the aim of generating more extensive discussion for assay performance. We believe that this will facilitate the process of translating new biomarkers from discovery into cancer diagnostics.

Assay development: analytical performance

General considerations

Once a promising cancer biomarker candidate is identified, the next step is to develop an assay with suitable analytical performance for diagnostic accuracy studies and for eventual use in routine clinical practice. Because results will be used to manage patients in real-time, assays should be accurate and highly reproducible, simple and easy to perform and, if possible, they should have high throughput. Technologies associated with biomarker discovery often do not meet these requirements, and the evaluation of alternate methodologies early on is highly advisable. The OVA1 test for ovarian cancer, for example, was initially developed on the SELDI mass spectrometry (MS) platform, because this platform had been used to discover the five proteomic biomarkers included in the test. However, despite significant efforts, the precision of the test could not be increased to

Biomarkers in Cancer Screening and Early Detection, First Edition. Edited by Sudhir Srivastava.
© 2017 John Wiley & Sons, Inc. Published 2017 by John Wiley & Sons, Inc.

clinically acceptable levels. The SELDI MS platform was therefore abandoned, and the test was eventually implemented using immunoassays [12].

The intended use, and the targeted country's regulatory requirements, should both be taken into consideration when determining the stringency of performance assessment. In order to develop an analytically robust cancer biomarker assay, however, at least the following parameters should be evaluated: precision, trueness, limit of quantitation, linearity and working range, specificity, carryover, and analyte stability upon storage and preparation. In general, Clinical Laboratory Standards Institute (CLSI) guidelines [13–21] provide excellent starting points for designing these experiments, and are becoming a widely used resource by clinical laboratories, assay developers, and *in vitro* diagnostics companies.

Precision

Precision refers to the closeness of agreement between a series of measurements obtained for the same sample under a specified set of conditions. Precision evaluates random error, and sources of random error include inadequately mixed reagents, unstable temperature or electrical supply, individual operator variation in sample handling, bubbles in reagents, and so forth. CLSI defines different kinds of precision [13], but repeatability and reproducibility are the most important for a clinical assay. Repeatability, also known as within-run precision, is determined from successive measurements obtained with the same method, in the same laboratory, by the same operator, using the same equipment, within a short interval of time [13].

In contrast, reproducibility, also known as within-laboratory precision, is based on measurements performed with the same method in the same laboratory but under different days, operators, reagent lots, ambient temperature, and so on [13, 22]. If the assay is to have a wide implementation, measurements from multiple laboratories may also be included in the evaluation [13]. Precision is quantitatively expressed in terms of standard deviation (SD), variance, or coefficient of variation (CV), and is often a function of the analyte concentration, with low concentrations resulting in poorer precision (i.e., larger CV) than high concentrations.

Precision should be evaluated across the entire reportable range of the assay during development of a new cancer biomarker assay. Particular care should be taken to assess it at the medical decision points of relevance to the intended clinical application of the cancer biomarker. Moreover, since cancer patients are often monitored over long periods of time, the evaluation of long-term stability is also of importance. Test materials for precision evaluation should simulate clinical samples as closely as possible [13]. Individual patient samples are not generally available in sufficient quantities for such experiments but pooled patient samples are a reasonable alternative. In the absence of the latter, certain commercially available materials may also be acceptable [13].

The decision as to what constitutes an acceptable level of precision is based on the effect of analytical performance on clinical decisions, published professional recommendations, performance goals set by regulatory agencies and External Quality Assessment schemes, and/or current state of the art [23]. The reader is referred to a number of excellent articles [24–26] for more details. Ultimately, whether assay precision is acceptable or not will be influenced, to a large degree, by the intended clinical use of the test. Decisions based on a single cancer biomarker result (for example, diagnosis or prognosis) will require high repeatability, while decisions based on time-related changes (for example, in the monitoring of therapy) will require high long-term reproducibility.

Trueness

Trueness refers to the closeness of agreement between the average value obtained from a large series of test results and a true or an accepted reference value [19]. Trueness evaluates systematic error, and sources of systematic error include improperly prepared reagents or reagent deterioration, changes in sample or reagent volumes due to pipettor misalignment, incorrect calibrator values, and so forth. Trueness is inversely related to bias – that is, the greater the bias, the greater the discrepancy between the average measured value and the true value. Constant bias yields results that differ from the true value by a fixed amount, while proportional bias yields results differing by an amount that is proportional to the concentration of the measurand.

Although the detrimental effect of assay bias on patient care is widely acknowledged, cancer biomarker assays without any bias are still lacking in clinical practice. Most immunoassays struggle with bias, due to a lack of antibody specificity. Immunoassays for prostate specific antigen (PSA), for example, detect both free PSA and PSA bound to α_1-antichymotrypsin (PSA-ACT), but differences exist as to the relative response elicited by each form [27, 28]. Equimolar assays generate identical signals for equal molar concentrations of free PSA and PSA-ACT, while skewed assays respond differently to the two forms. Similarly, human choriogonadotropin (hCG) exists in the intact form, as the free α- and β-subunits, as a nicked form of the β-subunit, as the core fragment, and as hypo- and hyperglycosylated forms [29]. However, not all forms exist in every type of body fluid, and the relative proportion of isoforms may vary among health and disease states [29–33]. The relative specificities of the antibodies used in an hCG assay are an important determinant of which hCG forms are measured and, therefore, of the reported hCG value [29, 34].

Bias is also problematic for molecular assays. For instance, tissue collection and preparation both exert a strong influence over the quality of extracted DNA and, therefore, on the final result. DNA isolated from formalin-fixed, paraffin-embedded (FFPE), for example, is often highly degraded, and is of poorer quality than DNA from fresh frozen tissue [35]. To date, collection and preparation procedures have not been standardized across different laboratories, and rely heavily on the subjective assessment and approval of pathologists. A few years ago, the College of American Pathologists highlighted this problem in a statement on KRAS testing for colorectal cancer [36]. Nowadays, many commercially available technologies for KRAS show better concordance, but differences in DNA quality may still lead to appreciable bias [37]. Although not yet used in clinical practice, currently available assays for circulating tumor cells (CTCs) also vary in how they enrich for and detect CTCs and thus yield discordant results [38].

While standardization efforts after the commercial release of a clinical assay can partially address bias-related issues, such efforts are challenging and time-consuming (see [39] for an example). For this reason, it is advisable to evaluate and minimize bias as much as possible during the translational stage of assay development.

Analytical sensitivity

The limit of detection (LoD) represents the lowest amount of an analyte that can be reliably distinguished from zero. Terms used interchangeably with LoD include lower limit of detection, minimum detectable concentration, analytical sensitivity, and biological limit of detection. While a low LoD is desirable for many clinical applications of cancer biomarkers, including early detection and monitoring of recurrence, it is not sufficient for clinical use. As discussed earlier, the assay also needs to have acceptable precision and bias at these low levels of analyte – otherwise, any result near the LoD may have so much uncertainty associated with it that it no longer allows confident clinical interpretation and decision making. A performance indicator that incorporates such requirements is the limit of quantitation (LoQ), the lowest concentration at which the analyte is not only reliably distinguished from zero, but also meets certain specifications for bias and precision [20, 40].

Other terms that have been used interchangeably with LoQ include lower limit of determination, lower end of the measuring range, lower limit of quantitation, and limit of quantification [20]. In most instances, LoQ exceeds LoD, but it is possible for the two quantities to be equal. As mentioned previously, the decision as to what constitutes an acceptable level of precision and bias at low concentrations will be strongly influenced by the intended clinical use of the test. In general, tests that produce results leading to invasive follow-up require the most strict performance criteria. The reader is referred to reference [20] for additional considerations in establishing LoQ.

Owing to the qualitative nature of molecular tests, LoD and LoQ are defined slightly differently. LoD, in general, refers to the minimum quantity of tumor DNA (or tumor cells in some cases) that must be present, or a percentage of tumor DNA that must be present in the background of normal DNA to detect the cancer biomarker of interest with acceptable precision [41]. As for protein- and carbohydrate-based cancer biomarkers, the intended clinical use of the test is a key determinant of the definition of "acceptable precision". Of the technologies that are routinely used in present clinical practice, quantitative PCR has the best sensitivity, at $\approx$ 1%, while Sanger sequencing has the worst at > 10% [42]. Newer technologies, such as digital PCR, show promise in lowering this limit to less than 0.01%, but have yet to be incorporated into widespread clinical practice [41–44]. The term LoQ is infrequently used with molecular assays, and will not be discussed here.

Specificity and analytical interference

Analytical interference may be defined as the effect of a substance in a sample that alters the correct value of the result [45]. In today's clinical laboratory, protein- and carbohydrate-based cancer biomarkers in biological fluid are generally measured by two-site, non-competitive immunoassays ("sandwich immunoassays") [46]. This technique has a number of limitations that should be considered during assay development and validation. The lack of complete antibody specificity for a single molecular species has been discussed previously.

The hook effect, where a sample with a high analyte concentration gives a signal that is much lower than the theoretically expected value, is another important limitation of such assays [47]. This phenomenon arises because high concentrations of analyte saturate all antigen binding sites on both the capture and label reagent antibodies, and thereby interfere with sandwich-formation. A subsequent wash step removes all species not bound to the capture antibody (including analyte-label antibody complexes), and leads to a lower-than-expected signal during detection. The hook effect is most problematic when the falsely low result is within the values of the calibration curve. In such a case, one would not suspect any wrong results unless a dilution of the patient's specimen was made.

Cancer biomarker assays are especially prone to the hook effect, since the concentration of most cancer biomarkers ranges over several orders of magnitude and, in some cases, may even exceed millions of units per liter [48–51]. Case reports of the hook effect causing a falsely low result, and thereby leading to adverse patient outcomes, are not uncommon. For example, Jassam and colleagues described a two-month-old infant with a liver tumor whose diagnosis and subsequent management was changed from hepatic hemangioendothelioma to hepatoblastoma after discovery of a falsely low alpha-fetoprotein (AFP) measurement [49]. To avoid such errors as best possible, the National Academy of Clinical Biochemistry recommends that every testing laboratory have defined protocols in place for identifying specimens that have "hooked" [26].

Dilution and re-measurement of a specimen is one way to identify a hook effect, but financial and time considerations prevent this from being applied to every specimen that arrives in a laboratory. In some cases, strong clinical suspicion of an erroneous result will suggest that the dilution protocol be applied but, in many cases, the erroneous result may go unnoticed. For this reason, it is imperative that the potential for hook effect is minimized before the assay is implemented in the laboratory (i.e., during the development phase). Other common interferences that have been documented for sandwich immunoassays include anti-reagent antibodies which are found in patient samples (e.g. human anti-mouse antibodies and rheumatoid factor) and nonspecific interferences [52–55]. To best characterize these possible sources of interference, a careful study with samples from the intended use population should be included as part of the assay validation.

Molecular assays also suffer from specificity and interference problems. DNA extracted from FFPE tissue, for example, has been associated with base modifications, as well as molecular jumping or template switching [56–58]. The latter refers to a phenomenon where polymerization continues after a prematurely terminated polymerization product jumps to another template, thereby creating an *in vitro* recombination product. Recent efforts to circumvent such problems include use of fresh frozen tissue instead of FFPE tissue, genotyping of cell-free tumor DNA, and characterization of CTCs [38, 42, 59–61].

An additional cause of interference problems is assay cross-reactivity with sequences other than the target sequence. Sources of such sequences include homologous genes and DNA carryover contamination of amplification products and primers from previous PCR. In general, such issues can be adequately addressed by careful primer design [62], inclusion of uracil DNA glycosylase in PCR reactions [64], unidirectional workflows [21, 64], the separation of pre- and postamplification areas and equipment [21, 64], and self-contained ("closed") assay design [21]. The reader is referred to several excellent articles and book chapters [41, 65, 66] for further discussions on specificity and interferences in molecular assays.

Carryover

Carryover refers to the materials, such as parts of a specimen or reaction reagent, that are unintentionally transferred from one reaction into subsequent reactions, thereby yielding erroneous results [17]. For protein- and carbohydrate-based cancer biomarkers, carryover is of particular concern when the clinically relevant concentration range spans several orders of magnitude and possibly even exceeds millions of units per liter (e.g., AFP, hCG, and carcinoembryonic antigen (CEA) [48]). In such instances, the transfer of even a small amount of a high-concentration sample into a subsequent reaction mixture may lead to serious adverse clinical consequences. Carryover in molecular assays is also of concern; the presence of even very small amounts of DNA from a previous amplification of the same target may lead to erroneous results [21, 65].

Owing to its serious repercussions, currently available commercial assays have multiple built-in features to minimize carryover, including the use of disposable pipette tips and sample cups, careful selection of sample and reagent probe materials, optimization of probe design and system wash procedures, and/or a self-contained ("closed") automated design [21, 67, 68]. Individual laboratories may also attempt to limit carryover and its downstream effects. Examples of such efforts include retesting of a sample that follows directly after a high-concentration sample [48], unidirectional workflows, and the separation of pre- and postamplification areas and equipment [21, 64].

Assay development: clinical performance

General considerations

Robust analytical performance is an essential but insufficient prerequisite for the successful clinical deployment of a novel cancer biomarker. Diamandis provided accounts of initially promising cancer biomarkers that failed to make it into clinical practice because of errors made during validation of the markers' clinical performance [4]. Ioannidis related similar stories and classified biomarker failures into four common types: type A (clinical reversal), type B (validation failure), type C (non-optimized clinical translation), and type D (promotion despite non-promising evidence) [5]. Of these four failure types, only one is related to the analytical performance of the cancer marker, with the other three being due to insufficient clinical validation. Clinical validation of a cancer marker is complex, time-consuming, and expensive; careful planning at every stage is, therefore, essential to avoid a waste of resources.

Intended use

When a cancer biomarker is being developed as a clinical diagnostics, its specific intended use is critical in defining the clinical performance criteria for the assay. Parameters that should be defined include: the disease of interest; the decision-making point along the disease progression path; the patient population for which the biomarker is intended; and the costs of true positive, true negative, false positive, and false negative results [9]. While defining an intended use is often the most challenging part of a project, close collaboration with clinical staff goes a long way in facilitating this process.

Clinical sensitivity and specificity

Clinical sensitivity and specificity are both measures of the intrinsic diagnostic accuracy of a test. Clinical sensitivity is the ability of the test to correctly identify those patients with the disease of interest, while clinical specificity is the ability to correctly identify those patients without the disease of interest [69]. An ideal assay demonstrates clinical sensitivity and specificity of 100%, but this is never achieved in practice, because an increase in sensitivity is only gained at the expensive of specificity, and vice versa. The decision to maximize sensitivity, specificity, or both depends on many factors, including the general course of the disease, the consequences of early versus late diagnosis, the consequences of a false positive or negative result and, to some extent, the financial costs associated with testing and subsequent patient care.

The proper study design for evaluating clinical sensitivity and specificity may be quite challenging. Careful consideration must be given to many issues including:

1 the availability (choice) of a technique for determining the true disease status of each individual;
2 identifying appropriate individuals to be included in the target populations;
3 the size of the study populations; and
4 appropriate and standardized interpretation of results from the test under evaluation.

An additional confounding issue is that cancer biomarkers may be used in applications other than diagnosis and, in these situations, it may be unclear how to define the target condition, or clinical sensitivity and specificity. For an in-depth discussion of these, and additional considerations, the readers are referred to several excellent articles [4, 70–76].

ROC analysis

Clinical sensitivity and specificity depend intimately on the decision threshold used for a test. A decision threshold is a predetermined, fixed value of an analyte that, when exceeded, indicates that a critical decision needs to be made with respect to the patient's care. Receiver operating characteristic (ROC) analysis is a powerful tool to evaluate diagnostic test performance, and is invaluable in the selection of a decision threshold that is appropriate for the intended clinical use of the test. Popular ways of selecting an optimal threshold include finding the point on the ROC curve closest to the coordinate ($x = 0$, $y = 1$), and calculation of the Youden index [77–79]. Both of these methods give equal weight to sensitivity and specificity, but fail to consider disease prevalence and the financial, emotional, and ethical costs of misdiagnoses. Although the latter considerations are very important in clinical practice, they are difficult to quantify and, as a result, they are rarely incorporated into ROC analyses.

One property of ROC curves that is extremely useful in the clinical validation of a cancer biomarker is the area under the curve (AUC). This parameter is a combined measure of the sensitivity and specificity of a test over all threshold values and is, thus, a useful indicator of the marker's overall diagnostic performance [80, 81]. A higher AUC indicates better performance, so an ideal assay (100% sensitivity and specificity) will have an AUC

of 1.0, while an assay with no power to discriminate diseased from healthy individuals will have an AUC of 0.5. In certain cases, however, the AUC will be too global of a summary measure, and will not accurately reflect the performance of the assay for the intended clinical application. A more meaningful way to evaluate the diagnostic accuracy in such cases is to calculate the partial area under the curve (PAUC) – that is, the AUC over a selected range of threshold values that covers the specificities of clinical interest [80, 81].

In addition to evaluating a single assay, ROC curves may also be used to compare multiple assays, or different generations of a single assay. In such instances, a visual examination of the ROC plot should always be done concomitantly with the assessment of quantitative parameters (e.g. AUC, PAUC), because assays can have identical AUCs or PAUCs and still perform differently over the range of threshold values examined [77, 80, 81].

While ROC analysis is very helpful in assessing the diagnostic performance of an assay, users need to be mindful of its limitations. For an in-depth discussion of common misuses of ROC curves, the reader is referred to a report by Obuchowski and colleagues [82].

Positive and negative predictive values

When evaluating the diagnostic performance of an assay, the prevalence of the disease in the target patient population also needs to be taken into account. The positive predictive value (PPV) and negative predictive value (NPV) combine prevalence with the test's clinical sensitivity and specificity. The PPV provides the likelihood that, given a positive test result, the patient actually has the disease in question. Similarly, the NPV provides the likelihood that, given a negative test result, the patient does not have the disease.

A test may have very high diagnostic accuracy and still have a low PPV or NPV, thereby limiting the test's adoption into clinical practice. Cancer antigen 125 (CA-125) clearly illustrates this problem; the sensitivity and specificity of CA-125 for ovarian cancer are $\approx 100\%$ and $\approx 99\%$ respectively but, owing to the low prevalence of ovarian cancer, the PPV of CA-125 for ovarian cancer is only 4%. Thus, out of every 100 positive test results, only four will signal the presence of real disease [83]. This problem exists not only for CA-125 but for most other cancer markers, and it is one reason for the current paucity in cancer screening assays. Therefore, some attempt should always be made to assess the PPV and NPV of a test during the evaluation of its clinical performance.

Conclusions

In this chapter, we have discussed the performance standards of cancer biomarker assays. The analytical requirements for a robust clinical assay include the concepts of precision, trueness, sensitivity, specificity and interference, and carryover. The clinical considerations include diagnostic accuracy, ROC analysis, and PPV and NPV. To translate biomarker assays into cancer diagnostics, ultimately, it is the test (device) for the cancer marker that will be evaluated and approved by regulatory agencies for clinical use. However, while we recognize that the road from biomarker discovery, validation, and regulatory approval to the translation into the clinical setting could be long and difficult, the reward for patients, clinicians and scientists could be rather significant.

List of abbreviations

MS – mass spectrometry; CLSI – Clinical Laboratory Standards Institute; SD – standard deviation; CV – coefficient of variation; PSA – prostate specific antigen; PSA-ACT – PSA bound to α_1-antichymotrypsin; hCG – human choriogonadotropin; FFPE – formalin-fixed – paraffinembedded; CTC – circulating tumor cell; LoD – limit of detection; LoQ – limit of quantitation; AFP – alpha-fetoprotein; CEA – carcinoembryonic antigen; ROC – receiver operating characteristic; AUC – area under the curve; PAUC – partial area under the curve; PPV – positive predictive value; NPV – negative predictive value; CA-125 – cancer antigen 125.

Competing interests

The authors declare that they have no competing interests.

Authors' contributions

All authors were involved in the drafting and revising of the manuscript. All authors read and approved the final manuscript.

References

1. Biomarkers Definitions Working Group (2001). Biomarkers and surrogate endpoints: Preferred definitions and conceptual framework. *Clinical Pharmacology & Therapeutics* **69**, 89–95.

2. Chan DW, Schwartz MK (2002). Tumor markers: Introduction and general principles. In: Diamandis EP, Fritsche HA, Lilja H, Chan DW, Schwartz MK (eds.). *Tumor markers. Physiology, pathobiology, technology, and clinical applications*, pp. 9–17. Washington: AACCPress.

3. Chan DW (2010). Will cancer proteomics suffer from premature death? *Clinical Proteomics* **6**, 1–3.

4. Diamandis EP (2010). Cancer biomarkers: Can we turn recent failures into success? *Journal of the National Cancer Institute* **102**, 1–6.

5. Ioannidis JPA (2013). Biomarker failures. *Clinical Chemistry* **59**, 202–204.

6. Pavlou MP, Diamandis EP, Blaustig IM (2013). The long journey of cancer biomarkers from the bench to the clinic. *Clinical Chemistry* **59**, 147–157.

7. Regnier FE, Skates SJ, Mesri M, Rodriguez H, Težak Ž, Kondratovich MV, Alterman MA, Levin JD, Roscoe D, Reilly E, Callaghan J, Kelm K, Brown D, Philip R, Carr SA, Liebler DC, Fisher SJ, Tempst P, Hiltke T, Kessler LG, Kinsinger CR, Ransohoff DF, Mansfield E, Anderson NL (2010). Protein-based multiplex assays: Mock presubmission to the US Food and Drug Administration. *Clinical Chemistry* **56**, 165–171.

8. Zhang Z, Chan DW (2005). Cancer proteomics: In pursuit of "true" biomarker discovery. *Cancer Epidemiology, Biomarkers & Prevention* **14**, 2283–2286.

9. Zhang Z, Chan DW (2010). The road from discovery to clinical diagnostics: Lessons learned from the first FDA-cleared *in vitro* diagnostic multivariate index assay of proteomic biomarkers. *Cancer Epidemiology, Biomarkers & Prevention* **19**, 2995–2999.

10. Vidal M, Chan DW, Gerstein M, Mann M, Omenn GS, Tagle D, Sechi S (2012). The human proteome – a scientific opportunity for transforming diagnostics, therapeutics, and healthcare. *Clinical Proteomics* **9**, 6–16.

11. Füzéry AK, Levin J, Chan MM, Chan DW (2013). Translation of proteomic biomarkers into FDA approved cancer diagnostics: issues and challenges. *Clinical Proteomics* **10**, 13–26.

12. Fung ET (2010). A recipe for proteomics diagnostic test development: The OVA1 test, from biomarker discovery to FDA clearance. *Clinical Chemistry* **56**, 327–329.

13. CLSI (2004). *Evaluation of precision performance of quantitative measurement methods; Approved guideline – Second edition.* CLSI document EP05-A2. Wayne, PA: Clinical and Laboratory Standards Institute.

14. CLSI (2003). *Evaluation of the linearity of quantitative measurement procedures: A statistical approach; Approved*

guideline. CLSI document EP06-A. Wayne, PA: Clinical and Laboratory Standards Institute.

15. CLSI (2005). *Interference testing in clinical chemistry; Approved guideline – Second edition*. CLSI document EP07-A2. Wayne, PA: Clinical and Laboratory Standards Institute.

16. CLSI (2013). *Measurement procedure comparison and bias estimation using patient samples; Approved guideline – Third edition*. CLSI document EP09-A3. Wayne, PA: Clinical and Laboratory Standards Institute.

17. CLSI (2014). *Preliminary evaluation of quantitative clinical laboratory measurement procedures; Approved guideline – Third edition*. CLSI document EP10-A3-AMD. Wayne, PA: Clinical and Laboratory Standards Institute.

18. CLSI (2005). *Evaluation of matrix effects; Approved guideline – Second edition*. CLSI document EP14-A2. Wayne, PA: Clinical and Laboratory Standards Institute.

19. CLSI (2005). *User verification of performance for precision and trueness; Approved guideline – Second edition*. CLSI document EP15-A2. Wayne, PA: Clinical and Laboratory Standards Institute.

20. CLSI (2012). *Evaluation of detection capability for clinical laboratory measurement procedures; Approved guideline – Second edition*. CLSI document EP17-A2. Wayne, PA: Clinical and Laboratory Standards Institute.

21. CLSI (2011). *Establishing molecular testing in clinical laboratory environments – Approved Guideline*. CLSI document MM19-A. Wayne, PA: Clinical and Laboratory Standards Institute.

22. Linnet K, Boyd JC (2008). Selection and analytical evaluation of methods – With statistical techniques. In: Burtis CA, Ashwood ER, Bruns DE (eds.). *Tietz fundamentals of clinical chemistry*, 6th edition, pp. 201–228. St. Louis: Saunders Elsevier.

23. Kenny D, Fraser CG, Hyltoft Petersen P, Kallner A (1999). Strategies to set Global Quality Specifications in Laboratory Medicine – Consensus agreement. *Scandinavian Journal of Clinical and Laboratory Investigation* **59**, 585–585.

24. Fraser CG (2001). *Biological variation: From principles to practice*. Washington: AACCPress.

25. Ricós C, Iglesias N, García-Lario JV, Simón M, Cava F, Hernández A, Perich C, Minchinela J, Alvarez V, Doménech MV, Jiménez CV, Biosca C, Tena R (2007). Within-subject biological variation in disease: collated data and clinical consequences. *Annals of Clinical Biochemistry* **44**, 343–352.

26. Sturgeon CM, Hoffman BR, Chan DW, Ch'ng SL, Hammond E, Hayes DF, Liotta LA, Petricoin EF, Schmitt M, Semmes OJ, Söletormos G, van der Merwe E, Diamandis EP (2008). National Academy of Clinical Biochemistry laboratory medicine practice guidelines for use of tumor markers in clinical practice: Quality requirements. *Clinical Chemistry* **54**, e1–e10.

27. Chan DW, Sokoll LJ (1999). Prostate-specific antigen: Advances and challenges. *Clinical Chemistry* **45**, 755–756.

28. Meany DL, Sokoll LJ, Chan DW (2009). Early detection of cancer: Immunoassays for plasma tumor markers. *Expert Opinion on Medical Diagnostics* **3**, 597–605.

29. Stenman UH, Tiitinen A, Alfthan H, Valmu L (2006). The classification, functions and clinical use of different isoforms of HCG. *Human Reproduction Update* **12**, 769–784.

30. Alfthan H, Haglund C, Roberts P, Stenman UH (1992). Elevation of free β subunit of human choriogonadotropin and core β fragment of human choriogonadotropin in the serum and urine of patients with malignant pancreatic and biliary disease. *Cancer Research* **52**, 4628–4633.

31. Cole LA (1997). Immunoassay of human chorionic gonadotropin, its free subunits, and metabolites. *Clinical Chemistry* **43**, 2233–2243.

32. Cole LA, Khanlian SA, Sutton JM, Davies S, Stephens ND (2003). Hyperglycosylated hCG (Invasive Trophoblast Antigen, ITA) a key antigen for early pregnancy detection. *Clinical Biochemistry* **36**, 647–655.

33. Saller B, Clara R, Spöttl G, Siddle K, Mann K (1990). Testicular cancer secretes intact human choriogonadotropin (hCG) and its free β-subunit: Evidence that hCG (+hCG-β) assays are the most reliable in diagnosis and follow-up. *Clinical Chemistry* **36**, 234–239.

34. Sturgeon CM, Berger P, Bidart JM, Birken S, Burns C, Norman RJ, Stenman UH (2009). Differences in recognition of the 1st WHO international reference reagents for hCG-related isoforms by diagnostic immunoassays for human chorionic gonadotropin. *Clinical Chemistry* **55**, 1484–1491.

35. Pant S, Weiner R, Marton MJ (2014). Navigating the rapids: The development of regulated next-generation sequencing-based clinical trial assays and companion diagnostics. *Frontiers in Oncology* **4**, 1–20.

36. CAP (2009). *Perspectives on emerging technology report: KRAS mutation testing for colorectal cancer*. College of American Pathologists: Northfield, IL.

37. Ross JS (2012). Clinical implementation of *KRAS* testing in metastatic colorectal carcinoma. *Archives of Pathology & Laboratory Medicine* **136**, 1298–1307.

38. Kin C, Kidess E, Poultsides GA, Visser BC, Jeffrey SS (2013). Colorectal cancer diagnostics: biomarkers, cell-free DNA, circulating tumor cells and defining heterogeneous populations by single-cell analysis. *Expert Review of Molecular Diagnostics* **13**, 581–599.

39. Birken S, Berger P, Bidart JM, Weber M, Bristow A, Norman R, Sturgeon C, Stenman UH (2003). Preparation

and characterization of new WHO reference reagents for human chorionic gonadotropin and metabolites. *Clinical Chemistry* **49**, 144–154.

40. Armbruster DA, Pry T (2008). Limit of blank, limit of detection and limit of quantitation. *Clinical Biochemistry Reviews* **29**(Suppl 1), 49–52.

41. Pont-Kingdon G, Gedge F, Wooderchak-Donahue W, Schrijver I, Weck KE, Kant JA, Oglesbee D, Bayrak-Toydemir P, Lyon E (2012). Design and analytical validation of clinical DNA sequencing assays. *Archives of Pathology & Laboratory Medicine* **136**, 41–46.

42. Diaz LA Jr, Bardelli A (2014). Liquid Biopsies: Genotyping circulating tumor DNA. *Journal of Clinical Oncology* **32**, 579–586.

43. Day E, Dear PH, McCaughan F (2013). Digital PCR strategies in the development and analysis of molecular biomarkers for personalized medicine. *Methods* **59**, 101–107.

44. Baker M (2012). Digital PCR hits its stride. *Nature Methods* **9**, 541–544.

45. Kroll MH, Elin RJ (1994). Interference with clinical laboratory analyses. *Clinical Chemistry* **40**, 1996–2005.

46. Rifai N, Gillette MA, Carr SA (2006). Protein biomarker discovery and validation: the long and uncertain path to clinical utility. *Nature Biotechnology* **24**, 971–983.

47. Chan DW (1987). *Immunoassay: A practical guide*. New York, NY: Academic Press.

48. Devine PL (1996). High dose hook effect and sample carryover in carcinoembryonic antigen assay performed on the Boehringer-Mannheim ES-300 automated immunoassay system. *European Journal of Clinical Chemistry and Clinical Biochemistry* **34**, 573–574.

49. Jassam N, Jones CM, Briscoe T, Horner JH (2006). The hook effect: a need for constant vigilance. *Annals of Clinical Biochemistry* **43**, 314–317.

50. Leboeuf R, Langlois MF, Martin M, Ahnadi CE, Fink GD (2005). Hook effect in calcitonin immunoradiometric assay in patients with metastatic medullary thyroid carcinoma: Case report and review of literature. *Journal of Clinical Endocrinology & Metabolism* **91**, 361–364.

51. O'Reilly SM, Rustin GJS (1993). Mismanagement of choriocarcinoma due to a false low HCG measurement. *International Journal of Gynecological Cancer* **3**, 186–188.

52. Emerson JF, Lai KKY (2013). Endogenous antibody interferences in immunoassays. *Laboratory Medicine* **44**, 69–73.

53. CLSI (2008). *Immunoassay interference by endogenous antibodies; Approved guideline*. CLSI document I/LA30-A. Wayne, PA: Clinical and Laboratory Standards Institute.

54. Sturgeon CM, Viljoen A (2011). Analytical error and interference in immunoassay: minimizing risk. *Annals of Clinical Biochemistry* **48**, 418–432.

55. Tate J, Ward G (2004). Interferences in immunoassay. *Clinical Biochemistry Reviews* **25**, 105–120.

56. Pääbo S, Irwin DM, Wilson AC (1990). DNA damage promotes jumping between templates during enzymatic amplification. *Journal of Biological Chemistry* **265**, 4718–4721.

57. Lamy A, Blanchard F, Le Pessot F, Sesboüé R, Di Fiore F, Bossut J, Fiant E, Frébourg T, Sabourin JC (2011). Metastatic colorectal cancer *KRAS* genotyping in routine practice: results and pitfalls. *Modern Pathology* **24**, 1090–1100.

58. Williams C, Pontén F, Moberg C, Söderkvist P, Uhlén M, Pontén J, Sitbon G, Lundeberg J (1999). A High frequency of sequence alterations is due to formalin fixation of archival specimens. *American Journal of Pathology* **155**, 1467–1471.

59. Schwarzenbach H, Hoon DSB, Pantel K (2011). Cell-free nucleic acids as biomarkers in cancer patients. *Nature Reviews Cancer* **11**, 426–437.

60. Yu J, Gu G, Ju S (2014). Recent advances in clinical applications of circulating cell-free DNA integrity. *Laboratory Medicine* **45**, 6–12.

61. Gevensleben H, Garcia-Murillas I, Graeser MK, Schiavon G, Osin P, Parton M, Smith IE, Ashworth A, Turner NC (2013). Noninvasive detection of *HER2* amplification with plasma DNA digital PCR. *Clinical Cancer Research* **19**, 3276–3284.

62. McCloskey C, Dunn ST (2012). Test validation. In: Hu PC, Hegde MR, Lennon PA (eds.). *Modern Clinical Molecular Techniques*, pp. 23–47. New York: Springer.

63. Longo MC, Berninger MS, Hartley JL (1990). Use of uracil DNA glycosylase to control carry-over contamination in polymerase chain reactions. *Gene* **93**, 125–128.

64. Sundquist T, Bessetti J (2014). *Identifying and preventing DNA contamination in a DNA-typing laboratory*. http://www.promega.com/~/media/Files/Resources/Profiles%20In%20DNA/802/Identifying%20and%20Preventing%20DNA%20Contamination%20in%20a%20DNA%20Typing%20Laboratory.ashx. Accessed June 19, 2014.

65. Robasky K, Lewis NE, Church GM (2014). The role of replicates for error mitigation in next-generation sequencing. *Nature Reviews Genetics* **15**, 56–62.

66. Verma S, Barkoh BA, Luthra R (2012). Pyrosequencing in cancer. In: Hu P, Hegde MR, Lennon PA (eds.). *Modern clinical molecular techniques*, pp. 295–306. New York: Springer.

67. Armbruster DA, Alexander DB (2006). Sample to sample carryover: A source of analytical laboratory error and its relevance to integrated clinical chemistry/immunoassay systems. *Clinica Chimica Acta* **373**, 37–43.

68. Laboratory instrumentation product guide: Automated immunoassay analyzers. In: *CAP TODAY* 2010, July Issue.

69. Lalkhen AG, McCluskey A (2008). Clinical tests: sensitivity and specificity. *Continuing Education in Anaesthesia, Critical Care & Pain* **8**, 221–223.

70. Linnet K, Bossuyt PMM, Moons KGM, Reitsma JH (2012). Quantifying the accuracy of a diagnostic test or marker. *Clinical Chemistry* **58**, 1292–1301.

71. Lijmer JG, Leeflang M, Bossuyt PMM (2009). Proposals for a phased evaluation of medical tests. *Medical Decision Making* **29**, E13–E21.

72. Zhou XH, Obuchowski NA, McClish DK (2002). *Statistical methods in diagnostic medicine.* New York: John Wiley & Sons.

73. Bachmann LM, Puhan MA, ter Riet G, Bossuyt PM (2006). Sample sizes of studies on diagnostic accuracy: literature survey. *BMJ* **332**, 1127–1129.

74. Bossuyt PMM, Reitsma JB, Linnet K, Moons KGM (2012). Beyond diagnostic accuracy: The clinical utility of diagnostic tests. *Clinical Chemistry* **58**, 1636–1643.

75. Van den Bruel A, Aertgeerts B, Buntinx F (2006). Results of diagnostic accuracy studies are not always validated. *Journal of Clinical Epidemiology* **59**, 559–566.

76. Weinstein S, Obuchowski NA, Lieber ML (2005). Clinical evaluation of diagnostic tests. *American Journal of Roentgenology* **184**, 14–19.

77. Zweig MH, Campbell G (1993). Receiver-operating characteristic (ROC) plots: A fundamental evaluation tool in clinical medicine. *Clinical Chemistry* **39**, 561–577.

78. Fluss R, Faraggi D, Reiser B (2005). Estimation of the Youden index and its associated cutoff point. *Biometrical Journal* **47**, 458–472.

79. Perkins NJ, Schisterman EF (2006). The inconsistency of "optimal" cutpoints obtained using two critera based on the receiver operating characteristic curve. *American Journal of Epidemiology* **163**, 670–675.

80. Park SH, Goo JM, Jo CH (2004). Receiver Opearting Characteristic (ROC) Curve: Practical Review for Radiologists. *Korean Journal of Radiology* **5**, 11–18.

81. Obuchowski NA (2005). ROC analysis. *American Journal of Roentgenology* **184**, 364–372.

82. Obuchowski NA, Lieber ML, Wians FH Jr. (2004). ROC curves in clinical chemistry: Uses, misuses, and possible solutions. *Clinical Chemistry* **50**, 1118–1125.

83. Scott MG (2010). When do new biomarkers make economic sense? *Scandinavian Journal of Clinical and Laboratory Investigation* **70**, 90–95.

CHAPTER 23

Bioethics and Cancer Biomarker Research

Nathan Nobis,[1] William E Grizzle,[2] and Stephen Sodeke[3]

[1] Morehouse School of Medicine and Morehouse College, Atlanta, GA, USA
[2] Department of Pathology, University of Alabama at Birmingham, Birmingham, AL, USA
[3] Tuskegee University National Center for Bioethics in Research and Health Care, Tuskegee, AL, USA

Introduction

The purpose of this chapter is to engage in some bioethical issues raised by cancer biomarker research. We will discuss concerns about some of the actual and potential *benefits* and *harms* from cancer biomarker research, concerns that individuals are treated with *respect* in the course of such research, and concerns that such research is *fair* and *just*. Our focus on bioethical issues specific to cancer biomarkers will include:

- the validation of biomarkers;
- confidentiality, specimen identification, and data protection; and
- the return of research results.

This focus necessitates a clear understanding of bioethics in its broadest sense, as well as in a contextual sense specific to cancer biomarker research that will claim our attention in this chapter. We shall not discuss any legal or regulatory aspects of cancer biomarker research. This is because law and regulations vary by place and time and, more importantly, laws and regulations are not a reliable guide to what is ethical. Laws can permit, and even require, immoral and unjust behaviors, and morally permissible and just actions can be illegal. Our discussion will focus, then, only on ethical or moral aspects of biomarker research.

What is bioethics?

To begin, we should explain what we mean by *bioethics*, both in the broadest sense and in a contextual sense. Bioethics has been broadly defined as "not ethics of biology, but *ethics in the service of the bios* – of a life lived humanly, a course of life lived not merely physiologically, but also mentally, socially, culturally, politically, and spiritually. This means that the practice of bioethics must involve undertaking a fundamental inquiry into the full human and moral significance of developments in biomedical and behavioral sciences and technology" [1].

This kind of broad orientation enables us to imagine the significant impact of any scientific activity, action or policies, of which cancer biomarker research is one, on human life and the demands of social justice. Contextually or operationally, then, we can define *bioethics* as the ethical or moral evaluation of actions and policies in biomedical research and healthcare. According to an influential approach to bioethics, the "Georgetown Mantra" [2, 3], moral or ethical issues exist when an action or policy results or will likely result in:

- **harms** – that is, making someone worse off than they were, in some important way;

Biomarkers in Cancer Screening and Early Detection, First Edition. Edited by Sudhir Srivastava.
© 2017 John Wiley & Sons, Inc. Published 2017 by John Wiley & Sons, Inc.

- **benefits** – that is, making someone better off than they were, in some important way;
- **disrespectful treatment**, which includes behaviors where someone might be seen as being "used" as a mere "thing," is taken advantage of, or is manipulated – that is, their power of choice and control over their own lives diminished or eliminated;
- **unfairness or inequality** – that is, differences in treatment and consideration that cannot be justified by any relevant reasons, and so are *unjust*.

Reflecting on cases of moral wrongdoing confirms the relevance of these factors. Many wrong actions result in harms to people, and the benefits are either limited or nonexistent. Many such actions also involve individuals being "used" as "mere means" – that is, treated in ways that they would not agree to be treated if their wishes were taken into account, or treated as mere things, without their preferences taken into account. Finally, many morally wrong actions involve the person doing the action treating *some* persons in ways he or she would not treat *other* persons, but for irrelevant reasons; for example, racists treat members of other races in ways they would not treat people of their own race, but for no good reasons. Racism, of course, *harms* the victim, lessens the victim's ability to seek *benefits* (and other goods), is *disrespectful*, and is *unfair* and *unjust*. Moral considerations often overlap, and an action or policy can be wrong for many reasons.

These moral factors, or their contrary factors, help also to explain why actions may be right and good. Right and good actions tend to benefit the recipient of the action. They also tend to lessen the harms that someone might have endured. When individuals are treated rightly, they are treated with respect, and their autonomy and self-determination is enhanced. Finally, right actions involve all individuals being treated fairly, with equal consideration and respect, which promotes justice for all. Our concern, then, is how these moral factors are relevant to aspects of cancer biomarker research.

Bioethics, ethics and the validation of cancer biomarkers

A biomarker is a biological or biologically derived indicator of a process, event or condition. For example, a biomarker may indicate the presence of a disease, or the likelihood of a disease outcome [4,5]. For a biomarker to be useful, it must accurately and reliably indicate the event, process or condition, so the marker must be validated [4, 5]. If it is not validated, benefits are unlikely and harms are likely, and so ethical problems are likely. Thus, if molecular markers (biomarkers) are used in medical care without rigorous validation, untoward consequences may ensue. If medical decisions are made based upon biomarkers that do not reliably aid in these decisions, then unneeded medical care may result or, alternatively, necessary medical care may be withheld. This will harm patients and increase medical costs.

Case study: prostate specific antigen

These concerns can be illustrated with the current use of prostate specific antigen for early detection of prostate cancer. This example demonstrates that validation of biomarkers is an ethical imperative that cannot be ignored. Since extensive resources are used for biomarker research, ethics requires that biomarkers be validated, in order to ensure that these resources are not wasted, and that the harms are reduced and the likely benefits increased.

Prostatic specific antigen (PSA) is an example of a biomarker that has been used clinically as a biomarker for the early detection of prostate cancer without definitive validation. PSA is an antigen specific for prostatic glandular tissue, and is not specific for prostate cancer. Thus, PSA can be elevated in the setting of several benign diseases/conditions of the prostate, as well as in prostate cancer. Patients who are evaluated for prostate cancer because of mildly elevated levels of PSA are just as likely not to have prostate cancer as to have prostate cancer. Therefore, the use of PSA as a screening biomarker for the early detection of prostate cancer can, at best, be beneficial to some patients – and, at worst, can be erroneous and have multiple detrimental consequences to other patients and society. The issue is that it is problematic if the benefits to some patients are cancelled out by harm done to other patients and, thus, to society overall.

For example, when an elevated PSA results in an evaluation to exclude prostate cancer, it could involve multiple biopsies of the prostate. Even if all initial biopsies are negative, they may be repeated, resulting in unnecessary costs to the patient and to society, and also needless anxiety. In addition, many indolent prostate cancers may be identified by biopsy, and these indolent prostate cancers may never have caused clinical disease in the patient. Yet, because these indolent cancers cannot be reliably separated by current methods from life-threatening cancers, they sometimes are treated by surgical removal of the prostate, or by radiation of the prostate – procedures that frequently have serious side-effects, including incontinence and impotence.

These problems have led to recommendations for discontinuing the routine use of a single PSA test as an early detection biomarker for prostate cancer [6–9] though this is still controversial in other populations [10]. However, society and patients cannot recover the wasted resources and medical consequences of almost four decades of the use of PSA, as well as the current controversy of trying to discontinue the use of a biomarker which has been sold as an important detection method for prostate cancer that saves lives. Based on this example, one could surmise that a rigorous validation is necessary before any clinical use of a biomarker. This involves several studies, leading to a prospective study that should demonstrate the cost-effectiveness of the use of such a biomarker in medical care [5].

Nevertheless, just as there are ethical issues in not validating a biomarker, there are ethical issues in the validation of a biomarker. These include ensuring that the use of the biomarker is adequately evaluated, the selection of populations tested as to its validity, and the methods used in testing. The requirements of validating biomarkers have been described in the literature. Even when these requirements have been adhered to, it is important to understand that the same biomarker can have multiple uses, and the validation for one use does not mean that a biomarker can be reliably used in another way in other settings. Validation of a biomarker is for one use, which may include the following: risk of disease; early detection and diagnosis; prognosis, prediction of therapeutic responses; or evaluation of therapies or of preventive approaches. For example, while PSA is

not a cost-effective biomarker for early detection of prostate cancer, it can be used more reliably to detect the recurrence of prostate cancer following prostatectomy or radiation of the prostate, and as an aid in the tissue diagnosis of metastatic lesions in males from an unknown primary.

Furthermore, each biomarker must be evaluated for determining a specific endpoint (e.g., prognosis) over a defined period of time (e.g., 10 years) and in a specific population. One other critical point to remember is that the cost-effectiveness for the use (e.g., to determine prognosis) of a biomarker may vary with race and ethnicity. Thus, it is important to ensure that the use of a biomarker is validated for use in minority populations. It is unacceptable to assume that a biomarker validated in a predominantly Caucasian American population can be used reliably in an African American population or even that a biomarker validated for use in an African American population would apply equally to the same use in a population from West Africa. Because prostate cancer is more frequent and aggressive in the African American (AA) population, screening of this population with PSA after a certain age may be more justified than screening in the Caucasian American (CA) population. More studies are needed in this area.

An example of how biomarkers may vary among racial/ethnic populations is the effort to treat lung cancers by targeting the signal pathway of the epidermal growth factor receptor (EGFR). The predicted success of this approach was, in part, based on results from the Japanese population; however, when this approach was tested in the population of the USA, it was not as effective as predicted. This is because the overexpression/mutations of EGFR that would be targeted effectively by this approach were primarily associated with the adenocarcinoma subtype of lung cancers which occur in Japanese females who have never smoked, but not in the general lung cancers that are typical of the population of the USA [11–13].

Bioethical conclusions about validation

In the validation and use of biomarkers, the main ethical issues involve benefits and costs to the individual. Society definitely needs to incorporate and evaluate biomarkers in minority populations, and more attention needs to be given to the education of populations about the costs, benefits and limitations of using specific biomarkers clinically.

Other ethical concerns include validation's effects on individual patients. Efforts at validation of biomarkers should not be undertaken without a clear benefit to individuals. One could argue that, in general, it would be a waste of limited research resources to validate a biomarker for the early detection of a sporadic deadly disease for which there is no treatment; however, for a heritable disease, such as Huntington's chorea, for which there is currently no cure, individuals may want to know if they will develop the disease, or if they are carriers of the disease, in order to make reproductive decisions. Thus, channeling resources toward validating a biomarker that could help in such decisions would be morally justified.

Finally, the last step in the validation of a biomarker ultimately requires analysis by an independent investigator (e.g., someone who did not develop the biomarker or initially test it) in an independent, prospective population. This is an effort that requires extensive resources. A waste of such resources negatively affects society. Thus, clear indications that a biomarker is likely to benefit medical care are necessary prior to most validation studies. Similarly, validation of a biomarker could occur, yet its use might benefit only a few individuals at a great cost to society. This is at odds with the utilitarian worldview of "the greatest good for the greatest number of people" and with the moral perspective that we should prioritize individuals who are worst off (i.e., the poorest of the poor), who would benefit most from receiving a greater share of the existing medical knowledge and care.

Thus, in a society in which resources are very limited, the question becomes whether the benefits to a few members of society justify a burden on society that may result in a shift of resources that harms another group of individuals. We must admit that, in some cases, the moral calculus may not be the morally justified framework if we hold that, regardless of status, each person has equal moral worth to all others; striking a balance would require the perspectives of all stakeholders and all things considered. But this is what social justice requires.

Data protection, confidentiality and the return of research results

Our remaining ethical discussion will be brief. While it may be scientifically desirable to retain research subjects' personal information and attach that to any biological samples or specimens (e.g., for follow-up or further study), it is risky for the research subjects. This is especially the case for cancer biomarkers, insofar as these data might fall into the wrong hands, resulting in harms to the research subjects. For example, it is possible that insurance companies or employers might unfairly discriminate against persons with certain cancer biomarkers, such as refusing cover to those deemed likely to develop certain cancer(s). This discrimination could occur whether these biomarkers are validated or not. Thus, any research participation and results must be protected and confidential.

On the other hand, individuals who participate in research might benefit if they learn their (well-validated) biomarker status regarding the development of a cancer. If a validated biomarker shows that it is unlikely that an individual will develop a cancer, he/she might wish that an employer and a health or life insurance company knows, to seek better rates or other benefits. Also, some individuals might like to know if a cancer is likely, based on a validated biomarker, so that the individual could act in ways to reduce specific risks – an action that would not have been taken without the knowledge provided by a biomarker.

These concerns raise the question of whether research results should be returned to individuals who participate in research [14, 15]. Doing this, of course, requires that individuals' data be identified and retained which, as explained above, poses risk for research subjects who might be harmed if their results were revealed. Setting aside that problem, however, we must keep in mind that to return research results to individual study participants requires a lot of resources. This may involve: retaining contact with research subjects; individual meetings with subjects; explaining research results to them, often at a stage where the long-term significance of the results is unclear, especially if the biomarker is not yet validated; referring subjects to clinicians and genetic counselors, and so forth.

Also, research assays are not performed using the same standards as clinical assays. Hence, research results may be wrong, and may not apply to all sub-populations.

While the desire to return research results to individual research subjects is noble, the practical difficulties and the amount of resources needed to do this makes it unfeasible in most cases. We do not merely mean to say that this task would be difficult, but that the complications in doing this would result in such expenses that researchers simply could not afford the costs. That is to say, if it is required that they return research results to individuals *in a responsible way*, investigators may wonder whether they could afford to do the research in the first place. It is possible to argue that, insofar as the research is morally justified, returning research results could typically prevent that research [15]. Thus, it is important to remind research subjects that they personally may not benefit from participating in research. We hope that others will benefit, and that research participants might even be among that group, but there is no such guarantee in medical research.

Conclusions

In sum, we have reviewed a number of bioethical issues that are unique to cancer biomarker research. Our discussion has been brief and, surely, there are many other issues to discuss. We hope, however, that our efforts to frame the issues in terms of asking about the actual or likely benefits, harms, fairness or unfairness, and respectful or disrespectful treatment have been instructive and insightful. To seek justice on these issues, we suggest that the ethics of any aspect of biomarker research be evaluated from what philosopher John Rawls called "the veil of ignorance": if you didn't know who you were, would you be willing for this research to be done? Asking this question, and answering it from any individual's point of view, will help ensure that research be done ethically.

References

1. Leon R. Kass (2003). *President's Council on Bioethics. Being human: chairman's introductory speech.* Washington DC: President's Council on Bioethics. p. 3.

2. Beauchamp TL, Childress JF (2012). *Principles of biomedical ethics*, 7th ed. London, UK: Oxford University Press.

3. Rachels J, Rachels S (2011). *The elements of moral philosophy*, 7th ed. New York: McGraw-Hill Humanities/Social Sciences/Languages.

4. Grizzle WE, Srivastava S, Manne U (2012). Translational Pathology of Neoplasia. In: Srivastava S, Grizzle WE (eds.). *Translational Pathology of Early Cancer*, pp. 7–20. Amsterdam: IOS Press BV.

5. Burke HB, Grizzle WE (in press). Clinical validation of molecular biomarkers in translational medicine. In: Srivastava S, editor. *Biomarkers in Cancer Screening and Early Detection.* Oxford (UK), Wiley.

6. Wallner LP, Frencher SK, Hsu JW, Chao CR, Nichol MB, Lee RK, Jacobsen SJ (2013). Changes in serum prostate-specific antigen levels and the identification of prostate cancer in a large managed care population. *BJU International* **111**(8), 1245–52.

7. Andriole GL, Crawford ED, Grubb RL 3rd, Buys SS, Chia D, Church TR, Fouad MN, Gelmann EP, Kvale PA, Reding DJ, Weissfeld JL, Yokochi LA, O'Brien B, Clapp JD, Rathmell JM, Riley TL, Hayes RB, Kramer BS, Izmirlian G, Miller AB, Pinsky PF, Prorok PC, Gohagan JK, Berg CD; PLCO Project Team (2009). Mortality results from a randomized prostate-cancer screening trial. *New England Journal of Medicine* **360**(13), 1310–9. Erratum in issue **360**(17), 1797.

8. Dahm P (2012). ACP Journal Club. Review: PSA-based screening does not reduce prostate cancer mortality or all-cause mortality. *Annals of Internal Medicine* **156**(8), JC4–02.

9. Chou R, Croswell JM, Dana T, Bougatsos C, Blazina I, Fu R, Gleitsmann K, Koenig HC, Lam C, Maltz A, Rugge JB, Lin K (2011). Screening for prostate cancer: a review of the evidence for the U.S. Preventive Services Task Force. *Annals of Internal Medicine* **155**(11), 762–71.

10. Schröder FH, Hugosson J, Roobol MJ, Tammela TLJ, Zappe M, Nelen V, Kwiatkowski M, Lujan M, Määttänen L, Lilja H, Denis LJ, Recker F, Paez A, Bangma CH, Carlsson S, Puliti D, Villers A, Rebillard X, Hakama M, Stenman U-H, Kujala P, Taari K, Aus G, Huber A, van der Kwast T, van Schaik R, RHN, de Koning HJ, Moss SM, Auvinen A, ERSPC Investigators (2014). The European randomized study of screening for prostate cancer – prostate cancer mortality at 13 years of follow-up. *Lancet* **384**(9959), 2027–2035.

11. Shigematsu H, Lin L, Takahashi T, Nomura M, Suzuki M, Wistuba II, Fong KM, Lee H, Toyooka S, Shimizu N, Fujisawa T, Feng Z, Roth JA, Herz J, Minna JD, Gazdar AF (2005). Clinical and biological features associated with epidermal growth factor receptor gene mutations

in lung cancers. *Journal of the National Cancer Institute* **97**(5), 339–346.

12. Shigematsu H, Gazdar AF (2006). Somatic mutations of epidermal growth factor receptor signaling pathway in lung cancers. *International Journal of Cancer* **118**, 257–262.

13. Cappuzzo F, Hirsch FR, Rossi E, Bartolini S, Ceresoli GL, Bemis L, Haney J, Witta S, Danenberg K, Domenichini I, Ludovini V. Magrini E. Gregorc V. Doglioni C, Sidoni A, Tonato M. Frankling WA, Crino L, Bunn, Jr, PA, Varella-Garcia M (2005). Epidermal growth factor recep-

tor gene and protein and gefitinib sensitivity in non-small-cell lung cancer. *Journal of the National Cancer Institute* **97**, 643–55.

14. Bledsoe MJ, Grizzle WE, Clark BJ, Zeps N (2012). Practical implementation issues and challenges for biobanks in the return of individual research results. *Genetics in Medicine* **14**(4), 478–483.

15. Bledsoe MJ, Clayton EW, McGuire AL, Grizzle WE, O'Rourke PO, Zeps N (2013). Return of research results from genomic biobanks: cost matters. *Genetics in Medicine* **15**(2), 103–105.

CHAPTER 24

Colon Cancer Screening

Molly Perencevich,[1,2] Jennifer Inra,[1,2] and Sapna Syngal[1,2]

[1]Division of Population Sciences, Dana-Farber Cancer Institute, Boston, MA, USA

[2]Division of Gastroenterology, Brigham and Women's Hospital and Harvard Medical School, Boston, MA, USA

Introduction

Colorectal cancer (CRC) is the second leading cause of cancer death in the United States. The lifetime risk of CRC in the United States is approximately five percent [1]. Incidence and mortality from CRC has gradually decreased during the past decade, which may be partially attributable to removal of adenomatous polyps or earlier stage at diagnosis of CRC, as a result of screening [2].

Molecular pathogenesis of colorectal cancer

Genetic changes within colonic cells are known to drive the sequence from normal tissue to CRC. Germline mutations are responsible for inherited CRC syndromes, such as familial adenomatous polyposis (FAP), Lynch syndrome, and MYH-associated polyposis (MAP). A stepwise accumulation of somatic mutations over time, however, is responsible for the majority of sporadic CRC cases.

The majority of CRCs are thought to arise from adenomatous polyps that eventually become increasingly dysplastic and gain invasive potential, due to a series of genetic alterations [3]. This process typically occurs over a period of about ten years in somatic CRCs, but is accelerated in inherited CRCs. The three types of genes involved in this process are oncogenes, tumor suppressor genes, and DNA mismatch repair (MMR) genes [4].

Genetic alterations in oncogenes can lead to a constitutively activated gene product, contributing to tumorigenesis. The oncogenes that have been identified to play a role in sporadic CRCs include *K-ras, src, c-myc* and *c-erbB-2* [5,6]. *K-ras* is often considered the most important oncogene in CRC, as mutations in *K-ras* are found in about 50% of sporadic CRCs, and in 50% of colonic adenomas larger than 1 cm [7,8]. *K-ras* mutations are usually not seen in smaller adenomas, suggesting that they are acquired later in the adenoma-carcinoma sequence [9].

Loss of function of tumor suppressor genes results in unregulated cell growth. The most important tumor suppressor genes involved in CRC are *APC* and *p53*. The *APC* gene is involved in FAP as well as sporadic cases of CRC; 40–80% of CRCs and adenomatous polyps have lost both copies of the *APC* allele [10,11]. Adenomas as small as 5 mm have also demonstrated loss of *APC* activity, suggesting that the loss of *APC* function is an early step in CRC tumor formation [12]. The *p53* tumor suppressor gene function is lost in 4–25% of adenomatous polyps, 50% of invasive foci within adenomatous polyps, and 50–75% of CRC, suggesting that loss of *p53* function occurs as a later step in the adenoma-carcinoma sequence [8,13–15].

Finally, MMR genes are responsible for correcting mismatched nucleotide base pairings during DNA replication [16]. These genes include *MLH1, MSH2, MSH6, PMS1,* and *PMS2*. When the

Biomarkers in Cancer Screening and Early Detection, First Edition. Edited by Sudhir Srivastava.

© 2017 John Wiley & Sons, Inc. Published 2017 by John Wiley & Sons, Inc.

repair processes are absent due to mutations, multiple mutations and errors can occur in oncogenes and/or tumor suppressor genes, which may lead to cancer. Most commonly, germline mutations in these MMR genes cause Lynch syndrome, although loss of function of the MMR genes can be seen in up to 15% of sporadic CRCs as well [16]. Sporadic CRCs with nonfunctional MMR genes, however, do not have a mutation in the MMR gene itself. Instead, the MMR genes in sporadic CRCs have undergone epigenetic changes that silence their expression, namely hypermethylation of the promoter region of the gene, and/or DNA hypomethylation with loss of imprinting [16–18].

Recent evidence has increasingly supported the existence of an alternative route for colorectal carcinogenesis through serrated polyps [19], in a pathway that appears to involve CpG island methylator phenotype [20] and mutation of the oncogene *BRAF* [21].

Current screening practice methodologies: approaches and limitations

Screening modalities

The goal of CRC screening is to detect and remove pre-malignant polyps and detect early-stage adenocarcinomas. There are several screening tests available, including stool-based tests (guaiac and immunochemical fecal occult blood tests) and structural exams (endoscopic or radiographic studies that look at the lining of the colon). Stool tests are generally more reliable for the detection of cancer than polyps, but occasionally they may assist in identification of advanced adenomas. Structural exams are better able to identify polyps and allow for subsequent removal, which has the potential for CRC prevention, in addition to early detection.

Fecal occult blood tests

The two types of fecal occult blood tests (FOBT) are guaiac-based tests and the newer immunochemical tests. Guaiac testing identifies hemoglobin in the stool by the presence of a peroxidase reaction. False positives can occur due to ingestion of red meat or peroxidase-containing foods, so patients must adhere to dietary restrictions. The newer immunochemical tests react with antibodies that are specific for the globulin component of hemoglobin, and do not require dietary restrictions.

FOBT has the benefits of being widely available, noninvasive, inexpensive (although the immunochemical tests are more expensive than guaiac-based tests), and can be performed at home. Consecutive stools are collected at home (three for guaiac, one or two for immunochemical), and are generally sent to the processing facility by mail. Samples obtained by digital rectal exam are not recommended. FOBT should be repeated annually and, if a test is positive, it should be followed with a colonoscopy.

Multiple studies of different FOBT have reported modest rates of sensitivity (generally less than 50%) and specificity for the detection of advanced adenomas and CRC, with immunochemical tests generally performing better than guaiac-based tests [22–26]. There have been concerns that FOBT may not identify right-sided lesions as well as those on the left side [22], and that patients with false positive FOBT may end up undergoing unnecessary colonoscopy procedures. Changing from guaiac to immunochemical tests may slightly increase CRC screening rates [27].

FOBT using guaiac-based testing has been shown in randomized controlled trials to reduce CRC incidence and mortality [28–34]. The reported reductions in mortality ranged from approximately 15–33%, with variations in study, annual versus biennial screening, and whether specimens were rehydrated or not (rehydration increases the false positive rate). There are no randomized controlled trials looking at the effect of fecal immunochemical testing on CRC incidence and mortality, but it is assumed to be equally or more effective, based on the improved performance characteristics.

Some of the ongoing randomized controlled trials evaluating colonoscopy for CRC outcomes also evaluate fecal immunochemical testing, so there may be more data available soon. There has been debate about whether the mortality benefit of fecal occult blood testing may be, in part, due to false positive FOBT tests that lead to colonoscopy, rather than the FOBT itself. Ensuring appropriate follow-up for a positive FOBT is a critical component of providing a mortality benefit from CRC screening.

Flexible sigmoidoscopy

Flexible sigmoidoscopy allows for direct visualization of the distal third of the colon (typically to the splenic flexure) and removal of identified polyps. Sigmoidoscopy is invasive, but generally less uncomfortable (sedation is not typically needed), and has a lower risk of complications compared to colonoscopy. It requires a simple preparation (generally an enema rather than an oral solution) and can be performed by a wider range of providers. It is recommended that sigmoidoscopy be performed every five years for average-risk individuals and, if polyps or CRC are found, a full colonoscopy should be performed.

Sensitivity and specificity for polyps and CRC are high for the area of the colon that is visualized. Several randomized control trials have shown both a reduction in CRC incidence (18–23%) and mortality (22–31%) from sigmoidoscopy [35–38]. Notably, these studies varied in enrollment criteria, screening frequency, whether polyps were removed, referral for follow-up colonoscopy, compliance with exams, use of screening outside the protocol, and use of screening in the control group.

Colonoscopy

Colonoscopy allows for direct visualization of the entire colon and removal of identified polyps. A full oral preparation to cleanse the colon is required for adequate visualization. It generally requires conscious sedation for comfort, which necessitates that patients be accompanied home after the test. It has a higher risk of complications, and is more expensive than FOBT and sigmoidoscopy.

Despite the lack of results from randomized controlled trials, colonoscopy has been considered by many to be the gold standard for colon cancer screening tests. It has been shown to detect proximal lesions that would have been missed by sigmoidoscopy [39–41]. Large prospective studies have shown substantial reductions in the expected risk of CRC during long-term follow-up after screening colonoscopy. The National Polyp Study showed that removing polyps decreases the incidence of CRC, and made projections on reductions of mortality [42, 43]. Large randomized controlled trials

evaluating colonoscopy are in progress, including two in Europe and one in the USA.

Colonoscopy is considered the most sensitive screening exam, but missed and incompletely removed lesions can occur, which may result in interval CRC. There are several factors that may impact the effectiveness of colonoscopy. Colonoscopy may be less effective for proximal lesions [44–46], which may be related to technical issues and cleanliness of the preparation, as well as biologic features that make these polyps more difficult to see, or cause them to grow more quickly [47,48].

The quality of the colonoscopy may also have an impact on the effectiveness. The adenoma detection rate of the colonoscopist has been identified as an independent predictor of the risk of interval CRC after screening colonoscopy [49]. Longer withdrawal time (greater than six minutes) is associated with higher adenoma detection rates [50], but an institution-wide policy of colonoscopy withdrawal time greater than or equal to seven minutes had no effect on colon polyp detection [51]. Other quality indicators that may impact the effectiveness of colonoscopy include cecal intubation rate and adequate colon cleanliness [52].

Double-contrast barium enema

Double-contrast barium enema (DCBE) involves the instillation of barium and air into the rectum, to evaluate the surface of the colon with multiple X-ray images. It does require an oral preparation, but does not require sedation. There are no randomized controlled trials of its use as a form of CRC screening, but it appears to have modest sensitivity and specificity for CRC and large polyps, and is less effective than colonoscopy [53]. An abnormal test must be followed up with a colonoscopy. Utilization of DCBE has declined significantly over the past years, especially with increased use of computed tomographic colonography.

Computed tomographic colonography

Computed tomographic colonography (CTC) involves taking images of the colon to create two- and three-dimensional imaging of the luminal surface of the colon. It is non-invasive and does not require sedation, but it does require air or carbon dioxide inflation through a rectal tube, to distend the colon to enhance imaging. It has traditionally required a preparation similar to colonoscopy, but newer technologies have used an oral contrast to tag stool, which is then electronically subtracted from the images. Radiologists must be specially trained to read CTC, and it may not be widely available. If CTC is abnormal, a colonoscopy should be performed as follow-up for removal of detected polyps.

The accuracy of CTC is thought to be similar to colonoscopy for larger polyps and CRC [54–56]. There is concern that CTC may miss more flat polyps that harbor malignant potential. Patient preference is generally in favor of CTC over colonoscopy [56, 57]. A cost-effectiveness analysis in 2010 found that CTC could be a cost-effective option for CRC screening, if the cost was substantially less than colonoscopy, or if a large proportion of otherwise unscreened persons were to undergo screening by CTC [58].

A summary of studies evaluating CRC screening modalities can be found in Table 24.1.

Table 24.1 Studies supporting the use of various methods of CRC screening.

Studies	Type of study	Results
Fecal occult blood test (FOBT)		
Guaiac-based test (GT)[¶]		
Mandel, 1993 [32] & Mandel, 1999 [34]	RCT (US)	• Annual GT ↓ CRC mortality by 33% at 13 years and 33% at 18 years. Biennial GT↓ CRC mortality by 6%* at 13 years. And 21% at 18 years No difference in CRC incidence at 13 years
Mandel, 2000 [28]		• Annual GT ↓ CRC incidence by 20% at 18 years. Biennial GT↓ CRC incidence by 17% over 18 years.
Hardcastle, 1996 [31]	RCT (UK)	Biennial GT ↓ CRC mortality by 15% over a median of 7.8 years. No difference in CRC incidence.
Kronborg, 1996 [30] & Jørgensen, 2002 [33]	RCT (Denmark)	Biennial GT ↓ CRC mortality by 18% at 10 and by 15% at 13 years. No difference in incidence.
Faivre, 2004 [29]	RCT (France)	Biennial GT↓ CRC mortality by 16% at 11 years. No difference in incidence.
Lieberman, 2001 [24]	Prospective[#] (US)	Sensitivity of GT for advanced neoplasia was 23.9%.
Immunochemical test (FIT)		
Morikawa, 2005 [22]	Prospective[#] (Japan)	Sensitivity of FIT for advanced neoplasia was 27.1% and 65.8% for invasive cancer.
Allison, 2007 [23]	Prospective[#] (US)	Sensitivity for cancer was 82% for FIT and 64% for GT. Sensitivity advanced adenomas was 29.5% for FIT and 41% for GT.
Levi, 2007 [26]	Prospective[#] (Israel)	Sensitivity of FIT for cancer was 94% and 67% for clinically relevant neoplasm.
Hundt, 2009 [25]	Prospective[#] (Germany)	Performance characteristics of 6 FIT varied widely. The two best-performing FIT had sensitivity for advanced adenomas of 25% and 27%.
Flexible sigmoidoscopy [&]		
Hoff, 2009 [38]	RCT (Norway)	• Intention-to-screen: No difference in CRC incidence at 7 years. ↓ CRC mortality by 27%* at 6 years. • Per-protocol: ↓ CRC mortality by 59% at 6 years.
Atkin, 2010 [37]	RCT (UK)	• Intention-to-screen: ↓ CRC incidence by 23% and mortality by 31% at 10.5 years. • Per-protocol: ↓ CRC incidence by 33% and mortality by 43% at 10.5 years. • ↓ incidence distal CRC but not proximal CRC.
Segnan, 2011 [36]	RCT (Italy)	• Intention-to-screen: ↓ CRC incidence by 18% and mortality by 22%* at 11 years. • Per-protocol: ↓ CRC incidence by 31% and mortality by 38%* at 11 years. • ↓ incidence distal CRC but not proximal CRC.

Table 24.1 (Continued)

Studies	Type of study	Results
Schoen, 2012 [35]	RCT (US)	• Intention-to-screen: ↓ CRC incidence by 21% and mortality by 26% at 11.9 years. • ↓ incidence in proximal and distal colon CRC, but ↓ mortality in distal CRC only.
Colonoscopy Winawer, 1993 [43] and Zauber, 2012 [42]	Prospective# (US)	Followed individuals who had colonoscopy with polypectomy: • ↓ CRC incidence (76–90%) at 6 years. • ↓ CRC mortality by 53% in individuals who had adenomas removed compared to the expected CRC mortality rate in the general population (based on SEER data).
Double-contrast barium enema Winawer, 2000 [53]	Prospective# (US)	• Sensitivity was 39% for polyps. • Rate of adenoma detection dependent on size (32% if all polyps < 0.5 cm; 53% if largest 0.6–1 cm; 48% if largest >1 cm).
CT colonography (CTC) Pickhardt, 2003 [54]	Prospective# (US)	Sensitivity for adenomas was 94% for polyps ≥ 1 cm, 94% for polyps at least 0.8 cm, and 89% for polyps at least 0.6 cm.
Johnson, 2008 [55]	Prospective# (US)	Sensitivity for large (≥ 1 cm) adenomas and cancers was 90%.
Zalis, 2012 [56]	Prospective# (US)	Sensitivity of laxative-free CTC for adenomas was 91% for adenomas ≥ 1 cm, 70% for polyps at least 0.8 cm, and 59% for polyps at least 0.6 cm.
Fecal DNA test Imperiale, 2004 [93]	Prospective# (US)	Sensitivity of fecal DNA test was 52% for cancer (vs 13% for GT) and 18% for advanced neoplasia (vs 11%).
Ahlquist, 2008 [94]	Prospective# (US)	• Sensitivity of fecal DNA test 1 was 20% for neoplasms (advanced and curable cancers) (vs 11% and 21% for GT). • Sensitivity of fecal DNA test 2 was 46% for neoplasms (advanced and curable cancers) (vs 16% and 24% for GT).

RCT, randomized controlled trial.

* Not statistically significant.

¶ RCT varied in enrollment criteria, dietary restrictions, specimen rehydration, screening frequency, compliance with exams, use of screening outside the protocol, and use of screening in the control group.

Prospective studies compared the test modality to colonoscopy.

& RCT varied in enrollment criteria, screening frequency, whether polyps were removed, referral for follow-up colonoscopy, compliance with exams, use of screening outside the protocol, and use of screening in the control group.

Screening recommendations according to risk stratification

Risk stratification of asymptomatic individuals is based on their risk of developing CRC, and is used to make recommendations regarding methods and intervals of CRC screening. The information needed to perform risk stratification includes the individual's age, personal and family history of CRC and polyps (including the age at diagnosis and polyp details if possible), and any conditions or other malignancies that may be associated with hereditary CRC syndromes. Individuals are generally categorized as average, moderate, or high risk for development of CRC (Figure 24.1).

There are a number of other factors, such as race, gender, diabetes mellitus, obesity, smoking, and alcohol use, that have been associated with increased CRC risk in observational studies. However, their causal relationship is unknown, or the relative risk is considered too small, such that these factors generally do not influence screening guidelines.

Average Risk	Moderate Risk	High Risk
• Age ≥ 50 • No risk factors	• Personal history of adenomas • Personal history of CRC • Family history of adenomas • Family history of CRC	• Hereditary CRC syndromes • Inflammatory bowel disease

Figure 24.1 Stratification of average, moderate, and high-risk individuals for CRC screening.

Average risk

An average risk individual has no personal or family history of polyps or cancer. All men and women of average risk are recommended to begin CRC screening at age 50, and there are several modalities that can be used. As discussed previously, screening average-risk, asymptomatic individuals has been shown to decrease CRC incidence and mortality, either by randomized controlled trials (FOBT and flexible sigmoidoscopy), or inferred due to equal or greater sensitivity for polyps and early CRC than these tests (colonoscopy and CTC).

Multiple organizations have issued guidelines for CRC screening in average-risk individuals. In 2008, a joint statement from the American Cancer Society (ACS), US Multi-Society Task Force (MSTF) on Colorectal Cancer, and American College of Radiology (ACR) listed several options for CRC screening (Table 24.2), but recommended that CRC screening should focus on CRC prevention [59]. Therefore, structural tests that are able to detect adenomatous polyps as well as early stage

Table 24.2 CRC Screening recommendations for average-risk individuals.

Tests that detect adenomatous polyps and cancer
• Flexible sigmoidoscopy every five years, or
• Colonoscopy every ten years, or
• Double contrast barium enema every five years, or
• Computed tomographic colonography every five years

Tests that primarily detect cancer
• Annual guaiac fecal occult blood test with high test sensitivity for cancer, or
• Annual fecal immunohistochemical test with high test sensitivity for cancer, or
• Stool DNA, with high sensitivity for cancer, interval uncertain

From Levin *et al.*, 2008 [59].

adenocarcinomas should be encouraged, if individuals are willing to undergo more invasive tests. If individuals are unwilling or unable to undergo these exams, stool tests should be performed.

Other organizations have issued CRC screening guidelines that vary in their recommended and preferred modalities. The US Preventive Services Task Force (USPSTF) guidelines in 2008 did not recommend barium enema, CTC, or fecal DNA testing, and did not express a preference for structural exams over stool-based tests [60]. The American College of Gastroenterology (ACG) guidelines in 2009 were similar to the ACS, MSTF and ACR recommendations, with the exception that they also recommended initiating screening at age 45 for African-Americans [61].

Over the past decades, the proportion of average-risk patients choosing specific screening modalities has changed in the United States. Flexible sigmoidoscopy rates have declined, colonoscopy rates have increased, stool blood tests rates have remained relatively constant, and the rates of double-contrast barium enema have become extremely low [62].

Despite evidence that CRC screening can decrease incidence and mortality from CRC, screening rates remain lower than desired. Although it has been slowly increasing over time, the national rate of any form of CRC screening in 2010 was 58.6%, based on the National Health Interview Survey [63], and 64.5%, based on the Behavioral Risk Factor Surveillance System [64], which is lower than rates for cervical and breast cancer screening. Risk factors for lack of screening include lower levels of income and education, lack of health insurance or usual medical care, non-white race, and underserved populations.

For patients who are at average risk of CRC, as there are currently multiple choices for CRC screening that all appear to have benefit over no screening, patient preference should also be considered, as it may improve adherence to CRC screening [65]. Other interventions, such as a patient navigator, can also improve CRC screening rates [66].

Moderate risk

Family history of CRC (not including familial syndromes)

Approximately 5% of US adults report a family history of CRC [67]. The magnitude of risk due to family history is directly related to three factors: the number of family members with CRC, the number of first-degree relatives with CRC, and the age at CRC diagnosis in the affected member(s) [68–70]. Non-first-degree relatives with CRC and family members who developed CRC after the age of 60 are also associated with a slightly increased risk of CRC. However, the magnitude of risk is not great enough to change screening recommendations, and these individuals are still considered to be average risk if no other cancer family history exists [68].

It is also thought that individuals with a family history of adenomatous polyps are at increased risk for CRC [71]. However, documentation and reporting of family history of adenomatous polyps is often very inaccurate. Therefore, individuals with a documented family history of an advanced adenoma (> 1 cm, high grade dysplasia, villous architecture) are screened as increased risk, while those individuals with a family history of non-advanced adenomas are screened as average risk [61].

Personal history of adenomatous polyps

Individuals with a personal history of adenomatous polyps are considered to be at moderate risk, and recommended colonoscopy intervals are based on their examination findings [72]. Individuals with one or two adenomas all less than 1 cm in size, and no high-grade dysplasia or villous features, are at a lower risk of developing advanced adenomas or CRC, and should have a follow-up colonoscopy in five to ten years. Higher risk individuals are those that have three or more adenomas, have one adenoma with a size greater than or equal to 1 cm, or have high-grade dysplasia or villous features. It is recommended that they have a follow-up colonoscopy in three years, provided that the polyps were not removed piecemeal, when closer follow-up is needed initially to ensure adequate removal. Current guidelines recommend that traditional serrated adenomas and sessile serrated polyps/adenomas be managed clinically like adenomatous polyps [73].

Personal history of CRC

Individuals with a history of resected CRC are at increased risk for recurrent and/or metachronous cancers and, therefore, need more intense surveillance intervals than average-risk individuals. Guidelines published by the US-MSTF on Colorectal Cancer and ACS in 2006 recommend that individuals who have had surgical resection of CRC at stage I, II, III or IV with intent to cure are candidates for surveillance [74]. Due to the higher rates of recurrence for rectal cancer, however, endoscopic examination of the rectum is performed at 3–6 month intervals for the first two to three years after resection. Rigid proctoscopy, flexible proctoscopy, or rectal endoscopic ultrasound are typically used. If CRC is resected endoscopically, it is reasonable to evaluate and biopsy the area 3–6 months after the endoscopic resection.

For the objective of identifying metachronous cancers, individuals who undergo curative resection should have their first surveillance colonoscopy at one year from the surgery (or at one year from the colonoscopy used to clear the colon of synchronous lesions). If that examination is normal, the next colonoscopy should be at three years and, if normal, the following colonoscopy should be at five years. If abnormalities such as adenomas are found, the intervals are shortened, as previously described. Colonoscopy is the recommended and preferred method of surveillance in individuals with prior CRC.

High risk

Familial colorectal cancer syndromes

Familial syndromes account for approximately 5% of CRC, with Lynch syndrome being the most common. Individuals have a much higher risk of CRC than the general population, but appropriate identification can permit intensive surveillance strategies to reduce the risk of CRC and other associated malignancies (which will not be discussed here).

Familial adenomatous polyposis (FAP) is an autosomal dominant syndrome due to mutations in the *APC* gene. Clinically, classic FAP is characterized by hundreds to thousands of colonic adenomas, and a lifetime risk of CRC of 100% if prophylactic colectomy is not performed. Individuals can have an attenuated phenotype, where they often have more than ten but less than 100 adenomas, with a later age of onset, and the lifetime risk of CRC is lower with a later age of onset. In classic FAP, 15% of patients will have colonic adenomas by age 10 and 90% of patients will have adenomas by age 30 [75].

It is recommended that, for individuals with FAP, colorectal screening should begin at age 10–12, with a flexible sigmoidoscopy. Once adenomas are detected, annual colonoscopy is recommended. Adenomas can be managed and resected endoscopically, as long as the polyp burden is not too numerous. Once the polyp burden becomes too great, prophylactic colectomy is recommended, given the high risk of CRC, and the preferred technique is total proctocolectomy with ileoanal anastomosis. If ileorectal anastomosis is preferred and rectal mucosa remains, annual endoscopic surveillance of that area is required, given continued adenomatous polyp formation. For individuals with attenuated FAP, it is recommended that screening start at age 20–25 years, and surveillance includes a colonoscopy every 1–3 years. Again, the polyp burden can be managed endoscopically, unless the burden of adenomatous polyps becomes too great. In that case, total colectomy with ileorectal anastomosis is often performed, as quality of life is often better, and the polyp burden in the rectum can often be managed endoscopically [76].

MYH-associated polyposis (MAP) is an autosomal recessive syndrome caused by biallelic mutations in the *MUTYH* gene. It may have a variable clinical presentation, resembling FAP, attenuated FAP, or early CRC without polyposis. Screening and colectomy guidelines are less clear for this syndrome, but colonoscopy is generally recommended, starting at age 25–30 years old.

Individuals with Lynch syndrome also have a high risk of developing CRC over their lifetime, although the lifetime risk is lower than for those individuals with FAP. Lynch syndrome is also an autosomal dominant syndrome, characterized by mutations in DNA mismatch repair genes (*MLH1, MLH2, MSH6, PMS2, EPCAM*). The lifetime risk of CRC in individuals with Lynch syndrome is 50–80% [77], with the average age of onset around 45 years. It is not unusual to have multiple synchronous lesions at the time of initial CRC diagnosis. Similar to sporadic CRCs, adenomatous polyps are the precursor lesions of CRC in individuals with Lynch syndrome. However, the adenoma-to-carcinoma sequence is significantly accelerated, such that progression from adenoma to carcinoma typically takes 2–3 years, compared to seven to ten years for average-risk individuals.

The recommendations for CRC screening in Lynch syndrome patients include a colonoscopy starting at age 20–25, with repeated colonoscopy every one or two years, given the high cancer risk, the subtle endoscopic appearance of tumors, and accelerated growth sequence from adenoma to carcinoma [78, 79]. One study of families with proven or suspected Lynch syndrome showed that a screening interval of two years or less was necessary, in order to diagnose CRC at an early stage [80].

Inflammatory bowel disease
Patients with inflammatory bowel disease (IBD) have a greater risk of developing CRC over their lifetime and, therefore, require intense surveillance. The risk of CRC in both ulcerative colitis (UC) and Crohn's disease (CD) is related to the duration and extent of disease [81].

In UC, patients with disease extending to the hepatic flexure, or those with pancolitis, have the greatest risk of developing CRC, and the risk of developing CRC begins 8–10 years after the start of UC symptoms [82]. The incidence of CRC after 30 years of disease is noted to be 12–20% in some studies [83], and even up to 30% in others [84]. Patients with isolated left-sided colitis also have an increased risk of CRC but, typically, the risk increases after 15–20 years of having UC symptoms [85]. Notably, patients with UC complicated by primary sclerosing cholangitis (PSC) have an increased risk of CRC, compared with those patients without PSC. The risk of CRC in CD is likely comparable to that in UC, but the exact magnitude of risk is not clear [84, 86, 87]. CRC in UC is more likely to be located in the sigmoid or rectum, while it is more evenly distributed between the right and left colon in CD.

In IBD, CRC is preceded by dysplasia, and dysplastic lesions may appear endoscopically diverse, presenting as flat or plaque-like lesions, nodules, polyps or masses, also known as dysplasia-associated lesion or mass (DALM). Individuals with UC and DALM lesions may also have an underlying malignancy, which may be missed by endoscopic biopsy and, therefore, these patients often require colectomy. CRC that develops in the setting of IBD are also more likely to have synchronous lesions, compared with sporadic CRC [88].

The American Gastroenterological Association (AGA) [89], ACG [90], and American Society for Gastrointestinal Endoscopy (ASGE) [91], recommend that colonoscopic surveillance begin after eight years of disease in patients with pancolitis, and after 15 years of disease in patients with left-sided colitis. Colonoscopy should be repeated every 1–2 years. Current recommendations are for four quadrant biopsies, obtained every 10 cm from the cecum to the rectum, regardless of mucosal appearance. In addition, suspicious lesions or masses should be biopsied. Novel imaging techniques, such as chromoendoscopy [92], are being investigated, and may have a role in achieving more targeted biopsies. Findings of adenocarcinoma, high-grade dysplasia, or any degree of dysplasia associated with a mass lesion, are indications for colectomy. If colectomy is not feasible, then intense surveillance every 3–6 months is recommended as an alternative.

Adoption of biomarkers in current screening practice: challenges and limitations

Molecular biomarkers have been developed in an effort to provide a non-invasive method of colorectal cancer screening which has the potential to improve screening compliance. Potential advantages of molecular markers over the current screening modalities are that they are non-invasive, do not require a bowel preparation or sedation, and do not require dietary restrictions. To date, fecal DNA testing has shown the most promise for CRC screening.

Fecal markers
CRCs shed cells that contain mutations and other markers of carcinogenesis. DNA tests have been

the most extensively studied, and will be discussed here, but other markers, such as RNA and proteins, have also been evaluated. Individual mutations in genes such as K-ras, $p53$, and APC can be detected. However, they are variably present in CRC and adenomas so, to improve sensitivity and specificity, multiple genetic mutations are usually targeted with panel testing. Additional stool DNA testing includes evaluation for microsatellite instability, long lengths of DNA (which occur more abundantly in stool in the setting of CRC), and aberrant DNA methylation (which can occur early in tumorigenesis).

An entire stool must be collected for fecal DNA testing, because human DNA accounts for a very small fraction of the total stool DNA (largely microbial), and because of marker heterogeneity within the stool. False negative tests can occur, due to insufficient recovery of fecal DNA, either due to an insufficient sample, or degradation of DNA due to transport and storage. Technologic advances in detecting molecular markers and stabilizing buffers that reduce degradation have increased sensitivity. False positives can occur, due to preneoplastic DNA alterations or, possibly, a gastrointestinal neoplasm proximal to the colon.

In a multicenter prospective trial of average-risk asymptomatic adults aged 50 years or older, an early-generation fecal DNA panel was compared to conventional guaiac-based FOBT and colonoscopy in a subgroup of 2507 subjects [93]. The fecal DNA panel consisted of 21 mutations (three in the K-ras gene, ten in the APC gene, eight in the $p53$ gene), the miscrosatellite-instability marker BAT-26, and a marker of long DNA. Fecal DNA testing was more sensitive than guaiac testing for cancer (52% versus 13%) and for advanced neoplasia (18% versus 11%), but both tests missed a substantial proportion of the cancers and advanced polyps that were detected by colonoscopy. The specificity in subjects with negative findings on colonoscopy was similar for the fecal DNA panel and guaiac testing at approximately 94% and 95%, respectively.

Another multicenter study prospectively compared two early-generation fecal DNA tests with guaiac-based FOBT and colonoscopy in 3764 subjects [94]. The first fecal DNA test was the same panel used in the previous study, and the second used three broadly informative markers

(*K-ras* mutations, scanning of *APC* mutator cluster regions, and methylation of the *vimentin* gene). Sensitivity for neoplasms (advanced adenomas and curable cancers) was 20% for the first fecal DNA test, 11% by conventional guaiac testing, and 21% by high-sensitivity guaiac testing, suggesting no improvement of the fecal DNA test over high-sensitivity guaiac testing. The second fecal DNA test had a sensitivity of 46% for neoplasms (compared with 16% and 24% for conventional and high-sensitivity guaiac testing, respectively), and it detected 46% of adenomas 1 cm or larger (compared with 15% and 17% for conventional and high-sensitivity guaiac testing, respectively). The second DNA test was not affected by neoplasm site, unlike both forms of guaiac testing. The rate of false positives was 16%, compared with 4% and 5% for the conventional and high-sensitivity guaiac tests, respectively.

Over the past several years, there have been several studies using next-generation fecal DNA tests, with varied panels of markers and technologies. A recent study used an advanced technique (quantitative allele-specific real-time target and signal amplification, or QuARTS) to analyze archived fecal specimens from 252 subjects with CRC, 293 colonoscopy-negative controls, and 133 subjects with adenomas 1 cm or larger [95]. The panel included four methylated genes (*NDGR4*, *BMP3*, *vimentin*, and *TFP12*), *K-ras*, and hemoglobin by fecal immunohistochemistry testing). The fecal DNA test had a sensitivity of 85% for CRC and 54% for adenomas = 1 cm, with 90% specificity. Detection rates increased with adenoma size with 54% = 1 cm and 92% > 4 cm, but no difference in sensitivity between proximal and distal lesions, or for the presence of dysplasia after adjustment for size. Validation studies of next-generation fecal DNA tests in the general screening population are in progress. If shown to be efficacious for screening, future research will need to focus on the optimal interval for these tests.

Fecal DNA testing for CRC screening was endorsed by the ACS, MSTF and ACR in 2008, although the recommended interval was uncertain [59]. Of note, the fecal DNA test that was available at the time this guideline was produced is no longer commercially available. The 2009 ACG guidelines also supported fecal DNA testing at an interval of three years, as an alternative screening approach [61]. The 2008 USPSTF recommendations for CRC screening did not support fecal DNA testing, due to insufficient evidence [60]. Future recommendations will incorporate more recent data on fecal DNA testing.

From a cost-effectiveness perspective, a 2010 analysis found that, at a cost of $350 per test, fecal DNA testing every three to five years would be cost-effective if the cost was decreased to $40 to $60 every three years, or at the current cost if the relative adherence to stool DNA testing were at least 50% better than that with other screening tests [96]. The cost of fecal DNA testing is expected to decrease with advances in technology [97], and future cost-effectiveness analysis will be needed to assess the role of fecal DNA testing in CRC screening.

Serum markers

Serum markers for CRC screening are not as close to clinical use as fecal DNA at this time, but they hold promise. Serum markers may be less sensitive for pre-malignant or early-stage CRC, as circulating levels tend to rise in advanced stages of disease. Several serum DNA markers have been evaluated, including DNA mutations and markers of aberrant methylation, as well as a variety of protein and RNA markers.

An example of a serum biomarker that has recently been explored is methylated *septin 9*, a test for aberrant methylation. It was compared to a fecal DNA panel test in paired samples from patients with CRC, large adenomas, and normal colonoscopies, and it was found that the fecal test was more sensitive than the serum test for non-metastatic CRC (91% vs 50%, respectively) and large adenomas (82% vs 14%, respectively) [98]. False positive rates were 7% for the fecal test, and 27% for the serum test.

A cost-effectiveness analysis of a serum methylated *septin 9* DNA test, compared with established CRC screening strategies, found that serum DNA test would need to achieve substantially higher uptake and adherence rates than the alternatives, in order to be cost-effective [99]. Combinations of protein markers have also been compared to FOBT, with mixed results [100, 101]. Further studies are needed to identify, evaluate, and validate serum biomarkers for CRC screening.

Summary

CRC is a common but preventable cancer. Current screening modalities are effective in reducing CRC incidence and mortality, but more work needs to be done to understand the best form(s) of screening and to improve screening compliance. Molecular biomarkers have the potential to contribute to improved CRC screening strategies, but more research is needed.

References

1. Siegel R, Naishadham D, Jemal A (2013). Cancer statistics, 2013. *CA: A Cancer Journal for Clinicians* **63**, 11–30.
2. Lieberman D (2010). Progress and challenges in colorectal cancer screening and surveillance. *Gastroenterology* **138**, 2115–26.
3. Fearon ER, Vogelstein B (1990). A genetic model for colorectal tumorigenesis. *Cell* **61**, 759–67.
4. Lynch JP, Hoops TC (2002). The genetic pathogenesis of colorectal cancer. *Hematology/Oncology Clinics of North America* **16**, 775–810.
5. Hamilton SR (1993). The molecular genetics of colorectal neoplasia. *Gastroenterology* **105**, 3–7.
6. Forgacs I (1988). Oncogenes and gastrointestinal cancer. *Gut* **29**, 417–21.
7. Takayama T, Ohi M, Hayashi T, *et al.* (2001). Analysis of K-ras, APC, and beta-catenin in aberrant crypt foci in sporadic adenoma, cancer, and familial adenomatous polyposis. *Gastroenterology* **121**, 599–611.
8. Vogelstein B, Fearon ER, Hamilton SR, *et al.* (1988). Genetic alterations during colorectal-tumor development. *New England Journal of Medicine* **319**, 525–32.
9. Pretlow TP, Brasitus TA, Fulton NC, *et al.* (1993). K-ras mutations in putative preneoplastic lesions in human colon. *Journal of the National Cancer Institute* **85**, 2004–7.
10. Lamlum H, Ilyas M, Rowan A, *et al.* (1999). The type of somatic mutation at APC in familial adenomatous polyposis is determined by the site of the germline mutation: a new facet to Knudson's 'two-hit' hypothesis. *Nature Medicine* **5**, 1071–5.
11. Spirio LN, Samowitz W, Robertson J, *et al.* (1998). Alleles of APC modulate the frequency and classes of mutations that lead to colon polyps. *Nature Genetics* **20**, 385–8.
12. Powell SM, Zilz N, Beazer-Barclay Y, *et al.* (1992). APC mutations occur early during colorectal tumorigenesis. *Nature* **359**, 235–7.
13. Scott N, Bell SM, Sagar P, *et al.* (1993). p53 expression and K-ras mutation in colorectal adenomas. *Gut* **34**, 621–4.
14. Ohue M, Tomita N, Monden T, *et al.* (1994). A frequent alteration of p53 gene in carcinoma in adenoma of colon. *Cancer Research* **54**, 4798–804.
15. Kaserer K, Schmaus J, Bethge U, *et al.* (2000). Staining patterns of p53 immunohistochemistry and their biological significance in colorectal cancer. *Journal of Pathology* **190**, 450–6.
16. Chung DC, Rustgi AK (1995). DNA mismatch repair and cancer. *Gastroenterology* **109**, 1685–99.
17. Veigl ML, Kasturi L, Olechnowicz J, *et al.* (1998). Biallelic inactivation of hMLH1 by epigenetic gene silencing, a novel mechanism causing human MSI cancers. *Proceedings of the National Academy of Sciences of the United States of America* **95**, 8698–702.
18. Herman JG, Umar A, Polyak K, *et al.* (1998). Incidence and functional consequences of hMLH1 promoter hypermethylation in colorectal carcinoma. *Proceedings of the National Academy of Sciences of the United States of America* **95**, 6870–5.
19. Leggett B, Whitehall V (2010). Role of the serrated pathway in colorectal cancer pathogenesis. *Gastroenterology* **138**, 2088–100.
20. Toyota M, Ahuja N, Ohe-Toyota M, *et al.* (1999). CpG island methylator phenotype in colorectal cancer. *Proceedings of the National Academy of Sciences of the United States of America* **96**, 8681–6.
21. Spring KJ, Zhao ZZ, Karamatic R, *et al.* (2006). High prevalence of sessile serrated adenomas with BRAF mutations: a prospective study of patients undergoing colonoscopy. *Gastroenterology* **131**, 1400–7.
22. Morikawa T, Kato J, Yamaji Y, *et al.* (2005). A comparison of the immunochemical fecal occult blood test and total colonoscopy in the asymptomatic population. *Gastroenterology* **129**, 422–8.
23. Allison JE, Sakoda LC, Levin TR, *et al.* (2007). Screening for colorectal neoplasms with new fecal occult blood tests: update on performance characteristics. *Journal of the National Cancer Institute* **99**, 1462–70.
24. Lieberman DA, Weiss DG (2001). One-time screening for colorectal cancer with combined fecal occult-blood testing and examination of the distal colon. *New England Journal of Medicine* **345**, 555–60.
25. Hundt S, Haug U, Brenner H (2009). Comparative evaluation of immunochemical fecal occult blood tests for colorectal adenoma detection. *Annals of Internal Medicine* **150**, 162–9.
26. Levi Z, Rozen P, Hazazi R, *et al.* (2007). A quantitative immunochemical fecal occult blood test for colorectal neoplasia. *Annals of Internal Medicine* **146**, 244–55.

27. Liles EG, Perrin N, Rosales AG, *et al.* (2012). Change to FIT increased CRC screening rates: evaluation of a US screening outreach program. *American Journal of Managed Care* **18**, 588–95.

28. Mandel JS, Church TR, Bond JH, *et al.* (2000). The effect of fecal occult-blood screening on the incidence of colorectal cancer. *New England Journal of Medicine* **343**, 1603–7.

29. Faivre J, Dancourt V, Lejeune C, *et al.* (2004). Reduction in colorectal cancer mortality by fecal occult blood screening in a French controlled study. *Gastroenterology* **126**, 1674–80.

30. Kronborg O, Fenger C, Olsen J, *et al.* (1996). Randomised study of screening for colorectal cancer with faecal-occult-blood test. *The Lancet* **348**, 1467–71.

31. Hardcastle JD, Chamberlain JO, Robinson MH, *et al.* (1996). Randomised controlled trial of faecal-occult-blood screening for colorectal cancer. *The Lancet* **348**, 1472–7.

32. Mandel JS, Bond JH, Church TR, *et al.* (1993). Reducing mortality from colorectal cancer by screening for fecal occult blood. Minnesota Colon Cancer Control Study. *New England Journal of Medicine* **328**, 1365–71.

33. Jorgensen OD, Kronborg O, Fenger C (2002). A randomised study of screening for colorectal cancer using faecal occult blood testing: results after 13 years and seven biennial screening rounds. *Gut* **50**, 29–32.

34. Mandel JS, Church TR, Ederer F, *et al.* (1999). Colorectal cancer mortality: effectiveness of biennial screening for fecal occult blood. *Journal of the National Cancer Institute* **91**, 434–7.

35. Schoen RE, Pinsky PF, Weissfeld JL, *et al.* (2012). Colorectal-cancer incidence and mortality with screening flexible sigmoidoscopy. *New England Journal of Medicine* **366**, 2345–57.

36. Segnan N, Armaroli P, Bonelli L, *et al.* (2011). Once-only sigmoidoscopy in colorectal cancer screening: follow-up findings of the Italian Randomized Controlled Trial – SCORE. *Journal of the National Cancer Institute* **103**, 1310–22.

37. Atkin WS, Edwards R, Kralj-Hans I, *et al.* (2010). Once-only flexible sigmoidoscopy screening in prevention of colorectal cancer: a multicentre randomised controlled trial. *The Lancet* **375**, 1624–33.

38. Hoff G, Grotmol T, Skovlund E, *et al.* (2009). Risk of colorectal cancer seven years after flexible sigmoidoscopy screening: randomised controlled trial. *BMJ* **338**, b1846.

39. Lieberman DA, Weiss DG, Bond JH, *et al.* (2000). Use of colonoscopy to screen asymptomatic adults for colorectal cancer. Veterans Affairs Cooperative Study Group 380. *New England Journal of Medicine* **343**, 162–8.

40. Imperiale TF, Wagner DR, Lin CY, *et al.* (2000). Risk of advanced proximal neoplasms in asymptomatic adults according to the distal colorectal findings. *New England Journal of Medicine* **343**, 169–74.

41. Lewis JD, Ng K, Hung KE, *et al.* (2003). Detection of proximal adenomatous polyps with screening sigmoidoscopy: a systematic review and meta-analysis of screening colonoscopy. *Archives of Internal Medicine* **163**, 413–20.

42. Zauber AG, Winawer SJ, O'Brien MJ, *et al.* (2012). Colonoscopic polypectomy and long-term prevention of colorectal-cancer deaths. *New England Journal of Medicine* **366**, 687–96.

43. Winawer SJ, Zauber AG, Ho MN, *et al.* (1993). Prevention of colorectal cancer by colonoscopic polypectomy. The National Polyp Study Workgroup. *New England Journal of Medicine* **329**, 1977–81.

44. Singh H, Nugent Z, Demers AA, *et al.* (2010). The reduction in colorectal cancer mortality after colonoscopy varies by site of the cancer. *Gastroenterology* **139**, 1128–37.

45. Baxter NN, Goldwasser MA, Paszat LF, *et al.* (2009). Association of colonoscopy and death from colorectal cancer. *Annals of Internal Medicine* **150**, 1–8.

46. Brenner H, Hoffmeister M, Arndt V, *et al.* (2010). Protection from right- and left-sided colorectal neoplasms after colonoscopy: population-based study. *Journal of the National Cancer Institute* **102**, 89–95.

47. Azzoni C, Bottarelli L, Campanini N, *et al.* (2007). Distinct molecular patterns based on proximal and distal sporadic colorectal cancer: arguments for different mechanisms in the tumorigenesis. *International Journal of Colorectal Disease* **22**, 115–26.

48. Soetikno RM, Kaltenbach T, Rouse RV, *et al.* (2008). Prevalence of nonpolypoid (flat and depressed) colorectal neoplasms in asymptomatic and symptomatic adults. *JAMA* **299**, 1027–35.

49. Kaminski MF, Regula J, Kraszewska E, *et al.* (2010). Quality indicators for colonoscopy and the risk of interval cancer. *New England Journal of Medicine* **362**, 1795–803.

50. Barclay RL, Vicari JJ, Doughty AS, *et al.* (2006). Colonoscopic withdrawal times and adenoma detection during screening colonoscopy. *New England Journal of Medicine* **355**, 2533–41.

51. Sawhney MS, Cury MS, Neeman N, *et al.* (2008). Effect of institution-wide policy of colonoscopy withdrawal time > or = 7 minutes on polyp detection. *Gastroenterology* **135**, 1892–8.

52. Rex DK, Petrini JL, Baron TH, *et al.* (2006). Quality indicators for colonoscopy. *American Journal of Gastroenterology* **101**, 873–85.

53. Winawer SJ, Stewart ET, Zauber AG, *et al.* (2000). A comparison of colonoscopy and double-contrast barium enema for surveillance after polypectomy. National Polyp Study Work Group. *New England Journal of Medicine* **342**, 1766–72.

54. Pickhardt PJ, Choi JR, Hwang I, *et al.* (2003). Computed tomographic virtual colonoscopy to screen for colorectal neoplasia in asymptomatic adults. *New England Journal of Medicine* **349**, 2191–200.

55. Johnson CD, Chen MH, Toledano AY, *et al.* (2008). Accuracy of CT colonography for detection of large adenomas and cancers. *New England Journal of Medicine* **359**, 1207–17.

56. Zalis ME, Blake MA, Cai W, *et al.* (2012). Diagnostic accuracy of laxative-free computed tomographic colonography for detection of adenomatous polyps in asymptomatic adults: a prospective evaluation. *Annals of Internal Medicine* **156**, 692–702.

57. Pooler BD, Baumel MJ, Cash BD, *et al.* (2012). Screening CT colonography: multicenter survey of patient experience, preference, and potential impact on adherence. *American Journal of Roentgenology* **198**, 1361–6.

58. Knudsen AB, Lansdorp-Vogelaar I, Rutter CM, *et al.* (2010). Cost-effectiveness of computed tomographic colonography screening for colorectal cancer in the medicare population. *Journal of the National Cancer Institute* **102**, 1238–52.

59. Levin B, Lieberman DA, McFarland B, *et al.* (2008). Screening and surveillance for the early detection of colorectal cancer and adenomatous polyps, 2008: a joint guideline from the American Cancer Society, the US Multi-Society Task Force on Colorectal Cancer, and the American College of Radiology. *Gastroenterology* **134**, 1570–95.

60. Screening for colorectal cancer: U.S. Preventive Services Task Force recommendation statement (2008). *Annals of Internal Medicine* **149**, 627–37.

61. Rex DK, Johnson DA, Anderson JC, *et al.* (2009). American College of Gastroenterology guidelines for colorectal cancer screening 2009 [corrected]. *American Journal of Gastroenterology* **104**, 739–50.

62. Meissner HI, Breen N, Klabunde CN, *et al.* (2006). Patterns of colorectal cancer screening uptake among men and women in the United States. *Cancer Epidemiology, Biomarkers & Prevention* **15**, 389–94.

63. Cancer screening – United States, 2010 (2012). *Morbidity and Mortality Weekly Report (MMWR)* **61**, 41–5.

64. Joseph DA, King JB, Miller JW, *et al.* (2012). Prevalence of colorectal cancer screening among adults – behavioral risk factor surveillance system, United States, 2010. *MMWR Surveillance Summaries* **61**, 51–6.

65. Inadomi JM, Vijan S, Janz NK, *et al.* (2012). Adherence to colorectal cancer screening: a randomized clinical trial of competing strategies. *Archives of Internal Medicine* **172**, 575–82.

66. Holden DJ, Jonas DE, Porterfield DS, *et al.* (2010). Systematic review: enhancing the use and quality of colorectal cancer screening. *Annals of Internal Medicine* **152**, 668–76.

67. Ramsey SD, Yoon P, Moonesinghe R, *et al.* (2006). Population-based study of the prevalence of family history of cancer: implications for cancer screening and prevention. *Genetics in Medicine* **8**, 571–5.

68. Johns LE, Houlston RS (2001). A systematic review and meta-analysis of familial colorectal cancer risk. *American Journal of Gastroenterology* **96**, 2992–3003.

69. St John DJ, McDermott FT, Hopper JL, *et al.* (1993). Cancer risk in relatives of patients with common colorectal cancer. *Annals of Internal Medicine* **118**, 785–90.

70. Butterworth AS, Higgins JP, Pharoah P (2006). Relative and absolute risk of colorectal cancer for individuals with a family history: a meta-analysis. *European Journal of Cancer* **42**, 216–27.

71. Winawer SJ, Zauber AG, Gerdes H, *et al.* (1996). Risk of colorectal cancer in the families of patients with adenomatous polyps. National Polyp Study Workgroup. *New England Journal of Medicine* **334**, 82–7.

72. Lieberman DA, Rex DK, Winawer SJ, *et al.* (2012). Guidelines for colonoscopy surveillance after screening and polypectomy: a consensus update by the US Multi-Society Task Force on Colorectal Cancer. *Gastroenterology* **143**, 844–57.

73. Rex DK, Ahnen DJ, Baron JA, *et al.* (2012). Serrated lesions of the colorectum: review and recommendations from an expert panel. *American Journal of Gastroenterology* **107**, 1315–29; quiz 4, 30.

74. Rex DK, Kahi CJ, Levin B, *et al.* (2006). Guidelines for colonoscopy surveillance after cancer resection: a consensus update by the American Cancer Society and the US Multi-Society Task Force on Colorectal Cancer. *Gastroenterology* **130**, 1865–71.

75. Kastrinos F, Syngal S (2011). Inherited colorectal cancer syndromes. *Cancer Journal* **17**, 405–15.

76. Jasperson KW, Tuohy TM, Neklason DW, *et al.* (2010). Hereditary and familial colon cancer. *Gastroenterology* **138**, 2044–58.

77. Chung DC, Rustgi AK (2003). The hereditary nonpolyposis colorectal cancer syndrome: genetics and clinical implications. *Annals of Internal Medicine* **138**, 560–70.

78. Dove-Edwin I, Sasieni P, Adams J, *et al.* (2005). Prevention of colorectal cancer by colonoscopic surveillance in

individuals with a family history of colorectal cancer: 16 year, prospective, follow-up study. *BMJ* **331**, 1047.

79. Lindor NM, Petersen GM, Hadley DW, *et al.* (2006). Recommendations for the care of individuals with an inherited predisposition to Lynch syndrome: a systematic review. *JAMA* **296**, 1507–17.

80. de Vos tot Nederveen Cappel WH, Nagengast FM, Griffioen G, *et al.* (2002). Surveillance for hereditary non-polyposis colorectal cancer: a long-term study on 114 families. *Diseases of the Colon & Rectum* **45**, 1588–94.

81. Rutter MD, Saunders BP, Wilkinson KH, *et al.* (2006). Thirty-year analysis of a colonoscopic surveillance program for neoplasia in ulcerative colitis. *Gastroenterology* **130**, 1030–8.

82. Collins RH, Jr., Feldman M, Fordtran JS (1987). Colon cancer, dysplasia, and surveillance in patients with ulcerative colitis. A critical review. *New England Journal of Medicine* **316**, 1654–8.

83. Lennard-Jones JE, Melville DM, Morson BC, *et al.* (1990). Precancer and cancer in extensive ulcerative colitis: findings among 401 patients over 22 years. *Gut* **31**, 800–6.

84. Ekbom A, Helmick C, Zack M, *et al.* (1990). Ulcerative colitis and colorectal cancer. A population-based study. *New England Journal of Medicine* **323**, 1228–33.

85. Greenstein AJ, Sachar DB, Smith H, *et al.* (1979). Cancer in universal and left-sided ulcerative colitis: factors determining risk. *Gastroenterology* **77**, 290–4.

86. Friedman S, Rubin PH, Bodian C, *et al.* (2001). Screening and surveillance colonoscopy in chronic Crohn's colitis. *Gastroenterology* **120**, 820–6.

87. Rubio CA, Befrits R (1997). Colorectal adenocarcinoma in Crohn's disease: a retrospective histologic study. *Diseases of the Colon & Rectum* **40**, 1072–8.

88. Itzkowitz SH (1997). Inflammatory bowel disease and cancer. *Gastroenterology Clinics of North America* **26**, 129–39.

89. Farraye FA, Odze RD, Eaden J, *et al.* (2010). AGA technical review on the diagnosis and management of colorectal neoplasia in inflammatory bowel disease. *Gastroenterology* **138**, 746–74, 74 e1–4; quiz e12–3.

90. Kornbluth A, Sachar DB (1997). Ulcerative colitis practice guidelines in adults. American College of Gastroenterology, Practice Parameters Committee. *American Journal of Gastroenterology* **92**, 204–11.

91. Leighton JA, Shen B, Baron TH, *et al.* (2006). ASGE guideline: endoscopy in the diagnosis and treatment of inflammatory bowel disease. *Gastrointestinal Endoscopy* **63**, 558–65.

92. Kiesslich R, Fritsch J, Holtmann M, *et al.* (2003). Methylene blue-aided chromoendoscopy for the detection of intraepithelial neoplasia and colon cancer in ulcerative colitis. *Gastroenterology* **124**, 880–8.

93. Imperiale TF, Ransohoff DF, Itzkowitz SH, *et al.* (2004). Fecal DNA versus fecal occult blood for colorectal-cancer screening in an average-risk population. *New England Journal of Medicine* **351**, 2704–14.

94. Ahlquist DA, Sargent DJ, Loprinzi CL, *et al.* (2008). Stool DNA and occult blood testing for screen detection of colorectal neoplasia. *Annals of Internal Medicine* **149**, 441–50, W81.

95. Ahlquist DA, Zou H, Domanico M, *et al.* (2012). Next-generation stool DNA test accurately detects colorectal cancer and large adenomas. *Gastroenterology* **142**, 248–56; quiz e25–6.

96. Lansdorp-Vogelaar I, Kuntz KM, Knudsen AB, *et al.* (2010). Stool DNA testing to screen for colorectal cancer in the Medicare population: a cost-effectiveness analysis. *Annals of Internal Medicine* **153**, 368–77.

97. Lidgard GP, Domanico MJ, Bruinsma JJ, *et al.* (2013). Clinical Performance of an Automated Stool DNA Assay for Detection of Colorectal Neoplasia. *Clinical Gastroenterology and Hepatology* **11**(10), 1313–8.

98. Ahlquist DA, Taylor WR, Mahoney DW, *et al.* (2012). The stool DNA test is more accurate than the plasma septin 9 test in detecting colorectal neoplasia. *Clinical Gastroenterology and Hepatology* **10**, 272–7 e1.

99. Ladabaum U, Allen J, Wandell M, *et al.* (2013). Colorectal Cancer Screening with Blood-Based Biomarkers: Cost-Effectiveness of Methylated Septin 9 DNA vs. Current Strategies. *Cancer Epidemiology, Biomarkers & Prevention* **22**(9),1567–76.

100. Tao S, Haug U, Kuhn K, *et al.* (2012). Comparison and combination of blood-based inflammatory markers with faecal occult blood tests for non-invasive colorectal cancer screening. *British Journal of Cancer* **106**, 1424–30.

101. Wild N, Andres H, Rollinger W, *et al.* (2010). A combination of serum markers for the early detection of colorectal cancer. *Clinical Cancer Research* **16**, 6111–21.

Index

Biomarkers in Cancer Screening and Early Detection, First Edition. Edited by Sudhir Srivastava.
© 2017 John Wiley & Sons, Inc. Published 2017 by John Wiley & Sons, Inc.